Introduction to
Health Science
Pathways to Your Future

Dorothy J. Winger, BS, MS
Health Science Teacher
Madison, Wisconsin

Susan Blahnik, BS, ME
Educational Consultant
Sun Prairie, Wisconsin

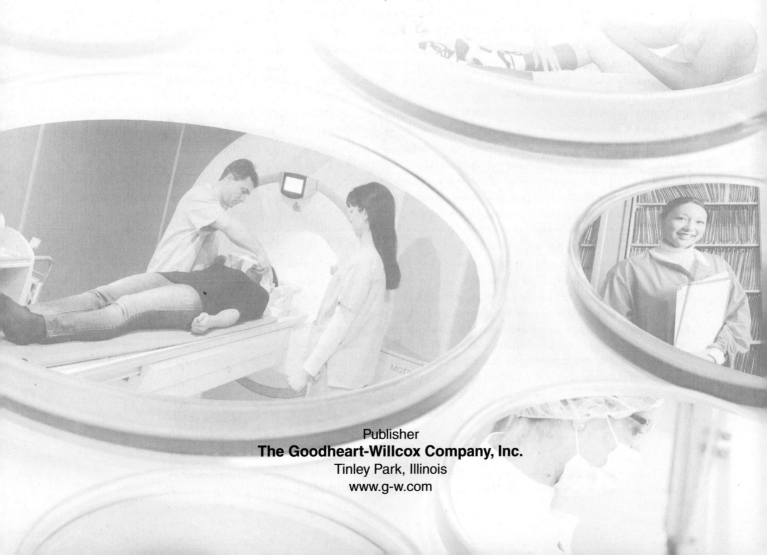

Publisher
The Goodheart-Willcox Company, Inc.
Tinley Park, Illinois
www.g-w.com

About the Authors

Dottie Winger, BS, MS, has 21 years of experience in teaching and curriculum development for health science and family and consumer science. She has dedicated the last 17 years to building the Health Science program at Madison East High School, where she is the Nursing Assistant program coordinator and has taught Health Science Occupations, Body Structure and Function, Medical Terminology, and Health Information Office Assistant. She also serves as a HOSA advisor, Red Cross blood drive coordinator, and Youth Health Service Corps advisor. Dottie has written statewide curricula, served as president of Wisconsin Health Occupations Professional Educators, sat on the Wisconsin Governor's Task Force on the Health Care Worker Shortage, and served on the leadership team to develop the Wisconsin Standards for Health Science. She has spoken at both national and state conferences on various educational topics. As an education consultant and mentor, Dottie continues to serve as a teacher leader.

Sue Blahnik, BS, ME, is a dedicated educator whose teaching career spans 40 years. Focusing on secondary education, she has taught career and technical coursework in health science as well as family and consumer education. She developed the health science career pathway for her local school district and taught Introduction to Medical Occupations, Body Structure and Function, and Medical Terminology. She established and managed the nursing assisting program, supervised youth apprentices, and advised the HOSA chapter. Sue has written statewide curriculums and recently served on the leadership team to develop the Wisconsin Standards for Health Science. She has presented at both national and state conferences and served as the first president of the Wisconsin Health Science Occupations Professional Educators. An avid supporter of service learning, Sue has mentored both students and fellow educators, and has received several grant awards to support health science instruction and service learning projects. Sue continues her commitment to children and learning as an educational consultant and author.

Contributors and Reviewers

Goodheart-Willcox Publisher would like to thank Mary Kennedy, who wrote the Recall Your Reading and Chapter Review sections in this book. Mary Kennedy is a national presenter, educational consultant, STEM/STEAM trainer, and veteran teacher of 34 years. She coauthored the *Goals for Living* textbook with Goodheart-Willcox.

Thanks also to Jane Heibel, who carefully reviewed the manuscript before publication. Special thanks to those who completed interviews and posed for pictures that appear in the unit openers.

Goodheart-Willcox Publisher would also like to thank the following instructors who reviewed selected manuscript chapters and provided valuable input into the development of this textbook program.

Susan DeVane
Health Science Instructor
McKenzie Center for
  Innovation and Technology
Indianapolis, IN

Joni Ferguson
Health Science Instructor
Barren County Area
  Technology Center
Glasgow, KY

LeeAnn Fountain
Health Science Instructor
TBAISD Career-Tech Center
Traverse City, MI

Kim Goins
Health Science Instructor
Sparkman Medical Academy
Ardmore, AL

Gail Pucker, RN
Health Science Educator
South Plantation High School
Plantation, FL

Michelle Quinn
CTE Instructor
Pine Forest High School
Fayetteville, NC

Kathleen Rocha
Health Science Instructor
Northside ISD
San Antonio, TX

Precision Exams Certification

Introduction to Health Science: Pathways to Your Future explores the knowledge and skills needed for successful careers in the five health science career pathways; therapeutic services, diagnostic services, health informatics, support services, and biotechnology. Goodheart-Willcox is pleased to partner with Precision Exams by correlating *Introduction to Health Science* to Precision Exams' Health Science Standards. Precision Exams' Standards and Career Skill Exams were created in concert with industry and subject matter experts to match real-world job skills and marketplace demands. Students who pass both the written and performance portions of the exam can earn a Career Skills Certification™. To see how *Introduction to Health Science* correlates to the Precision Exams Standards, please see the *Introduction to Health Science* correlations at www.g-w.com. For more information on Precision Exams, please consult the accompanying *Introduction to Health Science* Instructor Resources or go to www.precisionexams.com.

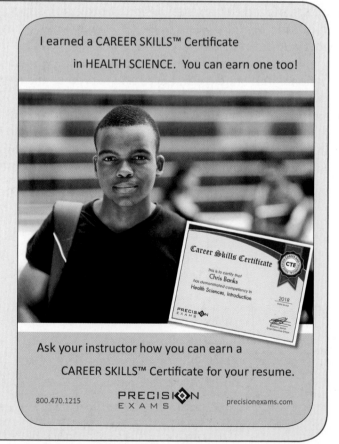

I earned a CAREER SKILLS™ Certificate in HEALTH SCIENCE. You can earn one too!

Ask your instructor how you can earn a CAREER SKILLS™ Certificate for your resume.

800.470.1215   PRECISION EXAMS   precisionexams.com

Contents in Brief

Contents

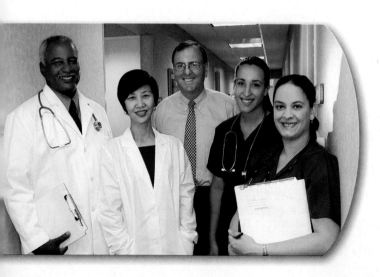

Chapter 4
Professional Knowledge
in Health Informatics 114

Chapter 5
Academic Knowledge:
Medical Terminology and
Body Organization 144

Unit 2
Therapeutic
Career Pathway 172

Chapter 6
Career Skills
in Therapeutic Services 174

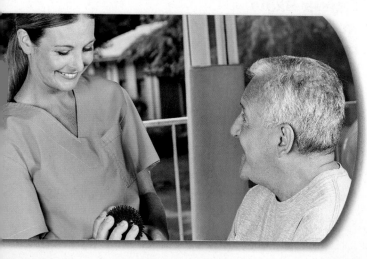

Unit 3 Diagnostic Career Pathway 328

Chapter 10 Career Skills in Diagnostic Services 330

Chapter 11 Fundamental Skills in Diagnostic Services 378

Chapter 12 Professional Knowledge in Diagnostic Services 414

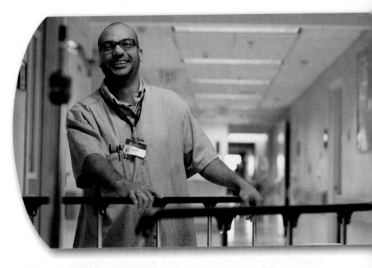

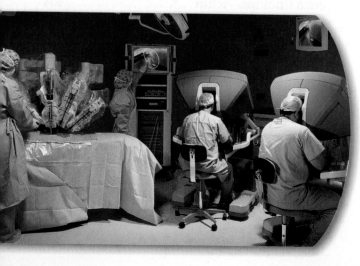

Skills and Procedures

The following skills and procedures are covered in chapters throughout this book. These skills, which are designated by the icon above, are important to learn if you wish to join the healthcare field.

Quick Search

Knowledge and Skills Guide

Pronunciation Guide

Spelling	Sounds Like	Phonetic Representation	Example Phonetic Spellings
a	all	aw	AWL
ä	father	ah	FAH-ther
a (long)	age, gate	ay	AYjh, GAYt
a (schwa)	amoeba	uh	uh-MEE-buh
a (short)	hat, map	a	HAT, MAP
ai (long)	fair, hair	ay	FAYr, HAYr
ai (short)	captain	a	KAP-tan
are	care, bare	air	KAIr, BAIr
au	Paul	aw	PAWl
au	luau	ow	LOO-ow
augh	caught	aw	KAWt
aw	crawl	aw	kRAWl
c (hard)	cat, cycle	k	KAT, SI-kuhl
c (soft)	cell, cilia, cycle	s	sel, SIHL-ee-uh, SI-kuhl
ch	child, much	ch	CHI-ld, MUch
ch	chrome	k	KROHm
ch	chef	sh	shEHf
ci	special, precious	sh	SPESH-uhl, PREH-shuhs
ck	suck	k	sUHk
dge	edge	j	EHj
e	entrepreneur	ah	ahn-truh-pruhn-NUR
é	résumé	ay	REH-zuh-may
e (long)	equal	ee	EE-kwuhl
e (schwa)	entrepreneur	uh	ahn-truh-pruhn-NUR
e (short)	let, best	eh	LEHt, BEHst
ea	break	ay	brAYk
ea	plead, flea	ee	PLEEd, FLEE
ea	bread	eh	brEHd
ear	heard, learn	er	HERd, LERn
eau	chateau	oh	sha-TOH
ed	played	d	pLAYd
ed	jagged	ehd	JAG-ehd
ee	need	ee	NEEd
ei	conceive	ee	kahn-SEEv
eigh	weigh	ay	WAY
er	keratin	air	KAIR-uh-tin
er	term	er	TERm
eu	neutral	oo	NOO-trahl

(continued)

Spelling	Sounds Like	Phonetic Representation	Example Phonetic Spellings
eu	Fr*eu*d	oy	frOYD
eu	*eu*thanize	yu	YU-thuh-nlz
eur	entrepren*eur*	yur	ahn-truh-pruhn-NUR
ew	s*ew*	oh	SOH
ey	wh*ey*	ay	WAY
g (hard)	*g*arage, *g*ust	g	gah-RAHJ, GUHst
g (soft)	*g*iant	j	JI-ant
gh	lau*gh*	f	LAf
gh (silent h)	*gh*ost	g	GOHst
gn	*gn*at	n	NAt
i (long)	*i*ris, h*i*ve	I	I-rihs, hIv
i (schwa)	penc*i*l	uh	PEHN-suhl
i (short)	*i*t, p*i*n	ih	IHt, PIHn
ia	cil*ia*	ee-uh	SIHL-ee-uh
ia	g*ia*nt	I	JI-ant
ia	pneumon*ia*	yuh	noo-MOHN-yuh
ie	f*ie*ld	ee	FEEld
ie	d*ie*	I	dI
igh	s*igh*	I	sI
ine	mach*ine*	een	muh-SHEEN
ir	s*ir*	er	SER
k	loo*k*	k	LUHWk
kn	*kn*ife	n	NIf
le	fidd*le*, puzz*le*	uhl	FIH-duhl, PUH-zuhl
ng	ra*ng*e	nj	RAYnj
nk	i*nk*	ngk	IHngk
o (long)	*o*pen, y*o*ke	oh	OH-pehn, YOHk
o (ȯ)	wr*o*ng	aw	RAWng
o (schwa)	tensi*o*n	uh	TEHN-shuhn
o (short)	h*o*t, r*o*ck	ah	HAHt, RAHk
oa	cl*oa*k	oh	KLOHk
oe	am*oe*ba	ee	uh-MEE-buh
oi	*oi*l, v*oi*ce	oy	OY-l, VOYs
oo (long)	m*oo*n, f*oo*d	oo	MOOn, FOOd
oo (schwa)	bl*oo*d	uh	BLUHd
oo (short)	b*oo*k	uhw	BUHWk
or	w*or*k, doct*or*	er	WERk, DAHK-ter
or	*or*der	or	OR-der
ou	y*ou*	ew	Yew
ou	ac*ou*stic	oo	uh-KOO-stihk
ou	h*ou*se, *ou*t	ow	HOWs, OWt

(continued)

Spelling	Sounds Like	Phonetic Representation	Example Phonetic Spellings
ou (schwa)	tough	uh	TUHf
ough	thought	aw	THAWt
ough	cough	awf	KAWf
ough	through	ehw	thREHw
ough	though	oh	THOH
ous	mucous	uhs	MYU-kuhs
ow	grow	oh	GROH
oy	boy	oy	BOY
ph	phone	f	FOHn
pn	pneumonia	n	noo-MOHN-yuh
qu	quick	kw	KWIHk
s	say, mist	s	SAY, MIHst
s	bones	z	BOHnz
s	pleasure	zh	PLEH-zher
si	tension	sh	TEHN-shuhn
si	Asia, abrasion	zh	AY-zhuh, uh-BRAY-zhuhn
tch	match	ch	MACH
ti	motion	sh	MOH-shuhn
u (long—1)	cute	yu	KYUt
u (short/schwa)	cup	uh	KUHp
u (long—2)	rule	oo	ROOl
ue	blue	oo	BLOO
ui	guide	I	GId
ui	build	ih	BIHld
ui	fruit	oo	fROOt
ur	burn	er	BERn
ur	urinalysis	yur	yur-ih-NAL-ih-sihs
uy	buy	I	BI
wh	what, which	w	WAHt, WIHch
wr	wrong	r	RAWng
x	ax	ks	AHks
x	xylophone	z	ZI-loh-fohn
y (consonant)	yes	y	YEHs
y (long E)	reality	ee	ree-AL-ih-tee
y (long I)	cycle	I	SI-kuhl
y (short I)	hymn	ih	HIHm
yn	larynx	ngk	LAIR-ihngks
z	zoology	z	zoo-AH-loh-jee

To the Student

Welcome to the field of health science!

We hope you will enjoy learning from the experiences and insights of healthcare workers as you read about the wide variety of careers in healthcare. You will study the five health science career pathways and will learn professional skills and standards of behavior used by workers in each pathway.

As you use the reading supports provided in this text, including professional vocabulary, mapping your reading, connecting with and reflecting on your reading, you will improve your understanding of health science content. At the same time, you will strengthen your reading and comprehension skills.

Whether you have a specific career in mind or are just beginning your search, you will be excited to know that there are literally hundreds of healthcare occupations from which to choose. When you read about work personalities, leadership styles, and preferences for data, people, things, or ideas, take time to consider your own personal preferences, and you will discover satisfying career options for your future. Practicing the technical skills associated with each pathway will provide additional clues to your preferred career pathway.

Prepare for challenging health science coursework by sharpening your study skills. Use the memory techniques for learning vocabulary, try different methods for taking notes, and assess your personal learning style to improve your study habits. If you develop a plan for managing your time and learn skills for taking exams now, you will see the benefits throughout your school and work life.

Above all, we hope you will be excited to learn about the amazing variety of healthcare careers and will feel prepared to discover the pathway to your future career!

Dottie Winger

Sue Blahnik

Chapter 1
Welcome to the Field of Health Science

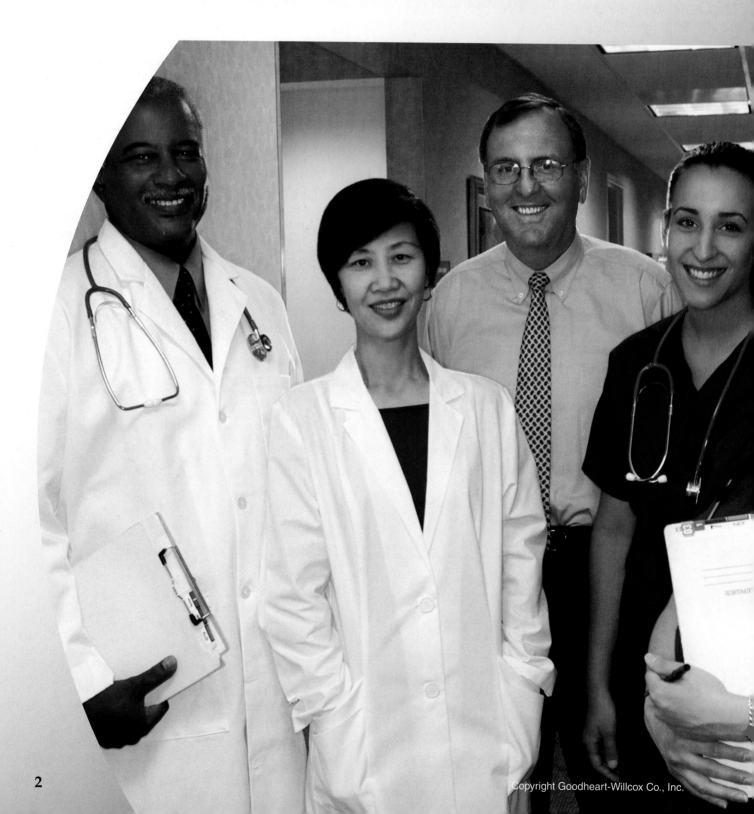

PROFESSIONAL VOCABULARY

 E-flash Cards

You will need to learn the essential terms listed below before you begin your reading. These terms will help you understand the main concepts of the chapter. These terms, which will be highlighted in yellow within the text, will become part of your professional vocabulary.

In addition to these essential terms, you will see bold terms throughout the chapter. The meanings of these terms are explained where the terms first appear. The bold terms, like the essential terms listed here, will become part of your professional vocabulary and deepen your understanding of the topics presented.

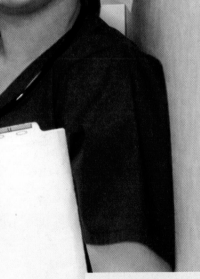

accreditation official recognition from a professional association that an educational program meets minimum educational standards for an occupation

alternative, complementary, integrative therapies healthcare practices and treatments that minimize or avoid the use of surgery and drugs

career clusters groups of similar occupations and industries that share a core set of basic knowledge and skills for all workers

career ladder a sequence of job positions progressing from entry-level to higher levels of responsibility and authority based on education, experience, and performance

career pathways smaller groups of specialized occupations within a career cluster that require more specific sets of knowledge, skills, and training

credentials documents proving a person's qualifications for a particular occupation

genomic medicine personalized medical care that uses a patient's unique combination of genes and chromosomes to prevent illness and maintain health

holistic care therapies that treat the patient as a whole person after assessing the individual's physical, social, mental, and spiritual well-being

nanotechnology a field of science that manipulates individual atoms and molecules to create devices that are thousands of times smaller than current technologies allow

National Healthcare Skill Standards standards determined by the National Consortium for Health Science Education, which describe the skills that workers need to succeed in healthcare careers

regenerative medicine a form of medical care that creates living tissue to replace tissue or organ functions lost due to age, disease, injury, or birth disorder

Western medicine the most common form of medical care in the United States, which uses medication and surgery to treat the signs and symptoms of illness

CONNECT WITH YOUR READING

Consider a medical problem or disease, perhaps one that affects members of your own family. What treatment would your grandparents have received for this illness? What treatment would you receive for this disease today? What treatment do you predict your grandchildren will receive if they are affected by this disease? Pair with another class member and share your thoughts.

MAP YOUR READING

On a separate sheet of paper, create a chart with five columns and six rows like the one shown here. Use the title of this chapter, "Welcome to the Field of Health Science," as the heading for your chart. List the following topics in the center column, with one topic in each row: *Evolution of Healthcare*, *Future Trends*, *Current Issues*, and *Career Pathways and Employment Opportunities*. As you read the chapter, list the main points related to each topic in the four boxes on either side of the appropriate heading.

Welcome to the Field of Health Science				
Point 1	**Point 2**	**Topic**	**Point 3**	**Point 4**
		Evolution of Healthcare		
		Future Trends		
		Current Issues		
		Career Pathways and Employment Opportunities		

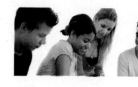

Healthcare Professions: Student Choices

Gerry's long stay in the hospital led her to appreciate the care she received from all types of healthcare professionals. June noticed the thoughtfulness shown to her dad by hospice personnel during his terminal illness. Fatou wants to return to her home country and work to improve healthcare there. Ron's dad, an athletic trainer, encouraged Ron to explore healthcare occupations in his career search. These students each have different situations and different experiences, but all of them are being led toward the same goal—a career in healthcare.

Think about your own life experiences. Can you identify the influences that have led you to consider a career in healthcare? Whether you have a specific career in mind or are just beginning your search, you will be excited to know that there are literally hundreds of healthcare occupations from which to choose. As you identify your personal skills and connect them to the job opportunities in this field, you will discover satisfying career options for your future.

In this chapter, you will learn how research findings have changed medical care and what changes may be on the horizon. You will also learn about challenges facing the healthcare industry in the United States. Finally, you will be introduced to the health science career cluster and its five career pathways. A general overview of the types of education, credentials, and skills that lead to employment in healthcare will prepare you to learn about each career pathway in the chapters that follow.

The Evolution of Healthcare

Only a hundred years ago, a physician had a small office in his home and made frequent visits to the homes of his patients. There weren't many treatments available, so he was able to carry all of his medical care supplies in a single black bag. Since then, there have been advancements in the world of medicine and acceptance of new attitudes and beliefs about healthcare guided by medical research and development.

Medical Advancements

A century ago, a physician studied the symptoms and courses of many diseases in medical school. He could diagnose an illness and tell his patients the likely outcome of their disease. He might be able to treat the pain involved with a disease, but he could not cure the disease itself. He provided personal care and support as well as advice to family members regarding care for the patient.

Patients sometimes recovered if they received good care at home. A physician might wish that more hospitals were available because he knew that good nursing care could improve patient outcomes. Often his job was to prepare patients for death from a disease that could not be treated.

Fifty years later, physicians were able to diagnose an illness, and it was far more likely that they could treat it. Medical research and scientific discoveries changed medical care. Sulfa drugs and penicillin shortened the course of infections and cured some that were previously fatal, such as meningitis. Insulin was now available to treat diabetes. X-rays were used to check for broken bones. Smallpox and tetanus vaccinations greatly reduced the incidence of illness.

During the past fifty years, technological advances have continued to change the methods and outcomes of medical treatment (Figure 1.1). Today, hospital patients experience life-saving treatments like heart bypass operations, heart valve replacements, and kidney transplants. An

Figure 1.1 A Century of US Healthcare

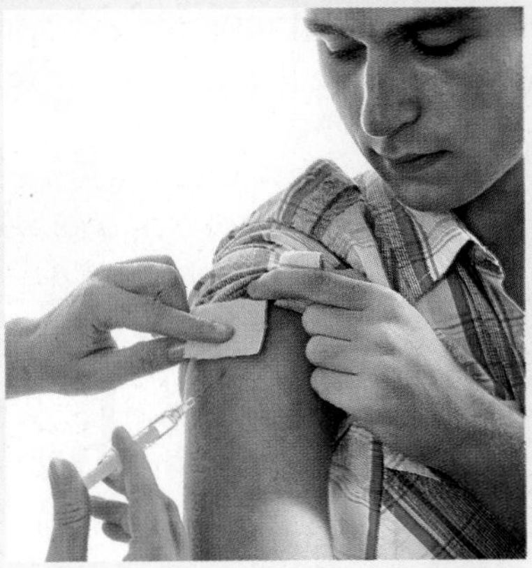

1900	1950	2000
Country Doctors	Vaccinations	Organ Transplants

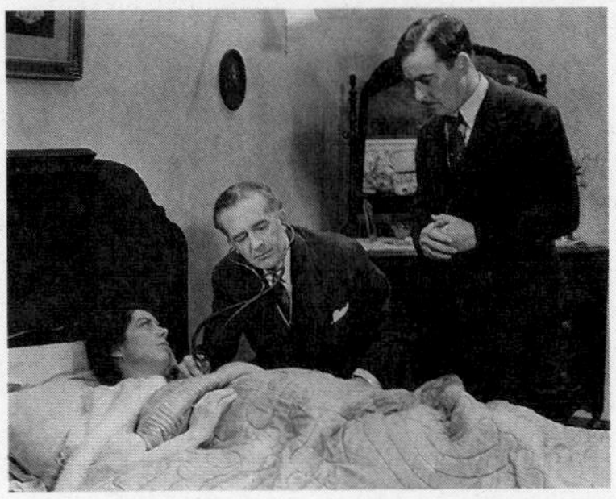

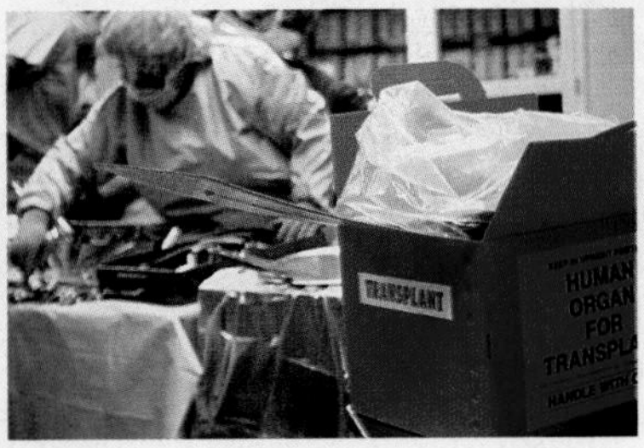

infusion of clot-busting drugs—which are injected directly into a vein—can reverse the paralysis caused by a stroke, and some cancers that were previously fatal are now treatable.

In the fast-changing field of healthcare, doctors are not the only ones who have seen the demands and capabilities of their profession grow. For example, many students today plan to pursue a career in nursing for the opportunity it provides to work in a wide variety of healthcare environments. Yet nursing as a profession has only existed for about 150 years. Florence Nightingale's early efforts to establish good nursing standards and practices in the 1800s have evolved into programs that train nurses in specialties such as informatics, patient education, organ transplantation, midwifery (mid-WIF-eh-ree), advanced practice nursing, and anesthesia (Figure 1.2).

New Attitudes and Beliefs

The evolution of healthcare is not limited to changes in patient care and treatment; it also includes changes in the current attitudes and beliefs of the people who will (or will not) benefit from those treatments. The discoveries of archeologists show that ancient cultures practiced medicine based on their spiritual beliefs and the use of herbal remedies. While the ancient practice of bloodletting is now rejected in favor of a hospital stay to treat appendicitis, not all spiritual and herbal treatments should be rejected in the practice of healthcare.

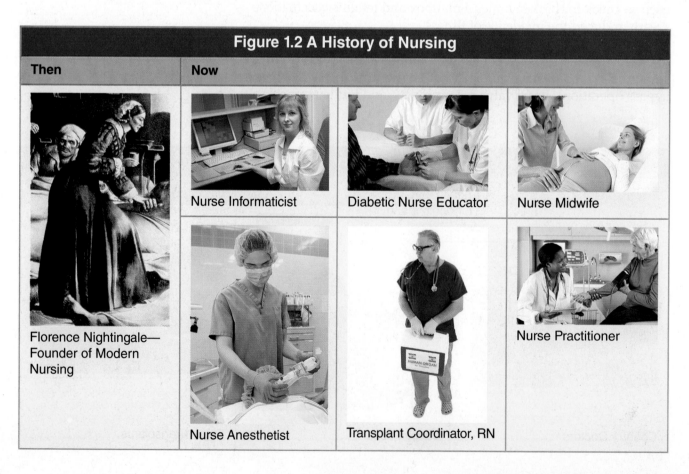

Figure 1.2 A History of Nursing

Then

Florence Nightingale—Founder of Modern Nursing

Now

Nurse Informaticist

Diabetic Nurse Educator

Nurse Midwife

Nurse Anesthetist

Transplant Coordinator, RN

Nurse Practitioner

For instance, the highly regarded neurosurgeon, Benjamin Carson, used prayer in his practice of medicine, and recent research is proving that green tea has many **antioxidant** (an-tee-AHK-suh-duhnt) benefits. Antioxidants promote good health by reducing cell deterioration and may contribute to disease prevention. History is a valuable tool for advancing medical care when helpful information is accepted and information that has proven harmful is rejected (Figure 1.3).

Figure 1.3 Highlights in the History of Medicine

Location and Period in History	Medical Practice	Beneficial/ Not Beneficial		Related Medical Practice Today
Many parts of the world (6000–3000 BC)	trepanning—removing part of skull to release bad spirits; some patients actually survived	👎	👍	Temporary removal of part of the skull is used to prevent brain damage due to brain swelling.
	use of plants and herbs, such as foxglove and opium poppy	👍	👍	Digitalis, which regulates heartbeat, is made from foxglove. Morphine, which is used for pain relief, is made from the opium poppy.
Egypt (3000–300 BC)	accurate health records	👍	👍	Accurate records are a legal requirement of medical care.
	bloodletting using leeches	👎	👍	Leeches are used to restore blood circulation to skin grafts.
China (1700 BC–220 AD)	acupuncture	👍	👍	Acupuncture successfully treats osteoarthritis, migraine headaches, and more.
Greece (1200–200 BC)	research into physical causes of disease	👍	👍	Research results form the basis for medical treatments.
Rome (700 BC–300 AD)	building of aqueducts and sewers to improve sanitation and prevent disease	👍	👍	There is a renewed focus on hand washing and hygiene practices to reduce infections.
Arabic/Islamic civilization (700–1500 AD)	universal health care and licensing for doctors and pharmacists	👍	👎	Many citizens have no health insurance and can't access regular medical care.
Europe (400–1400AD)	no medical advancements millions of deaths caused by epidemics	👎	👍	Rapid medical advancements are made. Vaccines prevent epidemics.
Europe (1400–1700 AD)	medical schools established	👍	👍	Educational training is established for more than 300 healthcare occupations.
Europe/America 17th and 18th centuries (1600–1800 AD)	study of anatomy and physiology through human dissection	👍	👍	Noninvasive imaging techniques can record anatomy and physiology.

(continued)

(continued)	Figure 1.3 Highlights in the History of Medicine		
Location and Period in History	**Medical Practice**	**Beneficial/ Not Beneficial**	**Related Medical Practice Today**
Europe/America (continued) (1600–1800 AD)	microscope invented; pathogens seen for the first time	👍 👍	Nanotechnology produces devices and particles too small to be seen by a microscope.
	many deaths caused by uncontrolled infections	👎 👎	"Superbug" infections remain a health problem.
	bifocals invented	👍 👍	Bifocals are still used, but laser surgery can correct vision problems.
Europe/America (1800–2000 AD)	first female physician	👍 👍	Females equal or outnumber males in medical school.
	first use of antiseptics and anesthetics	👍 👍	The use of antiseptic techniques and of general and local anesthetics is standard practice.
	discovery of penicillin	👍 👎	Overuse of antibiotics results in antibiotic-resistant bacteria.
	study of psychology and psychiatry	👍 👍	Therapies and medications treat "diseases of the mind."
	molecular structure of DNA modeled	👍 👍	The human genome is mapped.

Western medicine
the most common form of medical care in the United States, which uses medication and surgery to treat the signs and symptoms of illness

alternative, complementary, integrative therapies
healthcare practices and treatments that minimize or avoid the use of surgery and drugs

holistic care
therapies that treat the patient as a whole person after assessing the individual's physical, social, mental, and spiritual well-being

Traditionally, **Western medicine** has rejected forms of healthcare that don't focus on the physical signs of illness. Some of these ancient practices are considered **alternative, complementary, or integrative** (IN-tuh-gray-tihv) **therapies**. There is now a greater acceptance of the idea that wellness and the treatment of disease requires a holistic approach. This means that healthcare focuses not only on the physical needs of an individual, but also on his or her social, mental, and spiritual needs.

Holistic care works to maintain or restore wellness by promoting a balanced relationship between the mind, body, and spirit (Figure 1.4). People are most familiar with the components of physical wellness, which include a healthy diet, exercise, and routine medical care. However, other important components include the following:

- Mental/Intellectual wellness—intellectual curiosity, lifelong learning, creativity, and problem solving

- Social wellness—communicating and interacting well with others and maintaining positive personal relationships

- Spiritual wellness—living according to personal values, ethics, and morals; may incorporate religious practices

Our personal history and culture also affect our healthcare beliefs and practices. Your cultural heritage determines whether you say a prayer,

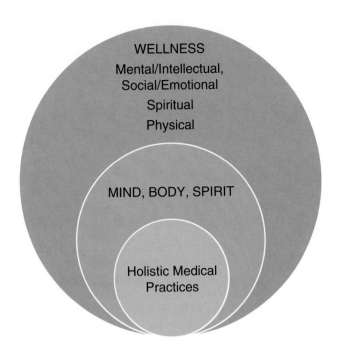

WELLNESS

Mental/Intellectual, Social/Emotional

Spiritual

Physical

MIND, BODY, SPIRIT

Holistic Medical Practices

Figure 1.4   Holistic medical practices can be found at the heart of preserving wellness by treating the mind, body, and spirit.

visit a shaman (SHA-muhn), or head to the health food store in times of illness. Do you have any home remedies? Gargling with salt water for a sore throat is a home remedy that has stood the test of time. However, research has shown both positive and negative results for using zinc lozenges (LAH-zuhnj-ez) to shorten the duration of a cold. When evaluating treatments for illness, Hippocrates's advice to "do no harm" is still the guideline used by medical care providers (Figure 1.5).

Accepting New Research

Although medical research may indicate the need for changes in healthcare practices, both healthcare workers and healthcare consumers must understand and accept the research before changes can be made. When they became new parents in the 1960s or 1970s, grandmothers of today were taught to place an infant facedown or on the side for sleeping. They were warned that sleeping on the back could result in possible death.

In contrast, today's parents are taught to always place an infant on the back for sleeping. They are warned that sleeping facedown greatly increases the risk for sudden infant death syndrome (SIDS). The basis for this turnaround was medical research showing that sleeping facedown significantly increased the risk of SIDS.

In 1994, a "Back to Sleep" campaign from the American Academy of Pediatrics (AAP) began to educate parents, caregivers, and healthcare providers about the ways to reduce the risk of SIDS. Since the start of this campaign, the percentage of infants placed on their backs to sleep has increased dramatically, and the overall SIDS rates have declined by 50 percent (Figure 1.6 on the next page).

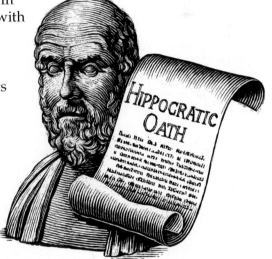

Figure 1.5   Hippocrates, known as *the Father of Medicine*, was a Greek physician who practiced medicine in 400 BC. His oath of medical ethics is still taken by physicians today. He believed in holistic care and promoted the wellness aspects of diet, rest, and cleanliness as part of the natural healing process. Who are some other important historical figures in the field of medicine?

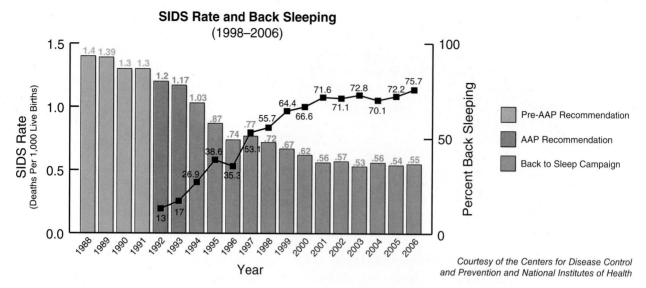

SIDS Rate and Back Sleeping
(1998–2006)

Figure 1.6   In the graph shown here, the bars represent deaths due to SIDS during different time periods. The black line represents the percentage of babies being put to sleep on their backs.

Courtesy of the Centers for Disease Control and Prevention and National Institutes of Health

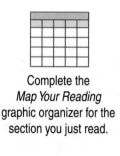

Complete the *Map Your Reading* graphic organizer for the section you just read.

RECALL YOUR READING

1. As recently as 100 years ago, doctors might have been able to _____ an illness, but they were often unable to _____ it.

2. After fifty years of medical advancements, physicians had _____ drugs and _____ to cure some previously fatal infections, and vaccinations prevented _____ and _____.

3. Today, medical care is changing rapidly because of advances in _____.

4. While Western medicine has often rejected _____ healthcare practices, many healthcare professionals are now embracing a _____ approach that considers more than the physical needs of a patient.

5. Healthcare practices change not only when research verifies the benefits, but also when both healthcare _____ and _____ understand and accept the research findings.

Future Trends

As you prepare for a career in healthcare, know that constant change is normal. It is entirely possible that someday you will work in a position that does not even exist today. Estimates show that current medical knowledge doubles every six to eight years. The healthcare and scientific communities are learning more every day, which means that teamwork and the sharing of medical knowledge will be more important than ever in the future. For a technically savvy generation of healthcare workers, global sharing of information will lead to even more rapid advances in healthcare.

Consider the experience of Addison, a surgical technologist at a major university hospital. She was hired before she graduated from her training program. During the first year of her job, Addison assisted the surgeons as they performed brain surgeries, and she observed the surgical procedures for treating patients with Parkinson's disease. The following year she was part of a medical team researching the installation of a magnetic resonance (REHZ-uh-nuhnts) imaging scanner within the surgical suite. This new technology improves the surgical experience for Parkinson's patients. Now, just three years out of school, she is a *preceptor* (prih-SEHP-tuhr) who trains future technologists in the use of magnetic resonance imaging during surgery.

What advances in medical care will you see? What issues will affect the practice and delivery of care? These are important questions for future healthcare workers. While the future cannot be predicted, current research can provide insight into how medical care may change (Figure 1.7).

Genomic Medicine

Future medical care will focus on predicting whether a specific person will develop a particular disease. Treatments will include methods for preventing this disease as well as improved methods for treating it. Medical care will also become more personalized when healthcare workers can determine which drug will be most effective for a particular patient based on that patient's unique combination of genes and chromosomes.

Genomic (jih-NOH-mihk) **medicine** identifies and studies the sequences in DNA, which carries the genetic information of organisms. A genome is the complete sequence of DNA for every chromosome in an organism—in this case, a human being. When scientists compare the genomes of human beings, they look at the genes on the DNA. While 99 percent of the genes are identical, a few are different. Those differences explain why one person will develop a disease or respond to a drug and another will not. Genomic medicine will allow doctors to make accurate predictions about how a patient's disease will progress and which

genomic medicine
personalized medical care that uses a patient's unique combination of genes and chromosomes to prevent illness and maintain health

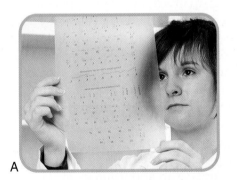

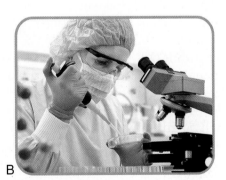

Looking at the Future of Healthcare

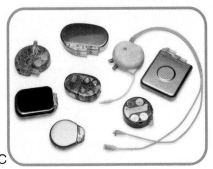

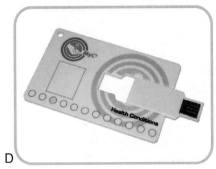

Figure 1.7   Recent advances in healthcare include genetic testing (A), stem cell research (B), miniaturization such as pacemakers (C), and chips that contain patients' medical history (D). *What other technological advances in healthcare can you name?*

medications will produce the best response with the fewest side effects. Drugs will be personalized to be effective and safe for a specific individual.

Genetic Variations

A person's genetic makeup affects how he or she responds to food. Consider that some people can eat whatever they want and never gain weight, while others gain weight more easily. Some can eat high cholesterol foods, but have no heart disease, while others use diet and medication to reduce cholesterol levels. These human variations are a result of genetic differences. Small differences in our genes affect how we **metabolize** (muh-TA-buh-lIz), or *process*, cholesterol. Using this knowledge, physicians will be able to recommend a low-fat, low-cholesterol diet for a specific patient before high cholesterol begins to clog his **coronary** arteries, which supply blood to the heart, and leads to a heart attack.

Genetic research is currently focusing on identifying gene variations that produce disease, predict the development of a disease, and tell how quickly a disease will progress. For example, knowing which patients will develop a particular cancer will allow doctors to begin treating patients earlier when there are only a few cancer cells present in the body. Individual genetic information will also help physicians select the type of cancer treatment that will be most effective.

Genetic tests are already being developed to predict the potential onset of a disease later in life. For example, some women carry a gene that greatly increases their risk for developing breast cancer. For these women, earlier and more frequent **mammogram** screenings will detect any developing cancer to treat in its earliest stages. Mammograms are X-rays that test for breast cancer.

Future Applications

In the future, designer vaccines may be developed for a specific person (Figure 1.8). Fragments of an individual's DNA might be used to create a vaccine that would prevent or treat an illness in only that person. Other vaccines will be developed to treat many infections that are not yet preventable. Vaccines may even be developed to prevent or treat long-lasting, or **chronic** (KRAH-nihk) illnesses like heart disease or cancer. Consider the benefits of the hepatitis B vaccine. Because chronic hepatitis B can lead to a form of liver cancer, the vaccine prevents both hepatitis B and the development of this specific type of cancer. In the future, many vaccines will be given by mouth, inhalation through the nose, or skin patches. In addition, often only one dose of each vaccine will be needed.

Eventually, genomic medicine may include **gene therapy**, which involves the insertion of a new gene to replace an abnormal gene. Research into gene therapy is ongoing with the goal of developing treatments for genetic diseases and disorders.

Figure 1.8 Individual genetic information will help physicians select the type of treatment that will be most effective for a specific patient. What types of illnesses might genomic medicine help treat?

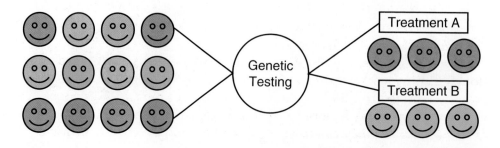

Regenerative Medicine

Stem cells may be increasingly important to medical care, especially in the field of **regenerative** (rih-JEH-nuh-ray-tiv) **medicine**. These basic cells have the power to develop into specific types of cells needed to create the tissues and organs of our bodies. The goal of regenerative medicine is to use a patient's stem cells to develop tissues and organs that replace damaged tissues and organs. Organs created through this process are developed from a patient's DNA, which should eliminate the current problem of organ rejection experienced by transplant patients today.

There are two types of stem cells—embryonic and adult. Embryonic (ehm-bree-AH-nihk) can become all types of cells found in the body. These stem cells come from discarded embryos created for infertile couples as part of the **in vitro**, or *test tube*, fertilization process. The use of embryonic stem cells is controversial.

Adult stem cells are found in tissues and are more limited in their ability to generate the various cells of the body. While researchers had believed that adult stem cells could only produce similar types of cells, newer evidence indicates that they may be more adaptable than previously thought. Despite some limitations, adult stem cells do appear to help repair damage caused by illness or injury. Today, adult stem cells are used for bone marrow transplants in the treatment of severe forms of blood cancer and anemia. In the future, stem cells could be developed to help heal heart tissue after a heart attack or to create pancreatic cells for patients with type 1 diabetes.

regenerative medicine a form of medical care that creates living tissue to replace tissue or organ functions lost due to age, disease, injury, or birth disorder

Technology and Medicine

Just as technology is causing major changes in our everyday lives, it is also fueling important advances in medicine. New technology produces shorter surgical recoveries and increased patient access to surgical specialists. Technology is even changing the way a healthcare facility keeps a patient's medical records on file.

Medical Imaging. The X-ray was a huge step toward seeing inside the human body without using surgery (Figure 1.9). But today's imaging technology can make an X-ray look like a faded photograph. Computed tomography (toh-MAH-gruh-fee) (CT) scans, magnetic resonance imaging (MRI), and ultrasound techniques can now provide extremely detailed images of human anatomy. These images are digitized so they can be rotated for a better view and accessed even after the patient has left the lab. Through these techniques, a physician can detect narrowed coronary arteries and diagnose lung cancers early, when they can still be treated successfully.

A virtual **colonoscopy** (koh-luh-NAHS-kuh-pee) or a DNA-based stool screening test may someday replace the more invasive optical procedure used currently. A colonoscopy examines the inner surface of the colon. People may be more willing to complete a virtual screening or a screening test they can use at home rather than the current invasive

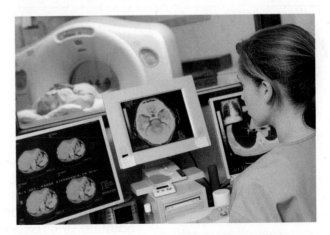

Figure 1.9   The digital images produced by this computed axial tomography (CAT) scan can be rotated or enlarged for a better view. Digital images are also easier to store than printed images.

procedure, which will mean early detection of more cases of colon cancer. As a result, researchers predict a drop in deaths caused by colon cancer. Traditional colonoscopies will only be required for the minority of patients who need to have polyps removed to prevent colon cancer.

Molecular (muh-LEH-kyuh-luhr) **imaging** provides detailed pictures of what is happening inside the body at the molecular and cellular level. This technique can show how the body is functioning and can track the progress of a disease. Doctors will be able to use this technique to learn where a cancer originated, if it has spread, and whether or not treatment has destroyed all of the cancerous cells. Molecular imaging can show how well blood is moving through the heart muscle and if the muscle has been damaged by a lack of blood flow. This is important information for the diagnosis and treatment of a heart attack.

Miniaturization in Medicine. The combined efforts of engineering and medicine are producing smaller and more powerful medical devices. Tubes called **stents** can keep arteries open. **Pacemakers**, which regulate heartbeats, used to be the size of a deck of cards. Now these devices are smaller than a matchbook. Other cardiac-assist devices currently being developed will help damaged heart muscles pump blood more effectively.

The science of **nanotechnology** (na-noh-tehk-NAH-luh-jee) is expected to develop devices so small they cannot be seen by a microscope (Figure 1.10). These tiny devices may be able to enter a cell to deliver a drug or kill cancer cells before a tumor forms. If these devices can deliver insulin directly to the blood, diabetics will not need multiple daily shots and oral tablets will replace insulin injections.

Surgery. Technological advances are also changing surgery. Fewer surgeries are needed when tiny tubes called **catheters**, guided by imaging machines, can be used to repair abdominal and even brain **aneurysms** (AN-yuh-rih-zuhms), which cause a weakening of blood vessels, before those blood vessels can burst. **Laparoscopic** (lap-uh-rahs-KAH-pihk) operations, which use tubes with cameras and tools attached to them, require very small incisions. This means that patients having a gallbladder or appendix removed will have much shorter hospital stays. Many surgeries are becoming **outpatient procedures**, which allow patients to leave the hospital shortly after a procedure has been completed. Hernia repairs, cataract surgery, and laser surgery to improve vision already require no hospital stay. One day, even hip replacements may be outpatient procedures.

Robots are being used to improve surgical procedures by providing an opportunity for surgery simulation. This type of simulation is an effective method for in-depth surgical training. When used with digital patient images, simulation allows the surgeon to "practice" on a specific patient and plan the best procedure for that patient. **Telesurgery** (TEHL-uh-suhr-juhr-ee) combines a reliable telephone line with robotic equipment and a skilled surgeon. In the future, an expert surgeon in another state

nanotechnology
a field of science that manipulates individual atoms and molecules to create devices that are thousands of times smaller than current technologies allow

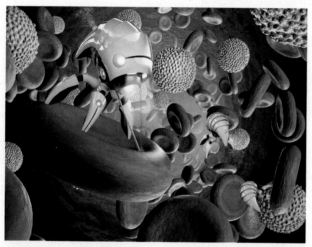

Figure 1.10   In the future, nanobots may move through the bloodstream to treat many diseases and conditions. For example, they might break up kidney stones or help blood to clot.

or country will be able to perform surgery while a patient is in his or her hometown hospital.

Medical Records. Computer technology is leading to digitized patient records (Figure 1.11). These are also known as *electronic health records* (EHR). You may have already seen computers in hospital rooms or clinic exam rooms. Healthcare workers use these computer systems to access patient records and enter vital signs of and treatments administered to a specific patient. Prescription updates can be sent directly to the patient's pharmacy through these systems. Currently, access to these records is limited to specific healthcare facilities or networks.

Eventually a patient's complete health record, including images of diagnostic tests, should be available to access online at any time and from any location. For example, suppose you are spending a week in Paris and are involved in an accident. Emergency personnel could use online health records to immediately find out whether or not you have allergies to any medications or if you have any chronic diseases like diabetes or asthma that will affect your medical treatment. In the future, you may carry a medical card with a pin number or a chip that can be scanned to allow access to your records.

The US military is already putting some medical information on soldiers' dog tags. Medical personnel who treat a wounded soldier can use a tablet computer to access baseline medical data. These personnel can also add notes about treatment given as the soldier moves from the medic to the field hospital and then to a major medical center for continued care. Digitized health records will become a reality when there is a common system and location for storing all of a patient's healthcare history. A secure system for protecting patient information is also necessary. Digitized health records will improve the quality and safety of your medical care.

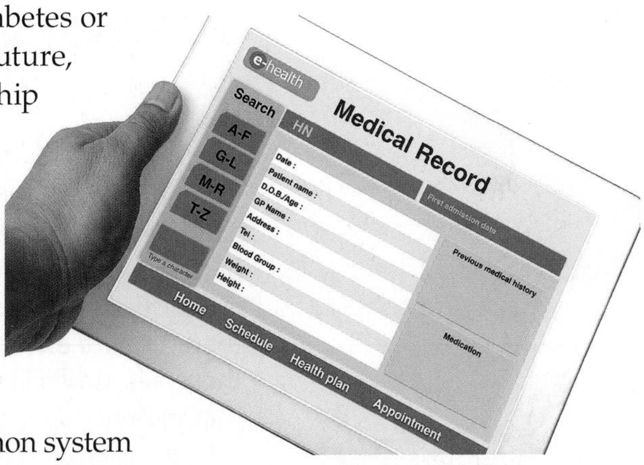

Figure 1.11   Electronic health records can be accessed online from different locations.

Back to Basics

Many patients are frustrated by a lack of personal attention in their medical care. As they move from one doctor to another, patients feel as though they are a set of symptoms or a disease to be cured rather than a valued person who is seeking relief. Patients are looking for medical care that is more holistic and pays attention not only to their physical requirements, but also to their emotional, social, and even spiritual needs (Figure 1.12 on the next page).

A growing number of patients are turning back to ancient healthcare practices, such as acupuncture (AK-yu-puhnk-cher) and homeopathy (hoh-mee-AH-puh-thee). Patients are finding relief from pain while using fewer medications and surgeries. Many of these alternative healthcare practices are not covered by insurance, so patients must be finding them effective. If these techniques were not working, patients would not be willing to pay for the treatment. Western medical providers are taking note of this trend, however, and many of the nation's hospitals, universities, and medical schools have established centers for

Figure 1.12   Other CAM practices include movement therapies such as Pilates, and the Feldenkrais method. Traditional healers including the Native American medicine man are considered CAM practitioners. The energy practices of magnet therapy, light therapy, qi gong, and Reiki are also considered CAM therapies.

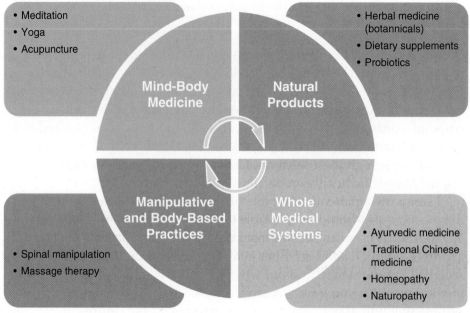

- Meditation
- Yoga
- Acupuncture

Mind-Body Medicine

- Herbal medicine (botannicals)
- Dietary supplements
- Probiotics

Natural Products

Manipulative and Body-Based Practices

- Spinal manipulation
- Massage therapy

Whole Medical Systems

- Ayurvedic medicine
- Traditional Chinese medicine
- Homeopathy
- Naturopathy

Data courtesy of the NCCAM

integrative medicine. These centers offer conventional Western medical care combined with alternative and complementary therapies.

The National Institutes of Health (NIH) has created a National Center of Complementary and Alternative Medicine (NCCAM). This organization is conducting multiple scientific studies to determine which alternative therapies are effective. As research confirms the benefits of particular therapies, medical doctors will begin to include or integrate those therapies into patient care plans. In many cases, research has shown that a particular therapy is effective, but the reason why it works is still unknown. As with any other kind of treatment, doctors must first know both the pros and cons of alternative therapies before fully adopting them (Figure 1.13).

Figure 1.13 Alternative Therapies	
Benefits of Select Alternative Therapies	**Precautions for Select Alternative Therapies**
Acupuncture has proven beneficial in treating pain caused by osteoarthritis, dental surgery, migraine headaches, and other causes.	Choose a reputable and experienced practitioner who can provide credentials. Be aware that insurance may not cover treatment costs.
A combination of glucosamine and chondroitin sulfate has proven beneficial for some patients with severe osteoarthritis pain. Omega 3 supplements can reduce the risk factors for heart disease.	Herbal remedies are regulated for safety but not for effectiveness. Natural products may interfere with other medications. Not all natural compounds are safe for use.
Massage benefits the development of premature infants, and it can provide relief from stress, anxiety, and the pain of migraine headaches.	Select a therapist who is trained and licensed. Avoid massage therapy if you take blood thinners or have a history of blood clots.
Meditation can reduce anxiety, depression, and chronic pain symptoms.	People with physical limitations may not be able to participate in meditative practices involving physical movement. Research is needed to determine if meditation can worsen symptoms in people who have certain psychiatric problems.

RECALL YOUR READING

1. Advances in mapping the human _____ hold promise for the development of _____ medicine that designs medical treatments for the individual patient.

2. _____, a serious drawback of organ transplantation, could be eliminated when a patient's own _____ are used to _____ new organ tissue.

3. Extreme miniaturization produced by scientists in the field of _____ could one day deliver medicine to individual cells, allowing doctors to treat a disease without damaging healthy tissue.

4. Through the practice of _____, a physician can use a robot to perform surgery on a patient in another city or possibly even another country.

5. As medical care has become more specialized, many patients want care that is more personalized. They are seeking more _____ medical therapies. The NIH has established the _____. This organization studies the _____ of alternative medical treatments.

Complete the *Map Your Reading* graphic organizer for the section you just read.

Current Issues in Healthcare

Affordability and access are the big issues challenging healthcare today. People in the United States are finding it increasingly difficult to pay for their healthcare costs. This means that more people are at risk of dying earlier due to lack of medical care. Efforts are being made, however, to address these important healthcare issues.

Affordable Healthcare

Healthcare costs in the United States have been rising for several years. As a result, the United States surpasses most other industrialized countries in terms of dollars spent on healthcare per resident (Figure 1.14 on the next page). Healthcare costs are rising faster than the rate of inflation and faster than the growth in national income. Employers and workers are finding it more and more difficult to afford health insurance, with premiums rising by more than 100 percent in the past decade. This trend of rising costs is expected to continue. Cost control, therefore, is a critical consideration for healthcare reform efforts.

Why are healthcare costs rising so rapidly? There is no simple answer because many factors are influencing this trend. One factor is the cost of newly developed healthcare technologies. The research and development costs of medications and new medical technologies increase the costs of newly developed treatments. As more consumers require or demand newer, more expensive treatments and procedures, overall spending increases.

In addition, Americans are living longer as a result of better treatments for chronic illnesses. This means that people receive more medical care for more years of life, which increases their total healthcare costs. As the baby boomer generation (people born between 1946 and 1964) ages, a larger number of people will need increased healthcare services.

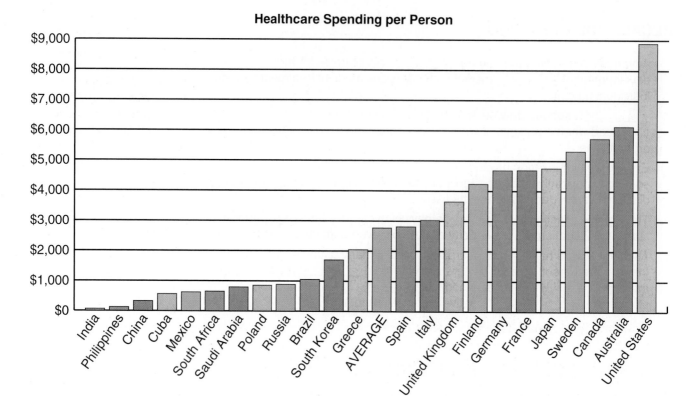

Figure 1.14   This chart shows how much money different countries spend on healthcare per person. Why do you think the US spends so much money on healthcare?

Some researchers also cite poor lifestyle choices as a factor in rising healthcare costs. For example, poor diet and lack of exercise have led to increasing obesity rates, most notably in children and teens. As a result, there has been an increase in the number of diagnosed diabetes cases. Because a higher number of newly diagnosed diabetics are young, they will require many years of healthcare treatment.

Accessible Healthcare

The cost of health insurance and out-of-pocket costs not paid by insurance create a barrier to accessing healthcare. As the cost of health insurance increases, some employers increase the amount that employees must pay to receive insurance, or simply stop offering health insurance.

Healthcare costs for an average family of four equal more than $20,000 per year (Figure 1.15). A family's out-of-pocket costs for healthcare are often greater than the amount spent on food, clothing, or transportation. In some cases, these costs are almost as much as a family spends on housing. When insurance is offered through an employer, the average worker pays $400 to $500 per month for insurance premiums. In addition, people must pay other healthcare costs, such as insurance deductibles and co-pays for prescriptions. You will learn more about these insurance terms in chapter 4.

While low-income families can qualify for Medicaid insurance and older individuals can sign up for Medicare, a growing number of middle class individuals and families are unable to afford health insurance. In 2013, about 50 million Americans lacked basic health insurance and

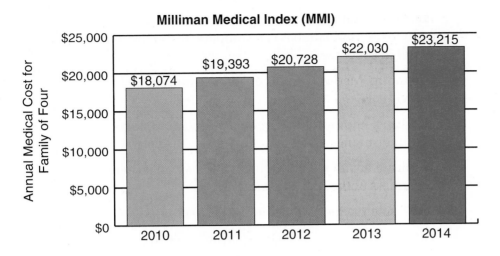

Milliman Medical Index (MMI)

Annual Medical Cost for Family of Four

- $25,000
- $20,000
- $15,000
- $10,000
- $5,000
- $0

$18,074 (2010)
$19,393 (2011)
$20,728 (2012)
$22,030 (2013)
$23,215 (2014)

Figure 1.15   This chart from Milliman, a statistical consulting firm, shows how much the average family spent on healthcare in recent years.

accessed care only in an emergency. This emergency care is expensive and most people cannot pay for it without help. As a result, hospitals and taxpayers are spending about $43 billion dollars each year to cover the costs of those who were treated but could not pay.

A shortage of primary care physicians, especially in rural areas, creates another healthcare accessibility problem. Many American physicians choose to specialize in a specific area of medicine. As a result, foreign-born physicians have filled many primary care positions in the United States. While this helps to alleviate the physician shortage, it can create a different kind of roadblock for those accessing healthcare. Imagine an elderly patient with hearing loss communicating with her soft-spoken physician who speaks English with a strong accent.

Addressing the Issues

Many cost-containment measures have already been tried in the healthcare industry. For example, treatments are classified into diagnostic-related groups (DRGs) that limit the amount paid to a hospital for a patient with a specific diagnosis. Health maintenance organizations (HMOs), which aim to provide lower-cost healthcare through contracts between insurance companies and healthcare providers, often provide preventive care free or at little cost. This system is based on the belief that prevention of illness reduces potential treatment costs.

In contrast, preferred provider organizations (PPOs) require members to choose from a select group of medical providers who have agreed to provide services for a specific cost. The use of home healthcare services and outpatient surgical centers reduces hospital costs. None of these measures, however, has been able to control the rising cost of healthcare.

On March 23, 2010, a national healthcare reform bill called the *Patient Protection and Affordable Care Act*, or the *Affordable Care Act*, was signed into law. The law calls for major changes to the healthcare system in an attempt to provide insurance for a larger number of Americans (Figure 1.16). Examples of major provisions of this law include the following:

- requiring most Americans to have health insurance by 2014

Figure 1.16   Provisions of the Affordable Care Act require most Americans to have health insurance. What are some other provisions of this law?

- creating a healthcare exchange or marketplace in each state where individuals and families can compare health insurance plans and enroll in coverage

- expanding Medicaid to cover a larger number of low-income individuals

- requiring employers with more than fifty employees to offer health insurance

- requiring health insurance plans to cover all individuals, regardless of their health status

- increasing payments for primary care services

- eliminating co-payments for specific preventive care services

- increasing support for prevention, wellness, and public health services

The specific requirements of this new law are still being implemented, and changes to regulations and processes are ongoing. While everyone agrees on the need to control healthcare costs and make healthcare affordable for all Americans, not everyone agrees with the requirements of this law. The changes required by the Affordable Care Act face strong political and policy challenges. As a result, the implementation of the law will continue to change the delivery and accessibility of healthcare for the foreseeable future.

Complete the
Map Your Reading
graphic organizer for the
section you just read.

RECALL YOUR READING

1. The cost of healthcare is outpacing Americans' ability to pay for it. In fact, health insurance _____ have risen by more than 100 percent in the past decade.

2. Many factors contribute to increasing healthcare costs, including the development of new _____, the increasing _____ of American citizens, and the rising rate of _____ among young people.

3. Rising insurance rates limit _____ to healthcare for many Americans. Even when an employer provides insurance coverage, the costs paid by the _____ are greater than all other family expenses except for housing.

4. A shortage of _____ restricts access to healthcare, especially in _____ areas of our country.

5. The Patient Protection and Affordable Care Act is bringing changes to healthcare with the goal of providing _____ for more Americans.

Career Pathways and Employment Opportunities

How will you find your future career in healthcare? While the path to your career is not always a direct route, your journey begins by learning about as many opportunities as you possibly can. National organizations that focus on career and technical education have developed a system for organizing all of the identified jobs and careers that exist today. The result is sixteen groups called **career clusters** (Figure 1.17). You will begin your search by looking at these clusters.

career clusters
groups of similar occupations and industries that share a core set of basic knowledge and skills for all workers

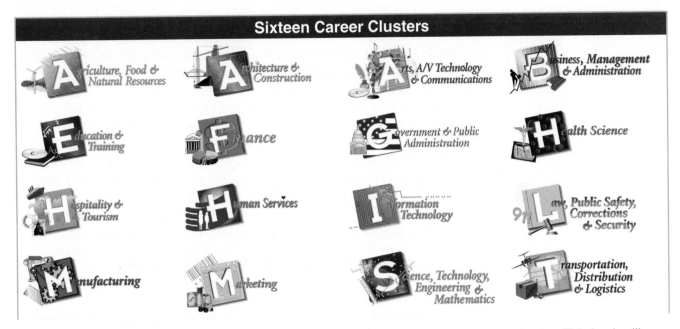

Sixteen Career Clusters

Figure 1.17   All occupations in the US workforce are addressed within these 16 career clusters. This book will discuss many possible careers within the Health Science cluster. What are some occupations you know that would fall under the category of Health Science?

Career Clusters and Pathways

Each career cluster contains a specific group of occupations and industries based on the similar knowledge and skills that they require. High schools and colleges use the clusters to develop courses that will prepare students for career success. You will use the career clusters to discover your personal interests and preferences. The clusters can help you to choose an occupational area that will lead you toward a satisfying career.

Identifying Your Interests and Strengths. Taking a career cluster survey will identify your top occupational interest areas. Sometimes students with a strong interest in health science are surprised when the health science cluster is not their top choice in the survey results. Career interests often come from life experiences, which are powerful motivators. But a person's anticipated career choice may not fit his or her personal preferences and strengths when the daily tasks of that career are examined.

Career Choice: Angie

When Angie was in elementary school, her beloved grandma became ill with cancer. Through many months of treatment, Angie observed several different nurses who provided care for her grandmother. She was impressed and moved by their compassionate care. As a result of this experience, she decided to become a nurse. As a high school student, she took every available health science class. The science and math courses were not her favorites, but she worked hard to learn the skills needed for a nursing career. When it came time to take a nursing assistant course, Angie found the clinical practice agonizing. Her stomach clenched each time she thought about going back to work with the patients. One night she broke down in tears in the employee lounge. It was time to reconsider her choice.

Angie still had a strong desire to help people but found that she did not enjoy the close physical care aspects of the nursing profession. She thought about the classes she enjoyed in school and remembered how much she liked the business projects in her marketing class. Her health science teacher reminded her that she did an excellent job leading the HOSA–Future Health Professionals service-learning project. The teacher also identified some of Angie's natural strengths, including recruiting and training fellow student volunteers, developing and delivering a healthcare presentation to 300 students, and designing and producing hands-on activities for the students to use. Angie also had a positive attitude and could always get fellow students excited about HOSA activities.

Though her life experiences had motivated Angie to become a nurse, she soon realized that her personal strengths did not fit that chosen career. Eventually, Angie decided that she was better suited to a career in marketing than one in nursing. When she finishes her degree, she hopes to do marketing or public relations work for a healthcare organization.

---

career pathways
smaller groups of specialized occupations within a career cluster that require more specific sets of knowledge, skills, and training

Within each career cluster, you will find individual pathways (Figure 1.18). A **career pathway** includes a smaller set of specialized occupations. Each career cluster has a core set of basic knowledge and skills used by all workers in that cluster. Each pathway contains a more specific set of knowledge, skills, and training that will build on the cluster's core knowledge.

Knowing the career cluster and pathway you are interested in pursuing helps you create a program of study for high school and college. As a health science student, for example, a program of study based on your chosen career pathway can help you understand why math and science courses are important to your future. Knowing your program of study may also offer opportunities to earn college credit while you are still in high school. Many high schools offer dual credit and advanced placement college coursework that is relevant to a student's career goals. In some cases, students actually attend courses at a college located near their high school. Following the sequence of courses outlined in your program of study will prepare you for employment in your chosen career.

As you research your healthcare career, include career clusters other than health science in your search. You may be surprised to learn that many occupations found in other career clusters are part of the healthcare industry (Figure 1.19 on page 24).

Health Science Career Cluster. To understand the wide variety of available healthcare careers, you will want to explore the entire health science cluster. The health science career cluster includes five distinct career pathways:

- **Health Informatics Services**—occupations focused on documenting patient care

- **Therapeutic** (thair-uh-PYU-tihk) **Services**—occupations that change the health status of a patient over time

- **Diagnostic Services**—occupations that create a picture of a patient's health status at a single point in time

- **Support Services**—occupations that create a therapeutic environment for providing patient care

- **Biotechnology Research and Development**—occupations involved in biotechnology research and development that applies to human health

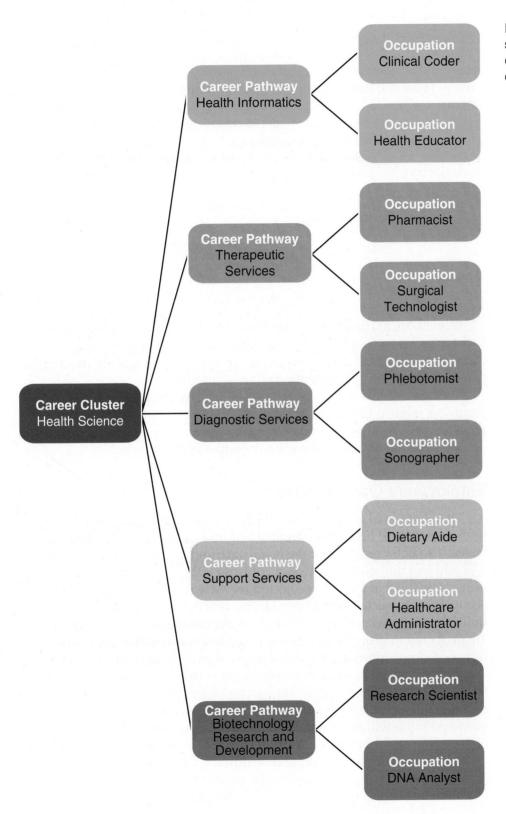

Figure 1.18   This flowchart shows different healthcare occupations organized by cluster and pathway.

Figure 1.19 Health Occupations in Other Career Clusters	
Cluster	**Healthcare Occupation**
Agriculture, Food, and Natural Resources	• dietitian • biochemist • food scientist
Education and Training	• adaptive physical education specialist • athletic trainer
Government and Public Administration	• epidemiologist • social worker • public health manager
Law, Public Safety, Corrections, and Security	• emergency medical technician • paramedic
Science, Technology, Engineering, and Mathematics	• biomedical engineer • biophysicist • medical scientist • microbiologist

More than 300 different occupations are spread out over these five pathways. Sometimes the tasks of a particular occupation fall into more than one pathway. Consider the physician who both diagnoses (diagnostic pathway) and treats (therapeutic pathway) an illness.

Each unit of this text focuses on one of the five health science career pathways (Figure 1.20). Studying the unique knowledge and skills required for a healthcare worker in each pathway will help you find the pathway that is the best fit for your strengths and interests.

Employment Opportunities

The Bureau of Labor Statistics (BLS) is a national agency that keeps track of statistical data about occupations and industries in the United States. The BLS predicts that the healthcare and social assistance sector will add five million jobs between 2012 and 2022. This accounts for nearly one-third of the total projected increase in jobs. Fourteen of the 30 occupations projected to have the largest percentage increase during this time period are related to healthcare. Healthcare support occupations are projected to grow by 28.1 percent, and healthcare practitioner and technical occupations are projected to grow by 21.5 percent.

This growth in healthcare employment is driven by two of the same factors that affect healthcare costs—an aging population and longer life expectancy. As the baby boomer generation ages, this large segment of our population will need additional healthcare services. The result is an increased need for healthcare workers.

Due to improved nutrition and healthcare, life expectancy for Americans has increased dramatically in the past century. People born in 1900 could expect to live an average of 49 years. People born just a

Figure 1.20 Example Healthcare Occupations by Pathway

Pathways	Therapeutic Services	Diagnostics Services	Health Informatics	Support Services	Biotechnology Research and Development
Sample Career Specialties/Occupations	Acupuncturist Art/Music/Dance Therapist(s) Athletic Trainer Audiologist Certified Nursing Assistant Chiropractor Dental Assistant Dental Hygienist Dentist Dietitian/Nutritionist Emergency Medical Technician Home Health Aide Licensed Practical Nurse Massage Therapist Occupational Therapist Occupational Therapy Assistant Orthotist/Prosthetist Paramedic Pharmacist Pharmacy Technician Physical Therapist Physician (MD/DO) Physician Assistant Psychologist Registered Nurse Rehabilitation Counselor Social Worker Speech Language Pathologist Veterinarian	Audiologist Cardiovascular Technologist Clinical Laboratory Technician Computer Tomography (CT) Technologist Electrocardiographic (ECG) Technician Exercise Physiologist Genetic Counselor Magnetic Resonance (MR) Technologist Mammographer Medical Technologist/ Clinical Laboratory Scientist Nuclear Medicine Technologist Nutritionist/ Dietitian Occupational Therapist Optometrist Phlebotomist Physical Therapist Positron Emission Tomography (PET) Technologist Radiologic Technician Respiratory Therapist	Admitting Clerk Clinical Account Manager Clinical Account Technician Clinical Coder Clinical Data Management Specialist Data Quality Manager Epidemiologist Ethicist Health Educator Health Information Administrator Health Information Technician Healthcare Administrator Information Security Officer Medical Assistant Medical Illustrator Medical Librarian Patient Advocates Patient Information Coordinator Project Manager Quality Data Analyst Reimbursement Specialist Risk Management Transcriptionist Unit Coordinator	Biomedical/Clinical Engineer Biomedical/Clinical Technician Clinical Simulator Technician Central Service Manager Central Service Technician Dietary Manager Dietary Aide Environmental Services Facilities Manager Health Care Administrator Maintenance Engineer Industrial Hygienist Interpreter Materials Manager Transport Technician	Biochemist Bioinformatics Associate Bioinformatics Scientist Bioinformatics Specialist Biomedical Chemist Biomedical/Clinical Engineer Biomedical/Clinical Technician Biostatistician Cell Biologist Clinical Data Management Associate/Consultant Clinical Pharmacologist Clinical Trials Monitor Clinical Trials Research Coordinator Geneticist Laboratory Technician Medical Editor/Writer Microbiologist Molecular Biologist Pharmaceutical Sales Representative Pharmaceutical Scientist Pharmacologist Processing Technician Quality Assurance Technician Quality Control Technician Regulatory Affairs Specialist Research Assistant Research Scientist Toxicologist

Cluster Knowledge and Skills

Cluster K&S

• Academic Foundation • Communications •Systems • Employability Skills • Legal Responsibilities • Ethics
• Safety Practices • Teamwork • Health Maintenance Practices • Technical Skills • Information Technology Applications

hundred years later, in 2000, can expect to live an average of 77 years, and a person born in 2010 can expect to live 78.7 years. Longer lives mean a longer time to maintain health. Again, the result is an increased need for healthcare workers.

Career Education and Training

Jobs in healthcare require different levels of education and training. Some entry-level workers receive on-the-job training, but most jobs require education beyond a high school diploma. Education past high school, which is called **postsecondary education**, can be obtained at community colleges, vocational or technical colleges, public and private colleges and universities, institutes of technology, and career colleges.

When you enter a postsecondary training program, you will earn college credit for the courses you complete (Figure 1.21). A class that meets for three hours each week usually earns you three credits. While that sounds easy compared to high school, college programs expect students to complete about two hours of homework for every hour of class time. So a full-time student taking 15 credits is expected to attend 15 hours of class time and complete 30 hours of homework time, for a total of 45 hours per week. Clearly, knowing how to read efficiently and study independently is important for college success.

When choosing your college program, look for one that is accredited. This means that the program has been approved by an agency that makes sure the program has quality standards and truly prepares its students for employment.

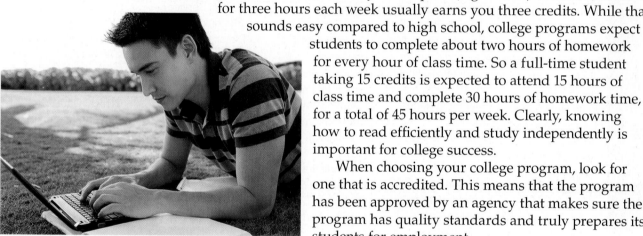

Figure 1.21 College students are expected to complete many hours of independent study.

accreditation
official recognition from a professional association that an educational program meets minimum educational standards for an occupation

The Importance of Accreditation: Liam

Liam learned about the importance of accredited programs the hard way. He happily enrolled in the new nursing program at a local career college when he learned that there was no waiting list. While the school cost more than the local technical college, Liam figured getting finished faster would make the higher cost worthwhile.

Everything went well until graduation, when Liam learned that the school had applied for **accreditation**, but had not yet been approved by the accrediting agency. This meant that Liam and his fellow graduates were not eligible to take the national certification test and, as a result, could not legally work as registered nurses.

Fortunately, this story has a happy ending. The school did receive accreditation within a few months. Liam passed the certification test and now works at a local hospital. Nevertheless, he had many anxious moments during those months after graduation when he wondered if he would ever be able to work as a registered nurse. Be sure to check that your chosen school or training program is accredited.

Postsecondary programs award different types of degrees based on the number of credits earned. The occupation you choose will determine the type of degree you need. For example, an occupational therapy assistant needs an associate's degree, but an occupational therapist must have a master's degree. Different schools offer different degrees. Figure 1.22A shows the types of degrees healthcare workers can earn. Figure 1.22B shows three medical professions and the level of education needed for each.

Figure 1.22A Postsecondary Program Degrees

Length of Program	Degree Awarded	Educational Institution
4 or more additional years	Doctor of Philosophy (PhD)	university/graduate school
2 or more additional years	master's degree (MS or MA)	university/graduate school
4-year academic program	bachelor's degree (BS or BA)	university/undergraduate school
2-year technical program	associate's degree	community or technical college
1-year technical program	diploma	community or technical college
less than 1 year technical program	certificate	community or technical college
on-the-job training	none	none

Figure 1.22B Education and Training Required for Medical Professionals

Medical Professional	Training Needed
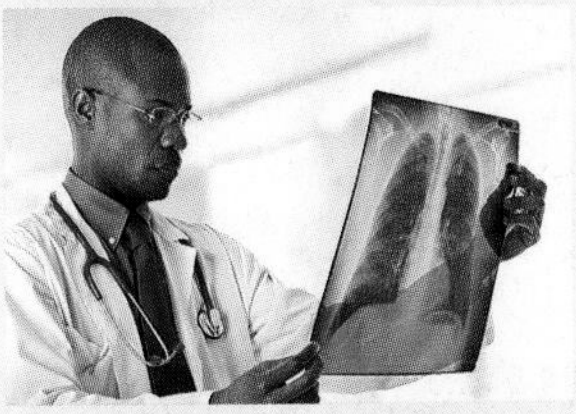 Medical Doctor—MD	• completion of a bachelor's degree followed by four years of medical school • completion of 3 or more years of residency after medical school
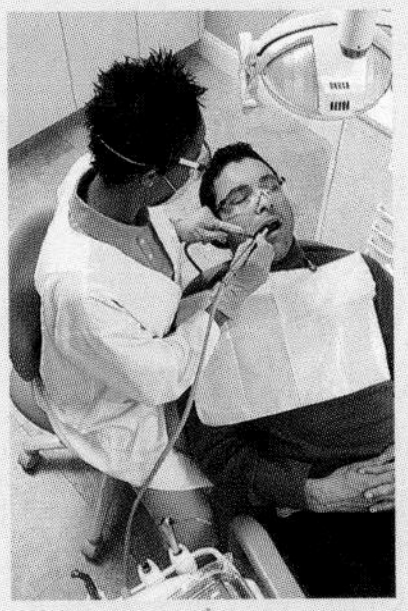 Dentist—DDS or DMD	• completion of a bachelor's degree followed by four years of dental school • completion of an additional two–four years for a specialty
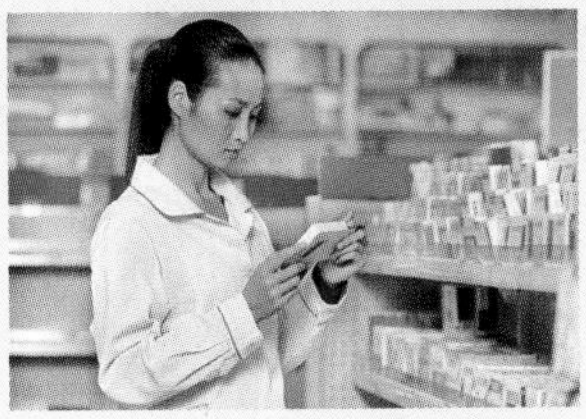 Pharmacist—PharmD	• completion of an associate degree or more commonly a bachelor's degree • completion of four years of pharmacy school

Job Titles and Credentials

credentials
documents proving a person's qualifications for a particular occupation

Healthcare organizations want to hire credentialed workers. This means that, in addition to earning a degree, a worker needs to pass a special test that further proves he or she is skilled in performing the duties of a specific healthcare occupation. After passing such a test, the worker has the credentials to perform the job for which he or she has been trained.

The terms *certification, licensure,* and *registration* all refer to a healthcare worker's **credentials**. While these terms have slightly different meanings, they all tell a future employer that a worker is qualified (Figure 1.23). Certification is awarded after a person has completed a course of study. Licensure is given after a person passes a licensure exam that proves he or she meets the qualifications for a particular occupation. Registration refers to the official record of individuals who have passed an examination and are qualified to perform the tasks of a specific occupation.

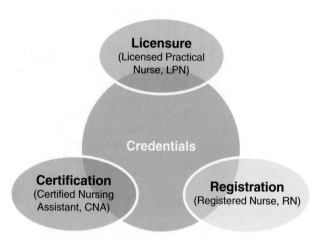

Figure 1.23 These are the different types of credentials available and examples of healthcare occupations that require credentials. Why are credentials important?

The titles of healthcare jobs can often tell you the level of education and training required to do each job (Figure 1.24). Entry-level titles such as *aide* or *assistant* indicate occupations that require fewer years of training and education. Advanced titles such as *technologist* or *therapist* indicate the need for several years of training and education.

As you determine how many years of training and education you want to pursue, you may want to compare the duties of an aide, a technician, and a therapist within an occupation such as physical therapy or medical lab careers.

Figure 1.24 Education and Training Requirements			
Job Title	**Education and Training**	**Examples**	**Exceptions**
technologist or therapist	bachelor's degree; often master's degree	occupational therapist medical lab technologist	respiratory therapist surgical technologist (both can be associate degree programs)
technician	associate's degree	dental lab technician biomedical technician	pharmacy technician healthcare technician (both require one year or less of education and training)
aide or assistant	diploma or certificate program requiring one year or less of education and training	medical assistant dental assistant therapy aide	occupational therapy assistant physical therapy assistant (both are associate degree programs)

Career Ladders

Due to the rising cost of college, students are looking for ways to make postsecondary education more affordable. Many are choosing to use a **career ladder** approach to their education (Figure 1.25). A career ladder represents the progression of jobs within a specific occupation or a particular work setting. The bottom of the ladder is the entry-level position that requires the least amount of training. As you move up the ladder, the job titles indicate increased education and training as well as increased responsibility.

career ladder
a sequence of job positions progressing from entry-level to higher levels of responsibility and authority based on education, experience, and performance

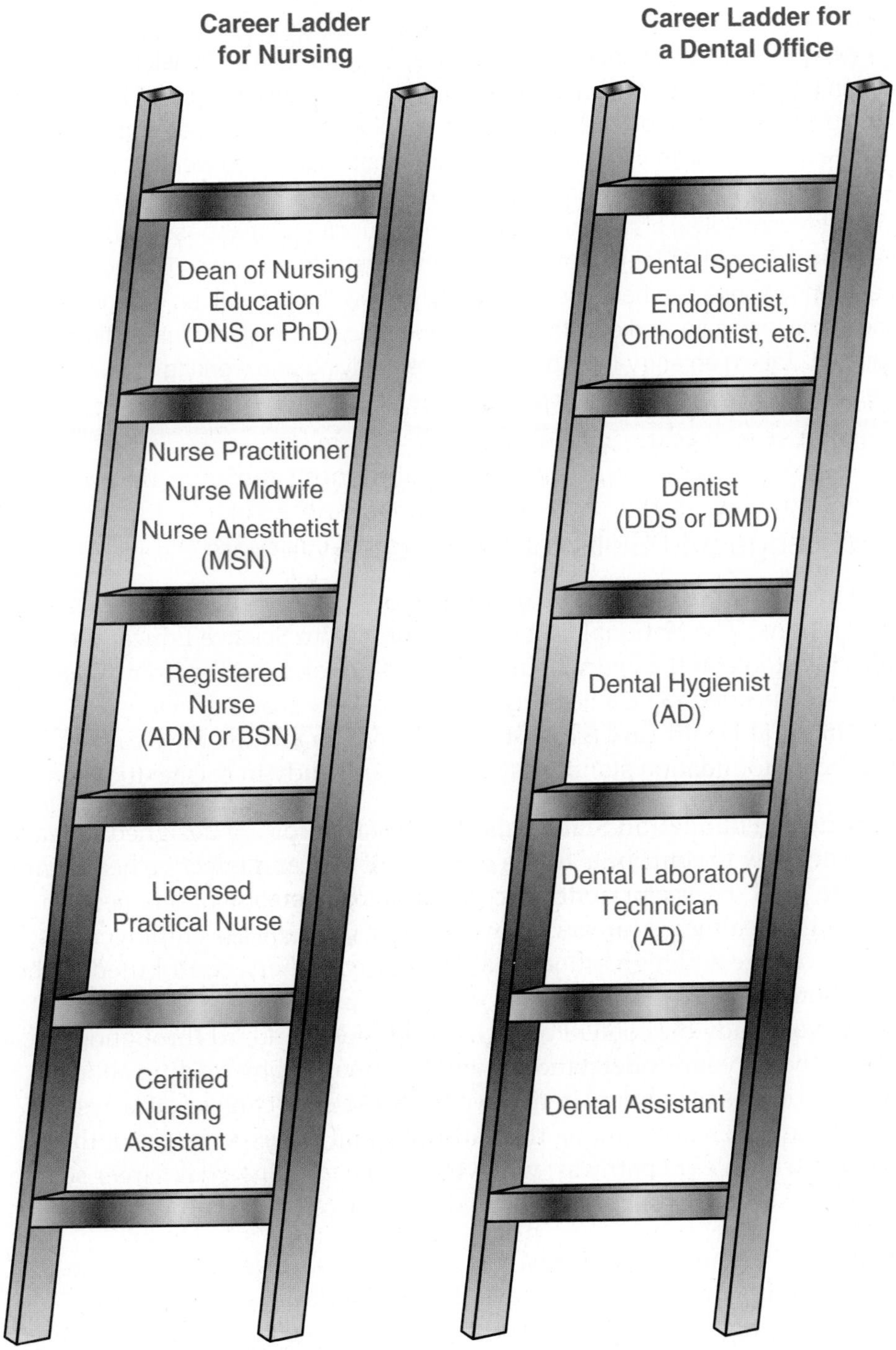

Figure 1.25   Entry-level jobs appear at the bottom of the career ladder. As you "climb the ladder," additional education and training are required. Jobs within the same occupation "piggyback" on each other. For example, you need to have an RN license before training to become a nurse anesthetist. However, jobs within the same work setting may have completely different education and training requirements. For example, you do not have to train as a dental hygienist before studying to become a dentist.

Career Ladder for Nursing

- Dean of Nursing Education (DNS or PhD)
- Nurse Practitioner Nurse Midwife Nurse Anesthetist (MSN)
- Registered Nurse (ADN or BSN)
- Licensed Practical Nurse
- Certified Nursing Assistant

Career Ladder for a Dental Office

- Dental Specialist Endodontist, Orthodontist, etc.
- Dentist (DDS or DMD)
- Dental Hygienist (AD)
- Dental Laboratory Technician (AD)
- Dental Assistant

Using the Career Ladder: Lamar

Lamar used a career ladder approach to his education by taking health science classes in high school. While he thought he would like to become an X-ray technician, he decided to take a nursing assistant course so he could get an entry-level job in healthcare. After high school, Lamar enrolled in the local community college and lived at home to save money. He continued to work at a local nursing home and learned that he enjoyed the tasks involved in the nursing profession.

The next year, Lamar transferred to the state university in a nearby city and continued to live at home. He found a nursing assistant job in a hospital close to his new school and continued to work while studying for his bachelor's degree in nursing. Lamar's employer helped to pay some of the tuition costs of his classes. Employers often support the education of employees who are seeking advanced degrees or certification. Since they want to maintain a skilled workforce, employers may forgive student loans or reimburse tuition for employees.

After completing his bachelor's degree in nursing, Lamar passed the national examination for nurses and became a registered nurse. The hospital was happy to hire him because they already knew that he was an energetic and compassionate worker with strong communication skills for interacting with patients. Taking an entry-level position while studying and working his way up the career ladder was a good strategy for Lamar.

Knowledge and Skills for Healthcare Workers

How do you begin to prepare for one of the 300 different healthcare occupations? The National Consortium for Health Science Education (NCHSE) took on the overwhelming task of organizing the knowledge and skills needed to be a healthcare worker. This group developed the **National Healthcare Skill Standards**, which include the eleven healthcare foundation standards that you will study in this textbook.

Healthcare Foundation Standards. These standards are designed to teach students how to contribute to the delivery of safe and effective healthcare (Figure 1.26). They represent the core set of skills most workers need to succeed in healthcare careers. More than 1,000 healthcare employers, as well as college and high school health science teachers, contributed to the development of the standards.

As you study the content of each foundation standard throughout this textbook, your understanding will be enhanced by reading about the experiences of workers in the five health science career pathways. By noting the differences among the pathways and the experiences of the workers within each pathway, you will be able to refine your career search and learn the core skills you will need for a successful healthcare career.

Healthcare Pathway Standards. The NCHSE also developed standards for each of the five career pathways. These standards advance your knowledge in a specific pathway after you have mastered the foundation

National Healthcare Skill Standards
standards determined by the National Consortium for Health Science Education, which describe the skills that workers need to succeed in healthcare careers

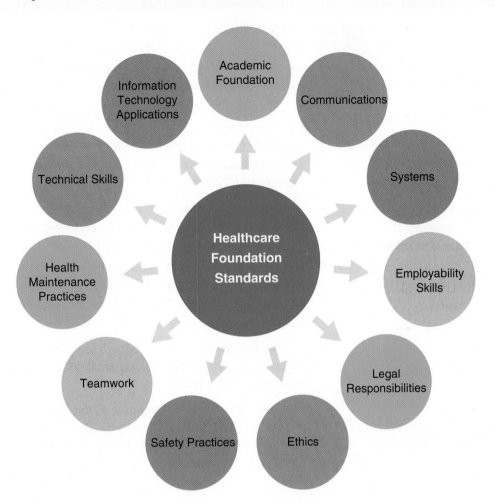

Figure 1.26   These categories of healthcare standards are all important for students to learn.

standards. While you might address the pathway standards in upper-level high school health science courses or in youth apprenticeship work programs, they are mainly the focus of postsecondary training programs.

RECALL YOUR READING

1. Taking a career cluster survey will help you to identify general career areas of interest to you. Looking at the smaller groups of occupations called _____ within the clusters you identified will help you narrow your search to specific _____ with similar sets of skills and knowledge.

2. Most healthcare jobs require further _____ after you finish high school.

3. In addition to completing a specialized training program, healthcare workers often need to obtain _____, which mean that they have passed a test of their knowledge and skills.

4. As individuals gain experience or complete additional education, they can move up the _____ in their occupation.

5. The _____ Standards include the eleven healthcare foundation standards you will study in this textbook.

Complete the *Map Your Reading* graphic organizer for the section you just read.

Welcome to the field of health science. Keep your eyes and ears open on this journey through the amazing variety of careers you will encounter in this field. Who knows? Maybe you will discover the pathway to your future.

SUMMARY

 Assess your understanding
with chapter tests

- Both the practice of and attitudes toward healthcare have evolved over the centuries.

- Healthcare is rapidly changing due to technological advances.

- A holistic approach to medical care works to maintain or restore mental, spiritual, and social wellness in addition to physical wellness.

- The National Center of Complementary and Alternative Medicine oversees scientific research studies to determine the effectiveness of alternative therapies.

- The cost of medical care in the United States is rising faster than the rate of inflation.

- Access to healthcare is a problem for many Americans, either because they can't afford health insurance or because there is no physician practicing in their community.

- The Patient Protection and Affordable Care Act calls for major changes to the US healthcare system to provide care to a larger number of citizens.

- All careers and industries can be grouped into one of sixteen clusters.

- The health science career cluster includes five occupational pathways: health informatics services, therapeutic services, diagnostic services, support services, and biotechnology research and development.

- Employment opportunities in healthcare are growing due to an aging population and the increasing life spans of US citizens.

- Healthcare workers earn credentials by completing specialized training programs and passing a licensing test before they are certified to work.

- Healthcare workers often progress to more advanced positions by seeking additional education and training.

- Students learn how to contribute to the delivery of safe and effective healthcare by studying course content that is based on the healthcare foundation standards.

MAXIMIZE YOUR PROFESSIONAL VOCABULARY

 Build vocabulary with
e-flash cards, games,
and audio glossary

Listed below are the essential, yellow-highlighted terms and the additional professional vocabulary terms that you encountered in this chapter. Complete the activities that follow the list to make all of these terms part of your everyday professional vocabulary.

accreditation

alternative, complementary,
    integrative therapies

aneurysms

antioxidant

career clusters

career ladder

career pathways

catheters

chronic

colonoscopy

coronary

credentials

gene therapy

genomic medicine

holistic care

infusion

in vitro

laparoscopic

mammogram

metabolize

molecular imaging

nanotechnology

National Healthcare Skill
    Standards

outpatient procedures

pacemakers

postsecondary education

regenerative medicine

stent

telesurgery

Western medicine

VOCABULARY DEVELOPMENT

Matching. Match each essential term from this chapter with the correct definition below by writing the letter of the definition next to the number of the essential term on a separate sheet of paper.

1. accreditation

2. alternative, complementary, integrative therapies

3. career clusters

4. career ladder

5. career pathways

6. credentials

7. genomic medicine

8. holistic care

9. nanotechnology

10. National Healthcare Skill Standards

11. regenerative medicine

12. Western medicine

a. standards determined by the National Consortium for Health Science Education, which describe the skills that workers need to succeed in healthcare careers

b. official recognition from a professional association that an educational program meets minimum educational standards for an occupation

c. documents proving a person's qualifications for a particular occupation

d. a form of medical care that creates living tissue to replace tissue or organ functions lost due to age, disease, injury, or birth disorder

e. groups of similar occupations and industries that share a core set of basic knowledge and skills for all workers

f. therapies that treat the patient as a whole person after assessing the individual's physical, social, mental, and spiritual well-being

g. a field of science that manipulates individual atoms and molecules to create devices that are thousands of times smaller than current technologies allow

h. the most common form of medical care in the United States, which uses medication and surgery to treat the signs and symptoms of illness

i. a sequence of job positions progressing from entry-level to higher levels of responsibility and authority based on education, experience, and performance

j. healthcare practices and treatments that minimize or avoid the use of surgery and drugs

k. personalized medical care that uses a patient's unique combination of genes and chromosomes to prevent illness and maintain health

l. smaller groups of specialized occupations within a career cluster that require more specific sets of knowledge, skills, and training

13. **Stand Up/Sit Down Terms Review.** Form two rows of chairs and stand in front of them with one student per chair, facing each other to form two teams. A leader, chosen by the class, will walk between the rows asking students for either a term or a definition. A correct answer allows the student to sit down. The first team with all students sitting wins.

14. **Target Practice Terms Review.** Draw a target shape with two rings and a bull's-eye in the center on a separate sheet of paper. In the outer ring, list vocabulary terms that refer to illness or the delivery of healthcare. In the middle ring, list the five career pathways in the field of healthcare. In the bull's-eye, list

terms that are connected to occupations and employment. Start with the outer ring and define each term. Circle each term you can't define. Continue defining terms until you hit the bull's-eye.

REFLECT ON YOUR READING

15. Review the disease treatment predictions you made before reading this chapter. How have your predictions changed now that you have finished reading the chapter? Select one healthcare trend that interests you. Why do you think that trend is significant? Reconnect with your class partner and share your thoughts.

BUILD CORE SKILLS

16. **Writing.** After reading this chapter, write a paragraph describing at least one way in which the costs of healthcare impact our country's economy.

17. **Critical Thinking.** Review Figure 1.3 and note the discoveries that are still important in today's delivery of healthcare. Use the Internet to search for important people in the history of medicine. Select one individual and list his or her main accomplishment, when it occurred, and its importance to healthcare today. Form groups based on the periods in history identified in Figure 1.3. As you share your findings with the class, note the number of students in each group. Can you use this information to draw a conclusion about the rate of medical advances made throughout history?

18. **Math.** Refer to Figure 1.6 to answer the following questions.

   a. Why are some bars green, some blue, and some purple?

   b. What do the numbers at the top of each bar tell us?

   c. What is the purpose of the black line?

   d. According to the data in the chart, what was the effect of the "Back to Sleep" campaign on the incidence of SIDS?

19. **Critical Thinking.** In this chapter you learned about the ways in which technology is affecting health sciences. You also learned that health science careers can be organized into five pathways. Do some research to identify at least one technological advancement in each of the five career pathways. Report your findings to the class.

20. **Math.** Complete the table at the bottom of this page to determine the monetary value of more education in the field of nursing. Your goal is to find the total dollar amount earned in a ten-year period minus the cost of education for each of the nursing credentials in the table. Remember to calculate using compounded percentage increases for salary and round totals to the nearest dollar amount. Does more education equal more income? Is further education worth the cost? Discuss with your classmates.

21. **Problem Solving.** Research the number of primary care physicians per resident in your community. Do you have a shortage? Across the United States, the average number of primary physicians per 1,000 residents ranges from 0.9 to 2.8. According to the chapter, what is one factor contributing to the shortage of primary physicians in the United States? Suggest ways to solve this problem.

22. **Critical Thinking.** Complete a career clusters survey. You can find many different surveys online. One possible survey can be found at the website for the National Association of State Directors of Career Technical Education Consortium, under *Career Clusters* and *Resources*. After completing the survey, identify your three top clusters of career interest. What factors will you consider as you choose a healthcare career if health science is not your first choice in the cluster quiz?

23. **Critical Thinking.** Select two of your own healthcare experiences from the following list. For each experience, identify a healthcare worker who played a role in that experience. Identify that worker's health science pathway and describe the credentials required for that healthcare career.

   Healthcare experiences: eating hospital food, having hearing checked, having a blood test, having vision checked, receiving oxygen, having teeth cleaned, reading a medical bill, taking a sick pet to a doctor, taking a

	Certified Nursing Assistant	Licensed Practical Nurse	Bachelor's of Science–Nurse	Master's of Science–Nurse
Cost of education for tuition and fees	$500 (1 course)	$3,000 (1 year)	$34,000 (4 years)	$54,000 (6 years)
Beginning yearly salary	$22,000	$31,000	$52,000	$80,000
Total 10-year income assuming annual 4% raises				
Total income minus the cost of education				

prescription medication, seeing a baby on a sonogram

24. **Speaking and Listening.** Locate an article about a future healthcare trend in the newspaper or online. Use any of the topics in the chapter or research a future healthcare trend that interests you. Cut out or print the article and type up a two-paragraph summary. In the first paragraph, summarize the main points of the article. In the second paragraph, include your personal thoughts about and reactions to what you have read. Be prepared to discuss your summary with your fellow students.

25. **Critical Thinking.** Match each medical advance in the left column with its corresponding example in the right column.

1. genomic medicine
2. nanotechnology
3. alternative therapies
4. regenerative medicine
5. surgical advances
6. computer technology
7. medical imaging
8. robotics

a. stents
b. telesurgery
c. virtual colonoscopy
d. laparoscopy
e. online medical records
f. lab-grown organ tissue
g. gene therapy
h. acupuncture

26. **Math.** Figure 1.15 indicates that US healthcare costs continue to rise. How much have they increased compared to income? Using the chart data and the following information, calculate the percentage of income spent on healthcare in 2010 and 2013.

The US median household income in 2010 was $51,144 and in 2013 it was $52,250. Budget experts recommend spending 25 to 30 percent of your income on housing and 15 percent each on food and transportation. Their recommendation for healthcare is 10 percent. Using the information given here and in Figure 1.15, what problems do you foresee in the budgets of the average American families?

ACTIVATE YOUR LEARNING

27. Pick one of the healthcare careers listed in Figure 1.20. Research this career and write 10 brief factual statements about the career you chose. Be prepared to play "Who Am I?," in which students take turns being the Mystery Career Contestant. As the contestant, you will give one statement from your list and let the rest of the class guess the career. Continue reading statements until someone guesses correctly. You may collect points for correct guesses and for stumping the class.

28. Use an 8 1/2 x 11-inch sheet of paper to create a career ladder for a healthcare occupation or a healthcare work setting of your choice. List the education and training required and the average salary for each career on your ladder. Display your drawing in a location assigned by your instructor. Complete a "gallery walk" to review all your classmates' drawings. Keep the following questions in mind:

a. What is the relationship between years of education and training and the average salary of these careers?

b. What is the salary comparison for different career ladders? What are the occupations or work settings with the highest and lowest salary ranges?

THINK AND ACT LIKE A HEALTHCARE WORKER

29. Suppose your best friend tells you she is disappointed and frustrated. She has always had her heart set on a healthcare career, but her career cluster assessment results don't list the health science cluster. The results say she is well suited for careers in Agriculture, Food, and Natural Resources; Government and Public Administration; or Science, Technology, Engineering, and Mathematics. You know she does well in all of her science classes and loves to help people. What will you say to her about pursuing a career in healthcare, and what steps will you encourage her to take as she plans for her future career?

GO TO THE SOURCE

30. Use the NCCAM website to research an alternative therapy of your choice. Write a one-paragraph case study about the experiences of a patient who uses that therapy. In your account, include one result that is factual and one result that is a myth or untrue. Review your case studies as a class to see if your fellow students can recognize the myths.

Unit 1
Health Informatics

Chapter 2

Career Skills in Health Informatics

Chapter 3

Fundamental Skills in Health Informatics

Chapter 4

Professional Knowledge in Health Informatics

Chapter 5

Academic Knowledge: Medical Terminology and Body Organization

---

While studying, look for the online icon to:

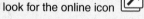

- **Listen** to the audio Glossary and review e-flash cards
- **Assess** learning with quizzes and online exercises
- **Expand** knowledge with animations and activities
- **Simulate** healthcare tasks and employability skills

www.g-wlearning.com/healthsciences

Study on the Go
Use your mobile device to practice vocabulary and assess learning
www.m.g-wlearning.com

Career Pathway

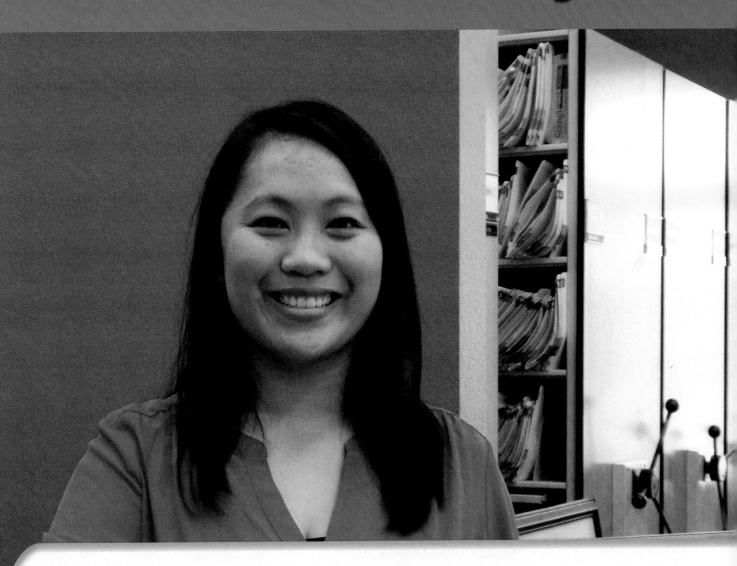

Healthcare Insider:
P. M. Xiong, Bachelors of Science
Health Care Management—Patient Care Coordinator

"I find my job to be very rewarding! The opportunity to meet new people and get to know them is the best part of my job. Making patients feel comfortable while they are visiting the dental office is essential. Many people are afraid of the dentist due to bad experiences. While working at the dental office, I realized that I wanted to manage my own office one day. I made the decision to go back to school to continue my education while working full time. It was very difficult to work full time, go to school full time, and be a mom to two young kids. But it was all worth it in the end."

Chapter 2
Career Skills in Health Informatics

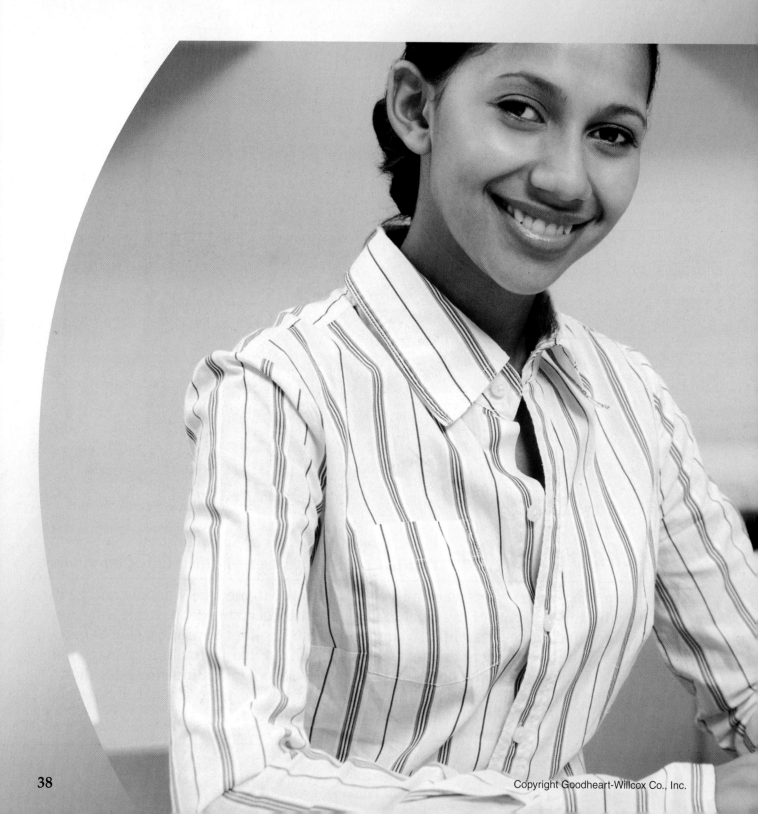

PROFESSIONAL VOCABULARY

E-flash Cards

You will need to learn the essential terms listed below before you begin your reading. These terms will help you understand the main concepts of the chapter. These terms, which will be highlighted in yellow within the text, will become part of your professional vocabulary.

In addition to these essential terms, you will see bold terms throughout the chapter. The meanings of these terms are explained where the terms first appear. The bold terms, like the essential terms listed here, will become part of your professional vocabulary and deepen your understanding of the topics presented here.

career portfolio   a written record of career planning and preparation

confidentiality   the legally protected right of patients to have their personal and medical information kept private

employability skills   skills related to choosing a career, acquiring and keeping a job, changing jobs, and advancing in a career

health informatics services   career pathway that involves methods, devices, and resources used to acquire, store, retrieve, and work with healthcare and biomedical information

HOSA–Future Health Professionals   a career and technical student organization for future healthcare workers

interdisciplinary healthcare team   a group of professionals from different health science training backgrounds working in coordination toward a common goal for the patient

internship   practical work or training experience that allows students to apply what they have learned in class

medical coding   the act of assigning numbers to descriptions of a patient's diseases, injuries, and treatments according to established codes

personal traits   an individual's unique combination of qualities and characteristics

professional look   the standards of appearance normally expected of a qualified person in a work environment

technical skills   the ability to perform tasks in a specific healthcare discipline or department

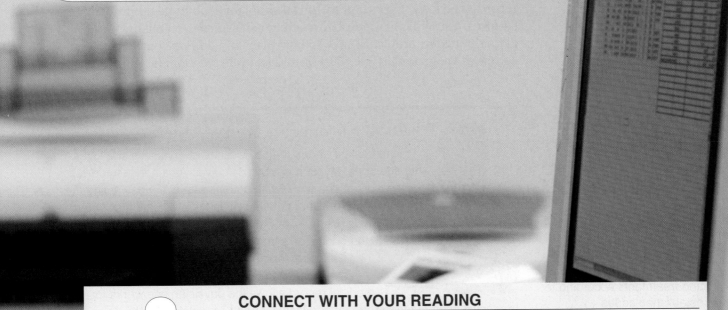

CONNECT WITH YOUR READING

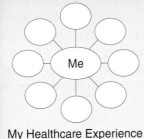

Me

My Healthcare Experience

Before you read this chapter, take time to think about a past experience you have had with healthcare. Create a bubble diagram in which the center bubble represents you. In each surrounding bubble, list a healthcare worker you saw or talked to during that healthcare experience. What seemed to be the main job of each person? Did each person work mostly with people, equipment, or information? Indicate what you believe to be the answer to this question in each person's bubble. Also draw lines or arrows to show how you believe all of the workers' jobs were connected. Share and discuss your diagram with a classmate.

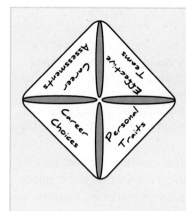

MAP YOUR READING

Create a visual summary for this chapter. Begin with a square sheet of paper—an 8 1/2-inch square works well. Fold each of the four points of the square to the center. Label each of the four resulting flaps with one of these topics: *Personal Traits*, *Career Choices*, *Effective Teams*, and *Career Assessments*. When you finish reading each of these sections in the chapter, open the corresponding flap and draw a picture or symbol to illustrate what you have read. Ask yourself what each topic looks like, how you could draw it, and what graphic or symbol best represents it. Finally, for each of the four topics, write two words that explain how the topic relates to you personally in the center square of your visual summary.

When considering healthcare careers, most people think of becoming doctors or nurses. Yet there are hundreds of different jobs in the field of healthcare. Some of those jobs fall into the career pathway of health informatics services. If you have a desire to help others, and you enjoy learning about the latest technology, you should consider a health informatics career.

In this chapter you will learn about job opportunities in **health informatics services** and begin to assess your personal career interests and aptitudes. You will also see how teamwork unfolds in a medical office and study the qualities of effective teams. You will learn the guidelines for effective correspondence and for maintaining a patient's medical record, which are important technical skills for a job in health informatics services. You will also complete a career assessment, establish your career portfolio, and learn how to improve your skills by participating in activities sponsored by HOSA–Future Health Professionals.

health informatics services
career pathway that involves methods, devices, and resources used to acquire, store, retrieve, and work with healthcare and biomedical information

medical coding
the act of assigning numbers to descriptions of a patient's diseases, injuries, and treatments according to established codes

The Health Informatics Worker: Myesha

When asked about her job, Myesha always says she loves what she does. Myesha is a puzzle solver. As a health informatics services worker, she works with patient data every day, doing the **medical coding** for every patient visit in the medical office where she works. Myesha has a strong background in anatomy. She understands the origins of, symptoms and signs of, diagnostic tests for, treatments for, and outcomes of diseases.

The information Myesha provides for a patient's medical record allows the physician she works for to receive payment for treatment services. Correctly coded information also allows the patient to receive health insurance benefits for those services. One of Myesha's favorite parts of her job is working with Medicare patients to arrange treatment plans that meet complex insurance requirements. Patients with serious illnesses feel a tremendous sense of relief when they find out that their medical costs will be reimbursed.

Myesha likes to help people, but she doesn't provide direct, hands-on care. Instead, she helps patients by ensuring their medical records contain accurate information. Myesha is a worker in the health informatics services career pathway.

Personal Traits

Are you well organized? Are you thorough and attentive to detail when you work? Is correct spelling important to you? If you possess these **personal traits**, then you might enjoy a career in the health informatics services pathway.

As you might guess from the name, information is the main focus of the health informatics worker. Because a patient's health can depend upon the accuracy of his or her medical record, health informatics workers must be thorough, reliable, and trustworthy.

Workers protect the privacy of patient information by maintaining **confidentiality**. Keeping information confidential requires more than avoiding talking about a patient's condition in a public place. Health informatics workers maintain confidentiality by

- not sharing computer passwords;

- closing any computer screen that shows patient information before leaving their work area;

- making sure that medical documents are not left in a fax machine where other people can see them;

- knowing who is able to receive a patient's medical information and which parts can be shared; and

- providing only facts and not making judgments or assumptions about the information.

Do you enjoy working with computers? Do you like learning new things? Medical records are quickly evolving from paper to electronic systems, so the computer is the constant companion of the health informatics worker.

Adjusting to new equipment, updated technologies, and revised software is common for health informatics workers. Workers must interpret rules and detailed instructions and keep up with constantly changing guidelines for coding and recording information. Health informatics workers welcome the challenge of adjusting to these changes because they want to improve the process for keeping accurate medical records.

personal traits
an individual's unique combination of qualities and characteristics

confidentiality
the legally protected right of patients to have their personal and medical information kept private

Professionalism: Kia

When you visit your local medical clinic, Kia's bright smile welcomes you. She is the medical assistant who greets you at the reception desk. As a health informatics worker, Kia accesses your account to update your personal information and checks information about your insurance coverage. She schedules your appointments and forwards your phone call to the correct worker when you call the clinic.

Kia's appearance and attitude must leave patients with a positive impression of the clinic. Without a good first experience, patients may assume that the clinic's medical care is poor and choose to find a different medical provider. A medical office is like any other business: it can't stay open if it doesn't make money.

Although Kia loves fashionable clothes, she is careful to wear business-like clothing at work. She chooses skirts and tops that are not too revealing, low heels, minimal jewelry, and light makeup to create a **professional look**.

Kia understands that she needs to look mature and **competent**, or *capable*, to patients of all ages. Appearing skilled and experienced projects an image of professionalism. In her office, visible tattoos are not allowed, and piercings are limited to her ears. Her clothing is neat, clean, and in good condition. For Kia, the way she looks is just as important as the way she acts.

Kia conveys a positive attitude naturally. She admits it was a challenge, however, to learn the practical steps for maintaining confidentiality in a medical clinic. She reminds herself to speak quietly so that patient information can't be heard by others. She is careful not to use a patient's name when calling coworkers over the intercom for a phone call. She has learned to avoid conversations about patients when she is in the elevator or the cafeteria.

professional look
the standards of appearance normally expected of a qualified person in a work environment

Health Informatics Services Career Choices

Jobs in health informatics services don't focus on direct interaction with patients or hands-on patient care. These jobs would appeal to people who are more interested in the data and information involved in healthcare than in patient interaction. If you enjoy both technology and healthcare, you might consider a career in health information management, health information technology, or health informatics (Figure 2.1).

Health Information Management

Health information management (HIM) workers assemble and organize a patient's health information to create a medical record. This document includes a **medical history** that lists all of the diseases and surgeries a patient has had, his or her current symptoms, results of examinations and diagnostic tests, treatments, and other health services. The record also lists the patient's **family medical history** because some

Figure 2.1 Health informatics services is an umbrella pathway for different types of career options that increasingly combine health information and technology. Which of the three career categories listed most interests you?

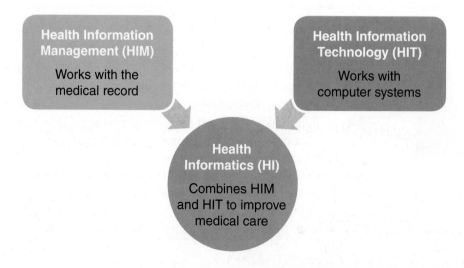

health concerns are genetic. The presence of a genetic marker for cancer or heart disease can shed light on a patient's illness or set of symptoms. Finally, the medical record contains **personal identifying information** such as a Social Security number to connect a patient to the correct record.

Increasingly, HIM employees work with electronic health records, which are stored on a computer database instead of in paper files. HIM workers understand the flow of information within healthcare facilities, from large hospital systems to a physician's private practice. HIM workers are vital to the daily collection, management, and protection of health information.

People who work in the field of health information management are called *health information technicians*. Health information technicians can specialize in particular kinds of information and data. For example, some—like Myesha, whom you read about at the beginning of the chapter—learn to code diagnoses and procedures using a numbering system. Each numerical code determines the payment the healthcare provider receives from Medicare, Medicaid, or other insurance programs. Other health information technicians may specialize in cancer registry data collection. This data is used to track treatment, survival, and recovery rates for research purposes.

Technicians work in all types of medical facilities, from dental offices to medical clinics to hospitals. Day shifts are common, with evening and night shifts available in facilities that are open 24 hours a day. A two-year associate's degree is the most common educational requirement for a health information technician.

Employers prefer to hire credentialed technicians. To become credentialed, a worker must pass a test to become certified and will continue to take classes each year to keep that certification up-to-date. There are separate certifications for health information technicians and medical coders (Figure 2.2).

Technology is changing the work and job titles of some health information technicians. For example, the medical **transcriptionist** used to type medical record information from a physician's recorded **dictation**, a verbal recording describing a patient's symptoms and the treatment given. This was a special skill that involved listening, pausing the recording, and accurately typing what was said. Recent improvements in computerized speech recognition software have made typing almost completely unnecessary.

Figure 2.2 Certifications for Health Information Technicians

Registered Health Information Administrator (RHIA®)	manages patient health information and medical records
Registered Health Information Technician (RHIT®)	ensures that medical records are complete, accurate, and entered in the correct format
Certified Coding Associate (CCA®)	qualified to code in both hospitals and physician practices
Certified Coding Specialist (CCS®)	skilled in coding patient medical record data in the hospital setting

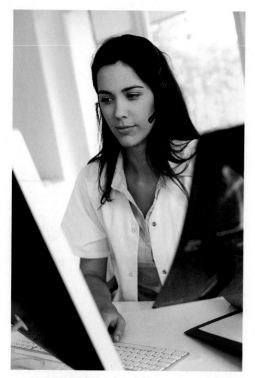

Figure 2.3 Transcriptionists, or *speech recognition editors*, utilize technology in their job every day. Many work from home and provide an important service to a healthcare facility.

Transcriptionists may now be called *speech recognition editors* (Figure 2.3). Their job is to correct errors made by speech recognition software. The work is often done at home, and the technician may be located far away from the facility. Sometimes these workers are located in a different state or even a different country from the facility for which they work.

Advancing in a health informatics career usually means getting more education and experience. With a bachelor's or a master's degree, experienced technicians can become compliance or privacy officers, medical records managers, or administrators. Those who advance typically possess strong business and management skills. Work in more advanced positions can involve long hours, and managers may have to respond to problems at all hours of the day. They must adapt to changing technology, interpret complex regulations, and work to improve efficiency while maintaining quality care.

Health Information Technology

Health information technology (HIT) focuses on the systems that are used to manage health information and the secure exchange of health information in a digital format. HIT workers understand the software and hardware used to manage and store patient data. These workers train in computer science and provide support for the electronic health records that HIM workers use to document a patient's health information.

Your fascination with computers and computer systems could lead you to an HIT career as a data analyst, systems analyst, or clinical information system specialist. All of these jobs are centered on computer data. Healthcare facilities need workers who can develop computer programs to collect, share, and store patient information. Some workers are needed to update programs and repair glitches in software. Others make sure that the correct information is collected, and develop security systems for maintaining the privacy of information. These jobs generally require a bachelor's degree. This occupational area is experiencing a high rate of growth, so job opportunities should be plentiful in the coming years.

Health Informatics

A new group of careers—**health informatics (HI)**—is emerging at the intersection of health information management and health information technology. Health informaticists (workers in health informatics) design and develop information systems that improve the quality, effectiveness, and efficiency of patient care. For example, they may study electronic health data to document patient safety concerns, patterns of disease, or the outcomes of various treatments. While the health informatics services pathway is broad, including all of the careers within the pathway, the emerging field of health informatics focuses on the science of using computer technology and health information management to advance medicine.

Students interested in informatics can consider four focused areas for research:

- **Medical informatics,** or *bioinformatics*, is based on physician research and is of interest to medical students.

- **Nursing informatics** focuses on clinical research and attracts nursing students.

- **Public health informatics** includes public health and bio-surveillance (tracking disease patterns and threats to the health of humans, animals, and plants) and is of special interest to public health students (Figure 2.4).

- **Applied informatics** examines how medical information moves in an electronic environment. It studies processes, policies, and technological solutions, and it attracts HIM students.

Unlike many other healthcare workers, biomedical and health informatics professionals possess a level of expertise in more than one field. Most health informatics jobs require a combination of computer and data science knowledge as well as some type of healthcare or business background. A bachelor's or master's degree in medical informatics, computer science, public health, or another field related to health science is a common requirement for employment.

Job titles in the health informatics field vary widely. Some examples include *nursing informatics director, director of IT informatics, regional informatics manager, health information systems analyst, clinical informatics specialist, informatics outreach architect,* and *pharmacy informatics specialist.*

As you might expect, health informaticists work in hospitals with research programs and large healthcare provider organizations, but they are also employed by government agencies, insurance companies, and software development and production organizations. Individuals with an informatics background might also find employment in the rapidly expanding area of **telemedicine**. In this field, communication and information technologies are used to provide medical services to patients in remote locations. Telemedicine virtually brings the medical specialist to the patient.

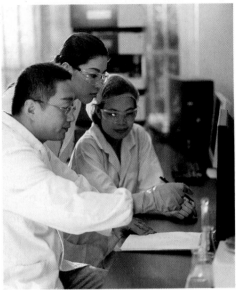

Figure 2.4   People working in public health informatics—a specific focus within health informatics—track disease patterns that might threaten humans. Would you be interested in this type of work?

Related Careers

If you want more contact with patients than you would have in traditional HIM, HIT, and HI jobs, consider becoming a medical assistant or health educator. Both of these jobs require the use of health information, but they also allow for interaction with patients.

Medical Assistants

If you would like more contact with patients than you would have in the jobs already described, you may want to consider becoming a medical assistant. Medical assisting is one of the fastest growing occupations, which means that many jobs should be available. Medical assistants work in a medical office for physicians, chiropractors, or other healthcare professionals. Their job is to keep the office running smoothly by performing a variety of tasks. If you are looking for variety, you will find it as a medical assistant (Figure 2.5 on the next page).

Figure 2.5 Tasks of a Medical Assistant	
Administrative/Clerical	**Clinical**

scheduling
  • hospital admissions
  • clinic appointments
  • laboratory services
filing insurance forms
answering the telephone
greeting patients
writing letters and memos
updating patient records
processing billing
	taking medical histories
	recording vital signs
	assisting with examinations
	performing basic lab tests
	collecting and preparing laboratory specimens
	instructing patients about medication and special diets
	authorizing prescription refills as directed
	drawing blood

internship
practical work or training experience that allows students to apply what they have learned in class

Medical assistants usually complete a one- or two-year training program that includes an **internship**. Interns spend time at a healthcare facility performing the skills they have learned in school. This work is part of their training program and is usually unpaid. They are supervised by a healthcare employee and by a school instructor. Graduates of medical assistant programs can become certified and choose a specialty area such as podiatry (puh-DI-uh-tree)—a medical practice concerning the feet—or ophthalmology (ahf-thal-MAH-luh-jee), a medical practice concerned with the eyes. Experienced assistants can advance to other occupations, such as office management, nursing, or laboratory technology, through additional training or education.

Health Educators

Helping patients use information to prevent illness and manage chronic conditions is becoming more important as healthcare costs increase. Health educators have at least a bachelor's degree and work with both individual patients and groups of people in a variety of locations. In medical offices, they educate patients about their diagnoses. On college campuses, they teach students about healthy lifestyle choices. As public health workers, they give out information to the media and the public during an emergency. Think about a past outbreak of an illness like influenza (the flu) in your community. Did you see signs about vaccination clinics or hear advice about hand washing to reduce infections? These were produced by a public health worker.

Health Educators and the Public: Adam

Health educators help people by providing health-related, scientific information. Adam loves science and chose biology as his major in college. He became a biotechnology (bI-oh-tehk-NAH-luh-jee) research scientist and worked to develop new products to prevent and treat disease.

Over the years, Adam noticed how much he enjoyed explaining new processes to his fellow employees and how frequently he volunteered to develop training programs for other workers. Eventually he realized that he had a strong interest in working with the public. Since that was missing from his research job, Adam transferred to an institute for biotechnology education and became an education specialist. Now he trains science teachers and educates science students about biotechnology and its research methods.

Other health informatics services career paths include medical librarians, illustrators, and historians. Health informatics workers can also be found in the finance or accounting departments of healthcare facilities. These workers, like all of those described in this section, are focused on information. If you love medical language and want to work in healthcare, but touching patients and handling body fluids is not for you, search the health informatics services pathway for your future career.

RECALL YOUR READING

1. Unlike doctors and nurses, who mostly see patients, health informatics workers focus on _____ rather than on direct patient care.
2. Informatics workers are accurate, organized, and alert to maintaining _____.
3. Health informatics workers frequently use computers and must adapt to ongoing changes in _____.
4. Health informatics services professionals work in health information _____, health information _____, or a newer field called health _____.

Complete the *Map Your Reading* graphic organizer for the section you just read.

Teamwork in the Medical Office

Healthcare workers know that they must have top-notch job skills and perform their duties accurately. They may not realize that they also need to be highly skilled at working in a team. The healthcare industry is increasingly using teams of workers to improve healthcare delivery (Figure 2.6).

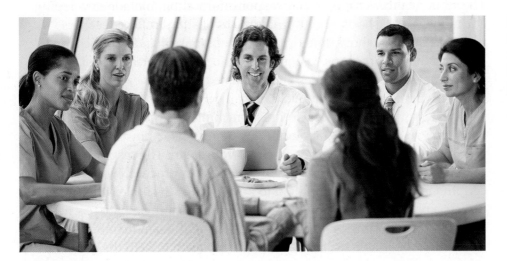

Figure 2.6   Each member of a medical team has roles and responsibilities that contribute to improved patient care.

The use of teams helps to improve patient safety, quality of patient care, and even customer service. Teams also reduce the cost of patient care by employing workers with different levels of training. For example, a nursing team that includes a registered nurse, a licensed practical nurse, and a certified nursing assistant is able to care for a larger group of patients than a single registered nurse can. As a healthcare worker, you need to know your roles and responsibilities within a team and understand how to be an effective team member.

Roles and Responsibilities

Myesha, whom you read about earlier in this chapter, is part of an **interdisciplinary** (ihn-ter-DIH-suh-plih-nair-ee) **healthcare team** in her medical clinic. The team members include doctors, nurses, therapists, medical assistants, insurance representatives, and even the housekeepers she works with in the office. Each member of the team has different skills and knowledge and contributes to the patient's care in a different way. Myesha knows that she must code patient procedures in a reasonable amount of time so that the clinic will receive payment for its services. She knows which people are responsible for each part of patient care and whom to ask if the medical records lack the information needed.

As part of a diverse interdisciplinary team, Kia—the medical assistant—organizes appointments so that patients do not wait for long periods of time and the doctor does not have to wait for the next patient to arrive. When there is an emergency or a delay, Kia adjusts the schedule and continues to meet the needs of patients. Calming a frustrated patient can be a challenge. As the first person who answers the phone, Kia must quickly assess the level of each caller's need. If every call went directly to the doctor, the doctor's day would be spent on the phone instead of assessing and treating patients. Sometimes Kia calls 911 if there is an emergency, but often she can have a nurse return the patient's call. In spite of many interruptions to her work, Kia is also careful to keep accurate and complete patient records so that the billing process goes smoothly.

You also read about Adam, the education specialist. All of the people on Adam's team are from the same discipline—they are all educators. The team members have similar responsibilities that include developing educational workshops, scheduling groups of students and teachers to attend the workshops, and organizing equipment and supplies for teaching these workshops. When the members of this team meet, they coordinate teaching schedules and evaluate the outcomes of their teaching methods to make improvements. They all benefit from working together.

Knowing your own roles and responsibilities is the first step in becoming an effective team member. You must also know the roles and responsibilities of the other members of your team. The responsibilities of each team member are part of his or her scope of practice, which includes certain tasks he or she is qualified to perform. For example, when Kia directs a phone call to the nurse, she is communicating a patient's need that she is not qualified to meet. By knowing each team member's scope of practice, she is able to choose the correct person to help the patient.

interdisciplinary healthcare team
a group of professionals from different health science training backgrounds working in coordination toward a common goal for the patient

Effective Teams

Directing information to the correct person is a teamwork-related skill. Skilled team members monitor the activities of other members, know their strengths and weaknesses, and organize tasks with each person's strengths in mind. For example, Kia knows that the doctor on her team is excellent at assessment and diagnosis of a patient but has a hard time remembering names. She is always careful to prompt the doctor's memory by introducing a patient at the beginning of an exam.

When a group of people works closely together, there will always be differences of opinion, which can create conflict within the team. Effective team members are able to handle disagreements without damaging their working relationships. Some people are naturally good at this type of cooperation and collaboration. Most of us, however, learn conflict resolution skills in the same way we learn our medical skills—through training and experience. You will learn about conflict resolution skills in chapter 6.

Members of effective teams remain positive in spite of personal differences. A positive attitude is critical to the success of a team. In addition to knowing the strengths and weaknesses of other members, everyone on the team must know how to fit their different personalities together to create a comfortable work environment. Understanding and respecting the feelings and beliefs of each team member is just as important as performing the duties of your job correctly.

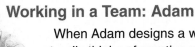

Working in a Team: Adam

When Adam designs a workshop for students, he naturally thinks of creative activities that students will enjoy. Another team member considers the information that must be presented for students to learn a scientific concept. A third team member creates a schedule and determines what lab supplies will need to be ordered. By using the personal strengths of each team member, the team can work efficiently. Team members rely on each other to complete different tasks when preparing for the workshop and are happy to focus on the tasks they enjoy most. A positive attitude toward teamwork and mutual trust among team members make this team successful.

RECALL YOUR READING

1. Healthcare facilities use teams of workers to improve patient _____ and the quality of patient _____ and to reduce _____.
2. Knowing the _____ and _____ of each team member makes a team more effective.
3. Effective team members are skilled at cooperating and handling _____ without damaging their working relationships.
4. Each team member's responsibilities are part of his or her _____.

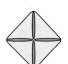

Complete the *Map Your Reading* graphic organizer for the section you just read.

Technical Skills in Health Informatics

technical skills
the ability to perform tasks in a specific healthcare discipline or department

Technical skills are the practical functions and tasks that a worker performs in his or her job. For a health informatics worker, being able to write is an **indispensable** technical skill that is highly desirable in the workplace. Since all patient communication and treatment must be documented, writing accurately and clearly is an important part of a job in health informatics services. In fact, healthcare workers in all career pathways need technical writing skills. Written documents connect all of the workers providing care for a patient (Figure 2.7).

Notice the technical writing tasks that each type of healthcare worker performs to create documents in a typical patient experience:

- The *medical assistant* takes a patient's complete medical history.

- The *physician* uses the medical history to determine a possible diagnosis.

- The *medical lab technician* records lab test results.

- The *radiologist* reads the images taken by the *radiologic technician* and sends a written report to the *physician*, who uses it to confirm the diagnosis.

- The patient receives a letter showing the results of the lab tests.

- The *pharmacist* follows a written prescription to provide medication to treat the patient.

- The *physical therapist* writes a therapy plan and sends written reports to tell the *physician* about the patient's progress.

All of these documents become part of the patient's medical record. The health information technician uses the medical record to code the patient's diagnosis and treatment and to send a billing statement to the insurance company. At all of these stages, technical writing skills are important because accurate and clear documents improve patient care.

Letters

As a health informatics worker, you will write **business letters** for a variety of purposes (Figure 2.8). For example, business letters may tell a patient the results of a test or provide consultation reports to

Figure 2.7 Effective Correspondence	
Characteristics	**Purpose**
no unnecessary words	avoids wasting the reader's time
accurate and complete information	avoids mistakes and misunderstandings
professional appearance (uses Block Style Format and Standard English)	makes you and your employer appear competent
logical organization of information	avoids frustrating or confusing the reader

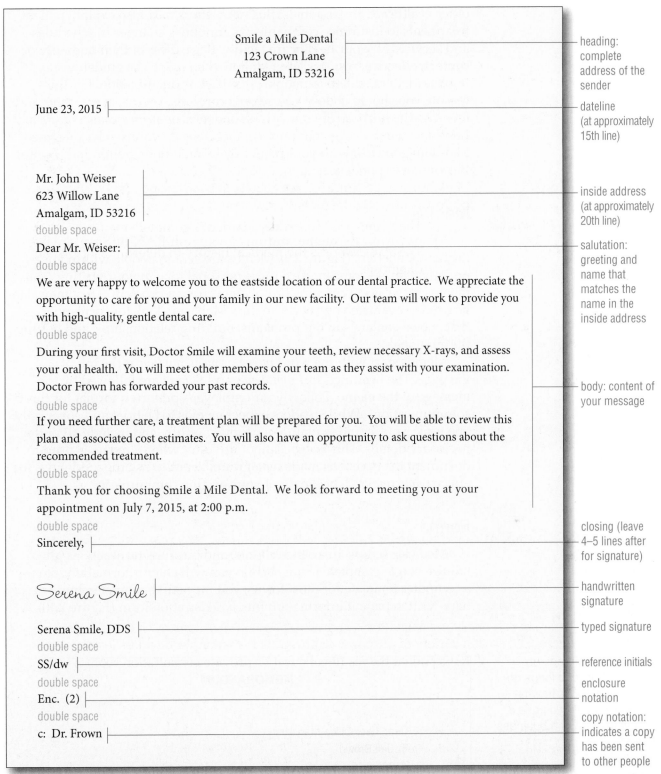

Smile a Mile Dental
123 Crown Lane
Amalgam, ID 53216 — heading: complete address of the sender

June 23, 2015 — dateline (at approximately 15th line)

Mr. John Weiser
623 Willow Lane
Amalgam, ID 53216 — inside address (at approximately 20th line)
double space

Dear Mr. Weiser: — salutation: greeting and name that matches the name in the inside address
double space

We are very happy to welcome you to the eastside location of our dental practice. We appreciate the opportunity to care for you and your family in our new facility. Our team will work to provide you with high-quality, gentle dental care.
double space

During your first visit, Doctor Smile will examine your teeth, review necessary X-rays, and assess your oral health. You will meet other members of our team as they assist with your examination. Doctor Frown has forwarded your past records. — body: content of your message
double space

If you need further care, a treatment plan will be prepared for you. You will be able to review this plan and associated cost estimates. You will also have an opportunity to ask questions about the recommended treatment.
double space

Thank you for choosing Smile a Mile Dental. We look forward to meeting you at your appointment on July 7, 2015, at 2:00 p.m.
double space

Sincerely, — closing (leave 4–5 lines after for signature)

Serena Smile — handwritten signature

Serena Smile, DDS — typed signature
double space

SS/dw — reference initials
double space

Enc. (2) — enclosure notation
double space

c: Dr. Frown — copy notation: indicates a copy has been sent to other people

Figure 2.8   A business letter includes specific components, some of which are explained here. The inside address of a letter should consist of the title, name, and complete address of the person to whom you are writing. The closing should always be friendly, but business-like. Never use "thank you" as your closing. Reference initials consist of the uppercase initials of the letter's sender and lowercase initials of the letter's typist. How does the above letter exemplify the guidelines to effective correspondence?

Simulate EHR

other healthcare professionals. Business letters may also explain patient treatments to insurance companies or announce changes in schedules and services for your healthcare facility. Regardless of their audience or content, effective business letters follow the same basic guidelines.

Your letters will go to people outside your organization. For this reason, you should choose your words carefully, keep a formal tone, and focus on the purpose of your correspondence, or *written communication*. Provide enough background information to keep your reader informed. Maintain goodwill with your reader by being honest, polite, and prompt in your correspondence.

Memos

Memos, short for **memorandums** (meh-muh-RAN-duhms), are less formal than letters (Figure 2.9). Memos are sent to people within your organization, so you can use a more personal tone in your writing. Your memos serve as a written record of an event or a problem. They may also be used to evaluate your performance. Managers look for correspondence that shows you are solving problems, building relationships, and getting the job done.

Memos start with the word *memo* or *memorandum* at the top of the page. The headings *To, From, Date,* and *Subject* are followed by the message of the memo. Follow your employer's preferred format for these communications. While readers expect memos to be brief and cover only one topic, you should explain your topic carefully and include all of the necessary details. This is especially important when a memo is used to document the decisions made by a group. Learn to use the guidelines for effective correspondence in all of your written communication.

Forms

Medical records, insurance claims, and business transactions all require you to complete forms. While you will enter information into a computer template for most forms, you may still be transferring handwritten patient information into a registration form (Figure 2.10).

Figure 2.9 Memos are usually short and focus on a particular topic. In what situations might you use a memo instead of a business letter?

Simulate
EHR

MEMORANDUM

To: Jean Lee, Office Manager
From: Jeff Brown
Date: 06/03/15
Re: Vacation leave

I would like to use vacation time on September 1, 2, and 5 to attend my sister's wedding. Please let me know at your earliest convenience if you can meet this request. I will need to make airline reservations for the trip.
Thank you for your help.

SUN VIEW MEDICAL — NEW PATIENT REGISTRATION FORM

PATIENT INFORMATION

PATIENT'S LAST NAME	FIRST NAME	M.I.	DATE OF BIRTH	PRIMARY CARE PHYSICIAN
Wolf	Bryan	J.	01-10-1999	Dr. Nolan

MAIDEN NAME	NAME YOU GO BY	MARITAL STATUS
N/A	B.J	☒ S ☐ M ☐ D ☐ W

STREET ADDRESS	APT. NO.
1025 Sun City Dr.	Ø

CITY	STATE	ZIP	HOME PHONE
Star Prairie	TX	74260	123-701-6529

SOCIAL SECURITY NUMBER	AGE	GENDER	CELL PHONE
000-00-0000	13	☒ Male ☐ Female	123-217-2220

EMPLOYER	OCCUPATION	WORK PHONE
N/A	Student	N/A

EMERGENCY CONTACT (NOT LIVING WITH YOU) / RELATION TO PATIENT	EMERGENCY CONTACT PHONE
Charmayne Prue – Grandmother	123-701-3507

SPOUSE OR PARENT / RESPONSIBLE PARTY INFORMATION

LAST NAME	FIRST NAME	M.I.	RELATIONSHIP TO PATIENT
Ohman	Melissa	K	☒ Parent ☐ Legal guardian ☐ Other _____

STREET ADDRESS	APT. NO.	HOME PHONE
1025 Sun City Dr.	Ø	123-701-6529

CITY	STATE	ZIP	CELL PHONE
Star Prairie	TX	74260	123-217-0472

SOCIAL SECURITY NO.	DATE OF BIRTH
000-00-0000	02-15-1977

RESPONSIBLE PARTY EMPLOYER	OCCUPATION	RESPONSIBLE PARTY WORK PHONE/EXT.
RNR Associates	Accountant	123-701-6000

SECOND PARENT INFORMATION

LAST NAME	FIRST NAME	M.I.	RELATIONSHIP TO PATIENT
Wolf	Marvin	J	☒ Parent ☐ Legal guardian ☐ Other _____

STREET ADDRESS	APT. NO.	HOME PHONE
425 Monroe St.	2	123-701-5490

CITY	STATE	ZIP	CELL PHONE
Star Prairie	TX	74260	123-217-3320

SOCIAL SECURITY NO.	DATE OF BIRTH
000-00-0000	06-22-1970

RESPONSIBLE PARTY EMPLOYER	OCCUPATION	RESPONSIBLE PARTY WORK PHONE/EXT.
MJW Electric	Electrician	123-701-2000

INSURANCE INFORMATION

PRIMARY INSURANCE COMPANY	COPAY	EFFECTIVE DATE
Whole Health Care	$25.00	01-01-2011

ID (POLICY NO.)	GROUP NO.
000100623	67018X

SUBSCRIBER	RELATIONSHIP TO SUBSCRIBER	SUBSCRIBER'S DATE OF BIRTH
Melissa Ohman	Child	02-15-1977

SUBSCRIBER'S EMPLOYER	SUBSCRIBER'S SOCIAL SECURITY NO.
RNR Associates	000-00-0000

SECONDARY INSURANCE COMPANY	COPAY	EFFECTIVE DATE
N/A		

ID (POLICY NO.)	GROUP NO.

SUBSCRIBER	RELATIONSHIP TO SUBSCRIBER	SUBSCRIBER'S DATE OF BIRTH

SUBSCRIBER'S EMPLOYER	SUBSCRIBER'S SOCIAL SECURITY NO.

Insurance payment and records release authorization: I authorize my insurance benefits to be paid directly to Sun View Medical. I am financially responsible for any unpaid balance. I authorize the release of any information requested by my insurance company.

Signature of Patient or Responsible Party_____ Date_____

PLEASE BRING INSURANCE CARD(S) TO YOUR APPOINTMENT. THANK YOU!

Figure 2.10 A registration form contains a patient's personal information, such as contact details, age, and full name. Why is it important to protect patients' personal information?

Simulate EHR

Accuracy and clarity are the most important considerations when completing forms, but a few guidelines can make this task easier.

- Speak privately with the patient to clarify information given on the form.

- Fill in all the spaces on the form. Use Ø, N/A, or None when a question does not apply to the patient.

- Recognize symbols or abbreviations often used in patient records. Abbreviations for marital status include S, M, W, and D, which stand for *single*, *married*, *widowed*, and *divorced*, respectively. "Living and well" is abbreviated as *l and w*. "Died" is abbreviated *d*, followed by the year of death.

- Family history includes the current health status and past conditions or diseases of the patient's parents, grandparents, sisters, and brothers.

- *Present illness* or *current complaint* requires a clear description of the patient's current signs and symptoms.

- *Responsible party* means the person who will be in charge of payment for the healthcare services the patient receives.

All written forms become part of the patient's medical record. This record communicates information about the patient's medical status to healthcare workers. It is also a legal document that provides evidence of the care the patient has received. In addition, medical records can be used for research, public health initiatives, or patient education. Because they are critical to patient care, these records must be easy to locate, well organized, accurate, and complete, but also brief.

Often called the patient's *chart* or *file*, each medical record contains two types of information—personal and clinical. Personal information, which may be included in a registration form, tells the doctor's office personnel how to contact a patient. It usually includes a photocopy of the patient's insurance card. **Clinical information** begins with the patient's medical history and includes all of the information about his or her health, medical conditions, and treatment (Figure 2.11). The personal and clinical information are separated in a patient's chart.

Remember that protected health information (PHI) must remain confidential. All written files must be protected from unauthorized access. You cannot leave files in areas where others may see them.

When a new patient makes an appointment, a medical clinic or office will often send forms for the patient to complete and bring to the appointment. This is more efficient than having the patient fill out forms while waiting to see the doctor. The patient has time to gather information and think carefully about the questions at home. As a result, the medical office receives a more accurate and complete medical history.

Many medical offices maintain a website where patients can download and print these forms or establish a private account and complete them online. If the office uses electronic health records, all handwritten forms are scanned into the patient's chart, and the paper forms are shredded to protect the privacy of the patient.

In addition to personal information and a medical history, the office needs permission to bill an insurance company. The office also needs permission to share confidential information with any other individual chosen by the patient. The office must give every patient a notice of privacy practices that explains how his or her protected health information is kept confidential and under what circumstances the information can be released to others.

Maintaining Accuracy: Kia

Kia makes sure that patient information is complete and clarifies any handwriting that is difficult to read. Using a private area to consult with patients, or making sure others can't hear the discussion is a legal requirement. Kia double-checks the forms for all required signatures so that bills for service can be sent to the insurance company. Accurate registration avoids future problems.

Figure 2.11 A medical history form contains clinical information, such as a patient's past diagnoses and treatments. Why is it important to protect patients' clinical information?

Simulate
EHR

SUN VIEW MEDICAL — MEDICAL HISTORY FORM
(please print/type)

Last Name	First Name	Middle Name

Date of Birth	Sex/Gender	Country of Birth ( )

Permanent Address	City	State	Zip Code	Telephone ( )

Local Address	City		Zip Code	Preferred Local Telephone

HAVE YOU HAD:

	YES	NO		YES	NO		YES	NO
Head Injury with Unconsciousness			Sexually Transmitted Disease			Counseling/Mental Health Treatment		
Asthma			Malaria			Recreational Drug Use		
Recurrent Headaches			Chicken Pox			Tobacco Use		
Seizure Disorder			Scarlet Fever			Alcohol Use		
Hearing Loss			Hay Fever			# times per week		
Recurrent Ear Infections			Rheumatic Fever			amount per session		
Visual Problems (other than glasses)			High Cholesterol			Exercise: # times per week		
Thyroid Problem			Hepatitis A, B, or C			Operations / Dates:		
Heart Problem/Murmur			Diabetes					
Kidney/Urinary Tract Problem			High Blood Pressure			Chronic Health Problems:		
Gynecology Problem(s)			Digestive Tract Problem					
Recent Weight Change			Cancer/Tumor/Cyst					
Bleeding/Blood Disorder			Spinal Cord Disruption			Alternative Medicine Practices:		
Tuberculosis			Eating Disorder					

ALLERGIES to Drugs/Medications: (write NONE if none)	OTHER ALLERGIES (i.e., environmental): (write NONE if none)	Routine Medications Taken: (write NONE if none)

Family Health History (List father, mother, siblings, spouse/partner and children)

Family Member	Age	If no longer living, cause of death and age of death

HAS ANY FAMILY MEMBER EVER HAD:

(parent, sibling, or grandparent)	YES	NO	Relationship		YES	NO	Relationship
Tubercolosis				Asthma			
Drug/Alchohol Use				Thyroid Disease			
Diabetes				Seizure Disorder			
Kidney Disease				Blood Disorder			
Heart Disease				Cancer			
High Blood Pressure				Stroke			
Arthritis				Obesity			

OTHER CONCERNS/INFORMATION:

SKILLS PROCEDURES

Filing

While most medical records are stored electronically these days, workers may still need to access paper records that are maintained as a back-up storage system. Patient records must be easy to store and find so that patient care and treatment can run smoothly on a day-to-day basis. Proper filing of records can also help avoid potential lawsuits by keeping all necessary information available for review. Medical records are stored either alphabetically or by number (numerically).

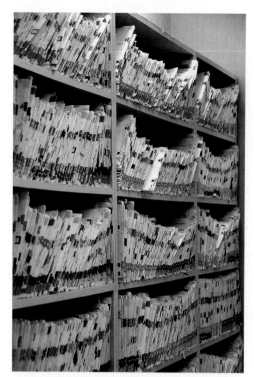

Figure 2.12   Color-coding is one effective method of organizing files.

The alphabetic system files records in order according to the patient's last name. File tabs or folders with a different color for each letter group—for example, A to F is green, G to L is yellow—can be used to quickly spot files that are out of order (Figure 2.12). In this system, files are alphabetized by the patient's last name and then by the first name when two patients have the same last name. Electronic records systems save time by automatically alphabetizing charts for storage. The alphabetical system can cause confusion when two patients have the same name. In such cases, the correct chart can be retrieved by using the patient's name and by checking the date of birth and other personal information (Figure 2.13).

Numeric filing systems give each patient a unique number. Most systems use six digits and charts are filed in numerical order. This avoids the problem of name duplication and helps to protect patient privacy. It is important to write numbers clearly, or type them onto labels, so that charts are not misfiled. A poorly written 7 can easily look like a 1. This system also requires a master index of patient names and numbers so you can find the correct chart when a patient comes in for an appointment.

Healthcare facilities choose the system of filing that best meets their unique needs. Systems other than alphabetic or numeric include geographic, chronologic, and by subject. A geographic system organizes files by location, such as state or city. This works well for a mobile clinic whose patients live in several different areas. Chronologic (krah-nuh-LAH-jik) filing is organized according to dates, such as years or months. Research studies often use this system to record their progress. Filing by subject, such as personnel files, inventory records, or accounts payable, may be used for storing information other than patient charts.

Figure 2.13 Alphabetic Filing Tips

Tip	Patient Name	File As
File by last name, then first name, then middle initial.	Jon C. Byers	Byers, Jon C.
Hyphenated names should be treated as one word.	Gabriel Garcia-Marquez	Garcia-Marquez, Gabriel
Abbreviated parts of names are filed as if spelled out.	Susan St. Cyr	Saint Cyr, Susan
Put professional titles and initials at the end of the name. They are not part of the system.	Dr. Mai Vang, MD	Vang, Mai, MD
Use birth dates for patients with identical names. Usually, the most recent date is first.	Nicole M. Grimm DOB: 10/22/1951	1. Grimm, Nicole M. 03/15/1979
	Nicole M. Grimm DOB: 03/15/1979	2. Grimm, Nicole M. 10/22/1951

Scheduling

An efficient schedule avoids long wait times for patients and maintains a consistent flow of appointments for physicians (Figure 2.14). Effective scheduling is a skill that requires practice and experience. Most clinics and offices use a computerized scheduling program, but paper and electronic scheduling systems both use the same guidelines.

Each page of the schedule is divided into segments of time, often 15 minutes. Each column can be used for a different physician, dentist, or other healthcare provider. There may be a separate column for scheduling lab appointments. The page must have enough space to list the patient's name, reason for appointment, and contact phone number.

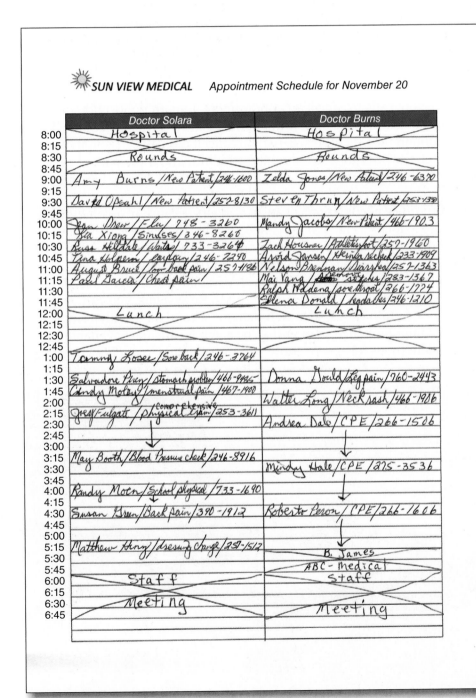

Figure 2.14   This patient appointment book notes when a healthcare worker should expect his or her patients.

The process of scheduling begins with blocking off times when providers are not seeing patients. Examples of blocked times include lunchtime, attendance at a conference, or time spent seeing patients in the hospital. The standard time allowed for each type of appointment should be determined ahead of time. Many appointments are 15 minutes in length, but a physical exam may last one hour. Leave a few open appointment times in the morning and in the afternoon. This allows for emergencies and for catch-up time if the scheduled appointments run late.

When scheduling a patient's appointment over the phone, you should learn the reason for the appointment and the patient's full name (Figure 2.15). Ask for the spelling if you are unsure. You should also list the patient's current phone number. Ask the patient for his or her preferred appointment time. It may take a few attempts to find an available appointment at a time that is convenient for the patient. Once you have set an appointment, repeat the day, date, and time for the patient before ending your call. If the appointment is made while the patient is in the clinic, provide a reminder card with these details as well as the name of the physician.

If a patient calls to cancel an appointment, remain polite and positive and ask why the appointment needs to be canceled. Record the cancellation in the schedule and list the cancellation and reason in the patient's chart. Offer to reschedule the appointment. If the patient needs continuing care, you may need to call back to remind him or her to reschedule.

If your office needs to cancel appointments because of an emergency or because a doctor is ill, you don't need to give the specific reason. Contact the patient as soon as you know about the schedule change, and try to reschedule while you have the patient on the phone.

Computerized scheduling systems have some advantages over handwritten schedules (Figure 2.16). With these systems, you can easily block certain times, such as lunch, for several days with a single entry. A computerized system will also search for the next available appointment times for you or show you the schedule for a date you have

Figure 2.15   Accuracy is important when scheduling appointments over the phone. Be sure to verify the patient's name and reason for coming in so that your appointment book is accurate.

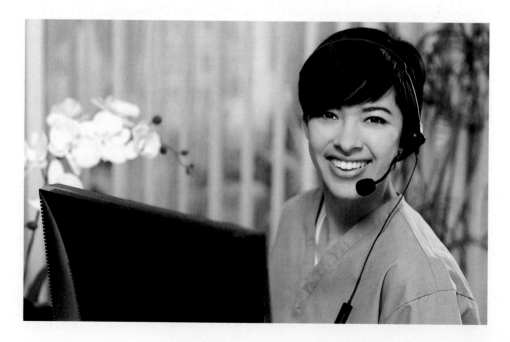

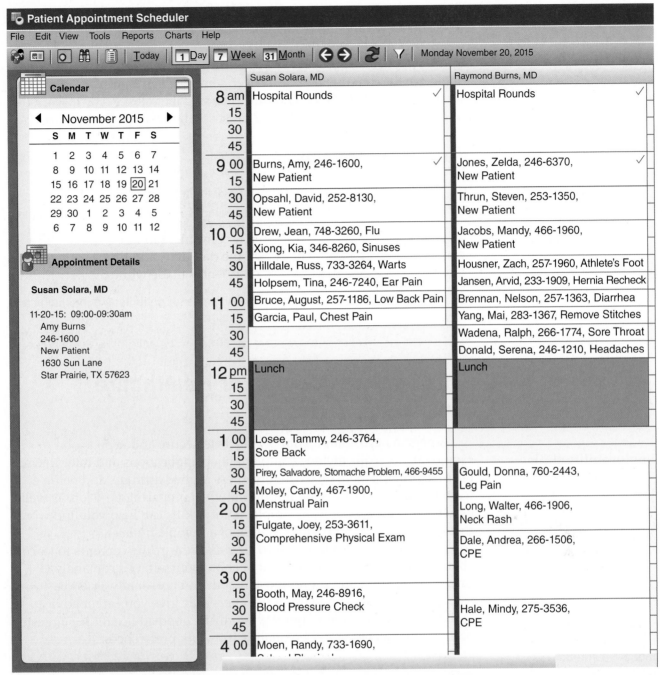

Figure 2.16   A patient appointment book may also be computerized. What do you think are the advantages of computerized patient appointment books? Can you think of any disadvantages?

Simulate EHR

entered. It is easy to print the day's schedule for each provider with these computerized systems.

Some offices may even use online scheduling systems. These allow patients to view available times and book their appointments online. Doctors can access online schedules from any computer at any time.

To make an appointment, a patient must set up an account with a secure user name and password. The patient selects the clinic location, his or her specific doctor, and the type of appointment needed. The software program calculates the amount of time required for the appointment and displays available dates and times. Once the patient selects a time, the appointment is added to the doctor's schedule, and the screen shows the patient pre-visit instructions, if applicable.

Many patients appreciate the opportunity to schedule an appointment even when the clinic is closed. However, some patients report frustration with online systems when they spend time accessing the website only to learn that the type of appointment they need must still be scheduled by phone.

Complete the *Map Your Reading* graphic organizer for the section you just read.

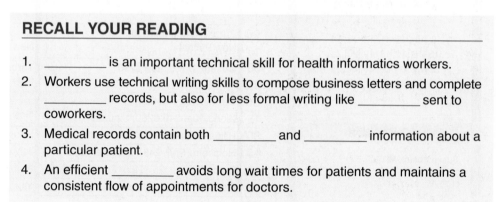

RECALL YOUR READING

1. _____ is an important technical skill for health informatics workers.
2. Workers use technical writing skills to compose business letters and complete _____ records, but also for less formal writing like _____ sent to coworkers.
3. Medical records contain both _____ and _____ information about a particular patient.
4. An efficient _____ avoids long wait times for patients and maintains a consistent flow of appointments for doctors.

Employability Skills for Healthcare Workers

employability skills
skills related to choosing a career, acquiring and keeping a job, changing jobs, and advancing in a career

A person needs **employability skills** to secure and keep a job. Employability skills include completing job applications and interviews, but also professionalism, trustworthiness, a good attitude, and being a team player. These skills are important when preparing for a job, as well as getting and keeping a job. Employability skills can help you find work that is satisfying and provides a sense of accomplishment.

The first step in finding a satisfying and rewarding career is to learn about yourself. Once you know more about yourself, you can analyze career opportunities and find those that fit you personally. Friends, teachers, counselors, and family members may give you career advice with the best of intentions, but it will only be good advice if the suggested occupation matches your personality and work preferences.

Career Assessments

Career assessments are tools such as questionnaires and surveys that you can use to find careers that will match your individual needs. If you completed a career cluster quiz as suggested in chapter 1, you know your top career clusters. Even if health science was not one of your top clusters, you can find ways to use your chosen career in the healthcare field. For example, computer scientists, public relations personnel, and accountants all come from different career clusters, yet all of these people can work in healthcare facilities.

Career clusters are organized according to different jobs within an industry. Since the clusters are not organized according to work interests, you will want to narrow your career search based on your own interests. By identifying your work interests, you can determine your career personality.

Career psychologist John Holland identified six basic personality types through many years of work and research in the field of psychology. Review the chart in Figure 2.17 to identify your top three personality types. Then, consider careers that match those personality types. Matching your personality to your career can lead to job satisfaction and success.

As you investigate careers that interest you, look for those that match your work preferences as well as your personality type. Do you prefer to work indoors or outdoors? Are you willing to work only on weekdays and only during the daytime? How long do you want to attend school? How much income do you want to earn? These preferences regarding the practical parts of a career are also important to your job satisfaction. Compare each of the careers you are interested in with your list of personal preferences as you develop your career plan.

Career Portfolios

Your **career portfolio** records the work you have done to prepare for a career or to get a specific job. You can use the contents of your portfolio to plan your high school course schedule, apply to college programs, complete scholarship applications, or apply for a specific job. Preserving your portfolio and keeping it up-to-date makes these tasks easier because you have all the information you need in one organized location.

career portfolio
a written record of career planning and preparation

Figure 2.17 Health Science Careers by Personality Type

John Holland Personality Type	Characteristic	Health Science Career Examples
realistic doer	likes mechanical hands-on activities	central supply worker electrocardiograph technician surgeon
investigative thinker	is an analytical problem solver	medical laboratory technician nurse practitioner psychologist
social helper	is cooperative and people-oriented	certified nursing assistant health science educator physical therapist
enterprising persuader	is a competitive leader	pharmaceutical sales representative healthcare administrator dean of nursing at a college or university
conventional organizer	pays attention to detail	dental assistant medical coding specialist operating room nurse
artistic creator	likes creative activities	medical photographer music therapist community health nurse

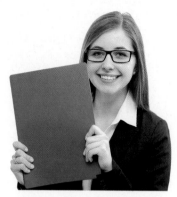

Figure 2.18   Keep your career portfolio on hand when applying for jobs. Your portfolio should contain all the information you might need for a job application.

Build
Portfolio

A quality portfolio highlights your knowledge, experiences, skills, and abilities (Figure 2.18). Your portfolio should contain the following information:

- an introductory letter or essay
- your résumé (REH-zuh-may)
- letters of recommendation
- records of paid and volunteer work experiences
- samples of projects and presentations that illustrate your skills
- health certifications you have earned
- a list of school and community activities in which you have participated
- scholastic and professional awards you have received

An introductory letter or essay reflects your personality, passions, and goals for your career and your life. This letter should answer some basic questions about you, your life, and your career goals. What experiences and interests have led you to this career? Why is this work important to you, and what do you think you can contribute to this career? What goals have you set for yourself in this career? Include an example of one of your positive characteristics. You may use information from this introductory letter as you fill out job applications and prepare for interviews. This is not a letter you send out to potential employers. This letter exists to help you consider your priorities as you begin your career journey.

A **résumé** is a short, one-page document that contains your accomplishments and experiences and explains how these relate to a job in which you are interested. A computer template can make it easy to create and revise your résumé. You should take care to adjust the document to fit the requirements of a specific job. List your name and contact information at the top of your résumé. Include your educational background, employment history, extracurricular activities, employment certifications, and special awards or honors. Keep a separate list of references to include when specifically requested.

Your résumé must be easy to read, so use the same font throughout the document. Use phrases separated into bullet points rather than complete sentences. Since you may be applying online, format your résumé so that it can be posted easily to a website; sent by e-mail; or printed, mailed, and then scanned by a potential employer (Figure 2.19).

You should also keep the results of your career assessments in your portfolio so you can review them when considering a new job. These results will help you determine if a job is a good fit for you. Your portfolio is a tool you will use throughout your work life.

HOSA Connections

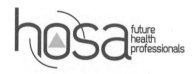

HOSA–Future Health Professionals
a career and technical student organization for future healthcare workers

HOSA–Future Health Professionals is a career and technical student organization (CTSO). Through CTSOs such as HOSA for health science students, FBLA for business students, and SkillsUSA for a variety of industries, students can develop leadership skills, learn more about career training programs, and participate in service-learning and other volunteer opportunities.

Figure 2.19 Tips for Readable Electronic Résumés

Recommendation	Reason
use a plain font like Arial	scanners can't read fancy fonts
avoid boldface, italics, and underlining	scanners don't interpret these correctly
use 10- to 12-point font size	scanners can't read small fonts
use one column lined up on the left margin	scanners will put multiple columns in the wrong order
use capital letters to show headings	scanners recognize capital letters
use the space bar instead of tab keys	scanners have trouble reading tabs correctly
use wide margins with lines of 60–65 characters	scanners can read 65 characters and won't chop off any of your words

HOSA provides professional development opportunities designed for health science students. Being a member of HOSA will benefit you and your career development, and participating in HOSA's competitive events can strengthen both your general career skills and your health informatics skills. Look at the *Competitive Events* section of the HOSA website for descriptions of the various events (Figure 2.20).

Figure 2.20 HOSA Competitive Events

Event Name	Event Description
Medical Spelling	written test and "spelling bee" competition
Medical Terminology	written test
Clinical Specialty	presentation of a career portfolio about and demonstration of a skill common to a chosen health career
Health Career Display	tabletop display featuring one healthcare career
Public Health	presentation about a public health concern
Health Education	student participation in planning and teaching a health-related concept
Extemporaneous Writing	written essay about a health-related topic or HOSA

RECALL YOUR READING

1. Examples of _____ include questionnaires and surveys.
2. A _____ documents the work you have done to prepare for a career or specific job.
3. A one-page document that contains your accomplishments and experiences and explains how they relate to a specific job is called a _____.
4. HOSA is a _____ and _____ student organization designed for developing the career and leadership skills of health science students.

Complete the *Map Your Reading* graphic organizer for the section you just read.

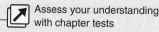

SUMMARY

Assess your understanding with chapter tests

- Health informatics careers focus on information rather than hands-on patient care.

- Health informatics workers must be accurate, organized, and able to protect the privacy of patient information.

- Those working in health informatics services frequently use computers and must adapt to ongoing changes in technology.

- Health information technicians maintain patient medical records and assist with patient scheduling.

- Health informatics services professionals include educators, computer specialists, and data analysts.

- Health informatics workers are part of the healthcare team. Knowing the roles and responsibilities of each team member and maintaining a positive attitude are critical to the success of the team.

- Health informatics workers must be skilled technical writers who can compose letters, establish and organize medical records, and schedule patient appointments.

- Career assessments and career portfolios document your career research and preparation. They are useful tools for completing college, applying for scholarships, and filling out job applications.

- HOSA is the career and technical student organization for health science students. HOSA activities promote the development of career and leadership skills.

MAXIMIZE YOUR PROFESSIONAL VOCABULARY

Build vocabulary with e-flash cards, games, and audio glossary

Listed below are the essential, yellow-highlighted terms and the additional professional vocabulary terms that you encountered in this chapter. Complete the activities that follow the list to make all of these terms part of your everyday professional vocabulary.

business letters
career assessments
career portfolio
clinical information
competent
confidentiality
dictation
employability skills
family medical history
health informatics (HI)

health informatics services
health information management (HIM)
health information technology (HIT)
HOSA–Future Health Professionals
indispensable
interdisciplinary healthcare team
internship

medical coding
medical history
memorandum
personal identifying information
personal traits
professional look
résumé
technical skills
telemedicine
transcriptionist

VOCABULARY DEVELOPMENT

1. Dice Roll Review. Number each professional vocabulary term listed above from one to six. Continue numbering until all terms have been assigned a number from one to six. Form groups of four to six students. One student starts as the "caller." Each player takes a turn to roll the die. The caller asks for the definition of any term matching the number rolled. A point is awarded for each correct response.

   At the end of the first round, a new student has the caller job and play continues.

2. Terms Tabloid. Write a fictional story about healthcare using at least 10 professional vocabulary terms. Replace the terms with blank spaces. Trade papers with another student and try to fill in the blanks in each other's stories. Have you used the vocabulary terms correctly?

Matching. Match each essential term from this chapter with the correct definition below by writing the letter of the definition next to the number of the essential term on a separate sheet of paper.

3. technical skills

4. internship

5. confidentiality

6. personal traits

7. career portfolio

8. interdisciplinary healthcare team

9. medical coding

10. professional look

11. employability skills

12. health informatics services

13. HOSA

a. the act of assigning numbers to descriptions of a patient's diseases, injuries, and treatments according to established codes

b. an individual's unique combination of qualities and characteristics

c. a written record of career planning and preparation

d. the standards of appearance normally expected of a qualified person in a work environment

e. a career and technical student organization for future healthcare workers

f. the legally protected right of patients to have their personal and medical information kept private

g. practical work or training experience that allows students to apply what they have learned in class

h. a group of professionals from different health science training backgrounds working in coordination toward a common goal for the patient

i. career pathway that involves methods, devices, and resources used to acquire, store, retrieve, and work with healthcare and biomedical information

j. skills related to choosing a career, acquiring and keeping a job, changing jobs, and advancing in a career

k. the ability to perform tasks in a specific healthcare discipline or department

REFLECT ON YOUR READING

14. Review the bubble diagram you created in the *Connect with Your Reading* activity. Pick one health informatics worker from the bubble diagram you created at the beginning of this chapter. Revise your diagram, if needed, to include a health informatics worker. Was this person a competent health informatics worker, or not? Use evidence from your reading to support your conclusion.

My Healthcare Experience

BUILD CORE SKILLS

15. **Writing.** Suppose that you are the administrator of a hospital, clinic, or other healthcare facility. Write a paragraph describing your ideal health informatics worker. What are the personal traits, characteristics, and interests that would lead someone to succeed in a health informatics services career?

16. **Critical Thinking.** Review the health informatics services careers that were discussed in this chapter. Which health informatics services career area—health information management, health information technology, or health informatics— has the best opportunities for employment? Would you consider a career in this area? Be prepared to explain the reasons for your choice.

17. **Problem Solving.** Suppose that you have a summer internship organizing the filing system for your professor's research project. Describe the type of filing system you will use and explain the reasons for your choice.

18. **Speaking and Listening.** Suppose that you are a college student studying health information management. You are speaking at your former high school and want to encourage the high school students to join HOSA. What will you say to explain the benefits of membership in HOSA?

19. **Reading.** Suppose that you have recently graduated from a medical coding training program. You know that employers like to hire

credentialed workers, so you decide to seek certification as a certified coding associate (CCA). Your program instructor mentioned that the American Health Information Management Association (AHIMA) offers certification testing and credentials. Visit the AHIMA website to find answers to the following questions about the certification process:

a. Besides completion of a training program, what other requirement is necessary to be eligible for certification?

b. How much does the exam cost, and how long is the exam?

c. The exam will cover coding and reimbursement procedures. What are the other four topics included in the exam?

d. Once certified, how will you keep your certification current?

ACTIVATE YOUR LEARNING

20. Prepare a sample business letter using the topic described here. Follow the guidelines for effective correspondence and correct formatting in Figure 2.8.

    Letter topic: Introduce patients to Dr. James Brace, who will be joining the Smile a Mile dental practice. Dr. Brace's specialty is orthodontics. Let patients know what services he will provide and how this will improve the dental practice. Include the date on which he will begin seeing patients, and explain how patients can schedule an appointment. This letter is written by you on behalf of Dr. Serena Smile.

21. Prepare a sample memorandum using the topic described here. Follow the guidelines for effective correspondence and use the correct format in Figure 2.9.

Memorandum topic: Announce to the staff that Smile a Mile employees will have holidays on both July 4 and July 5 this year. This memorandum comes from you as the office manager.

22. Create a new patient file using the patient data provided here. Select a name for your patient. For the patient's medical history, create several more family members. While Rita (patient's mother) has diabetes, the rest of the family is pretty healthy. Include a registration form and a medical history form based on Figures 2.10 and 2.11. Label your file folder with your patient's name. File your folder in a class file cabinet with the patient records created by your fellow class members.

Your patient [Insert chosen name]

• Your patient is a 17-year-old junior in high school. He or she recently moved to Star Prairie and is seeing a new doctor today to get a physical to play hockey.

• The patient's mother, Rita, works as a preschool teacher at Playtime Child Care Center at 14 Ruby Lane in Star Prairie, TX 74260.

• Rita has rented a condo at 400 S. Main Street. The phone number is 123-701-0197. Rita provided an insurance card (see below).

• The patient experienced congestion during the months of March and April. The patient wishes his or her acne would clear up, and Rita is worried about hockey season because the patient suffered a concussion during a game last year.

23. Complete a patient schedule for Dr. Solera using 15-minute increments between 8:00 a.m. and 5:00 p.m. Dr. Solera will be seeing patients at the hospital until 9:00 a.m. and the time between 12:30 and 1:30 p.m. will be

DC Health Plan

Group number 06172   Member number 03654

Member name: Rita James 01

(Your fictitious name) 02

1600 Allen Blvd   Washington, DC 65432

Claims questions: 1-800-789-6756

Dr. Solera's lunchtime. Enter the following appointments with this information in mind. Remember to leave room for emergency appointments and provide enough time for each type of appointment. Use Figure 2.16 to help you estimate appropriate times for each type of appointment.

Jane Brooks—school physical

Lamar Smith—back pain

Ali Sims—complete physical exam

Jim Sykes—skin rash

Barb Engles—insect bite

Martel Brown—fever and flu symptoms

Gina Downs—pelvic pain

Robert Alquist—new patient

Josh Oines—remove stitches

Noah Collins—sports physical

Betty Franks—knee pain

Hannah Jacobs—sore throat

Kerry Long—blood pressure check

Marquis Linton—complete physical exam

Angie Olson—back pain

Quinton Zelman—new patient

Review the section on patient scheduling. Check your schedule and add any information you may have missed. What factor makes actual clinic scheduling more difficult than the schedule you created?

Angie Olson has called to cancel her appointment. Make the necessary notations in your schedule.

THINK AND ACT LIKE A HEALTHCARE WORKER

24. Liam graduated from college with a degree in biology and will start medical school in the fall. He has been working as a personal care assistant in the internal medicine department at a medical clinic during the summer. One of his patients requires an ear cleaning. Liam has never done this procedure. He asks Jesse, a fellow personal care assistant, to do the ear cleaning procedure. Jesse, who has been trained and has performed many ear

cleanings, completes the procedure while Liam observes. Review the professional vocabulary list for this chapter. Select two terms that relate to this scenario and explain how they apply.

GO TO THE SOURCE

25. Use the Internet to learn more about careers in health informatics services. Select two careers of interest to you and complete a career profile page for each career. Use at least one site that ends in .gov and one site that ends in .org. Record the following information for each career:
    - name of career
    - tasks involved in this career
    - personal traits and abilities needed
    - educational requirements
    - type of credential needed and how it is obtained
    - work conditions
    - wages and benefits
    - job outlook for the future
    - list the websites you accessed

    How do the two careers compare? Why might you prefer one to the other?

DEVELOP YOUR HEALTH SCIENCE CAREER PORTFOLIO

26. Create a résumé and introductory letter for your career portfolio. Follow the guidelines described on page 62. Then ask for feedback on these documents from someone who knows you well, and who has good writing skills, such as an English or business education teacher. Revise your work according to their feedback. Place these items in your career portfolio.

27. Review the personality types chart in Figure 2.17. Which two types are most like you? Search the O*NET website for the two careers you researched in the *Go to the Source* activity. Do the interest types listed for these careers match your selected personality types? What conclusions can you draw based on your findings?

28. Research HOSA competitive events listed in this chapter. Use the HOSA website for this activity. Select and note your top choice event. List the reasons for your choice.

Chapter 3
Fundamental Skills in Health Informatics

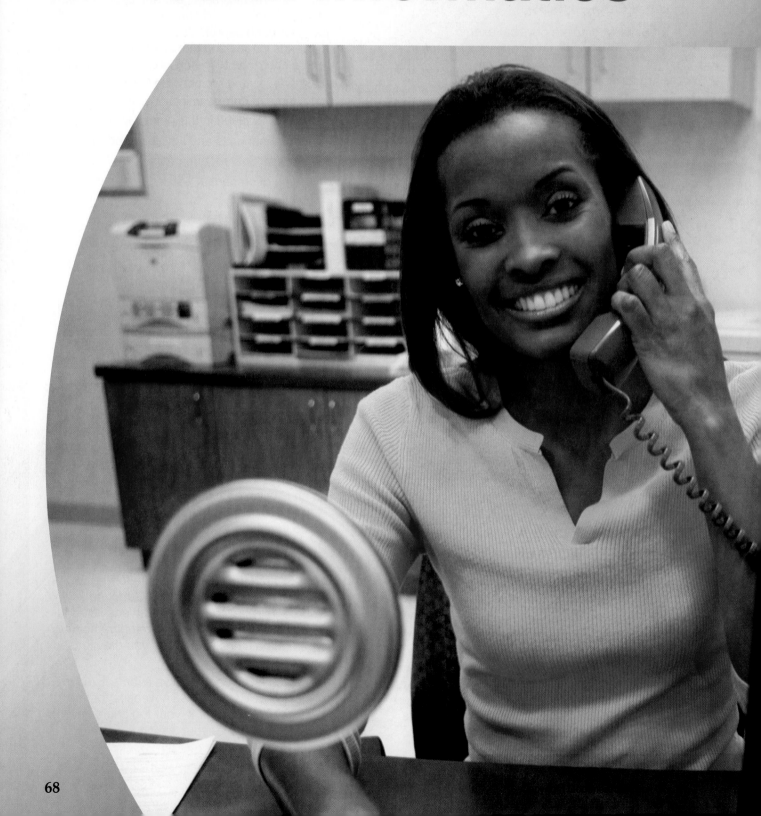

PROFESSIONAL VOCABULARY

 E-flash Cards

You will need to learn the essential terms listed below before you begin your reading. These terms will help you understand the main concepts of the chapter. These terms, which will be highlighted in yellow within the text, will become part of your professional vocabulary.

In addition to these essential terms, you will see bold terms throughout the chapter. The meanings of these terms are explained where the terms first appear. The bold terms, like the essential terms listed here, will become part of your professional vocabulary and deepen your understanding of the topics presented.

body language   nonverbal communication that occurs through conscious or unconscious gestures and movements

claims process   the procedure for submitting costs for medical services so that payment can be collected or denial can be determined

communication   the act of sharing a message, thought, or idea so that it is accurately received and understood

copay   an out-of-pocket fee paid by a person with health insurance at the time a covered service, such as an office visit or a prescription, is received

data   facts about a specific topic, which are used for reference or analysis

electronic health record (EHR)   a medical document that contains information from all of the clinicians involved in a patient's care and which can be created and managed by authorized clinicians and staff across more than one healthcare organization

etiquette   term for a code of polite behavior among members of a profession or group

explanation of benefits (EOB)   a detailed account of each claim processed by an insurance plan, which is sent to the patient as notification of claim payment or denial

facsimile machine   a machine used to transmit pictures or written documents using the public telephone network

feedback   the response of an audience to a message

health literacy   a person's ability to obtain and understand health-related information and make informed decisions using that information

medical documentation   written reports of observable, measurable, and reproducible findings from examinations, supporting laboratory or diagnostic tests, and assessments of a patient

medical record   a file that contains documents that describe a specific patient's medical history and medical care within one healthcare organization; also known as a *chart* or *file*

statistics   term for the science that includes the collection, organization, and interpretation of numerical data

triage   an evaluation process in which a group of patients is sorted according to the urgency of their need for care

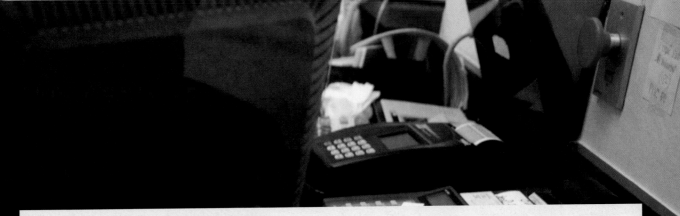

CONNECT WITH YOUR READING

Think about your last visit to a healthcare facility such as a medical clinic, dental office, or hospital. What new equipment did you see? What procedures had changed from what you knew before? How was patient information recorded? Share your observations with your classmates and discuss what caused the changes or why the changes may have been implemented.

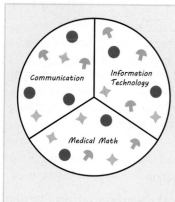

MAP YOUR READING

Create a visual summary by drawing a large circle on a blank sheet of paper. Divide the circle into three pizza slices. Label one slice *Communication*, another *Information Technology*, and the third *Medical Math*. As you finish reading each section of the chapter, place the following "toppings" on your pizza:

- Draw "pepperoni" circles containing the main ideas, or the "meat" of the information.
- Draw "mushroom" shapes containing bits of information that are new or interesting for you and kept you from "vegging out" as you read.
- Draw "mystery" toppings (you create the shapes) that contain questions you still have about your reading.

In this chapter, you will read about fundamental skills that health informatics workers need to do their job well. You will learn about the process of communication and how healthcare workers use listening, speaking, reading, observation, and writing skills to communicate effectively. You will also learn the guidelines for documenting information in a medical record and for triaging telephone calls to identify medical emergencies.

This chapter includes an introduction to the topic of health literacy, which highlights the importance of checking for patient understanding. As you read about the development of the electronic health record, you will begin to understand the role that information technology plays in health informatics services. You will learn the correct format for healthcare e-mails and fax transmissions, which will build your information technology skills. Finally, you will apply your math skills to the health informatics tasks of interpreting graphs and charts, coding diagnoses and procedures, completing insurance claims, and receiving patient payments.

The Communication Process

Oftentimes, communication mistakes are minor or simple. Other times, however, they can lead to serious errors in patient care with devastating results for patients and their families. Because patient information is shared with multiple healthcare workers during the process of diagnosis, treatment, and payment, communicating with care and accuracy is critical to patient outcomes. Healthcare facilities need effective systems for documenting, managing, and sharing patient information, and healthcare workers need effective communication skills for interacting with patients, patients' family members, and fellow healthcare workers (Figure 3.1).

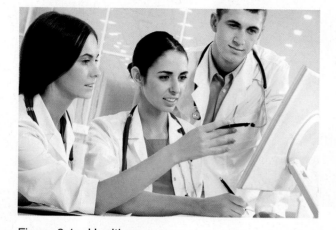

Figure 3.1   Healthcare workers must have excellent communication skills. Why is it important to communicate effectively about patient records?

Communication Error: Abby

Abby left work in a rush to make a late afternoon appointment at the medical clinic. With a full-time job and three grandchildren to care for, she was always on the run. This is why she didn't think much about the clicking noise and fluttery feeling in her ear when she first noticed it. Now, however, it was happening almost every day and she wanted to make sure it wasn't a serious problem.

After a short wait at the clinic, the medical assistant took Abby back to the exam room. Following some initial questions, she waited about 15 minutes for the doctor. When he arrived, the doctor looked in her ears and told her the audiologist (aw-dee-AH-luh-jihst) would give her a hearing test. Following the test, the audiologist took her back to the exam room to wait.

Abby assumed the doctor would return to discuss the hearing test with her. She waited about 30 minutes, but it was getting later and quieter in the clinic. When she noticed the lights turning off in the hallway, Abby left the room to find the assistants closing the office for the day. They were embarrassed about forgetting her and blamed the audiologist for not telling them that she was waiting in the exam room. She headed home without any idea whether her symptoms were serious or not.

This was just a minor misunderstanding—a simple mistake in communication. Although this situation was frustrating for Abby, it wasn't a critical problem. She learned the next day that her hearing was fine and her symptoms were caused by stress.

Communication is the process of sharing a message, thought, or idea. The key element in communication is understanding. Effective communication shares meaning and understanding between the person sending the message and the person or persons receiving it.

The sender begins the communication process by creating the message. Effective communicators consider their audience, or those receiving the message. The information being communicated must be organized, relevant to the receiver, and delivered in a format and language that the receiver understands.

The sender of a message determines the best format for the message. He or she may choose a written form, such as a letter, memo, or report. Alternatively, the sender may choose spoken communication, as in a presentation, performance, conversation, or verbal instructions. He or she may also choose to communicate the message in the form of pictures, charts, or video.

The sender also decides the best method for delivering the message. Messages can be delivered in face-to-face conversation or by telephone. Written communications can be mailed, e-mailed, faxed, texted, or posted in a place where receivers can access the information. Websites, books, magazines, and brochures are only a few of the media outlets available for distributing written material to a large group of people. The sender considers several factors when deciding the best method for delivering a message:

communication
the act of sharing a message, thought, or idea so that it is accurately received and understood

- How many people will receive the message?
- How close (in distance) is the sender to the receiver?
- Is it important to have a written record of the information?
- How quickly does the receiver need to have the information?
- How much formality is required for the message to follow the guidelines of protocol?

Protocol (PROH-tuh-kawl) refers to the appropriate conduct, etiquette, or procedures for communication. Healthcare communication follows many protocols that seek to provide accurate patient information to providers and insurers while preserving the privacy of the patient's health information.

The receiver physically takes delivery of a message in whatever format and method the sender has chosen. However, communication does not end at this point. The communication process is a cycle or a loop that eventually returns to the sender (Figure 3.2).

The receiver is obligated to participate in the communication process. Paying attention to the message and the sender is not only courteous (KER-tee-uhs), or polite, but is also necessary to sustaining the communication process. Unless the receiver understands the message and responds in some way, there is no communication.

feedback
the response of an audience to a message

When the receiver responds to the message, he or she provides **feedback** that closes the communication loop. Through feedback, the sender learns that the receiver has understood the message as it was intended. If there is no feedback, the sender doesn't know if the message was even received, much less understood. When the receiver responds with questions, the communication continues in its cycle of sender-message-receiver-feedback until a clear understanding is achieved.

Effective communication requires listening, speaking, reading, observing, and writing skills. As you read the following sections, think about ways you can improve your own communication skills and note how healthcare workers use these skills to improve job performance.

Listening

Listening is the most neglected of all the communication skills, yet it is the most vital skill for understanding a message.

Figure 3.2   The communication cycle is shown here. The sender begins the communication process, and the receiver provides feedback to show understanding of the message. Why is feedback so important for communication?

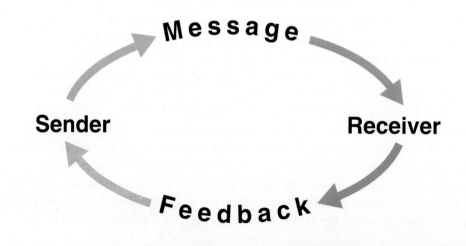

Because we can hear or process words at a much faster rate than they are spoken, our minds can easily wander while we are listening to someone. Good listeners pay attention and concentrate on understanding what a speaker is saying. When they notice a distraction, they purposefully refocus their attention on the speaker.

Poor Listening Skills: Jeff and Kara

Jeff approached his boss, Kara, for some advice on how to complete his written report. Kara assured him that she was happy to answer his questions. However, she was trying to complete her own reports before the final deadline. Since she was proud of her multitasking skills, she continued to type while attempting to answer Jeff's questions. After a couple of minutes, Jeff excused himself and went back to his office. It seemed clear to him that Kara was busy with her own work and didn't have time to answer his questions. He did the best he could on his report, but he made a couple of mistakes that cost the company extra time and money to correct.

Obvious factors such as a noisy environment, a phone call, or an interruption from another person can interfere with good listening. However, an effective listener must also be alert for personal reactions that disrupt attention. Do you avoid listening carefully because you think you already know what the speaker is going to say? Do you focus on what you will say in response rather than paying attention to the speaker's message, especially if you disagree with him or her? Good listeners practice the following steps to improve not only listening, but also understanding a message:

- Face the sender.

- Maintain eye contact if this is comfortable for the speaker.

- Eliminate, or at least limit, outside distractions.

- Keep your attention on the speaker and not on your reaction to his or her words.

- Wait for the speaker to finish before responding. Don't interrupt or finish the speaker's sentence.

- Be comfortable with a brief silence. This allows the speaker to gather his or her thoughts and encourages him or her to provide further information.

- Keep track of information that needs clarification so you can provide feedback by asking further questions to improve your understanding.

Speaking

Effective speaking requires more than a large vocabulary. The manner in which you speak counts just as much as the words you use. Consider the following techniques used by effective speakers and practice them to improve your healthcare communication skills:

- **Always speak clearly and distinctly.** You may not realize that you speak more softly at the beginning or end of your sentences, or that you run words together. Maybe you talk very quickly, making it difficult to understand everything you are saying. Try recording your voice in conversation. How clear and distinct is your speech?

- **Speak to the listener.** Look at your audience, whether that's one person or a crowd of many people. Making eye contact will help you hold the attention of your audience and show your interest in them.

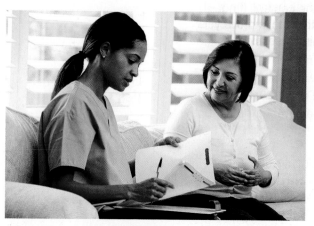

Figure 3.3   Using Standard English is especially important when giving information to patients who speak a language other than your own. How can you effectively communicate with these patients?

- **Carefully choose words that your audience will understand.** Use Standard English, including correct grammar and pronunciation, in the work setting. This level of formality is appropriate in healthcare facilities and indicates worker competence (Figure 3.3).

- **Talk "with" your listener rather than "at" your listener.** Speak in a friendly and courteous tone of voice. Use positive language, and keep your messages short and clear. Introduce a constructive idea rather than focusing on criticism. Then check for understanding by asking for opinions so that the listener can provide feedback.

Reading

Can you think of a healthcare job that doesn't require reading? Reading and comprehension skills are vital to workplace success. It is important that workers comprehend, or understand, what they are reading. Effective employees not only read, but also understand the memos, reports, directions, and records associated with healthcare documentation and procedure.

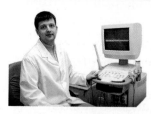

Reading Instructions: Manny

As part of his job, Manny will be using a new piece of imaging equipment. He plans to read the instruction manual even before he begins orientation and training on the new machine. The ability to read and comprehend printed materials helps workers find information quickly so they can operate equipment safely and accurately. Manny uses the following guidelines to improve his speed in reading and to help him remember more of what he has read:

- **Read with a purpose.** Ask why you are reading this document. Manny is reading an instruction manual so he can operate a machine safely. Your purpose might be to learn new information or find answers to your questions. Think about what you already know about the subject of your reading and what questions or predictions occur to you. Manny already knows how to operate an earlier version of this machine. He predicts that the new machine will provide improvements in image quality, but he wants to know if its operation will be as simple and efficient as that of the older machine.

- **Read actively.** Review the section headings of the entire document and decide if you will read for main ideas or for details. Concentrate as you read each section. Ask yourself questions, make comparisons, or visualize what you are reading. Mark sections to read again if they seem confusing. Manny skims over the parts of the manual that describe processes similar to those for the machine he used to use. He reads slowly through the sections about changes and improvements in the operation of the machine. Finally, he uses sticky notes to mark sections that are unclear and writes his questions on the notes.

- **Recall or retell what you have read.** If you can tell another person about what you have read, you probably have a good grasp of the content. If not, reread some sections and discuss the information with others to improve your understanding and memory. When Manny attends the training session, he knows what questions to ask by referring to his sticky notes. As he learns to operate the new machine, he visualizes the steps that are in the manual and uses this mental picture of his reading to operate the imaging machine safely and accurately.

- **Conquer new vocabulary.** The technical readings used in healthcare contain vocabulary terms that are specific to the health science field. Learning medical terminology is similar to studying a foreign language. Be prepared to study vocabulary terms and continue to learn new terms as you encounter them. Experiment with different study methods until you find the ones that work best for you. Manny knows that simply making flash cards won't help him remember information. He needs to see a picture, so he creates an image to help him visualize a new term and its meaning.

Observing

Observation is a skill that involves looking for the messages that are not spoken, but can be found in nonverbal signals. Effective communicators pay attention to **body language** as well as what a person is saying. A smile or sneer, a raised eyebrow or a frown, a shrug or a clenched fist—all of these expressions and gestures communicate a message as clearly as if words had been spoken. Be aware of the nonverbal signals you send and receive, or you may communicate the wrong message.

Healthcare workers use observation when assessing their patients. They look for obvious signs of illness or distress, but are also alert to situations in which a patient's verbal and nonverbal messages don't match. Body language is usually the expression of what the sender truly feels and thinks because it takes place as a result of subconscious thought. A patient may say she's fine, but her clenched teeth and shallow breathing send a different message.

In addition to observing the unconscious body language of patients, healthcare workers also consciously use their own body language to improve patient care. Effective healthcare workers make sure to look at the patient, but also turn and lean slightly toward him or her to convey interest and caring. They nod or say *yes* to acknowledge what the patient

body language
nonverbal communication that occurs through conscious or unconscious gestures and movements

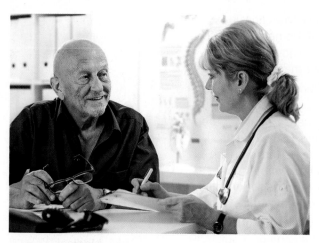

Figure 3.4   Healthcare workers should maintain eye contact and be as friendly as possible as they talk to patients.

is saying, and they practice showing a warm and open facial expression to encourage the patient to speak freely (Figure 3.4).

In certain situations, healthcare workers might even need to use gestures and facial expressions to indicate to a patient that they are currently busy but are aware of the patient's needs. For example, if Kia is talking on the phone when a patient arrives for an appointment, she will greet the patient with a smile, nod her head, and make a quick hand gesture to indicate that she will speak with the patient as soon as she can. This type of body language reassures the patient, who might otherwise feel ignored.

Writing

Effective writing is clear, concise, and accurate. When writing, you must organize your thoughts and present your ideas in a logical manner. In a healthcare setting, the accuracy and clarity of a written document can affect the life and well-being of patients. You have already practiced writing-related tasks that are common in medical offices, including writing letters and memos and completing forms. As you practice new technical writing skills related to healthcare, you will learn the guidelines or rules to follow when recording patient care. Following these rules creates an accurate medical record that becomes a legal document showing the medical care a patient has received.

Complete the *Map Your Reading* graphic organizer for the section you just read.

RECALL YOUR READING

1. The most important element in communication is _____ the message.
2. The communication loop is closed when the receiver provides _____ to the sender.
3. _____ is the most vital skill for understanding a message.
4. Healthcare workers must understand _____ as well as what people are saying.
5. A medical record is a _____ that provides evidence of the care a patient has received.

Communicating Healthcare Information

When caring for patients, the smallest piece of information is potentially important. Therefore, healthcare workers learn to communicate and record patient information by documenting it in a patient's medical record. Since telephone conversations can communicate information about a patient's symptoms or an emergency, phone calls are also documented. Checking that the patient understands all information provided is a goal of every patient interaction, and this check is also recorded in the chart.

Communicating through the Medical Record

A **medical record** is an important form of communication in the healthcare setting. All caregivers and support staff must be able to locate a patient's chart quickly and find information in it easily (Figure 3.5). This information is critical to providing consistent patient care and coordinating care and treatment between different caregivers and settings. For this reason, high-quality medical records are vital to the smooth operation of any medical facility. These records are the official documentation of

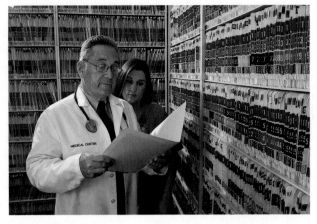

Figure 3.5   Medical records must be organized and accessible. What information does a medical record document?

- the physician's **assessment**, or *evaluation*, of the patient's health;

- treatments the patient receives;

- changes in the patient's health; and

- communication between the patient and healthcare workers.

Traditionally, each patient has a paper folder in which forms and reports from a visit to the healthcare provider are organized. Each facility keeps a record of every patient it sees, so individuals will have several medical records if they visit multiple healthcare facilities. Though these paper folders still exist in some offices, healthcare offices are rapidly converting to electronic records systems. Regardless of the type of system used, patient information must always be well organized, accurate, and complete.

medical record
a file that contains documents that describe a specific patient's medical history and medical care within one healthcare organization; also known as a *chart* or *file*

Information Contained in the Medical Record. While both personal and clinical information are kept in a patient's medical record, clinical information accounts for the largest amount of data. Many different forms provide the **clinical data** recorded in a patient chart. The following are some of the forms that may be found in a medical record at a healthcare clinic or office, and examples of the information included on those forms:

History and Physical

- The chief complaint provides the patient's reason for seeing the physician. Using the patient's own words in the form of a direct quote is most accurate.

- The medical history, also called the *family and personal history*, shows the patient's major illnesses and surgeries, as well as those of close relatives, including parents, grandparents, aunts and uncles, and siblings.

- The review of systems and physical examination includes the results of examining the patient's major body systems to look for undiagnosed problems.

- The diagnosis, or *medical impression*, is the physician's opinion of the medical problems experienced by the patient. A *differential diagnosis* includes all the possible problems to be ruled out to identify the correct diagnosis.

Progress Notes

These notes describe what happens each time the patient sees a healthcare provider. The notes start with the history and physical information and include the recommended tests and treatment plan, including new prescriptions or refills. They provide a summary of each conversation with the patient, whether by telephone, through e-mail, or in person. Progress notes use an organized format such as SOAP so a healthcare provider can quickly understand the patient's situation and concerns (Figure 3.6).

Narrative Nurse's Notes

These notes describe the patient's complaints or symptoms and the actions of the nursing staff in response.

Reports

- Radiology reports contain information about X-rays, MRIs, CT scans, sonograms (SAH-nuh-grams), and other imaging studies completed in the office or in another facility.

- The laboratory (including pathology) results section contains copies of the results of any blood tests, urine tests, or biopsies completed in the office or in another facility.

- The results of specialized tests such as EKGs, stress tests, or colonoscopies are included.

- Consultation reports come from other physicians who have examined the patient at the request of the patient's primary physician. Therapists also submit consultation reports on the patient's progress.

- Operative reports and discharge summaries are also common to hospital records.

Figure 3.6   The SOAP format is one communication technique used to document a patient visit. It was developed by Dr. Lawrence Weed, MD in the 1960s as part of the problem-oriented medical record. SOAP notes provide a structured and uniform method for communicating information to other healthcare providers and for allowing providers to retrieve all patient records for a given medical problem.

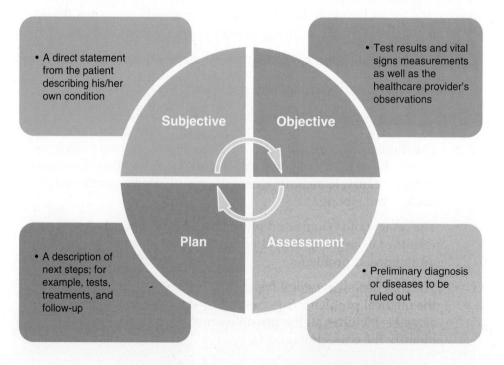

- A direct statement from the patient describing his/her own condition

- Test results and vital signs measurements as well as the healthcare provider's observations

Subjective

Objective

Plan

Assessment

- A description of next steps; for example, tests, treatments, and follow-up

- Preliminary diagnosis or diseases to be ruled out

Medication Administration

This section includes all of the medicines administered or prescribed to the patient. Injections and vaccinations are included in this section.

Correspondence

Correspondence includes copies of all letters and memos involving the patient; for example, letters sent to or received from the patient, or letters received from or sent to other physicians.

Additional Forms

- These include consent forms and the signed HIPAA privacy notice (see chapter 4 for more information on HIPAA).

- These may include copies of a living will, a healthcare power of attorney, or organ donation forms, all of which should be kept in the record.

Organization of Medical Record Information. All documents in a patient's medical record follow a specific system of organization. (Figure 3.7 on the next page). Each document should be placed behind the appropriate tab. These tabs may include *imaging*, *laboratory*, and *pharmacy*. Tabs such as these are included in a **source-oriented medical record (SOMR)**, which is the most common paper-based system for organizing information in a medical record. An SOMR works especially well in the office of a specialist who treats a limited number of medical problems.

Physicians who treat a wide range of problems—such as a family practice physician, pediatrician, or internal medicine physician—may choose to organize information according to the patient's problem. A record organized under this system is called a **problem-oriented medical record (POMR)**. In a POMR, the patient's medical problems appear on the first page of the record. A number is assigned to each problem, and all information relating to that problem receives the same number. This system also works well in healthcare settings where the patient will see different providers due to rotating staff members. Each physician can quickly scan a POMR to review the patient's progress. The POMR system forms the basis for the organization of the electronic health record.

Regardless of the method used to organize information in a medical record, the most recent information is always filed first in each section. New pages are added on top of previous pages so that the information is in reverse chronological order, meaning newer items at the front and older items at the back. As soon as the physician has reviewed a patient's forms, he or she adds them to the medical record. This happens on a daily basis so the record is always complete and provides accurate information to guide patient treatment.

Functions of Documentation. Medical documentation refers to the forms and notes that healthcare workers add to a medical record by way of charting. **Charting** is the process of recording observations and information about patients. Many different healthcare workers complete the various aspects of charting. For example, a medical assistant may record demographic information about new patients or interview patients to complete a medical history form. Nurses routinely measure and record

medical documentation
written reports of observable, measurable, and reproducible findings from examinations, supporting laboratory or diagnostic tests, and assessments of a patient

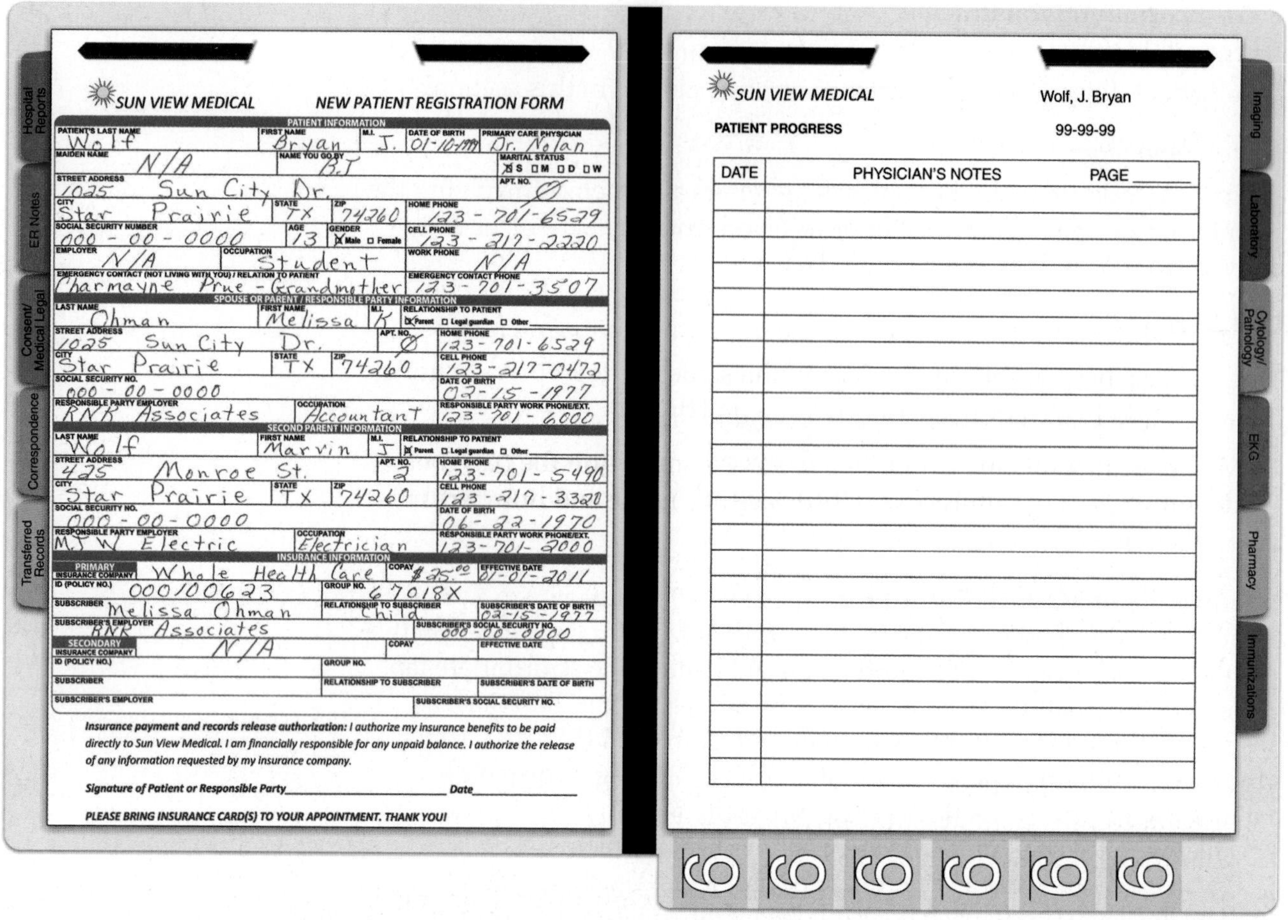

Figure 3.7   In a source-oriented medical record (SOMR), all information must be organized under tabs such as *Hospital Reports*, *ER Notes*, *Consent/Medical Legal*, *Correspondence*, *Transferred Records*, *Imaging*, *Laboratory*, *Cytology/Pathology*, *EKG*, *Pharmacy*, and *Immunizations*. The number tabs along the bottom of the file are the medical record number. This can also be found below the patient's name.

vital signs and specific care procedures they have performed, such as injections. Health information technicians code diagnoses and treatment procedures to facilitate payment from insurance companies.

While medical documentation promotes quality care, the medical record serves other purposes as well. For example, a medical record is a legal document that can be used as evidence in court to prove what care was provided to the patient. When records are incomplete or illegible, there is no proof that treatment was provided. The rule is, "If it wasn't documented, it wasn't done!"

Careful documentation saves money by reducing repetition of tests and avoiding unnecessary procedures. By providing complete information, documentation promotes preventive steps and early intervention to reduce serious outcomes. For example, a complete record of rising blood pressure readings could prompt a physician to recommend lifestyle changes or medication to prevent the blood vessel damage that leads to an increased risk for a stroke.

Careful documentation follows the guidelines of regulatory agencies or government programs such as Medicare. For a healthcare facility, **compliance** with these guidelines is necessary to receive reimbursement of costs for treatment and reduce denials of payment from insurance providers. Compliance means that guidelines are followed or observed.

Guidelines for Documentation. High-quality medical records meet three standards—they are accurate and complete; they are legible and easy to read; and they are timely, meaning that they are written when the procedure or treatment takes place. While these guidelines include the steps for hand-written documentation, you will learn in chapter 7 that many of the same principles apply to computer-generated medical records. Follow these guidelines to create high-quality documentation:

1. Use black or blue ink for all written notes.

2. Make sure your handwriting is neat and readable.

3. Verify the patient's name and identifying numbers on the page before documenting any information. The patient's name and numbers must appear on every page in the chart.

4. Since the patient's name is on the every page of the chart, you do not need to rewrite it in each chart entry.

5. Chart your own observations and actions only. Never chart or sign for another healthcare worker. You are personally liable for the care you provide, and the chart is the legal record of your care.

6. Leave no blank or empty lines between entries in the record. This prevents others from making entries that will be mistaken for part of your documentation (Figure 3.8).

7. Record the correct date and time for each entry. Only use military time.

   Example: *06/16/15–0830*

8. Do not erase, cover up, or cross out chart entries. If you make a mistake, draw a single line through the mistake, write "error," then date and initial the change.

   Example: *Ate 100% of ~~dinner~~ breakfast.*
                              ——error 06/16/15 TS

9. Record objective observations rather than your opinions. Record the patient's reactions using the patient's own words in quotation marks.

   Example: *Skin is red and moist to touch. States, "It itches like crazy!"*

10. Always record your verbal report to your supervisor.

    Example: *Temperature: 101.5—Reported to charge nurse.*

NURSE'S PROGRESS NOTES

DATE	TIME	NURSING CARE NOTES	SIGNATURE
06-16-15	0830	*Refused breakfast* —————————	*Tom Smith RN*
06-16-15	0900	*Complains of a sharp pain in shoulder*——	
		Skin appears red and warm to touch ———	*Tom Smith RN*

Figure 3.8   As shown here, you should never leave blank lines in a chart entry. Draw a line through any empty spaces so coworkers don't use that space.

Simulate EHR

11. Use correct spelling, terminology, punctuation, and grammar. Use only facility-approved abbreviations (Figure 3.9). This avoids confusion that could lead to treatment errors. For example, is "6IU of insulin" supposed to be *61 units* or *6 International Units*?

12. Write numbers and measurements in actual figures rather than using general terms such as "many" or "OK."

    Example: *BP 120/80*   is better than   *BP normal*.

13. Complete the record as soon as possible after the activity that is being recorded has occurred. However, you should never record activity *before* it occurs. If you record treatment, begin to give the treatment, and are suddenly called to an emergency, the record will show that the patient has already received treatment. This can lead to errors in procedures such as giving medication. Late entries can result in dates or times that are out of order. These gaps between entries are confusing for anyone accessing the information (Figure 3.10). Timely entries provide greater accuracy since the event is still fresh in your mind.

14. Sign your name and title at the end of each entry.

    Example: *Tom Smith, RN*

All contact made with patients should be included in the medical record. You should document all phone calls from patients, phone calls that give information to patients, and phone calls regarding prescriptions. These chart entries must contain the date and time of the call, what the patient said or asked for, your reply, and the actions you took in response to the call. Attach any forms used for recording patient phone calls to the progress notes in the medical record.

Figure 3.9 Official "Do Not Use" List of Abbreviations			
Chart Item	**Forbidden Abbreviation**	**Potential Problem**	**Use Instead**
unit	U, u	mistaken for *0* (zero), *4* (four), or *cc*	write the word *unit*
International Unit	IU	mistaken for *IV* (intravenous) or the number *10* (ten)	write the words *International Unit*
daily **every other day**	Q.D., QD, q.d., qd Q.O.D., QOD, q.o.d, qod	mistaken for each other period after the *Q* mistaken for *I*, and the *O* mistaken for *I*	write *daily* write *every other day*
X.0 **.X**	trailing zero (X.0 mg)[2] lack of leading zero (.X mg)	decimal point is missed	write *X mg* write *0.X mg*
morphine sulfate **magnesium sulfate**	MS MSO4 and MgSO4	can mean *morphine sulfate* or *magnesium sulfate* confused for one another	write *morphine sulfate* write *magnesium sulfate*

NURSE'S PROGRESS NOTES

DATE	TIME	NURSING CARE NOTES	SIGNATURE
06-16-15	0900	Complains of a sharp pain in shoulder———	
		Skin appears red and warm to touch ———	Tom Smith RN
06-16-15	0930	Late entry (06-16-15—0830) Refused	
		breakfast———————	Tom Smith RN

Figure 3.10   Notice how the out-of-order entry gives the impression that the patient's pain occurred before, rather than after the patient refused breakfast.

Communicating by Telephone

The telephone is typically the most common method of contacting a healthcare facility that patients have. You may have to answer the phone as part of your duties as a healthcare worker. Creating a positive experience for callers earns goodwill for your facility. More importantly, your telephone communication skills will affect health outcomes for patients as you quickly connect them to the correct healthcare resource, provide clear directions, or even respond to a medical emergency.

Telephone skills begin with appropriate **etiquette** (EH-tih-keht). In healthcare facilities, telephone skills also include screening, prioritizing, and documenting calls, tasks that all become part of healthcare delivery.

etiquette
term for a code of polite behavior among members of a profession or group

Courteous Conversation. The increasing use of instant communication that is not face-to-face means individuals don't have a chance to practice the art of conversation. A recent walk through a high school cafeteria showed most students sitting together but not talking to each other. Each student was engaged with the technology of a smartphone, cell phone, or media player. Occasionally, students showed images or messages to each other, but they didn't have a conversation.

Creating a positive telephone conversation is even more challenging than a face-to-face encounter because you can't observe nonverbal cues such as facial expressions or body language. As a result, your verbal skills become even more important.

Answer the phone with a smile (Figure 3.11). Surprisingly, smiling actually makes your tone of voice more cheerful and positive. Remember that your tone of voice sends a strong signal in a phone conversation. You may be very busy when the telephone interrupts your work, but you should not let your irritation come through in your voice. Instead, aim for a pleasant tone that is low in pitch. Speak at a moderate speed and more slowly if you are giving directions. Practice pronouncing words clearly and distinctly since people can't read your lips to improve their understanding. Eating, drinking, and chewing gum will ruin your conversation. Avoid them when you communicate by phone.

Basic telephone etiquette requires you to answer the phone as soon as possible. You should answer no later than the third ring. Remember, you are working in a healthcare facility and this may be an emergency call. Use your facility's standard greeting to identify your facility and yourself. This lets callers know they have dialed correctly. A typical greeting might be, "Hello, Sun View Medical. This is April, the medical assistant. How may I help you?"

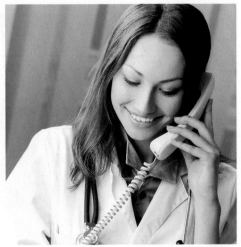

Figure 3.11   When talking on the phone, try smiling to convey a cheerful and positive attitude.

In larger facilities, automated messages will guide the direction of a call but will also provide a direct-dial number for emergency calls.

Use courteous phrasing when asking questions. "How may I help you?" is better than "What do you want?" Compare the following questions to note the difference courteous phrasing can make:

Original		Courteous
• "What's your name?"	becomes	"May I have your name, please?"
• "What did you say?"	becomes	"Would you repeat that, please?"

As a routine courtesy, you should thank callers before you hang up and allow them to hang up first to be certain they have finished speaking.

Courtesy also counts when using the "hold a call" feature on a telephone. First, make sure the call is not an emergency or another physician calling to speak to one of your physicians. Then ask for permission before placing a caller on hold. Take a callback number and a message if the person can't remain on hold.

While this sounds simple, in a healthcare setting, you will often be handling many phone calls and patients at once. Remember to check back every minute or two with the caller who is on hold. If you can't connect the call, continue to ask if the caller wants to remain on hold or leave a callback number.

Above all, you should understand how to use the telephone equipment in your office properly. There is nothing more frustrating than waiting on hold, being disconnected, and having to start the call process all over again. If you mistakenly disconnect a patient who is on hold, call the person back and apologize before completing the call.

Call Screening and Triage. Every call received at a healthcare facility must be screened to determine who will respond to the caller (Figure 3.12). Most calls involve scheduling an appointment and can be handled by the medical assistant or personnel working at a centralized appointment desk. Calls from other physicians or calls from the physician's family are handled according to the physician's preferences. You will need to learn these preferences to manage the calls appropriately. Follow your facility's policy for responding to calls from salespeople or insurance companies. In a smaller office, the medical assistant may respond to these calls, but in a larger facility they may be transferred to a specific department such as *Business Services*.

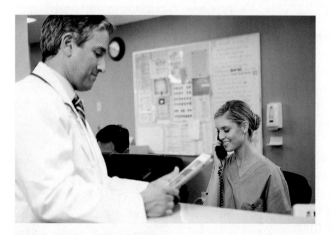

Figure 3.12 A medical receptionist often has to perform triage on a flurry of phone calls. What is the importance of triage?

Approved personnel, such as medical assistants or nursing staff members, can manage routine patient requests for prescription refills or test results, as well as progress reports from other healthcare personnel. Typically, a physician will review updated information in a patient's chart and speak with patients who do not report satisfactory progress. However, you should always tell the physician about calls in which the patient reports new symptoms or a seriously worsening condition. Do not wait for the doctor to discover this information in the patient's chart.

When a patient calls to report symptoms of illness, you must be able to tell the difference between a panicked caller and a medical emergency. To evaluate the different calls coming into a healthcare facility, you will need to use **triage** (TREE-ahj). In a clinic setting, triage may be handled by a specific triage nurse, or it may be part of the medical assistant's duties.

The process of triage includes asking a series of questions to determine whether emergency medical personnel should be called or if the patient can wait to see the physician at the next available appointment time. You will be most effective in triaging calls if you remain calm as you learn what happened and what symptoms the patient is experiencing. The following conditions represent true emergencies and require immediate care:

triage
an evaluation process in which a group of patients is sorted according to the urgency of their need for care

- chest pain or any other severe pain

- difficulty breathing

- loss of consciousness

- a fever above 102°F

- heavy bleeding

- severe vomiting or diarrhea

Privacy rules guide the phone conversations of healthcare workers. Remember to use care when discussing patient information so others can't overhear it. Know when and with whom patient information may be shared. For example, the patient must provide permission for information to be shared with family members. In some facilities, it is a breach of privacy to acknowledge that a specific person is even a patient. Be cautious about sharing test results over the phone. Is this within your scope of practice? Some facilities designate specific staff members to communicate test results and, in some cases, the physician will make such calls.

Simulate EHR

Documenting Phone Conversations. Since all phone communication with patients must be documented in their medical records, you will need an efficient system for recording messages and conversations. Facilities often use a form designed specifically for the unique needs of its patient care specialty. A phone message should at least include the following information:

- caller's name

- date and time of call

- phone contact number for the caller

- a short description of the caller's question or concern

- person to whom the message is directed

- your signature or initials so the message recipient can check with you if he or she has questions (Figure 3.13)

Message		
To: **Dr. Jones**		
Date:	**6/22/2015** Time:	**1430**
WHILE YOU WERE OUT		
Caller's Name: **Sharon Sims**		
Business: **Star Prairie Pharmacy**		
Phone Number: **123-701-9500**		
	Returned your call	Wanted to see you
X	Please return call	Stopped by
	Will call again	Rush
Message:		
Called for clarification of prescription #6540700 for patient Margaret Black. Generic form not available in 50 mg tablets. Can two 25 mg tablets be substituted or will prescription be rewritten for brand name medication?		
Taken by: **Jane Brown, MA**		**6/22/2015**

Figure 3.13   One efficient method for recording phone messages is shown above.

When a patient calls the healthcare facility, you should place a copy of the phone message you took in the patient's chart. When you contact a patient, write a summary of your conversation to document the call in the patient's chart. Remember that the medical record is a legal document of the care provided. As a result, you should be concise, accurate, and complete when documenting your phone calls with patients (Figure 3.14).

Improving Health Literacy

Consider the following situations. The doctor tells a female patient not to remove her dressing for 48 hours. Still medicated after her outpatient surgery, she wonders why she can't change into pajamas when she gets home.

A young mother brings her crying baby to the emergency room with an ear infection. The physician prescribes an antibiotic. Two days later, the mother returns with her crying baby and claims that the medicine is not working. When he examines the child, the doctor finds traces of the medicine in the child's ear.

A man receives medication for hypertension. He decides he doesn't need the medicine because he isn't feeling hyper. A physician seeks treatment for a fracture. As he leaves the clinic, he realizes that even though he treats similar injuries in his own practice, he can't remember most of the information and care instructions the staff has just told him to follow.

Message			Message	
To: **Dr. Jones**			To: **Dr. Jones**	
Date: **6/22/2015**	Time: **1430**		Date: **6/22/2015**	Time: **1430**
WHILE YOU WERE OUT			**WHILE YOU WERE OUT**	
Caller's Name: **Judy Bleeker**			Caller's Name: **Judy Bleeker**	
Business: **N/A**			Business: **N/A**	
Phone Number: **456-812-0611**			Phone Number: **456-812-0611**	
Returned your call	Wanted to see you		Returned your call	Wanted to see you
Please return call	Stopped by		Please return call	Stopped by
Will call again	Rush		Will call again	Rush

Message:

Pt called to cancel appt for ear recheck. Says child is feeling better. Advised to continue medication and keep appt to make sure eardrum is normal. Patient says, "That seems like a wasted trip. I'm not coming." Advised Dr. Brenner.

Taken by: **Jane Brown, MA**   **6/22/2015**

Message:

Pt called to cancel appt.

Taken by: **Jane Brown, MA**   **6/22/2015**

Figure 3.14   Which of these entries was probably made shortly after the phone call? Which entry provides a better defense in a court case?

All of these situations illustrate health literacy concerns. **Health literacy** is just as important as the healthcare treatment you receive. In fact, research shows that literacy skills are the strongest predictor of health status. Your health literacy skills influence your health more than your age, income, employment status, education level, or racial and ethnic group.

Low health literacy is expensive for everyone. When patients don't understand explanations and instructions given by doctors and other healthcare workers, they often end up back at the healthcare facility. Billions of dollars are spent each year for additional treatment that is needed when patients fail to follow their doctor's care instructions. Patients may fail to follow instructions because they don't understand them or because they don't understand the consequences of not following them.

Health literacy influences all aspects of healthcare. It affects a person's ability to determine how much medicine to give a child, how to choose a health insurance plan, how to prepare for a surgical procedure, and even how to navigate a healthcare facility. For example, how many people going to the hospital for an X-ray will know that the department they're looking for is called *radiology* or *imaging*?

We all know that medical care is complicated. Yet understanding how to care for yourself is more important today than ever before. Today, patients are released from the hospital as soon as possible and more procedures are performed on an outpatient basis to keep costs down. As a result, the ability to understand any healthcare information being given to you is essential for when you return home. Healthcare workers have an obligation to provide high-quality care, and communicating effectively with patients is an important part of that care.

Poor reading skills limit a patient's ability to understand healthcare instructions, but the reasons for a lack of health literacy go beyond the ability to read. According to research, almost half of patients cannot read medication labels effectively. They may be able to read the words, but they can't interpret those words to understand how to properly take the medicine. Health literacy involves understanding and interpreting information as well as simply reading the words (Figure 3.15).

Oral language skills also play an important role in health literacy. Patients must be able to express their health concerns and describe their symptoms accurately. They need to ask questions and understand and remember spoken medical advice or treatment directions. Many patients, however, are embarrassed when they don't understand information, so they fail to ask questions. If the doctor said, "Your condition is known as *cholelithiasis* (koh-luh-lih-THI-uh-suhs)," would you wonder what that is? Would you ask the doctor to explain?

It is important to ensure that the information given to patients is actually understood. Healthcare workers can do this by assessing a patient's level of literacy and adapting their communication accordingly. They may need to use simpler language or hand gestures to explain care procedures or medication administration. Showing the

health literacy
a person's ability to obtain and understand health-related information and make informed decisions using that information

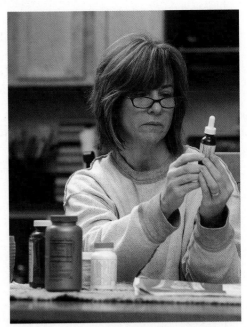

Figure 3.15   Improving health literacy leads to a better understanding of procedures and medication instructions.

patient how much medicine to take is more helpful than assuming that he or she knows how to calculate and measure dosage in the metric system.

Providing written instructions at a simple reading level, accompanied by illustrations, can improve understanding dramatically. This also helps patients remember and be able to follow care directions when they return home. Providing a direct contact number encourages patients to call with additional questions or concerns once they leave the facility.

There are additional health literacy skills that need to be addressed. Establishing educational programs to help patients navigate the complex healthcare system improves access to medical care. Patients can benefit from knowing more about the many different healthcare professionals they may see, as well as how to schedule appointments or pay for healthcare services. Learning how to prevent illness, take medication safely, and care for chronic conditions like diabetes helps patients maintain or improve their health status while reducing healthcare costs.

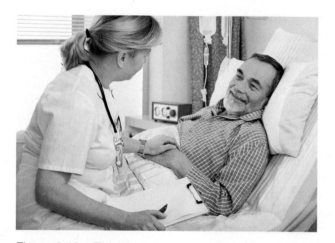

Healthcare workers need to learn cultural competency skills so they can recognize and effectively serve patients who are vulnerable due to limited health literacy. Cultural competency training can teach healthcare workers signs that may indicate that a patient does not have effective health literacy skills. Elderly patients, for example, are at high risk for hospitalization and rehospitalization because they have difficulty following complicated medication schedules (Figure 3.16). Culturally competent healthcare workers recognize that providing assistance with medication setup and scheduling might prevent the need for emergency care or rehospitalization.

Figure 3.16 Elderly patients may need extra help interpreting medication schedules.

Health literacy is not a passing concern. Rather, it is a complex issue that affects the health outcomes of a large segment of the patient population. Your ability to communicate with patients in a way that they can understand will go a long way toward improving their health status.

Complete the *Map Your Reading* graphic organizer for the section you just read.

RECALL YOUR READING

1. All patient care must be included in the patient's _____.
2. When healthcare facilities comply with medical documentation guidelines, they are more frequently _____ for patient services.
3. All telephone communication with patients becomes part of their _____.
4. _____ skills involve understanding health information and are the strongest predictor of health status.

Information Technology

Technology is changing the way we communicate. Computers and personal devices such as smartphones, tablets, and media players are at the heart of that change. We keep in touch with the activities of our friends by reading and responding to their posts, or connect with future jobs through online contacts. Even e-mails have become too slow for most personal communication.

Technology is also changing the way people communicate in the field of healthcare. Basic computer literacy is an expected skill for all healthcare workers because computers are rapidly replacing paper in both healthcare documentation and facility operation. Even jobs with the smallest connection to direct patient care or medical records must interact with computers. A housekeeper updates an inventory of cleaning supplies. A central services technician barcodes supplies for billing purposes. A maintenance engineer runs computer diagnostics (dI-ag-NAHS-tihks) on the air conditioning system to check for needed repairs. A hospital administrator uses a PowerPoint presentation to communicate the growth plan for her facility.

Nowhere is technological change more far-reaching than in the development of the **electronic health record (EHR)**. The electronic health record has the potential to speed up the documentation process, improve the accuracy of patient records, and expand access to complete medical records for all providers. While the process of converting paper records to electronic records is complex, the goal of improved care drives the efforts to implement effective electronic systems.

Electronic Health Records—Past, Present, and Future

Medical providers have long realized the advantages that computerization brings to medical records. As early as the 1960s, efforts to develop **computerized patient records**—early versions of the EHR— were ongoing at the Mayo Clinic in Rochester, Minnesota; at the Medical Center Hospital of Vermont; and at El Camino Hospital in California. During the next two decades, many similar systems were developed. With a computerized system, information about drug dosages and drug interactions could be accessed quickly and treatment plans could be communicated to everyone caring for the patient. The systems were limited, however, by the size and processing power of a mainframe computer.

Past Developments. During the 1990s, powerful new personal computers (PCs) and networking capabilities were developed. As the cost of computers decreased, several new companies entered the **electronic medical record (EMR)** market. EMRs were an earlier version of the EHRs that are now used. Using the EMRs, physician's offices and outpatient clinics began to convert their paper records to electronic formats. These less complex healthcare settings were able to use commercially available programs, but the complexity of a hospital environment—with its many departments and services—meant that adoption of electronic records systems could not happen yet. Many long-term care facilities and home health organizations also found the cost of computerization too high.

In addition to their limitations and high cost, EMRs had a slow start when they were first introduced because healthcare workers lacked confidence in their security and efficiency. Could these records be altered without the physician's knowledge or consent? Would a power outage cause a computer "crash" and a loss of vital information? Is typing really faster than writing? Many physicians who were used to writing all of

electronic health record (EHR)
a medical document that contains information from all of the clinicians involved in a patient's care and which can be created and managed by authorized clinicians and staff across more than one healthcare organization

their records were reluctant to learn computer skills. Often, computers were not at the point of care, meaning that staff had to leave patients to enter information on a computer.

Obstacles. As recently as 2010, fewer than 300 hospitals in the United States had fully implemented the use of electronic health records. By comparison, most countries with national healthcare systems such as the Netherlands (NETH), Sweden (SWE), and New Zealand (NZ) have fully implemented electronic records (Figure 3.17). Why has the process of converting to electronic records taken more than 30 years when the benefit of improved patient care seems so obvious?

First, converting to computerized programs is expensive. The cost of implementing an EHR system falls on the healthcare facility. Some hospitals have mortgaged their facilities to provide capital for investing in a records system, but not all healthcare facilities are able to do this.

Additionally, electronic record systems often make sharing information difficult. Healthcare is delivered in a competitive environment in the United States. As a result, companies develop **proprietary** (pruh-PRI-uh-tair-ee), or *private*, systems that can't communicate with other records systems. For example, the Cerner Power Chart cannot communicate with the Centricity record system. This limits the interoperability (ihn-ter-ah-per-uh-BIH-luh-tee) of the electronic record system, which means it cannot work with other systems in the healthcare provider network. A general practitioner using the latest system from one company can't send a patient's record to a specialist practicing in a different office down the hall if he uses a product from a competing company. To exchange information, the general practitioner has to print out the record and deliver it by hand. This counteracts any ease of use provided by the electronic record system.

Current Developments. Despite the obstacles involved, the United States continues to progress toward EHR implementation. Today, many

Figure 3.17   Between 2009 and 2012, the United States dramatically increased its use of electronic health records. Why does the United States still lag behind other countries in EHR use?

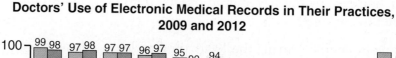

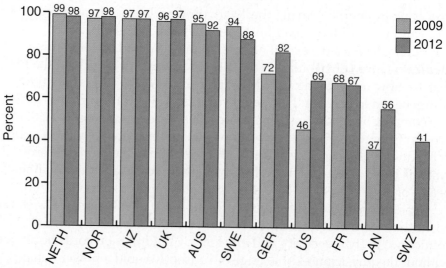

Source: 2009 and 2012 Commonwealth Fund
International Health Policy Survey of Primary Care Physicians.

healthcare facilities are exploring and using comprehensive programs that deliver all the functions of an electronic health record. The EHR includes information such as patient demographics and medical history, progress notes and problems, vital signs, medications, lab reports and radiology reports, chief complaints, care alerts, and preventive care guidelines. The functions of scheduling, transcription, e-prescribing, evaluation, and coding have also been incorporated.

Newly developed systems are beginning to improve interoperability by incorporating **continuity of care records (CCRs)**. These records contain a standardized summary of the most relevant and timely health information about a patient. Physicians can access and update these regardless of the records system being used. Personal health records (PHRs) invite patients to participate in their own health management. Using a secure Internet connection, patients can use PHRs to schedule appointments, review lab or radiology results, and communicate with their physicians.

Improvements in security, the development of mobile technologies such as the smartphone and tablet computer, and government-sponsored financial incentives are speeding the adoption of electronic records systems. In the past 10 years, the EHR usage rate for physicians increased from 18 percent to 57 percent, as reported to the Centers for Disease Control and Prevention. The Department of Health and Human Services has set a deadline of 2015 for EHR usage. After that time, Medicare and Medicaid healthcare providers who are not using electronic health records may have to pay penalties.

Physicians who use EHR systems are beginning to see improvements in care (Figure 3.18). One physician uses his electronic patient data to identify diabetic patients who are overdue for screening tests. Seconds later, he e-mails those patients a reminder or sends a letter to those without Internet access. Two years ago, just 40 percent of his diabetic patients were in their target range on a standard test for blood sugar. Since implementing data checks and e-mail reminders, that number has risen to 70 percent.

Consider how an EHR system improved patient care in the following scenario. The major healthcare organization that operates both the clinic where the physician works and the hospital she's calling has installed a

Figure 3.18 Benefits of Electronic Health Records	
Improved efficiency and reduced medical costs	• reduce time spent on paperwork • reduce duplication of medical tests
Improved care coordination	• give every provider access to the same information about a patient • up-to-date medication and allergy lists facilitate prescribing among physicians
Improved patient outcomes	• improved patient compliance through automated reminders for routine screening • reliable point-of-care information and reminders notifying providers of important health interventions
Improved quality and convenience	• accurate coding and billing facilitated by legible documentation • e-prescriptions sent electronically to the pharmacy

networked EHR system in every clinic and hospital it owns. The physician calls the emergency room (ER) at the hospital to ask if a patient with seizure-like symptoms should be sent to the neurology department or the emergency room. The ER physician checks the patient record, sees that the patient's symptoms are atypical for epilepsy, and has the patient transferred to emergency care. A cardiac monitor reveals an abnormal heartbeat that is corrected by implanting a pacemaker. Without the benefit of immediate access to an electronic record, this patient would likely have been referred to neurology, where a dangerous heart condition could not be diagnosed.

Health Informatics Services Applications

Electronic communication has dramatically increased the speed of personal and business correspondence. Sometimes, however, that speed can result in carelessness and loss of privacy for patients. Health informatics workers must always be attentive to protecting the privacy of patient information when using electronic systems for communication and other tasks. Workers must also use appropriate etiquette and follow facility procedures when using technology to communicate with patients, doctors, and fellow healthcare workers.

E-mail. Electronic mail (e-mail) communication has become vital to daily business operations in healthcare facilities (Figure 3.19). E-mail has largely replaced the traditional paper options for sending memos, announcements, and reports. It is increasingly being used to send secure, digital lab results and discharge summaries to the physician's office. Health informatics workers use electronic communication systems to code services and submit claims for payment to health insurance providers and to the Centers for Medicare and Medicaid Services.

E-mail is sent by means of a secure transmission process such as encryption to protect patient privacy. A secure web portal can also be used. In this case, physicians and patients both sign in to a secure website to send messages back and forth within that site.

Each healthcare organization stores, monitors, and manages its e-mail communications. Employers have the right to read any message sent through their computer system by an employee. Since e-mails belong to the organization, employees must use them for business purposes only. Many businesses also monitor Internet use by employees. Online shopping and writing negative posts about your employer while at work could cost you your job.

Managing e-mail communications has become challenging because employees may receive dozens of messages each day. Therefore, your e-mails must be clear and accurate, but also brief and to the point. Address only one concern in each e-mail so that recipients can organize their messages more easily. Because your recipient can't read your

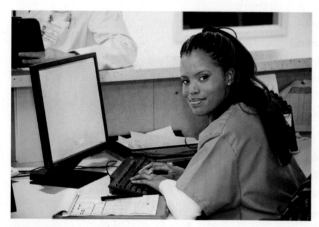

Figure 3.19   Health informatics workers communicate mainly through e-mails. They may receive dozens of messages each day. How quickly should you respond to an e-mail?

nonverbal signals, you should choose your words carefully to convey the correct message in a professional tone. Avoid sending a message when you are angry or frustrated. Since your e-mail may be forwarded to others, review your words before you hit the send button.

When you send an e-mail to a friend, your message's format may be unstructured and casual. As you reply to each other, you don't need to repeat your name as you would if writing a business letter. However, e-mail communication in a healthcare setting is more formal and follows the rules of business communication because it may become part of the legal record of patient care.

The format of an e-mail is similar to that of a printed memo. Follow these guidelines as you write an e-mail message:

- **To.** In this line, key in the names of your main recipients. These are the people who will be replying to your e-mail or those with a primary interest in your message.

- **Copy (CC).** Use this line to add people who will want to read the information but are not expected to reply.

- **Blind Copy (Bcc).** Generally, it is courteous to let the recipient know all the people who are receiving your message. However, you can use the Blind Copy, or *Bcc*, feature when your e-mail is being sent to a large number of people outside your organization. This courtesy protects the privacy of everyone's contact information and reduces clutter at the beginning of the message.

- **Subject.** Provide a clear and concise statement for your subject line. Avoid general statements such as *Hello* or *For Your Information*. Include a subject that reflects the topic or content of your e-mail so your readers can keep track of their replies.

- **Salutation.** Keep your salutations formal by using the word *Dear* in front of the recipient's name for all communication being sent outside your facility. If you are on a first-name basis with the intended recipient, you may use the first name in e-mail communication. However, in all communication, you should follow the guidelines set by your healthcare facility.

- **Message.** Format your message the same way you would a letter or memo. Use Standard English and check your spelling, punctuation, and grammar. Keep your message short and simple. Avoid using all capital letters, as this can be interpreted as shouting your message. Use an attachment to provide details, if necessary.

- **Closing.** Use a friendly but business-like closing such as *Sincerely* or *Cordially*. Less formal e-mails to coworkers may end with *Thanks* or *Thank you*.

- **Signature.** Include your full name and contact information, including your job title and department, at the bottom of your e-mail. Since many programs display only the sender's name, include your e-mail address in your signature. You can set up your program to insert this information automatically. Include a confidentiality footer with every e-mail. This statement is required for sensitive, confidential, or protected health information. It also adds privacy protection to e-mails that are sent to an incorrect address (Figure 3.20).

Before sending any patient information to another provider or an insurance company, be certain that you have a written release from the patient. When sending personal information to a patient, be sure to direct it to the correct e-mail address. Double-check the address before you send the message. If a mistake is made, unauthorized individuals may gain access to protected health information.

Follow professional etiquette guidelines for handling the e-mail you receive as well as the e-mail you send. Respond to incoming e-mails as quickly as possible, but at least within 24 hours. If you need more time to write your response, send a short message indicating that you will respond as soon as possible. Use the *out-of-office* feature when you are not at work. This feature will generate an automatic reply that lets people know when you will return.

When you respond to a message, stick to the original topic in your reply. To switch to a new topic, create a new e-mail and mention the new topic in the subject line. This allows both the sender and the recipient to organize and file the messages by topic.

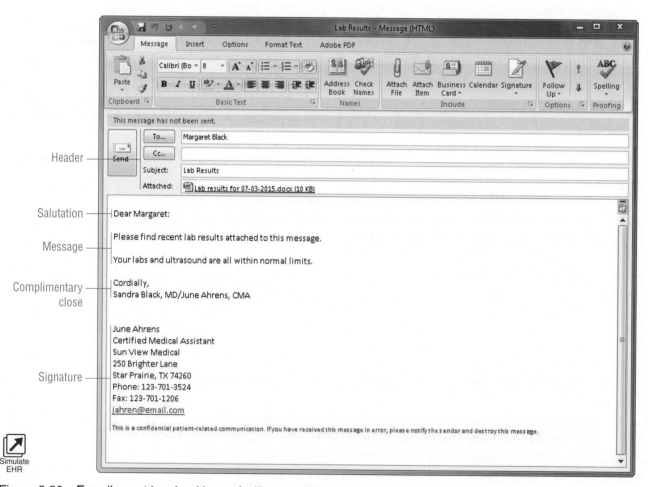

Figure 3.20   E-mails sent in a healthcare facility must follow specific guidelines.

Some healthcare facilities use a messaging system so employees can communicate with each other quickly via computer. These in-office messages tend to be far less formal than e-mails, but always follow your facility's guidelines (Figure 3.21).

Fax. Facsimile (fak-SIH-muh-lee) **machines**, or *fax machines* send paper documents via a phone line and reprint them on the recipient's machine or send them electronically to the recipient's e-mail inbox. The process is relatively easy and inexpensive. While e-mails are becoming the preferred method for sending documents, you may still encounter a fax machine at your place of employment.

facsimile machine
a machine used to transmit pictures or written documents using the public telephone network

Always use a cover sheet when sending a document through a fax machine (Figure 3.22 on the next page). The cover sheet is a standard form that is always the first sheet sent with a document. It forms a physical barrier to guard sensitive information and clearly identifies the recipient, or person receiving the fax. A cover sheet includes the following information:

- name and contact information of the office sending the fax

- name of the recipient

- telephone number of the recipient's fax machine

- date and time the fax is sent

- total number of pages, including the cover sheet

- confidentiality statement (required by law and similar to an e-mail confidentiality statement)

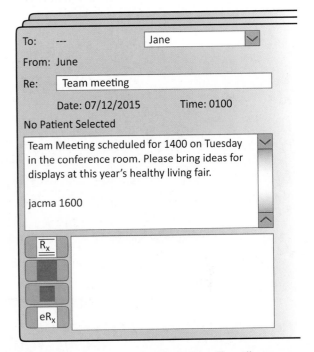

Figure 3.21   E-mail memos sent to coworkers can be written more casually than business e-mails.

Sending documents via a fax machine can create concerns about confidentiality, so certain procedures must be followed. You should always wait until the machine has processed your documents so you can take them with you rather than leave them in the machine. In that way, you can maintain confidentiality in your own office. It can be difficult, however, to maintain confidentiality once the documents are sent to another office. If the intended recipient works in a busy office, how can you be certain he or she will be the only person to see the documents? Always check to see that your cover sheet is the first page sent in your fax to provide some protection for sensitive information.

A simple error such as using the wrong phone number can send confidential documents to the wrong business. A furniture company may accidentally receive faxed documents intended for employees of a medical clinic, causing a breach of confidentiality. Always be sure that you have the correct phone number.

Figure 3.22   A cover sheet should always be included when sending a fax.

Simulate
EHR

SUN VIEW MEDICAL

For:

Fax number:

From:

Fax number:

Date: Time:

Regarding:

Number of pages:

Comments:

"Confidential Notice – This fax may contain protected health information of a personal and sensitive nature related to an individual's healthcare. If you have received this message by error, please notify the sender immediately to arrange for return or destruction of these documents."

Complete the
Map Your Reading
graphic organizer for the
section you just read.

RECALL YOUR READING

1. More healthcare facilities are using _____ because of improved security and government-sponsored financial incentives.
2. Follow the rules for business communication when sending _____ because they may become part of the legal record of patient care.
3. Respond to all e-mails within _____.
4. A fax cover sheet identifies the recipient and protects private information by creating a _____.
5. For legal reasons, include a _____ statement with every e-mail or fax.

Medical Math

From the most basic systems of measurement to the most complicated algorithms (AL-guh-rih-thuhmz) for computing research data, healthcare workers use math skills every day. The following applications demonstrate a few basic ways that health informatics workers use data analysis skills and work with numbers.

Understanding Numerical Data

The healthcare industry relies on the collection and interpretation of large amounts of **data** to direct effective patient care. Data also guides the business operations of the healthcare facility. Data usually consists of a group of facts that reveal information about a specific topic. The science of **statistics** is used to analyze and interpret data. Healthcare workers handle numerical data on a daily basis and must be able to understand, analyze, and interpret this information.

Comparing the mean, median, and mode in a set of data is one method of analysis. The **mean** is the mathematical average of your data. To find it, add all of the numbers in your data set and divide by how many numbers are in that set. **Median** describes the number found exactly in the middle when your data is listed in numerical order. In an even-numbered data set, you take the mean of the middle two numbers to determine the median. **Mode** is the number that occurs most frequently in your data set. If no number occurs more often than any other, then there is no mode. There can be zero, one, or multiple modes in a data set.

data
facts about a specific topic, which are used for reference or analysis

statistics
term for the science that includes the collection, organization, and interpretation of numerical data

Using Mean, Median, and Mode: Devon

Devon is collecting data to determine the average age of clients in his physical therapy practice. He does so by recording the ages of patients he sees on a given day. On the first day, he sees seven clients whose ages are 3, 13, 15, 45, 52, 57, and 75. The average, or *mean* age of his clients on the first day is 37.

Since your interpretations rely on the data collected, your statistics may vary when you collect sets of data in different circumstances. On the second day of data collection, Devon sees five clients whose ages are 17, 45, 48, 61, and 61. On this day, the average, or *mean* age of his clients is 46.

Client Ages in PT Practice		
	Day One	**Day Two**
patient ages	3, 13, 15, 45, 52, 57, 75	17, 45, 48, 61, 61
mean	sum (260) divided by the number of clients (7) = 37	sum (232) divided by the number of clients (5) = 46
median	45	48
mode	Since there are no duplicate numbers, there is no mode.	61

If Devon sees each client once a week, how many days of data should he collect to determine the average age of his current client group? Your first thought might be to collect seven days of data since there are seven days in a week. However, what piece of information or data do you need to know before you can answer accurately?

When interpreting data, people often refer to the *average*. Usually, but not always, they are talking about the mean of a data set. However, the term *average* can be confusing. Suppose 1000 people live in your hometown and all of them earn $50,000 per year. The mean and the median of this data are both $50,000. A new resident moves into town and earns $1 billion this year. The median stays the same because the middle number is still $50,000. The mean becomes $1.04 million. However, the "average" resident is not earning more than a million dollars each year.

Average Confusion: Tracy

Tracy has several friends and family members who work in the field of nursing. As a newly graduated practical nurse, Tracy wants to figure out whether a potential job is paying an "average" wage. To do this, Tracy makes a chart of the wages earned by each of her friends and relatives.

Nursing Wages of Family and Friends	
Family member/friend	**Wage per hour**
Aunt Sue, RN	$45
Barry, CNA	$15
Darien, CNA	$15
Uncle James, NP	$55
Mom, LPN	$20
Data Analysis	
Mean	$30
Median	$20
Mode	$15

Her potential employer has told her that the average wage for a practical nurse is $15 per hour and offers to pay Tracy $13 per hour. That offer sounds reasonable, but it is $2 below the mode, $7 below the median, and $27 below the mean of the data she has collected and analyzed.

What might account for the differences in the wages of Tracy's acquaintances? Years of work experience, specialized training, or specialized skills might be influencing Tracy's data. It would be more helpful for her to compare the wages paid to nurses with abilities and years of experience similar to her own.

Tracy's next set of data compares entry-level wages for practical nurses at a variety of healthcare facilities. How does her wage offer compare to this new set of data? What additional piece of data would help you to determine whether Tracy's potential employer is offering a reasonable wage?

Entry-Level Nursing Wages	
Healthcare facility	**Hourly wage for entry-level practical nurses**
Sun View Medical Clinic	$14
Angelic Skilled Nursing Facility	$15
Pine Acres Assisted Living	$13
Merciful Care Hospice	$18
Sun View Hospital	$18
Data Analysis	
Mean	$15.60
Median	$15
Mode	$18

Read and Interpret Charts and Graphs

Charts and graphs display data visually. When constructed carefully, charts and graphs make data easier to comprehend, compare, and use. Five basic types of charts include

- a simple **table**, which arranges data in rows or columns;
- a **line graph**, which shows the changes in data over time;
- a **bar graph**, which shows comparisons between categories of data;
- a **circle graph** (pie chart), which shows the relationship of parts of a data set to the whole; and
- a **pictograph**, which presents data using images.

The elements of a chart or graph must be drawn to scale so the data is accurately represented. Using computer software makes this task much easier.

A graph has three main elements: the vertical axis (the *y-axis*), the horizontal axis (the *x-axis*), and at least one line, set of bars, circle, or image. Follow these steps to read the information in a graph or chart:

1. Read the title of the graph.
2. Read the labels and range of numbers along the side (vertical axis) and the information on the bottom (horizontal axis).
3. Determine what units the graph uses. This information can be found on the axis or in the legend. In Figure 3.23 (on the next page) for example, the y-axis uses dollars earned per year and the x-axis uses numbers of people employed.
4. Look for patterns, groups, and differences.

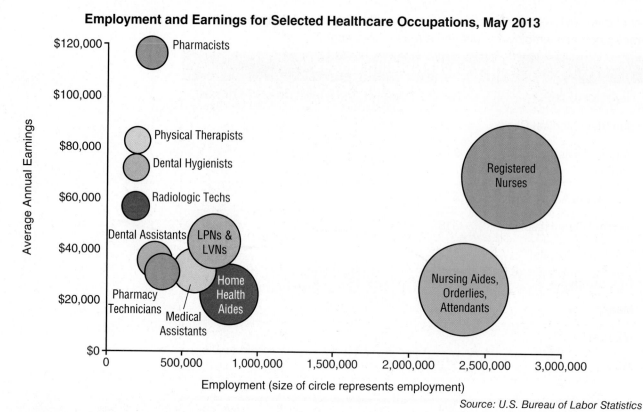

Employment and Earnings for Selected Healthcare Occupations, May 2013

Source: U.S. Bureau of Labor Statistics

Figure 3.23   This chart uses a pictograph format. The size of the bubbles provides a visual comparison of the number of people employed in a specific healthcare occupation. According to this chart, which healthcare occupation employs the most people?

For example, Figure 3.24 shows US healthcare expenditures. The graph tells us that residents of the southern and midwestern United States spend a higher percentage of their total expenses on healthcare costs than the residents in the northeastern or western states.

When displaying data, you should carefully consider which type of chart will provide the clearest visual representation of your information. Figure 3.25 shows two different ways of displaying data about the utilization of hospital beds per quarter. If you want to show which quarters have the highest utilization rates, the circle graph works better because it shows percentages of the whole. However, if you want to compare the actual utilization rates, the bar graph is the best choice because it shows the numerical value for each quarter.

Reimbursement Tasks

Health informatics workers complete several tasks that facilitate reimbursement for healthcare services. All diagnoses and procedures are given a numeric code. These codes are used when workers complete insurance claim forms so that insurance companies will pay, or *reimburse*, the provider for the services the patient received. In addition, healthcare workers collect payments directly from patients at the time of service. They must be able to handle money, give correct change, and issue receipts for payment.

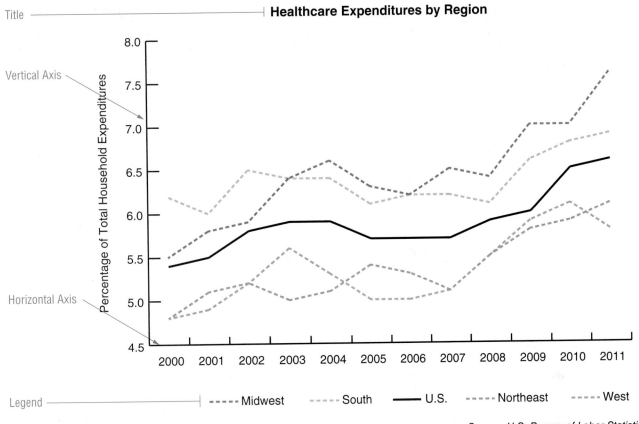

Figure 3.24   This chart uses a line graph format. Different components of a line graph include the vertical and horizontal axes and the legend.

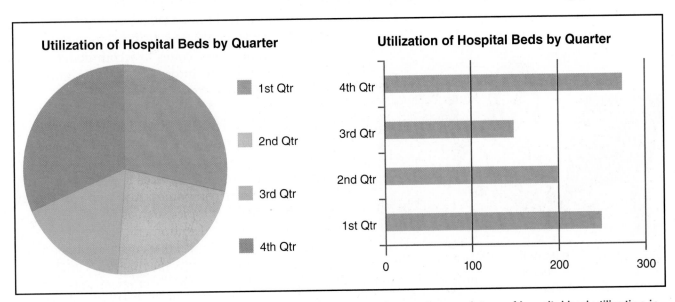

Figure 3.25   These charts display the same data. Which chart gives a clearer picture of hospital bed utilization in each quarter of the year?

Coding Diagnoses and Procedures. Medical coding is the process of translating written medical documentation into a numeric form. Coding has several purposes:

- **Reimbursement.** Codes are printed on insurance claim forms. Insurance companies reimburse the facility or the physician based on the codes for the diagnoses and the procedures or services performed.

- **Research.** Physicians access medical records using coded information. For example, a physician might request medical records for all patients who were treated for appendicitis (codes 540–543) in one hospital or all hospitals within a system. Records with those diagnosis codes could be quickly identified in a computer listing.

- **Public health.** Government public health agencies use coded diagnostic information to track the occurrence of certain diseases. For example, they may want to know the number of new cases of *pertussis* (whooping cough), code 033.0, diagnosed in a particular part of the state.

- **Patient care.** Recently, a manufacturer of an artificial hip replacement recalled its product. The manufacturer alerted surgeons who had used this product. The surgeons or hospitals then retrieved the names of patients who had undergone hip replacement surgery by searching for the procedure code 27130. The surgeons then contacted these patients to inform them of the product recall.

The World Health Organization (WHO) developed the coding system for diagnoses. Each year the Department of Health and Human Services (HHS) updates and publishes the **International Classification of Diseases Clinical Modifications (ICD-CM)**. Healthcare facilities transitioned from the ninth revision of ICD codes (ICD-9-CM) to the tenth revision (ICD-10-CM) on October 1, 2014. In the latest revision, WHO is using alphanumeric (letters and numbers) codes to accommodate more diseases and specific information. For example, appendicitis codes range from K35 to K35.9.

Each year, the American Medical Association (AMA) publishes the **Physician's Current Procedural Terminology (CPT)**. The numeric codes contained in this publication are used to report procedures and services to public and private insurance companies. Additional codes are published for other topics such as dental services, injuries, and medical equipment.

Medical coding specialists use their expertise to identify a patient's specific diagnosis and procedure from the medical record (Figure 3.26). These specialists can distinguish between the smallest of differences in codes. For example, a 27660 code indicates closed treatment of *patellar* (kneecap) dislocation without anesthesia, but a 27562 code is the same treatment *with* anesthesia. In this example, the cost would be higher for the treatment that requires

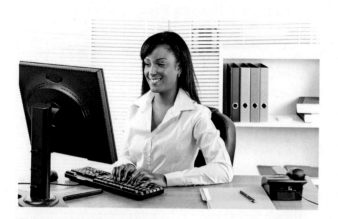

Figure 3.26   One type of health informatics worker is the medical coding specialist, who assigns a code to each diagnosis, procedure, and service listed in the medical record.

anesthesia. It is important for medical coding specialists to know these code differences because a misinterpretation of a code could mean more cost to the patient or reduced income for the provider.

Coders begin with the primary diagnosis and read for the specific details or location. The ICD codes are organized by disease or body system. This means that, when searching for appendicitis, coders begin by searching diseases of the digestive system.

Coders then move on to the specific treatments used for the primary diagnosis. This is where CPT codes are used. These codes are organized by the type of service given, such as anesthesia, surgery, radiology, or laboratory.

Errors in coding cost patients money when the insurance company denies a claim for a service that should be covered. Even bigger problems occur when a coding error causes a patient to be labeled incorrectly in an insurance database. For example, when the code for a "heart attack" is used instead of the code to "rule out a heart attack," a patient may be denied long-term care insurance or life insurance.

The complex process of accurate medical coding begins with the following steps:

- Use the latest edition of the ICD and CPT codes. Many errors result from using outdated editions.

- Always refer to the guidelines rather than relying on your memory.

- Check your codes to make sure that the diagnosis and service codes support each other. For example, coding for an appendectomy is an obvious error when the diagnosis is an ear infection.

- Never hesitate to ask the physician to clarify a code, procedure, or documentation in the medical record.

Completing an Insurance Claim Form. Insurance companies, or **third-party payers**, provide a large portion of a medical practice's income. Therefore, health informatics workers must understand the **claims process** through which the medical practice receives payment. Following a patient visit, the health informatics worker completes a claim form and submits it to the insurance carrier, which is the company through which a patient is insured (Figure 3.27 on the next page).

The top portion of a claim form lists all of the patient's identifying information along with an address, name, and ID numbers for the insurance company. If the patient is not the person who carries the insurance benefit, such as a child or spouse, the form will also show identifying information for the insured person. Because many people receive insurance benefits through an employer, the form may also ask for the name of the employer.

Adult patients sign the claim form, granting permission to release their medical information to the insurance company. The person carrying the insurance also signs the form, allowing payments to be made directly to the medical office. This process is called the **assignment of benefits**. Most offices have new patients sign a release form when they complete registration materials; then the office can simply type in the words *Signature on File* when submitting claims. This can also be used for the physician's signature.

claims process
the procedures for submitting costs for medical services so that payment can be collected or denial can be determined

HEALTH INSURANCE CLAIM FORM
APPROVED BY NATIONAL UNIFORM CLAIM COMMITTEE (NUCC) 02/12

☐☐☐ PICA   PICA ☐☐☐

| 1. MEDICARE ☐ (Medicare#) | MEDICADE ☐ (Medicade#) | TRICARE ☐ (ID#/DoD#) | CHAMPVA ☐ (Member ID#) | GROUP HEALTH PLAN X (ID#) | FECA BLK LUNG ☐ (ID#) | OTHER ☐ (ID#) | 1a. INSURED'S ID NUMBER   (For program in Item 1)   **03654** |

2. PATIENT'S NAME (Last Name, First Name, Middle Initial)
Brown, Kathleen J.

3. PATIENT'S BIRTH DATE   SEX
MM **06** DD **29** YY **1970**   M ☐   F **X**

4. INSURED'S NAME (Last Name, First Name, Middle Initial)
Brown, Kathleen J.

5. PATIENT'S ADDRESS (No., Street)
400 South Main St.

6. PATIENT RELATIONSHIP TO INSURED
Self **X**   Spouse ☐   Child ☐   Other ☐

7. INSURED'S ADDRESS (No., Street)

CITY **Star Prairie**   STATE **TX**

8. RESERVED FOR NUCC USE

CITY   STATE

ZIP CODE **74260**   TELEPHONE (Include Area Code) **(123) 701-0197**

ZIP CODE   TELEPHONE (Include Area Code) ( )

9. OTHER INSURED'S NAME (Last Name, First Name, Middle Initial)

10. IS PATIENT'S CONDITION RELATED TO:

11. INSURED'S POLICY GROUP OR FECA NUMBER
06172

a. OTHER INSURED'S POLICY OR GROUP NUMBER

a. EMPLOYMENT? (Current or Previous)
☐ YES **X** NO

a. INSURED'S DATE OF BIRTH   SEX
MM   DD   YY   M ☐   F ☐

b. RESERVED FOR NUCC USE

b. AUTO ACCIDENT?   PLACE (state)
☐ YES **X** NO

B. OTHER CLAIM ID (Designated by NUCC)

c. RESERVED FOR NUCC USE

c. OTHER ACCIDENT?
☐ YES **X** NO

C. INSURANCE PLAN NAME OR PROGRAM NAME
DC Health Plan

d. INSURANCE PLAN NAME OR PROGRAM NAME

10d. CLAIM CODES (Designated by NUCC)

d. IS THERE ANOTHER HEALTH BENEFIT PLAN?
☐ YES **X** NO   *If yes*, complete items 9, 9a, and 9d.

READ BACK OF FORM BEFORE COMPLETING & SIGNING THIS FORM.
12. PATIENT'S OR AUTHORIZED PERSON'S SIGNATURE I authorize the release of any medical or other information necessary to process this claim. I also request payment of government benefits either to myself or to the party who accepts assignment below.

SIGNED **Signature on File**   DATE **11/12/2015**

13. INSURED'S OR AUTHORIZED PERSON'S SIGNATURE I authorize payment of medical benefits to the undersigned physician or supplier for services described below.

SIGNED **Signature on File**

14. DATE OF CURRENT ILLNESS, INJURY, OR PREGNANCY (LMP)
07 30 2015 QUAL.

15. OTHER DATE
QUAL.   MM DD YY

16. DATES PATIENT UNABLE TO WORK IN CURRENT OCCUPATION
FROM MM DD YY TO MM DD YY

17. NAME OF REFERRING PROVIDER OR OTHER SOURCE

17a.
17b. NPI

18. HOSPITALIZATION DATES RELATED TO CURRENT SERVICES
FROM MM DD YY TO MM DD YY

19. ADDITIONAL CLAIM INFORMATION (Designated by NUCC)

20. OUTSIDE LAB? $ CHARGES
☐ YES ☐ NO

21. DIAGNOSIS OR NATURE OF ILLNESS OR INJURY Relate A-L to service line below (24E)   ICD ind.

A. **845.03**   B. **250.00**   C.   D.
E.   F.   G.   H.
I.   J.   K.   L.

22. RESUBMISSION CODE   ORIGINAL REF. NO.

23. PRIOR AUTHORIZATION NUMBER

24. A. DATE(S) OF SERVICE FROM MM DD YY	TO MM DD YY	B. PLACE OF SERVICE	C. EMG	D. PROCEDURES, SERVICES, OR SUPPLIES (Explain Unusual Circumstances) CPT/HCPCS MODIFIER	E. DIAGNOSIS POINTER	F. $ CHARGES	G. DAYS OR UNITS	H. EPSDT Family Plan	I. ID. QUAL.	J. RENDERING PROVIDER ID. #
1	07 30 15	07 30 15	11		99213	1	200 00	1		NPI	
2	07 30 15	07 30 15	11		82947	2	50 00	1		NPI	
3										NPI	
4										NPI	
5										NPI	
6										NPI	

25. FEDERAL TAX I.D. NUMBER   SSN ☐ EIN **X**
54-0000000

26. PATIENTS ACCOUNT NO.
0346

27. ACCEPT ASSIGNMENT?
X YES ☐ NO

28. TOTAL CHARGE
$ **250 00**

29. AMOUNT PAID
$

30. Rvsd for NUCC Use

31. SIGNATURE OF PHYSICIAN OR SUPPLIER INCLUDING DEGRESS OR CREDENTIALS
(I certify that the statements on the reverse apply to this bill and are made a part thereof.)

SIGNED **Signature on File**   DATE 11/12/2015

32. SERVICE FACILITY LOCATION INFORMATION
**Sun View Medical
250 Brighter Lane**
a.   b.

33. BILLING PROVIDER INFO & PH#
**Sandra Black, MD
Star Prairie, TX 74260
(123) 701-3524**
a.   b.

NUCC Instruction Manual available at www.nucc.org   **PLEASE PRINT OR TYPE**   APPROVED OMB-0938-0999 FORM CMS-1500 (08-05)

CARRIER   *PATIENT AND INSURED INFORMATION*   *PHYSICIAN OR SUPPLIER INFORMATION*

Figure 3.27   Health informatics workers fill out claim forms like this one so that facilities can be paid for services rendered.

Simulate EHR

The bottom portion of the claim form lists the identifying and contact information for the provider and healthcare facility. The dates of service and specific ICD and CPT codes for diagnosis and treatment are also listed. You may see a number in the *Place of Service* column. Different facilities have different numbers, so 01 indicates a pharmacy, 11 is a medical office, and 21 is a hospital. In addition, charges for each service, as well as a total charge and balance due from the insurance company, are listed.

When the *Accept Assignment* section is marked *yes*, the provider will accept an agreed upon amount as full payment. The costs of each service depend on the provider's contract with a particular insurance company. When the *Accept Assignment* section is marked *no*, the provider is free to charge any amount for services. If the charged amount is higher than the *insurance allowed amount* (the amount that will be paid by the insurance company), the patient must pay the difference.

Accuracy of claims directly affects income for a medical practice. When a claim is returned because of incomplete or incorrect information, the claim must be resubmitted and payment is delayed for several weeks. Taking the time to verify insurance coverage and to double-check for accuracy before sending a claim will save time and money that may have gone toward a correction (Figure 3.28).

The electronic health record speeds up the claims process considerably. Software programs can extract required data from the patient's record and transfer it to the claim form. Electronic signatures complete the process, and the forms are submitted electronically.

When the claims administrator settles a claim, the medical provider and the patient receive an **explanation of benefits (EOB)**. This report shows what, if anything, the insurance company is paying for; what it is not paying for; and why. The small numbers in the *Remarks* column align with a list of explanations. Always look at the bottom of the report to see the explanation of the charge (Figure 3.29 on the next page).

On an EOB, the words *amount allowed* and *network savings* mean that the medical provider has a contract with the insurance company. Under this contract, the medical provider agrees to accept the insurance payment as full payment for a given service, even if the provider normally charges more for the particular service. This reduces costs for insurance companies and brings new patients to providers who have contracts with the patient's insurance company.

The EOB is *not* a bill, but it does include information about deductibles and coinsurance as they apply to the claim. Patients should review services, dates of services, and charges for services on each EOB to make sure this information is accurate. When claims are denied or payment is delayed, patients can contact the insurance company to get answers to their questions.

After the claims process has been completed, the medical provider is ready to bill the patient for any amount unpaid by the insurance company.

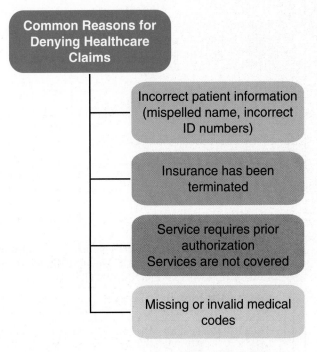

Common Reasons for Denying Healthcare Claims

- Incorrect patient information (mispelled name, incorrect ID numbers)
- Insurance has been terminated
- Service requires prior authorization Services are not covered
- Missing or invalid medical codes

Figure 3.28   These reasons for denying healthcare claims could be prevented by double-checking for accuracy.

explanation of benefits (EOB)
a detailed account of each claim processed by an insurance plan, which is sent to the patient as notification of claim payment or denial

1600 Allen Blvd
Washington, DC 65432

Forwarding Service Requested

RITA JAMES
1234 ANYPLACE DRIVE   ①
STAR PRAIRIE, TX 74260

②

	7/20/2015
Patient Name:	RITA JAMES
Group Number:	06172
Claim Number:	102345678910 DENTAL
Patient ID Number:	03654

EXPLANATION OF BENEFITS

Below is an explanation of your benefits with DC Health Plan.   **THIS IS NOT A BILL** ③
Please do not send money to DC Health Plan. Send any money owed to the provider of service.
④ PROVIDER NAME: **SV ENDODONTRICS**

Code	Description of Service	Date	Amount Charged	Amount Allowed	Deductible	Copay/ Coinsurance	Remark	Amount Paid
3330-03	Root canal	6/20/15	$1,105.00	$1,066.32		$213.27	45 02	$853.05
⑤	⑥	⑦	⑧	⑨	⑩	⑪	⑫	⑬

⑬   ⑭
Amount Paid by Plan: **$853.05**   Member Responsibility: **$251.95**

Remark Explanation(s):   ⑫
45—Charge exceeds maximum allowable fee.
02—Coinsurance amount. Your 20% coinsurance is $213.27.

If you are covered by more than one health benefit plan, you should file all your claims with each plan.
If you have any questions about this claim, please call your Customer Service Team at (123) 456-7890 or 1-800-123-4567,
or contact us at www.dchealthplans.org. Please see your member handbook or contract for claim appeal procedures. ⑮

>>PLEASE KEEP A COPY OF THIS DOCUMENT FOR YOUR RECORDS<<

1. name of the main subscriber for your health insurance policy
2. summary of patient information
3. the EOB is **not** a bill or request of payment
4. the name of the provider or facility that provided healthcare services
5. medical code for the service or procedure required
6. general description of the services you requested
7. the date on which you received this healthcare service
8. the amount your provider has billed your health insurance for each service

9. the amount that your health insurance allows for each service billed
10. the amount applied to your deductible
11. the copay or coinsurance amount you must pay after your deductible is applied
12. additional messages that may explain how your claim was processed
13. the amount your health insurance will pay the provider for services you received
14. the amount you owe the provider. Your provider will bill you separately
15. information on how to contact Customer Service

Figure 3.29   This EOB shows that the patient pays 20% of the total bill according to her insurance plan coverage. However, because the provider does not have a fee agreement with the health insurance plan, the provider has charged more than the amount allowed by the insurance plan. As a result, the patient owes $251.95 instead of $213.27.

A statement mailed to patients shows how much the physician's office billed the insurance company and how much the insurance company paid (Figure 3.30). After the insurance company's payment is deducted from the total cost for services, the patient pays the balance.

Receiving and Recording Office Payments. Medical providers often require copayments, or **copays**, before the patient sees the physician. They also have payment policies for individuals who do not have insurance coverage. The provider policy is typically displayed at the reception desk (Figure 3.31 on the next page) and may be explained in a brochure or on the provider's website. Medical assistants must be prepared to collect these payments at the patient registration desk and issue a receipt.

Patients pay at the time of service in one of three ways—cash, check, or credit or debit card. There are important procedures to remember for each of these three ways.

- **Cash.** Secure the cash in a locked drawer and provide a printed receipt showing cash payment.

- **Check.** Get two forms of identification from new patients. Do not accept a third-party check unless it is from an insurance company. Inspect the check for the correct date, amount, and signature.

copay
an out-of-pocket fee paid by a person with health insurance at the time a covered service, such as an office visit or a prescription, is received

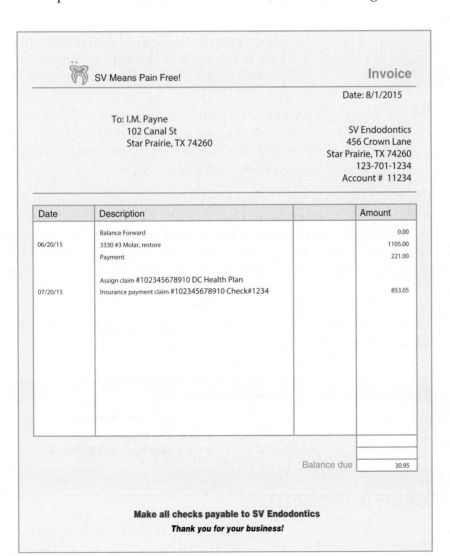

Figure 3.30 This invoice shows how much the patient owes after the insurance company has paid its share.

Invoice content:

SV Means Pain Free!   **Invoice**

Date: 8/1/2015

To: I.M. Payne
102 Canal St
Star Prairie, TX 74260

SV Endodontics
456 Crown Lane
Star Prairie, TX 74260
123-701-1234
Account # 11234

Date	Description		Amount
	Balance Forward		0.00
06/20/15	3330 #3 Molar, restore		1105.00
	Payment		221.00
	Assign claim #102345678910 DC Health Plan		
07/20/15	Insurance payment claim #102345678910 Check#1234		853.05

Balance due   30.95

Make all checks payable to SV Endodontics
Thank you for your business!

Figure 3.31 A placard such as this one would usually be displayed at the reception desk.

At your office visit today, you will be asked to:

- Pay your insurance copay.
- Pay a $100.00 deposit if you do not have insurance coverage.

(cash, check, debit card, or credit card accepted)

Sun View Medical   www.sunviewmed.com/policies

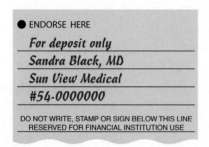

Figure 3.32 This check has been endorsed properly.

Endorse the check with a stamp that says *for deposit only* (Figure 3.32). Provide a printed receipt showing payment by check.

- **Credit or debit card.** This is a more secure form of payment, but it requires the provider to pay a fee to the credit card company. Provide a printed receipt showing a credit payment.

All receipts should list the name of the medical provider, the name and account number of the person paying, the current date, the amount of the payment, the purpose for the payment, and the form of payment (Figure 3.33).

Completing a Bank Deposit. Keep a record of each payment, either in a log with a copy of each receipt or in a computer file. Post the payments to the patients' accounts. Double-check to make sure you are posting the correct amount to the right account. At the end of each day, you will tally the payments received and prepare a bank deposit of the checks and cash received. Follow these steps to prepare a bank deposit:

1. Separate checks and cash. Make sure each check is endorsed.
2. Organize the bills by grouping $1s, $5s, $10s, and $20s together, all facing the same direction.

Figure 3.33 A receipt will be given to a patient after he or she has paid for services.

Simulate
EHR

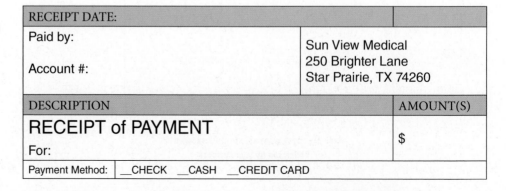

3. Count the cash and record the total amount on the **deposit slip** (Figure 3.34).

4. List each check separately with the name of the patient and the amount of the check.

5. Total the amount of cash and checks. Enter this number on the deposit slip. Make a copy of the deposit slip for the office records.

6. Place the cash, checks, and deposit slip in an envelope to take to the bank. Be sure to get a deposit receipt from the teller.

7. Enter the date and the amount of the deposit in the office checking account register.

The payments collected in a healthcare facility account for a significant portion of a medical provider's income. Follow your facility's payment policies, and use professional business practices when you receive and deposit payments.

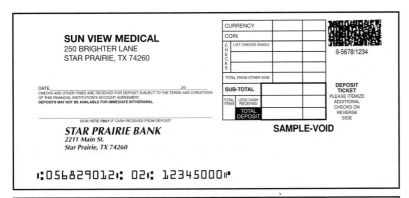

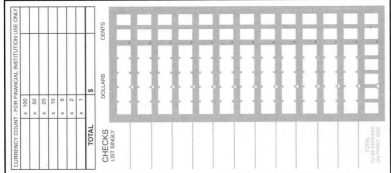

Figure 3.34   A sample deposit slip. Record multiple checks on the back of the slip and transfer total amounts to the front.

RECALL YOUR READING

1. Healthcare workers need skills for analyzing and interpreting the _____ they encounter on the job.

2. Data analysis begins by comparing the _____, _____, and _____.

3. Data is easier to understand when displayed in a _____ or _____.

4. _____ changes written medical documentation into numeric form.

5. Healthcare workers complete insurance _____ forms so that the insurance company can reimburse the provider.

6. _____ are often required before the patient sees the physician.

Complete the *Map Your Reading* graphic organizer for the section you just read.

Chapter 3 Review

SUMMARY

Assess your understanding with chapter tests

- Understanding is the key element in communication.

- While the sender initiates the communication process, the receiver provides feedback to close the communication loop.

- Listening is the most neglected communication skill.

- A medical record documents the medical care received by a patient.

- Compliance with medical documentation guidelines provides reimbursement of provider costs and reduces claim denials.

- All telephone communication with patients is documented in their medical records.

- Health literacy involves understanding information about your own health so that you know how to take care of yourself and can make good decisions about your health.

- Improvements in security, development of mobile technologies, and government-sponsored financial incentives are speeding the adoption of electronic records systems.

- E-mail communication in a healthcare setting follows the rules of business communication because it may become part of the legal record of patient care.

- A confidentiality statement is legally required to be included in every outgoing e-mail or fax communication.

- Healthcare workers handle numerical data on a daily basis and must be able to understand, analyze, and interpret this information.

- Charts and graphs display data visually and make it easier to comprehend, compare, and use.

- Medical coding is the process of translating written medical documentation into a numeric form.

- Medical assistants collect patient copays and issue receipts at the time of service.

MAXIMIZE YOUR PROFESSIONAL VOCABULARY

Build vocabulary with e-flash cards, games, and audio glossary

Listed below are the essential, yellow-highlighted terms and the additional professional vocabulary terms that you encountered in this chapter. Complete the activities that follow the list to make all of these terms part of your everyday professional vocabulary.

assessment
assignment of benefits
bar graph
body language
charting
circle graph
claims process
clinical data
communication
compliance
computerized patient record
continuity of care record (CCR)
copay
data
deposit slip

electronic health record (EHR)
electronic medical record (EMR)
etiquette
explanation of benefits (EOB)
facsimile machine
feedback
health literacy
International Classification of Diseases Clinical Modifications (ICD-CM)
line graph
mean
median
medical documentation

medical record
mode
Physician's Current Procedural Terminology (CPT)
pictograph
problem-oriented medical record (POMR)
proprietary
protocol
source-oriented medical record (SOMR)
statistics
table
third-party payer
triage

VOCABULARY DEVELOPMENT

Matching. Match each essential term from this chapter with the correct definition below by writing the letter of the definition next to the number of the essential term on a separate sheet of paper.

1. explanation of benefits (EOB)
2. claims process
3. triage
4. communication
5. health literacy
6. body language
7. etiquette
8. medical record
9. data
10. electronic health record (EHR)
11. copay
12. medical documentation

a. facts about a specific topic, which are used for reference or analysis
b. written reports of observable, measurable, and reproducible findings from examinations, supporting laboratory or diagnostic tests, and assessments of a patient
c. the act of sharing a message, thought, or idea so that it is accurately received and understood
d. the procedures for submitting costs for medical services so that payment can be collected or denial can be determined
e. term for a code of polite behavior among members of a profession or group
f. an evaluation process in which a group of patients is sorted according to the urgency of their need for care
g. nonverbal communication that occurs through conscious or unconscious gestures and movements
h. an out-of-pocket fee paid by a person with health insurance at the time a covered service, such as an office visit or prescription, is received
i. a medical document that contains information from all of the clinicians involved in a patient's care and which can be created and managed by authorized clinicians and staff across more than one healthcare organization
j. a person's ability to obtain and understand health-related information and make informed decisions using that information
k. a detailed account of each claim processed by an insurance plan, which is sent to the patient as notification of claim payment or denial
l. a file that contains documents that describe a specific patient's medical history and medical care within one healthcare organization; also known as a *chart* or *file*

13. **Pictionary Terms Review.** Work with a partner to illustrate the essential terms from this chapter. One person will select a term and sketch until his or her partner guesses the correct term from the illustration. Then you and your partner will switch roles and continue until all the essential terms have been used.

14. **Defend a Term.** Draw two columns on a blank sheet of paper. Write *Reimbursement* at the top of one column and *Medical Record* at the top of the second column. Under *Reimbursement*, list all the terms from this chapter that are related to providers receiving payment. Under *Medical Record*, list all the terms related to developing and maintaining a patient's chart. Be prepared to defend your additions to each list.

REFLECT ON YOUR READING

15. Consider your last visit to a healthcare facility. Select one example of changing communication technology from your experience or from the chapter. How might this communication influence the field of healthcare and the quality of patient care? List both positive and negative effects of the change.

BUILD CORE SKILLS

16. **Critical Thinking.** List three of the skills for effective listening described in the text. Rate yourself on each skill and provide an example to explain your rating.

17. **Critical Thinking.** Use the Internet to find photos of people expressing various emotions. Can you correctly identify the emotion shown in each photo by evaluating the person's nonverbal communication? Print three of the photos you selected and bring them to class. Ask your classmates to identify the emotion in each photo. Then discuss your responses.

18. **Writing.** Review the following chart entry. Then rewrite the entry using the guidelines for documentation explained on page 81.

12/16/15	1230	This crabby patient didn't eat any of her ~~breakfast~~ lunch.
12/16/15	1500	She is such a complainer—like her ankle is always hurting!
		Her vital signs are OK
		Susie Smith

19. **Speaking and Listening.** Review the following phone conversation and identify errors made by the speaker.

"Hi! Who do want to talk to? What's your problem? Say that again. Like, Dr. Jeffers won't be in till, like, tomorrow. What's your name? You'll have to come in then. Bye."

20. **Problem Solving.** Screen and triage the following list of phone calls in order of importance. Use numbers to indicate the level of importance of each phone call. Number one is most urgent and number four is least urgent.

- A mother calls to say her 4-year-old has a stomachache, but no fever.
- A man calls to say he has tightness in his chest and pain down his arm.
- A father calls to say his daughter was stung by a bee and her hand is beginning to swell.
- An elderly, crying woman calls saying that her husband fell in the bathroom and is slurring his words.

21. **Speaking and Listening.** Record a telephone conversation using the script given here. Then listen to the recording and evaluate your tone of voice. How clear and distinct is your speech?

Good afternoon, this is Sun View Medical (name) speaking. What can I do for you today? (Patient shares symptoms and indicates the need for a doctor's appointment.)

We can set up an appointment for you. Which day of the week works best for you? (Pause) I have a 10:00 a.m. or a 2:00 p.m. appointment available. What time works best for you? (Pause) Very good! Is there anything else I can do for you today? (Patient says no.)

Well, thank you for calling. We have your appointment set up for next Thursday, the 22nd, at 2:00 p.m. We will see you then.

22. **Writing.** Complete a phone message form after reading the following conversation. Use the phone message form from Figure 3.13 for reference.

The call comes in on today's date at 10:30 a.m.

Sally: Good morning! Better Medical Clinic, Dr. Seelas' office. This is his receptionist, Sally. May I help you?

Caller: I'd like to schedule an appointment to have my stitches taken out. But I need to talk to Dr. Seelas first.

Sally: To whom am I speaking?

Caller: Carl Turner.

Sally: What is the phone number you can be reached at?

Carl: (824) 762-1400

Sally: What is the best time to have him return your call?

Carl: Anytime today is good for me.

Sally: I will give him this message and Dr. Seelas should be able to call you this afternoon. Thank you, Carl!

23. **Reading.** Explain what is meant by "reading with a purpose." Then list three healthcare documents and give a possible purpose for their reading.

24. **Problem Solving.** Explain how the terms *proprietary* and *interoperability* relate to the implementation of the electronic health record.

25. **Math.** Better Medical Clinic is comparing the number of morning and afternoon medical appointments to adjust staffing. Read the data for each day on the next page. For each set of data, find the mean, median, and mode.

- Morning: 17, 30, 25, 35, 28
- Afternoon: 13, 20, 20, 25, 10

Consider what you learned about scheduling in chapter 2. Suggest a factor other than the number of appointments that will affect staffing.

26. **Math.** Create a chart or graph that compares estimated figures of rates for newly diagnosed cases of cancer in different states. Find a partner, share your data results, and discuss how your chart compares with your partner's chart. Explain why you used a certain method to display the data.

- MT: 5,550
- WI: 31,920
- CA: 165,810
- VT: 4,060
- TX: 110,470
- KY: 25,160
- NV: 13,780
- MS: 15,190

ACTIVATE YOUR LEARNING

27. Complete a copay receipt for your patient, Charles Kilgore, using the form from Figure 3.33 and the following information. Today, Charles Kilgore paid a $10 copayment for his doctor examination. He paid with check number 1407 to his account 87346.

28. Complete a deposit slip for the following group of payments using the form from Figure 3.34.

    Cash collected: $20, $15, $10, $5, $30

    Checks collected: $100 (Kerry Shaw), $10 (Joe Bradley), $50 (Jennifer Jones), $20 (Gary Lister)

29. Write a business e-mail using the following information and the correct format, as shown in Figure 3.20. The e-mail should be written on today's date to Greg Forenzo, MD, from Juanita Huerta, MA, regarding a staff meeting scheduled for next Tuesday to discuss safety precautions and confidentiality concerns within the department.

30. Prepare a fax cover sheet using the following information and Figure 3.22 as a reference. Use today's date and the current time. The four-page report that is being sent contains the lab results of Chris O'Connor's blood work. These results are being sent to Dr. John Krena (fax number 472-617-8379) from lab tech Sarah Westly (fax number 472-617-2424). Sarah is requesting to meet with Dr. Krena after he reads the results.

THINK AND ACT LIKE A HEALTHCARE WORKER

31. For each of the following circumstances, decide what is wrong with the situation or how a healthcare worker should react to the situation. Apply the principles of effective communication that you learned in this chapter.

- A doctor says, "I think your problem is cholelithiasis."
- The healthcare worker speaks in a very soft voice.
- The clinic receptionist says to a patient, "I don't got any appointments at that time."
- The healthcare worker interrupts the patient before he or she is finished speaking.
- A patient with limited English nods his head, but still seems confused as the healthcare worker explains a procedure.

GO TO THE SOURCE

32. Refer to the example in Figure 3.27 and use the following information to complete a health insurance claim form found on the companion website. Use the Internet to find the correct medical coding for this diagnosis and determine realistic charges for these services.

A male patient named Robert Blake first went to his doctor, Roy Blanchard, at Better Medical Clinic on January 10, 2015 for an office visit. Robert had a unilateral chest X-ray, which revealed a broken rib due to a car accident on January 8, 2015. There was a follow-up office visit on March 15, 2015. Robert lives at 2400 East Highland Drive, Boland, MN 84672. His phone number is (840) 672-3456. His wife, Shelly, drove him to the clinic. She does not work outside the home. Robert is insured with a signature on file through the Benefit Health Plan, group number 02635. The insurer's I.D. number is 04635. Robert was born November 11, 1984. The patient account number is 0429 with an accepted assignment federal tax I.D. number 38-0000.000. The billing provider's phone number is (426) 814-7639. Robert did not pay for any services yet.

Chapter 4
Professional Knowledge in Health Informatics

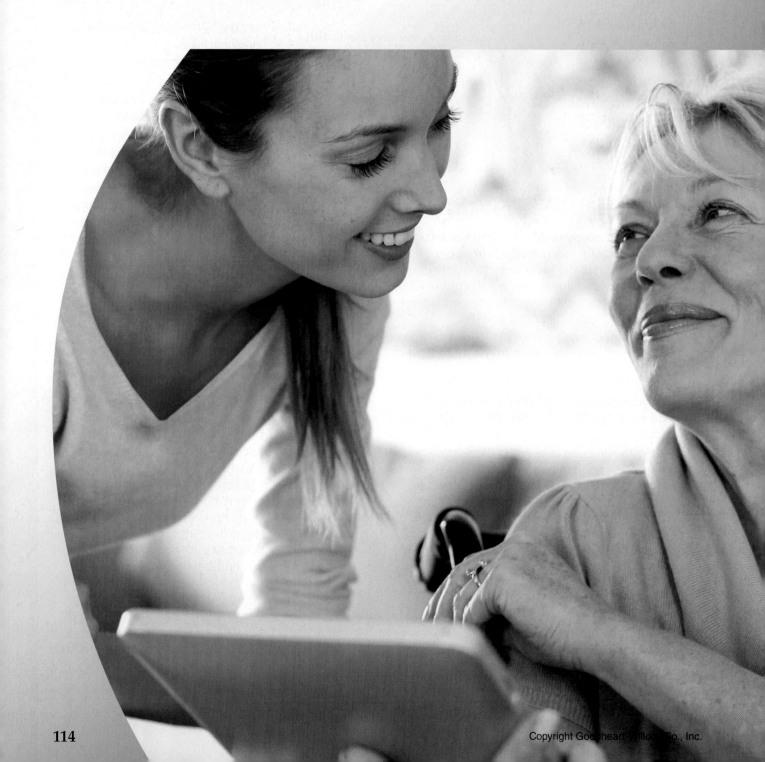

PROFESSIONAL VOCABULARY

 E-flash Cards

You will need to learn the essential terms listed below before you begin your reading. These terms will help you understand the main concepts of the chapter. These terms, which will be highlighted in yellow within the text, will become part of your professional vocabulary.

In addition to these essential terms, you will see bold terms throughout the chapter. The meanings of these terms are explained where the terms first appear. The bold terms, like the essential terms listed here, will become part of your professional vocabulary and deepen your understanding of the topics presented.

advance directive a legal document prepared by a patient before a health crisis occurs to guide healthcare decisions in situations when the patient is unable to speak for himself or herself

civil law the branch of law that establishes rules for business relationships between people or between individuals and businesses

contract a legally binding agreement between two or more people or agencies

criminal law the branch of law that aims to protect individuals and society by defining certain actions as crimes, or offenses against society

ethical a term used to describe an action that fits with someone's personal morals or professional rules of conduct

Health Insurance Portability and Accountability Act (HIPAA) a federal law that makes it easier to obtain healthcare coverage and protects personal health information

legal disability a condition that results in a person being unable to enter a contract, such as being under the age of consent, being ruled mentally incompetent, or having an altered mental state due to drugs or semi-consciousness

managed care a system that limits access to and use of healthcare to control costs

protected health information (PHI) all individually identifiable personal information obtained through healthcare

registration placement on an official list, or registry, of qualified workers

system an organized structure composed of many parts that work together and depend on each other to carry out a set of functions

tort an action that harms another person's body or property or takes away his or her freedom of action in some way

CONNECT WITH YOUR READING

Who is responsible for your healthcare? Consider that question as you read the following scenario.

Mr. Stake was dead on arrival at the hospital Monday morning. He had been complaining that he didn't feel like his usual self since he had lost his job. The previous Friday, he had paid out-of-pocket to see a general practitioner, who had recommended a stress test and referred him to a cardiologist.

Mr. Stake didn't have insurance and couldn't afford to see the cardiologist. The health information technician at the clinic said he didn't qualify for free care because his wife worked part-time. Mr. Stake wanted to research other payment options, so he scheduled the stress test for the following Friday, when he would again be able to use the car he and his wife shared.

Once he was home, Mr. Stake called the Public Health Department to ask about receiving financial assistance for his care, but they could only provide funds for blood tests and immunizations. On Sunday, he had chest pains and called the urgent care facility that was closest to his rural home. No one answered, however, because the urgent care facility had cut back their weekend hours to save money. Early the next morning, Mr. Stake set out on the long drive to the hospital in the nearest town, but he had a heart attack on the way and skidded off the road. By the time the paramedics arrived, Mr. Stake couldn't be saved.

Who or what is responsible for Mr. Stake's death? What legal and ethical issues are involved in this situation? What parts of the healthcare system have failed Mr. Stake? As you read this chapter, look for additional information to support or reject your answers.

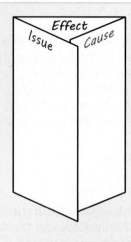

MAP YOUR READING

Use a sheet of paper to create a tri-fold visual summary. Divide the paper into thirds. Fold the right third of the paper in, then the left third. The results will look like a brochure. Once you have created this visual summary, write *Issue* at the top edge of one outside flap, *Cause* at the top of the other outside flap, and *Effect* at the top of the inside flap. As you read this chapter, identify at least one healthcare issue in each section that would be important for a health informatics worker to understand. List important points on each of the three flaps for the issues you identify. Use the following as an example:

Issue: What happens if a health informatics worker reveals private patient information to an unauthorized person?

Cause: The worker may not know the law or chose not to follow the law.

Effect: The healthcare worker could be reprimanded or lose his or her job; the patient could lose trust in his or her care provider and choose not to share important information in the future.

Think back to a time when you were inside a healthcare facility. Do you remember the different types of workers who were there? How did they all seem to fit together? Would you say that they were part of a larger system? How do you imagine this system works?

In this chapter, you will be introduced to systems theory and some of the ways it applies to healthcare provider and payment systems. Legal and ethical issues that affect these systems will also be explained. As you read, you will consider how systems theory and legal and ethical issues affect health informatics workers. In future chapters, you will see how these topics also apply to therapeutic, diagnostic, environmental, and biotechnology research and development careers.

Healthcare Delivery and Payment Systems

system
an organized structure composed of many parts that work together and depend on each other to carry out a set of functions

Today's complex, technological world is composed of many **systems**. Cell phone users rely on a system of cell towers to connect to friends. Drivers use a global positioning system of satellites to find out how to get from their homes to a new restaurant. The US educational system is organized by state and local governments to prepare individuals for future careers and participation in society. Every new problem or situation you encounter occurs within a larger system.

Two major systems are involved in American healthcare. One is the healthcare provider system. The other is the healthcare payment system. Before examining these two systems, however, this chapter will explain systems theory. This field of study examines the parts of a system and how they interact. Analyzing complex systems helps us understand them more easily.

Systems Theory

A system achieves its goals by maintaining a balance of its many parts. Each system is made up of five factors: input, throughput, output, feedback loop, and environment (Figure 4.1).

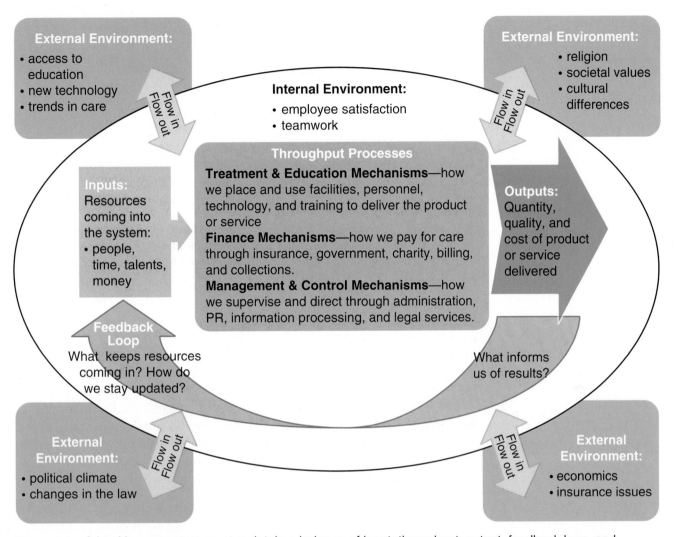

Figure 4.1 A healthcare system must maintain a balance of input, throughput, output, feedback loop, and environment. **How do health informatics workers contribute to throughput?**

- **Input** includes the population being served and why they need or want service through this system. Inputs also include the resources the system needs to function, such as workers, equipment, and financial resources. In the healthcare system, inputs are patients, healthcare workers, and diagnostic or treatment equipment.

- **Throughput** refers to how the system processes or uses the inputs. Patient care, staff management, and educational mechanisms are important throughputs for the healthcare system.

- **Output** refers to the results produced by the system's functioning. In healthcare, outputs include treated patients, costs, and gains in knowledge and information.

- The **feedback loop** involves responses to the functions that are used to keep the system going. What can be done differently to provide greater satisfaction? What will bring customers and resources back into the system?

- Finally, every system is affected by its **environment**. Internal environment factors, such as employee satisfaction, teamwork, equipment maintenance, and good fiscal management keep the system healthy. Changes in the external environment also affect the system. A change in resources, shift in demographics, creation of new laws, or development of new technology can have a huge impact on a healthcare system.

The five factors that make up systems theory can be used to analyze various systems. The parts of a system work together in a balanced way toward a common purpose. Analyzing a system and the relationship among its parts can help to anticipate and solve problems. Systems analysis can also be used to improve outcomes, reduce costs, or evaluate how the actions of participants contribute to achieving a system's goal or delay achieving it.

Healthcare Provider Systems

The healthcare provider system is a mix of individuals and institutions that deliver healthcare to patients, residents, or clients. Healthcare is one of the largest industries in the United States. Healthcare facilities provide services ranging from medication and consultations to surgery and around-the-clock care. These facilities include hospitals, long-term care facilities, doctor's offices, clinics, laboratories, emergency medical services, home health agencies, behavioral health organizations, rehabilitation services, and hospices. Healthcare facilities range in size from private offices to national organizations and provide preventive, curative, and rehabilitative services (Figure 4.2). These healthcare provider systems vary widely in their input, throughput, and output. They are also strongly impacted by the external environment in which they operate.

Government and Nonprofit Participants. Government agencies provide much of the research and regulation in the healthcare industry. For example, the **World Health Organization (WHO)** is an agency of the United Nations that is concerned with international public health. WHO monitors disease epidemics such as AIDS, provides assistance to people affected by disasters like earthquakes, and sets international standards such as water quality for safe drinking.

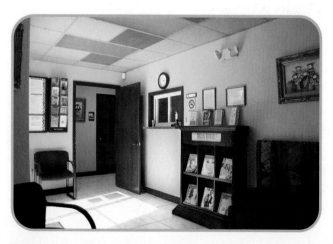 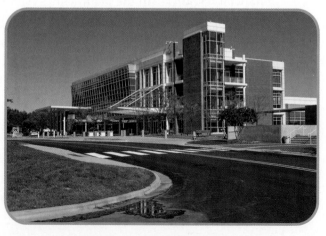

Figure 4.2   All healthcare facilities, whether one small office or a giant complex, can be described through systems theory.

In the United States, the **Department of Health and Human Services (HHS)** has 11 divisions that oversee many programs focused on improving the health of Americans. These programs include the following:

- *The Administration for Children and Families (ACF)* works to improve the well-being of children, families, and communities.

- *The Administration for Community Living (ACL)* provides older Americans and people with disabilities access to community support systems that allow them to live productive and satisfying lives.

- *The Agency for Healthcare Research and Quality (AHRQ)* carries out research aimed at improving the safety, quality, and efficiency of healthcare.

- *The Agency for Toxic Substances and Disease Registry (ATSDR)* protects Americans from exposure to hazardous substances in the environment, waste sites, and chemical spills.

- The **Centers for Disease Control and Prevention (CDC)** focuses on disease outbreaks and prevention in the United States.

- The **Centers for Medicare & Medicaid Services (CMS)** provides health insurance for 100 million Americans under the Medicare program for the elderly and the Medicaid program for the poor.

- *The Food and Drug Administration (FDA)* regulates medical products, tobacco, foods, dietary supplements, and cosmetics, as well as electronic devices that create radiation.

- *The Health Resources and Services Administration (HRSA)* oversees organ donations and focuses on improving access to healthcare services for people who are uninsured, isolated, or medically vulnerable.

- *The Indian Health Service (IHS)* focuses on providing access to comprehensive and culturally acceptable healthcare for Native Americans and Alaska Natives.

- The **National Institutes of Health (NIH)** conducts research and provides information toward improving public health through 27 different agencies.

- *The Substance Abuse & Mental Health Services Administration (SAMHSA)* works to reduce the impact of substance abuse and mental illness on American communities.

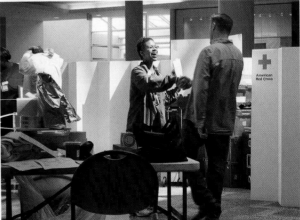

Figure 4.3 The American Red Cross is a nonprofit organization that provides disaster relief, CPR certification, first aid classes, and blood donation services.

In addition to these national healthcare departments, each state has its own public health department or agency. These local departments and health authorities conduct research, promote health, and enforce regulations to prevent disease and injury within the community. As government organizations, these agencies and facilities are funded by tax dollars.

Many **nonprofit organizations** also exist at national, state, and local levels (Figure 4.3). They have both paid staff and volunteers, and operate on donations and grants. Any profits these organizations make are used to achieve their charitable goals, such as research, education, and low-cost care. The March of Dimes, Red Cross, American Heart Association, and American Cancer Society are a few examples of nonprofit organizations dedicated to healthcare issues.

Healthcare Providers. A wide variety of facilities can be connected through a continuum of care to provide healthcare. **Hospitals** are typically large facilities that offer a wide range of services from inpatient care, surgery, and critical care to physical therapy, radiology, and laboratory services. Hospitals may provide general care or specialize in a particular age group or disease. They may be operated by government agencies, universities, nonprofit or religious organizations, or profit-making corporations. They range in size from limited services and just a few beds to numerous large departments with hundreds of beds. The size, focus, and funding of a hospital determine what technology and services it has available for its patients.

Emergency medical services (EMS) provide rapid response care for those experiencing sudden illness and injury. Ambulance and flight-for-life services make medical care available from the point of injury to the emergency room (Figure 4.4). These services and the advanced training of their providers can extend life, but they come at a high cost that may not be covered by health insurance.

Outpatient care that does not require hospitalization is offered through **ambulatory care** centers. These are walk-in clinics for nonemergency care. Many outpatient surgeries can be performed in a doctor's or dentist's private office. This avoids the financial cost and family stress caused by a hospital stay.

Clinics allow several practitioners to save resources by sharing an office and support staff. Practitioners in a clinic usually specialize in a particular field, like dentistry, or a particular condition, like heart disease. Some physicians still provide healthcare in independent offices, but more are doing so in group practices.

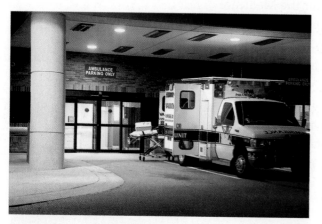

Figure 4.4   Ambulances transport patients to the emergency room when injury or illness occurs suddenly.

Behavioral healthcare is a huge field. These services can include substance abuse treatment, psychiatric evaluation, group therapy, eating disorder treatment, probation or parole services, and domestic violence programs. Services may be inpatient or outpatient and are often ongoing. The Mental Health Parity (PAIR-uh-tee) and Addition Equity Act of 2008 and the Affordable Care Act of 2010 prevent insurance from placing limitations on mental health treatment other than those that would normally apply to physical health provisions.

The continuum of care also includes facilities that provide different levels of support for people who are unable to live independently at home because they are frail, elderly, or disabled. Some of these individuals live with their families, whose care for them is supplemented by **home health care** or adult day care while family members are at work. The home health team often includes nurses, home health aides, clergy, and professionals who provide rehabilitation services. Physical therapy, occupational therapy, and respiratory therapy are common rehabilitation services that help people adjust to or heal from serious injuries and health issues. A case manager may be sent to the home to assess the client's needs. This person can direct the client to additional services, such as home medical equipment, Meals on Wheels, and transportation services. Senior centers provide elderly people with social activities and access to a support network. Respite care programs are also available to provide family members with a short-term, planned break from their role as caregivers. Without the support of these services, many more elderly and disabled people would end up in expensive long-term care facilities.

Long-term care facilities provide skilled nursing care and rehabilitation services for residents who will live in the facility for many months or years. Residents who require 24-hour care—such as those with dementia, severe illnesses, or incapacitating physical disabilities—may live in nursing homes. Some people stay in a skilled-care facility for rehabilitation after an injury or surgery. People who have less severe disabilities may use an assisted-living facility (Figure 4.5). This apartment-like setting includes services such as assistance with meals, laundry, medication, and housekeeping. Community-based residential facilities are group homes for people with particular support needs due to conditions such as Down syndrome or Alzheimer's disease. Long-term care insurance is available to help cover the costs of these facilities that are not included in traditional healthcare insurance.

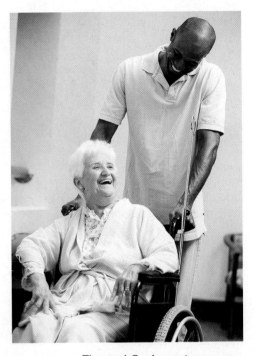

Figure 4.5   Long-term care includes nursing homes, assisted-living facilities, and community-based residential facilities. What is the difference between these long-term care settings?

Hospice (HAHS-puhs) **care** is available for clients who have been diagnosed with a terminal disease and generally have less than six months to live. This type of care focuses on trying to maintain quality of life as much as possible and prepare the patient and family for death. Palliative care helps dying patients make their last days as pain-free, meaningful, and dignified as possible. Hospice care includes support for family members, helping them find ways to cope with their loved one's imminent death and to grieve afterward.

A recent trend involves having satellite facilities bring healthcare to the public. For example, physical therapy clinics may be found in health clubs, pharmacies are common in grocery stores, and optometrists have offices in department stores. New healthcare services and massage therapies are being incorporated at day spas. You may receive a vaccination at your local pharmacy rather than going to a doctor's office. Satellite facilities are a cost-effective way to make healthcare more accessible.

Many of the same facilities and services that exist for people are also available to animals. Animal hospitals, veterinary offices, and doggie day spas provide a variety of healthcare services. Animal care may also require laboratory and medical imaging services. As a result of increased services and costs for animal care, insurance companies now offer pet health insurance.

Research and Testing. Biomedical research and testing facilities include laboratories, engineering companies, and pharmaceutical (far-muh-SOO-tih-kuhl) companies. Medical research through chemical, animal, and

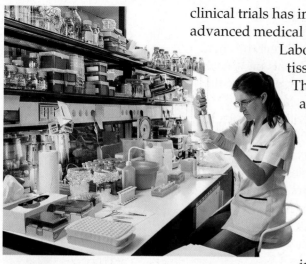

clinical trials has improved the safety of medications and treatments, advanced medical treatments for many diseases, and increased longevity. Laboratories perform tests on blood, body fluids, and tissues to help physicians diagnose disease (Figure 4.6). These labs may be freestanding entities or part of a healthcare facility such as a hospital or clinic. Pharmaceutical companies develop, test, and market new medications, while engineering companies make medical equipment for patient diagnosis and treatment, such as ultrasound machines and robotic surgical machines. Software firms develop medical records systems and electronic simulators to help train healthcare workers. Although these facilities may not provide hands-on healthcare, they are an important part of the healthcare system.

Figure 4.6   Healthcare workers in labs test blood, body fluids, and tissues to help diagnose illness.

Healthcare Payment Systems

Individuals, employers, insurance companies, and government agencies take part in various payment systems that cover the cost of healthcare. The Affordable Care Act of 2010 (ACA) requires all Americans to participate in health insurance plans provided by their employers or to purchase insurance through public health insurance exchanges to cover the cost of their healthcare. The government uses tax dollars to finance healthcare for certain groups of citizens. Large grants and donations may provide funding for healthcare focused on a specific goal, such as smoking cessation. People may also choose to pay for some elective healthcare procedures out of their own pockets. All of these payment systems bring money into the healthcare provider system, which absorbs the cost of some medical care for people who can't pay their medical bills.

Healthcare costs are steadily increasing, and they are likely to continue increasing into the future. Total healthcare spending in 2013, the last year for which data is available, was $2.9 trillion, double what it had been 10 years before. These rising costs have an impact on care provided and on the extent of publicly financed healthcare. Efforts to control these rising costs have not been effective.

Insurance Basics. Insurance is a risk pool because it groups together many people who face a risk. These individuals contribute money to the pooled funds, sharing the total cost. The monthly fees individuals pay into this money pool to receive insurance coverage are called **premiums**. When insured people use healthcare services, they make a claim on the money pool to cover their costs.

Typically, insurance companies require individuals to cover some of their own healthcare costs. Insurance companies often set an amount called a **deductible** that is the minimum amount a patient must pay out-of-pocket before the insurance company will pay for healthcare. Insurance companies send customers an explanation of benefits (EOB) for each claim to track expenditures, deductibles, insurer payments, and amounts owed by the insured. Some plans set limitations on the maximum amount they will pay for services such as home care or mental health visits in a year.

Some plans require pre-authorization or referrals to see a specialist. These restrictions reduce overuse but may also result in less effective healthcare.

An individual's share of the costs compared to the insurance company's share is called **coinsurance**. Coinsurance is expressed as a percentage or ratio, such as 80/20, which means that the insurance company pays 80 percent of qualified costs and the insured individual pays 20 percent. The insured individual may pay this amount as a set fee when he or she receives services. These payments are called *copayments*, or *copays*. For example, patients typically pay a copayment of $10 to $35 when seeing a primary care physician.

Laboratories and hospitals typically bill the insurance company and insured individual after providing care. At that time, the insurance company determines how much it will pay and what copayment is owed by the insured. There may be a maximum set on the amount you will pay in a year for coinsurance and copays. After that maximum is met, the insurance company will pay 100% of qualified costs through the end of the year.

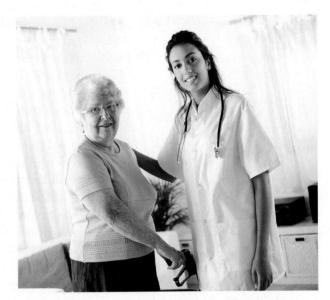

The federal government provides **Medicare** coverage for people 65 years of age and older (Figure 4.7). This program helps with the cost of healthcare, but it doesn't pay for all medical expenses or long-term care. Medicare is divided into parts that pay for different types of services. Part A covers hospital and skilled nursing costs, Part B provides medical insurance, Part C is Medicare coverage offered through private insurance companies, and Part D covers prescription drugs. Individuals must purchase private **Medigap** policies to cover costs not paid by Medicare.

Medicaid is another government-provided health insurance program. It provides hospital and medical insurance for people with low incomes, children in low-income families, and those who are disabled and cannot work. The program is administered by state governments, so it varies from state to state. To receive Medicaid, individuals must meet eligibility requirements set by the state. Some children in low-income families do not meet these requirements but belong to families that do not have health insurance. These children may be covered under another program called the *Children's Health Insurance Program (CHIP)*.

Two other government healthcare programs cover specific groups of people. **Worker's compensation** plans cover injuries that happen to people while they are working on a job. These programs also vary by state and can cover both healthcare costs and loss of income due to injury. TRICARE, formerly called *CHAMPUS*, is the government healthcare program that provides insurance for uniformed service members, former members of the armed forces, and their dependent families.

Figure 4.7   Medicare, a health insurance system funded by the government, provides insurance coverage to people 65 years of age and older. What does each part of Medicare cover?

Controlling Costs. In the past, insurance payments were made based on actual costs. Any covered procedure was paid for by the insurance company. This encouraged providers to recommend additional, sometimes unnecessary, procedures to keep business flowing. The result was increased costs for patients and insurance companies. Both the government and private insurers have developed **managed care** systems to limit overuse of healthcare services and reduce rising healthcare costs.

managed care
a system that limits access to and use of healthcare to control costs

The government effort to reduce costs centered on diagnostic-related groupings (DRGs). Using DRGs means that medical conditions are coded by diagnosis, procedure, and level of complication. The assigned DRG determines how much a government insurance program will pay the provider for services to treat a patient with a particular diagnostic code. If care is provided at a lower price than what is set based on the DRG, the provider can keep the difference. However, if the care is more expensive due to additional testing or procedures, the provider will have to pay the extra costs. This prospective payment system, which was adopted by most insurance providers in the 1980s, removes the incentive for healthcare providers to prescribe or approve more tests and treatments.

Private insurers have worked to reduce costs by developing several distinct categories of insurance in managed care systems. These include health maintenance organizations, preferred provider organizations, point of service plans, and exclusive provider organization plans (Figure 4.8).

Health maintenance organizations (HMOs) employ doctors, pharmacists, dentists, laboratories, and hospitals in an integrated and patient-focused network to cover all aspects of medical care for insured individuals. This insurance plan only covers care from providers within the network and generally has low deductibles or copayments, or none at all beyond the monthly premium. In this system, providers are paid according to the number of patients enrolled in the plan. They receive the same pay regardless of whether or not they see a specific patient each month. Bonuses may be paid to physicians for keeping costs down. This payment system encourages patients to see their providers more regularly to maintain good health, but it does not encourage providers to recommend more services than necessary to their patients (Figure 4.9).

Figure 4.8   There are several different choices of healthcare plans for people in the United States. How are these plans different?

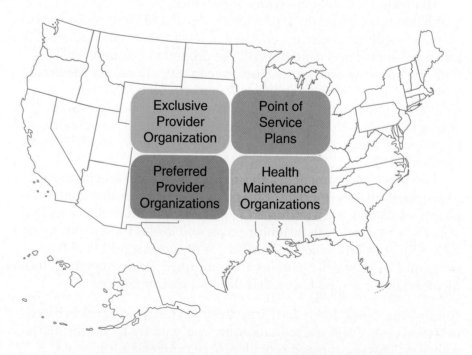

Many insurers use **preferred provider organizations (PPOs)**—which are more flexible than HMOs—to control costs. In a PPO, insurers contract with private physicians and hospitals to provide treatment and care at a reduced cost in return for an increased number of patients. The PPO pays providers only when they actually provide care. Insurance plans with PPOs have set copayments for insured individuals when they receive services, usually with an annual deductible. The insurance company typically charges lower monthly premiums for a PPO than for an HMO. This payment system creates an incentive for doctors to encourage patients to use more healthcare services but uses copays to discourage overuse by patients.

Two variations that combine elements of the HMO and PPO have emerged in the last ten years—point of service plans and exclusive provider organization plans. **Point of service (POS)** plans have smaller deductibles and copays than a PPO, but they require you to get a referral from your primary care provider before seeing a specialist, like an HMO does. Like a PPO, it is possible to see specialists outside of the network of providers, but the deductibles and copays are higher.

Exclusive provider organization (EPO) plans charge an access fee for a network of healthcare providers at reduced rates. The premiums of an EPO plan are usually lower than those of an HMO, but the choice of covered providers is more limited. Referrals from your primary care physician are required for specialists, and they must be part of the network of providers. Network providers are paid on a fee-for-service basis, and patients are charged small copays for use of a service to reduce any tendency to overuse the service.

Insurance companies and the government also try to control costs through the promotion of preventive care and healthful lifestyles. Preventive care includes such practices as routine physical exams, immunizations, and patient education. These practices are aimed at restraining costs by providing care before problems become more expensive to treat.

Many medical conditions, such as heart disease, type 2 diabetes, and lung cancer, are associated with unhealthy practices. By encouraging people to make wise behavioral decisions such as maintaining a healthy weight, getting adequate exercise, and avoiding smoking or alcohol use, public health officials hope to reduce the risk that Americans will develop these chronic conditions.

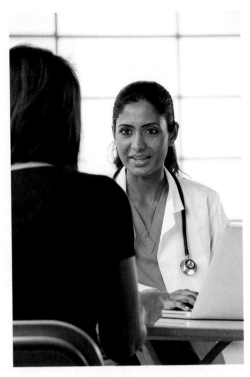

Figure 4.9   Having a healthcare plan like an HMO may mean that people see their doctors more often, leading to better health.

Applying Systems Theory to Healthcare Trends

Systems theory brings a new way of looking at and anticipating the effects of change on healthcare. Change may come at any point in the healthcare system. The needs and wants of patients change, available finances and technology change, and new laws and economic conditions continually change the environment within which healthcare provider and payment systems operate.

Insurance. One traditional issue in healthcare has been the growing number of Americans who are uninsured or underinsured. This has particularly been a problem for the unemployed and for young adults transitioning from their parents' healthcare coverage to their own. Millions of children are without adequate insurance as well.

Systems theory helps us think about the effect large numbers of uninsured people have on both the provider and payment systems. It affects the amount of resources, or input, coming into the healthcare system. Having a large number of uninsured young people keeps insurance costs high because young people tend to be healthier than older people. If those young people were contributing to the insurance pool, their premiums would help cover the cost of the services needed by older people. In addition, if uninsured individuals do have a health problem, they tend to wait until it is advanced before seeking medical care. This makes their treatment more difficult and costly, affecting the throughput of the system.

Children without healthcare may not have annual checkups or keep their immunizations up-to-date, meaning they can spread preventable diseases, such as measles (Figure 4.10). The growing epidemics of pertussis (puhr-TUH-suhs), or *whooping cough*, and tuberculosis (too-ber-kyuh-LOH-suhs) are evidence of this problem with system output. When people are uninsured, they also lack a connection with a particular care provider, creating an impact on the feedback loop.

The Affordable Care Act intends to solve these problems by creating a new system under which all Americans will have healthcare coverage. As the ACA's new provisions go into effect, the resulting changes will affect all areas of the healthcare provider and payment systems. The increased number of patients may result in healthcare worker shortages. Increased training capacity and cross training of workers will be important. The increased use of insurance will require a more efficient method for sharing information and making payments between care providers and insurers. It will take time to adjust to all these changes.

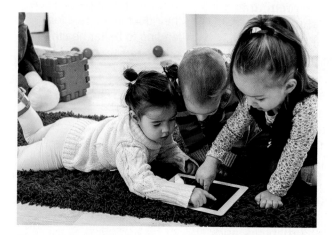

Figure 4.10   Germs can spread easily in large groups of children at school or a daycare.

Cost Management. Another issue in developing and maintaining an effective and manageable healthcare system involves how each person handles his or her individual responsibility for reducing healthcare costs. Just as patients can reduce the cost of healthcare by taking care of themselves and using their available care responsibly, healthcare workers can affect the system with their job performance. Good communication, accurate records, careful use of supplies, and effective education of patients can help keep healthcare costs down. Cross training can reduce the need for additional workers. Staff training to reduce medical errors, work injuries, and infections can also save money for healthcare providers and payers.

Facilities often use a variety of cost-saving measures. Combining several related services can save money by eliminating duplicate staff and facility costs. Bulk purchasing is usually cheaper than making many smaller purchases, as long as the supplies are used before their expiration date.

Hospital Stays. The aging of our population is having an impact on our healthcare systems as well. People are now living longer than in the past, and with more severe health problems. Insurance companies have responded to the increased demand for care by reducing the number of days paid for hospital stays and shifting care to cheaper outpatient, rehabilitation, and home health services. Hospitals need to be careful not to send patients home too early, however, or more expensive complications may result. This shift has also resulted in an increasing number of specialists who help diagnose and treat complex health problems. Specialists earn more money, so these areas seem to draw the interest of more young healthcare providers. These services are usually concentrated in large urban hospitals. As older family practice and general medicine doctors retire, a shortage of generalists and healthcare providers has occurred in rural areas.

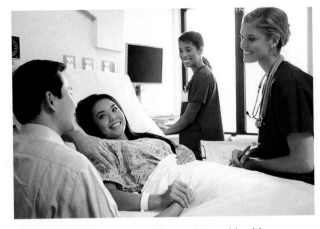

Figure 4.11   Healthcare workers may encounter language barriers when caring for multicultural patients. List some ways that this could affect all aspects of a system—input, throughput, output, and the feedback loop.

Diverse Patients. The influx of a multicultural population also creates new barriers and concerns (Figure 4.11). Patients may be reluctant to share their health questions with healthcare providers who are so different from themselves. Communication barriers and low health literacy make access to care more difficult. These issues may result in poor outcomes and unsatisfied customers. In this situation, nearly all areas of the system are affected—input, throughput, output, and the feedback loop.

RECALL YOUR READING

1. _____ can be used to think through the causes and effects of changes between related parts of healthcare provider and payment systems.

2. A change in input, throughput, _____, feedback, or the _____ will create a corresponding change in all of the other parts of a system.

3. Healthcare facilities include private _____, _____ organizations, and many other settings.

4. _____ care refers to a payment system that attempts to reduce healthcare _____.

Complete the *Map Your Reading* graphic organizer for the section you just read.

Legal and Ethical Issues in Health Informatics Services

Healthcare workers are affected by both legal and ethical issues. Whether you are a medical information technologist entering patient information into a hospital's database or a clinical coder applying appropriate codes to a patient's billing record, legal and ethical issues will influence your daily work. Health informatics workers also need to be aware of many laws affecting patient rights and the proper use of patient health information.

Legal Issues Affecting Healthcare Workers

Legal issues are defined by laws that are enforced by the government. Laws are written by the US Congress, state legislatures, and local government bodies. Sometimes laws provide guidelines that executive department agencies must implement by issuing detailed regulations. Those regulations are just as important and authoritative as laws. Where laws conflict, or where regulations are unclear, court decisions may clarify how the law is to be applied.

Many laws affect healthcare workers. The Emergency Medical Treatment and Active Labor Act (EMTALA) says that hospitals that receive federal funding cannot turn away patients who are unable to pay for their own emergency care (Figure 4.12). The Hill-Burton Act requires hospitals to meet the language needs of non-English-speaking patients. AIDS legislation addresses fair treatment for patients who already have this disease or have tested positive for HIV. Employment laws such as the Civil Rights Act, Americans with Disabilities Act, and Family Medical Leave Act (FMLA) affect healthcare workplaces just as they do other workplaces. Additional laws are passed and old laws can change each year, so it is up to you to stay informed.

The first step in staying informed is to understand the difference between the two main types of law—civil law and criminal law. **Civil law** deals with property rights, personal rights, contracts, and personal injury. Court cases involving civil law begin with a lawsuit, in which one party claims that another party has injured his or her rights, property, or person. A patient complaining about the unauthorized release of private medical information is one example of a case that would appear in a civil law court.

In a civil case, the person suffering the injury (the plaintiff) accuses the other party (the defendant) of causing him or her some harm. The case is decided by a judge or a jury. If the defendant is found guilty, he or she may be ordered to pay the plaintiff a specific amount of money, called *damages*. If the defendant is found not guilty, no payment is required.

civil law
the branch of law that establishes rules for business relationships between people or between individuals and businesses

Figure 4.12   The EMTALA ensures that patients in emergency situations receive care even if they cannot pay.

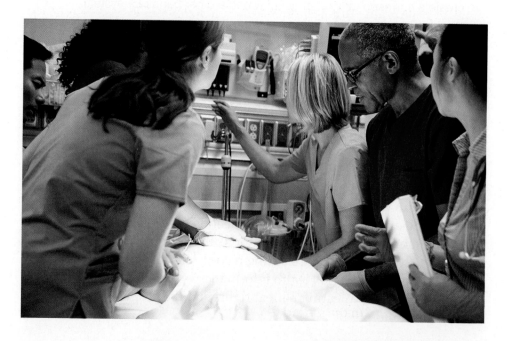

Federal, state, and local governments prosecute violations of **criminal law** against individuals. Practicing healthcare without the proper credentials and misusing narcotics are crimes. Insurance fraud, such as submitting a claim for payment to an insurance company for care that was not provided, is also a crime. In some cases, it is a crime *not* to perform an action. For instance, almost every state requires healthcare workers to report cases of suspected child abuse to state authorities. Failure to do so is defined as a crime by most states. Some states also make the person who failed to report possible abuse open to civil charges.

In criminal cases, the defendant is the person accused of the crime. The government, acting through a prosecuting attorney, brings the charges against him or her. A defendant who is found guilty is sentenced to some form of punishment, such as a fine or a period of time in prison. A defendant who is found not guilty goes free.

Contracts. Legal issues in healthcare typically fall under civil law because the doctor-patient relationship forms a **contract**. Contracts have four elements:

- Two parties enter into an agreement in which one promises to perform some action for the other. Employees of the healthcare provider may act as its agents to create such an agreement when they offer to arrange for or provide care.

- The contract must include consideration, meaning the transfer of something of value from the party benefiting from the action to the party performing it. This means paying a healthcare provider for treatment.

- The contract must be for a legal purpose. A contract to sell illegal drugs, for instance, is invalid.

- Both parties must be fully capable of entering into the agreement. A person with a **legal disability** is not considered capable of entering into a contract. Such individuals include minors who are under the age of consent, people ruled mentally incompetent, or anyone in an altered mental state due to drugs or semi-consciousness. In those cases, a parent or guardian must provide consent. Consent is assumed in emergency situations when the patient is unable to give it and a guardian cannot be reached.

Contracts can be either **expressed**, meaning the terms are spelled out in detail, or **implied**, meaning an agreement is assumed based on the actions of both parties. A person who purchases health insurance enters an expressed contract with the insurance provider. The terms and conditions of the contract are fully stated, as are exclusions from coverage. A physician and patient typically engage in an implied contract for care that meets an accepted standard of quality. The two parties do not need to sign a formal agreement for a contract to exist.

People who form a contract don't always provide the service or payment they promised. In these situations, the terms of the contract are broken, and a breach of contract takes place. For example, if a home health agency is paid to provide weekly nursing care and the nurse does not show up, a breach of contract has occurred. A patient who refuses to pay for an operation has committed a breach of contract as well. When this happens, the party who has suffered from the breach—the recipient of home nursing care in the first case or the surgeon in the second—can sue the other party, claiming injury.

criminal law
the branch of law that aims to protect individuals and society by defining certain actions as crimes, or offenses against society

contract
a legally binding agreement between two or more people or agencies

legal disability
a condition that results in a person being unable to enter a contract, such as being under the age of consent, being ruled mentally incompetent, or having an altered mental state due to drugs or semi-consciousness

tort
an action that harms another person's body or property or takes away his or her freedom of action in some way

Torts. A **tort** is a harmful action that causes injury, restricts someone's freedom or damages property. *Fraud*—a deceitful practice—is one example of a tort. A company that falsely and knowingly claims a product will cure a condition may be found guilty of committing a tort against a person who is harmed by using that product. The injured person has a right to payment for the damages the product causes.

For health informatics workers, tort cases are most likely to involve invasion of privacy. **Invasion of privacy** applies to a person's personal information as well as his or her body. Healthcare workers must be careful never to discuss a patient or his or her needs in a public area where personal details can be overheard or with people who are not involved in the patient's care (Figure 4.13). Workers also need to be careful about releasing information to others.

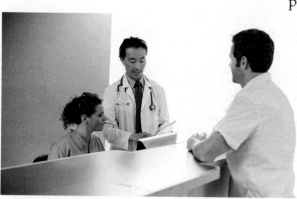

Figure 4.13   Personal information about patients must be kept private. Does the scene above show an area in which healthcare workers can discuss sensitive information? Why or why not?

Medical information can be released legally for several reasons, such as to send patient information to another healthcare provider, to file insurance claims, to comply with government requests for treatment information, or to respond to a court's request for medical records. In the first three situations, a signed patient authorization form must be on file to allow the release of the information. A patient release is not required when complying with court orders for medical records or disclosing reportable incidents and conditions, such as sexually transmitted infections to public health authorities or gunshot wounds to the police.

Exposing someone's personal information can cause great embarrassment and harm to a reputation. **Defamation** (deh-fuh-MAY-shuhn) of character means damaging someone's good name or reputation. Verbal defamation, such as gossip, is known as **slander**. When done in writing, defamation is called **libel**. You are guilty of libel if you e-mail a friend to talk about a patient's stay in rehab. Defamation and invasion of privacy can affect someone's personal life, social life, and career. You may be asked to sign a confidentiality agreement before you begin working in a healthcare facility.

Ethical Issues in Healthcare Careers

ethical
a term used to describe an action that fits with someone's personal morals or professional rules of conduct

While legal issues are defined by laws, **ethical** issues are defined by morals and values. These are beliefs about what is right or wrong. Morals are learned from family, friends, and experiences. They guide our ethical decision making and standards of appropriate behavior.

Ethical Codes. Some occupations have professional standards for ethics. These standards may be embodied in **codes of ethics,** which are formal statements of expected ethical behaviors. They describe the standards of conduct expected of members of the profession. The American Health Information Management Association (AHIMA) Code of Ethics is one example. This code applies to workers in health informatics services (Figure 4.14). Codes of ethics provide professionals with guidance to help them handle difficult decisions. These codes emphasize principles such as the importance of preserving life and not doing harm. They also push

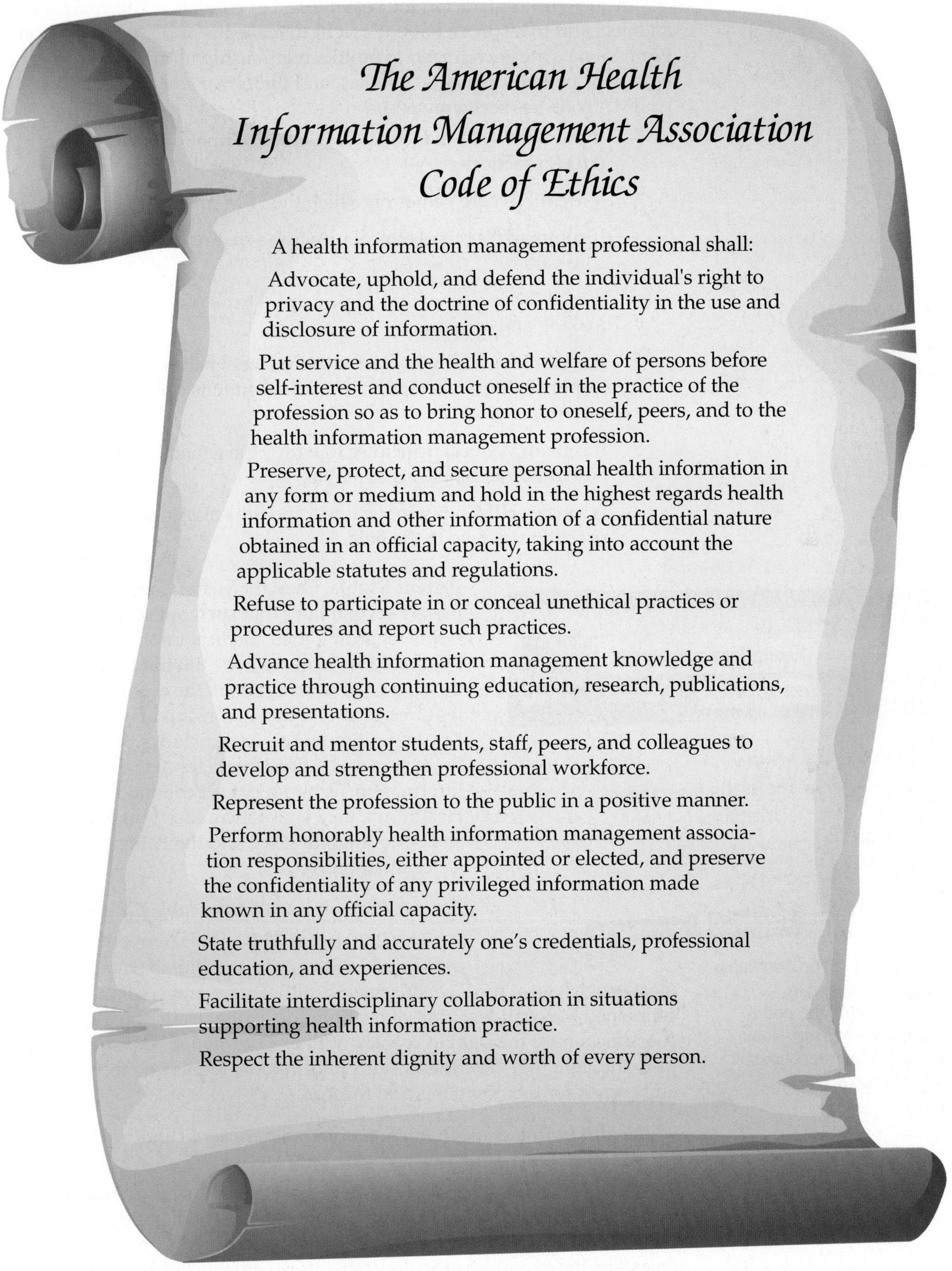

The American Health Information Management Association Code of Ethics

A health information management professional shall:

Advocate, uphold, and defend the individual's right to privacy and the doctrine of confidentiality in the use and disclosure of information.

Put service and the health and welfare of persons before self-interest and conduct oneself in the practice of the profession so as to bring honor to oneself, peers, and to the health information management profession.

Preserve, protect, and secure personal health information in any form or medium and hold in the highest regards health information and other information of a confidential nature obtained in an official capacity, taking into account the applicable statutes and regulations.

Refuse to participate in or conceal unethical practices or procedures and report such practices.

Advance health information management knowledge and practice through continuing education, research, publications, and presentations.

Recruit and mentor students, staff, peers, and colleagues to develop and strengthen professional workforce.

Represent the profession to the public in a positive manner.

Perform honorably health information management association responsibilities, either appointed or elected, and preserve the confidentiality of any privileged information made known in any official capacity.

State truthfully and accurately one's credentials, professional education, and experiences.

Facilitate interdisciplinary collaboration in situations supporting health information practice.

Respect the inherent dignity and worth of every person.

Figure 4.14   The AHIMA Code of Ethics describes the standards of conduct expected of health informatics workers.

healthcare workers to act in the best interest of patients, to do what is fair and just, and to respect a patient's right to make his or her own decisions. Professionals are encouraged to build a relationship of trust and respect with their patients, patients' families, and their own coworkers. The AHIMA code has seven purposes:

- It promotes high standards of health information management (HIM) practice.

- It identifies core values on which the HIM mission is based.

- It summarizes broad ethical principles that reflect the profession's core values.

- It establishes a set of ethical principles to be used to guide decision making and actions.

- It establishes a framework for professional behavior and responsibilities when professional obligations conflict or ethical uncertainties arise.

- It provides ethical principles to which the general public can hold an HIM professional accountable.

- It teaches HIM's mission, values, and ethical principles to practitioners new to the field.

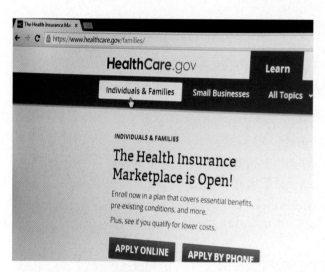

Figure 4.15   The Affordable Care Act, signed in 2010, affected the entire healthcare system. How did the ACA affect health information?

Patient Rights. Over the years, Congress has passed several laws that spell out patients' rights regarding their medical information (Figure 4.15). Workers in health informatics services need to be aware of the actions that are required or prohibited as a result of these laws. Key legislation in this area includes the Patient Protection and Affordable Care Act, the Health Information Technology for Economic and Clinical Health Act, the Health Insurance Portability and Accountability Act, and the Patient Self-Determination Act.

Patient Protection and Affordable Care Act (ACA)

This 2010 law significantly altered the healthcare landscape in the United States. While most provisions of the law addressed healthcare coverage, some parts concerned the confidentiality of health information. Under the ACA, consumers have the right to privacy of their information. Consumers also have the right to review their health information, request corrections to it, and copy it for their own medical records.

Health Information Technology for Economic and Clinical Health (HITECH) Act

The HITECH Act, passed in 2009, intended to improve healthcare through the increased use of health information technology (HIT). It is hoped that HIT will increase the quality of healthcare by ensuring that providers have complete and accurate information; by allowing different providers to better coordinate care; and by helping providers diagnose conditions sooner, which should help reduce the cost of care. In addition, HIT offers the promise of a greater ability to share information between providers and patients over the Internet or in other electronic formats. The HITECH Act provided funds for physicians and healthcare organizations like hospitals to shift to or improve their existing HIT systems. Many providers and organizations increased their use of HIT as a result of this law.

Health Insurance Portability and Accountability Act (HIPAA)

Technological advances have also caused new concerns about confidentiality. In 1996, President Bill Clinton signed into law the **Health Insurance Portability and Accountability Act**. HIPAA was intended to streamline the insurance coverage and reimbursement process while safeguarding healthcare records and protected health information. The 2003 Privacy Rule gave individuals rights over their personal health information and set rules and limits on who could look at and receive this information. The Privacy Rule required the Department of Health and Human Services to develop standards and rules for storing and sharing health information.

Protected health information (PHI) includes a patient's name, medical record number, birth date, Social Security number, address, telephone number, e-mail address, employer, and so on. This information may be obtained from conversations, e-mail messages, electronic files, printed files, observations during treatment, computer displays, faxed documents, and many other methods of display or communication. This individually identifiable information must be protected for both privacy and safety reasons. Under HIPAA, PHI may only be shared for treatment, payment, or other authorized purposes. Every health informatics worker should know what information is protected and how to protect it. The last section of this chapter suggests steps that workers should take to protect PHI.

Patient Self-Determination Act (PSDA)

Passed in 1990, the Patient Self-Determination Act was written to help healthcare consumers protect their right to make their own decisions. This act requires many healthcare institutions to provide information about decision-making rights and to ask patients if they have **advance directives**. These written legal documents state a patient's wishes for care when he or she is unable to communicate, such as during a loss of consciousness. There are several different types of advance directives, including a living will, do not resuscitate order, and a power of attorney. The rules for advance directives vary from state to state.

A **living will** is a patient's written document giving instructions about which procedures may or may not be used to sustain or prolong his or her life, such as feeding tubes or ventilation. To be legal, living wills must conform to state laws. Typically, these documents have to be signed by the patient and witnessed by another person. The patient or a family member should provide a copy of the living will to their doctor so the patient's wishes are known (Figure 4.16). In most states, a living will does not go into effect unless two doctors have certified that you are not able to make decisions for yourself. There may be other requirements, such as "terminal illness" or "permanent unconsciousness," in some states.

Health Insurance Portability and Accountability Act (HIPAA)
a federal law that makes it easier to obtain healthcare coverage and protects personal health information

protected health information (PHI)
all individually identifiable personal information obtained through healthcare

advance directive
a legal document prepared by a patient before a health crisis occurs to guide healthcare decisions in situations when the patient is unable to speak for himself or herself

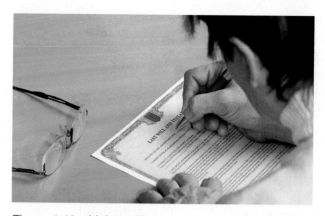

Figure 4.16 Living wills must be signed by the patient and witnessed by another person. What information does a living will contain?

Do-not-resuscitate (DNR) orders are advance directives that specifically state that a patient is not to be revived if his or her heart stops beating. DNR orders are issued by hospital staff at a patient's request. In some states, DNR may also be indicated on a living will, but this would not take effect unless the living will is in effect. A DNR order does not require the certification of two doctors. Some hospitals give patients with DNR orders special wristbands to indicate their wishes.

The **power of attorney (POA)** for healthcare appoints someone to make healthcare decisions for a person in the event that he or she is unable to make his or her own choices. Like living wills, these documents must be signed and witnessed to be legal. A power of attorney generally becomes active when two doctors declare a patient to be incapacitated or unable to make decisions. The patient's record should include any advance directives.

Rules vary from state to state, but without advance directives, family members may not be authorized to make decisions for adults who suffer from a severe accident, stroke, or Alzheimer's disease. Without an advance directive, decision making may legally be given to a guardian appointed by the court to determine what care is in the best interests of the patient. That guardian may have less flexibility and freedom in decision making than a person named in advance by the patient. Getting a court-ordered guardian can also be expensive, time-consuming, and emotionally draining for the family. The best way for patients to make sure their wishes are followed is to have advance directives in writing and discuss their wishes with their physician, family, and the person they appoint as an agent.

Some individuals have documents that say they are willing to donate usable organs when they die. Several states, for instance, allow drivers to state this willingness on their driver's licenses. Others carry organ donor cards in their wallets or purses. Organ donation preferences can also be stated in a living will.

Legal and Voluntary Professional Standards

Because healthcare workers have important responsibilities, many are required to prove their qualifications before they can work. Physicians, for instance, must pass licensing exams to obtain a doctor's license before they can see patients. Licenses are required by state law. Workers in other healthcare occupations have to demonstrate that they meet certain standards as well.

Certification is one way to demonstrate a healthcare worker's qualifications (Figure 4.17). Certification is not usually set by state law but is offered by professional associations. AHIMA, for instance, offers programs for certifying health information technicians, coders, data analysts, and other workers. The National Commission for Health Education Credentialing certifies health educators. Once certified,

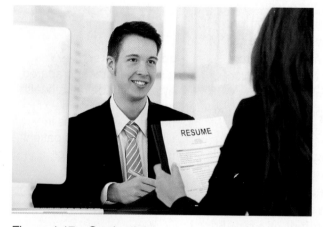

Figure 4.17 Credentials can be very important to those seeking a job in the field of healthcare. What are the different types of credentials?

workers will need to earn continuing education credits to recertify. Workers in some occupations are not required to earn certification in order to work, but employers tend to favor those who have done so. Gaining certification, then, is a wise career decision.

Some healthcare occupations have **registration** programs, in which workers enter an official list, or *registry*, of qualified workers. Some of AHIMA's certification programs give the title "registered" to workers who have earned certification. For instance, a worker could qualify as a registered health information technician (RHIT).

Certification and registration are typically earned through education and testing. To qualify for these programs, individuals usually have to graduate from educational programs accredited by the applicable professional association. Accreditation shows that a professional association has judged an educational program to meet minimum educational standards for the occupation. A majority of healthcare organizations choose to apply for accreditation from a body called *The Joint Commission* (formerly called *JCAHO*). This group reviews the quality of care provided by healthcare organizations before accrediting them.

registration
placement on an official list, or registry, of qualified workers

---

RECALL YOUR READING

1. Morals guide _____ decisions about right and wrong while laws guide _____ decisions that are enforced by the court.
2. The Affordable _____ Act and Health _____ Portability and _____ Act protect patients' personal health information.
3. Patients are encouraged to be involved in their care decisions and to plan ahead through _____.
4. _____ and _____ are usually voluntary, but may open job opportunities, while _____ is required by law.

Complete the
Map Your Reading
graphic organizer for the
section you just read.

Safety Issues in Health Informatics Services

Workers in health informatics services are generally not involved in direct patient care. The records they maintain, however, are a vital element of the patient care system, as these records include detailed information about a patient's condition, specific treatments, test results, and statements of the patient's wishes. This information comes into play not only in the delivery of care but also in billing and reimbursement.

Privacy of Health Information

Healthcare workers are responsible for protecting against the unauthorized use or disclosure of confidential patient information. Privacy notices are required to tell patients how their healthcare information will be used. This includes data used for treatment, billing, marketing, research, and reports to the Medical Information Bureau (MIB). The MIB maintains a database of health information on some individuals who apply for life or health insurance. Patients must authorize

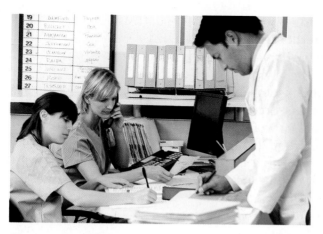

Figure 4.18 Protected health information must be kept private unless authorized for release by the patient. **What are the consequences of breaching a patient's confidentiality?**

any other uses or disclosures of their PHI, such as the release of a birth announcement to the newspaper or the posting of the patient's name outside the door of his or her hospital room. Any disclosure of PHI must be limited to the amount of information that is reasonably necessary. Healthcare workers have a responsibility to know who in the organization needs which information and when they need it (Figure 4.18).

The consequences of failing to safeguard patient information can be severe. Unauthorized release of a patient's health information can influence his or her work and home life. If information about heart disease or genetic testing for cancer is leaked from a company's human resources office, the company may look for a reason to fire that worker to avoid supporting his or her care. Theft of PHI can lead to identity theft, with someone accessing patients' bank accounts, making purchases on their credit cards, and stealing their Social Security numbers. Patients rely on healthcare workers to protect their information.

The consequences of breaching confidentiality can be severe for healthcare workers. HIPAA is a federal law, so financial penalties and jail time are possible consequences for serious and willful violations, such as selling patient information. Breach of confidentiality also violates professional ethics and can affect a healthcare worker's employability. Workers who commit such a breach may have a letter of reprimand placed in their personnel files or lose their jobs. Their actions also affect the reputation of their employer, leaving a provider open to lawsuits, penalties, and loss of business.

Ensuring Confidentiality

Patient safety and privacy should be protected in all aspects of communication. The first rule for ensuring the confidentiality of a patient's medical records is never to give that information to anyone who is not authorized to have it. If an unauthorized person asks you for patient information, you can say, "I'm sorry, but I can't discuss that because it is private patient information."

Health informatics workers should never provide PHI to another office unless the patient or his or her legal representative has specifically requested or approved the release. When legitimate information requests are received, workers should only supply the specific information requested. Patient information should never be shared outside of the patient care team. This is both illegal and unethical. Patient charts, electronic health records, e-mails, documents, conversations with the patient, phone calls, and messages concerning the patient are all considered confidential.

Reception areas should be arranged so that others waiting in line cannot hear conversations that may include PHI. If you see or hear someone else breaking the rules of confidentiality, you should remind the person that the information is private. You can say, "Your conversation can be overheard. Would you like to use a private room?"

Healthcare workers must accurately identify a patient before proceeding with the details of the reason for his or her visit. Updates on patient status or medical test results should be released only to the patient or guardian, the care team, or others specifically authorized by the patient. Only the minimum information required for a task should be released—never a patient's complete chart. The patient should indicate how he or she would like to receive information and whether or not a message can be left in a voicemail or an e-mail.

The increased use of technology and electronic records brings new concerns for keeping patient information private. Confidentiality can be breached when electronic health records are improperly stored, sent, or safeguarded. Some basic precautions to help keep electronic PHI safe include the following:

- Access to patient files must be restricted and confidential information should be destroyed, shredded, or otherwise made unreadable before being discarded.

- Encryption software should be used to protect the security of information that is stored on computers or sent in electronic files. Encryption uses a mathematical formula to change the information so that it cannot be understood if it is accessed without permission. All electronic health records containing PHI should be encrypted. Information technology departments set up the encryption processes, but all other healthcare workers are responsible for using these precautions correctly. Never send files containing PHI through e-mail or other means that are not encrypted.

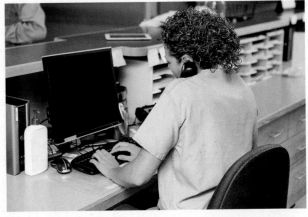

- Protect your computer monitor from view by unauthorized people (Figure 4.19). If you work in an area that is visible to patients, such as the reception desk, you must tilt the screen or use a screen cover that limits the viewing angle. You should log off whenever you walk away from your computer so that sensitive information does not remain displayed.

Figure 4.19 When working at the reception desk, healthcare workers must protect their computer screens from being viewed by unauthorized personnel.

- Computerized files must be protected from unauthorized access. Use safe password procedures. Create a strong password that cannot easily be guessed or figured out by others. It should be at least eight characters long and include upper- and lowercase letters, numbers, and symbols to make it more complex. Never use words that can be found in a dictionary, common abbreviations, or backward spelling because deciphering programs test for these. Remember that your password is like a signature. Never share your password with another person or write it down in an unsecured location.

- The use of smartphones and tablets has grown in the last decade. These devices create special safety concerns because they are small and more easily lost or stolen. If you use an electronic device while on your job, and it contains patient information, you are responsible for following the rules for encryption, passwords, and locking the device when it's not in use. If the device contains PHI and is lost or stolen, you will need to report the possible breach of confidentiality to your supervisor as soon as possible; patients must also be notified. Access to cameras and social media websites through smartphones are also an area of concern. Identifiable patient information and photos should not be captured or used without proper authorization and consent. Patients must sign a release if their picture will be used on a website for marketing purposes. Patient pictures and information should never be shared on your own social media sites. As discussed earlier, the HITECH Act addresses these computer and electronic security concerns.

Ergonomics of Computer Use

Ergonomics is the study of designing and arranging a workplace to increase productivity and safety. An office space should be arranged to reduce unnecessary movements from one place to another. A desk and chair should be set at heights that allow freedom of movement and reduce strain.

Repetitive motion injuries (RMIs) are becoming increasingly common workplace injuries. They are caused by the overuse of a specific body part or the poor positioning of a body part while it is under stress. Computer use is a common culprit in most RMI cases. Health informatics workers commonly have RMIs in the hands, wrists, elbows, and shoulders. For example, carpal tunnel syndrome can result from poor wrist position when typing or using a mouse. This condition causes pain, tingling, numbness, swelling, and a loss of strength in the fingers and wrists.

Lower back injury can also be caused by sitting, standing, or lifting with the back in poor position. The severity of the injury may be increased if the body is under stress from carrying a heavy weight such as a stack of files.

The risk of developing RMIs can be minimized by setting up your workstation so that your body is in good alignment (Figure 4.20). The following are guidelines for good alignment:

- Your hips and knees should form 90-degree angles while seated.

- Your back should be upright and supported.

- Your feet should be flat on the floor or supported on a footrest.

- Your lower arms should be supported and form a 90-degree angle to your upper arms.

- Your wrists should be supported at a natural angle where the thumb is in line with the lower arm. You may need to adjust your chair or table height to achieve good alignment.

Frequent stretches can help to reduce or prevent RMIs as well. Take a short break from your working position every 20 to 30 minutes. Stretch and flex your muscles to encourage circulation and range of motion. Make a fist, then spread your fingers wide. Arch your back and move your shoulders in circles. Shift your weight from side to side. Tighten your abdominal muscles to straighten your back. Stretch your arms above your

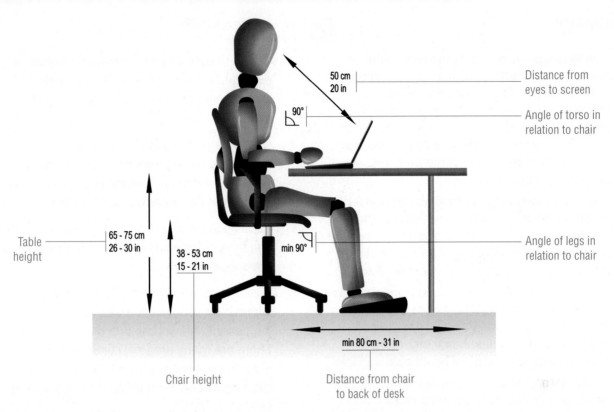

Figure 4.20   Paying attention to ergonomics and body alignment can help prevent repetitive motion injuries. When typing, how should your wrists be positioned?

head and out to the sides. Let your head hang down, then straighten up and rotate it from side to side. Taking a few moments to stretch will make you more productive and can prevent pain.

Computer screens can cause eyestrain, which may result in headaches. Be sure the top of your computer monitor is at eye level. If you type in information from paper forms, have a paper holder at the same level as the screen. Reduce glare on the screen by adjusting window blinds or the contrast on the computer's display. People who wear bifocals should consider using screen-reader glasses while on the computer. Take short breaks from the computer every 20 to 30 minutes to rest your eyes.

If you notice signs of RMI, speak with your supervisor about possible changes to your workstation that may help to prevent or relieve the strain. Federal regulations require employers to take actions to reduce these injuries. If you help to transport heavy materials, ask for a wheeled cart or other assistance. Also, consider ways to break your tasks down into smaller loads.

RECALL YOUR READING

1. A breach of _____ affects the patient, the worker, and their employer.
2. Increased use of technology and _____ records cause new concern for patient _____.
3. _____ injuries caused by overuse, _____ caused by computer screens, and _____ caused by poor position can all be prevented by proper arrangement of the workstation.

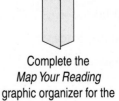

Complete the *Map Your Reading* graphic organizer for the section you just read.

SUMMARY

Assess your understanding with chapter tests

- Healthcare providers and payments both operate as systems. Systems theory can be used to analyze the causes and effects of changes between related parts of a system. A change in input, throughput, output, feedback, or the environment will have a ripple effect on all of the other resources, structures, processes, and end results in a system.

- There are many types of healthcare provider facilities and services at the national, state, and local levels. Each has a different purpose or serves a different group of people. The care they provide overlaps and is interconnected.

- Managed care refers to a payment system that attempts to control healthcare costs. HMOs, PPOs, Medicare, and Medicaid are common forms of healthcare insurance organized to manage cost and usage of healthcare services.

- Both laws and ethical values define appropriate behavior for healthcare workers. Health informatics workers need to be particularly concerned with invasion of privacy. Breaking these laws may result in financial penalties, jail time, and loss of a job.

- Codes of ethics outline the ethical behavior expected of healthcare workers. These statements serve as a reference point for making decisions.

- HIPAA helps to assure easy access to healthcare while protecting the privacy of patient information. Healthcare workers need to know what PHI includes and how to protect it.

- Patients are encouraged to be involved in their healthcare decisions and to plan ahead through advance directives.

- Privacy is a major safety issue in health informatics services. A breach of privacy affects the patient, the worker, and their employer. There are many areas of concern when guarding patient privacy. Electronic devices create new concerns for privacy and worker safety.

- Repetitive motion injuries and eyestrain can both be prevented by proper arrangement of the workstation.

MAXIMIZE YOUR PROFESSIONAL VOCABULARY

 Build vocabulary with e-flash cards, games, and audio glossary

Listed below are the essential, yellow-highlighted terms and the additional professional vocabulary terms that you encountered in this chapter. Complete the activities that follow the list to make all of these terms part of your everyday professional vocabulary.

advance directive

ambulatory care

Centers for Disease Control and Prevention (CDC)

Centers for Medicare and Medicaid Services (CMS)

civil law

code of ethics

coinsurance

contract

criminal law

deductible

defamation

Department of Health and Human Services (HHS)

emergency medical services (EMS)

environment

ethical

exclusive provider organization (EPO)

expressed

feedback loop

health maintenance organization (HMO)

Health Insurance Portability and Accountability Act (HIPAA)

home health care	managed care	premium
hospice care	Medicaid	protected health information (PHI)
hospital	Medicare	
implied	Medigap	registration
input	National Institutes of Health (NIH)	slander
invasion of privacy		system
legal	nonprofit organization	throughput
legal disability	output	tort
libel	point of service (POS)	worker's compensation
living will	power of attorney (POA)	World Health Organization (WHO)
long-term care facility	preferred provider organization (PPO)	

VOCABULARY DEVELOPMENT

Matching. Match each essential term from this chapter with the correct definition below by writing the letter of the definition next to the number of the essential term on a separate sheet of paper.

1. advance directive
2. civil law
3. contract
4. criminal law
5. ethical
6. Health Insurance Portability and Accountability Act (HIPAA)
7. legal disability
8. managed care
9. protected health information (PHI)
10. registration
11. system
12. tort

a. the branch of law that establishes rules for business relationships between people or between individuals and businesses

b. all individually identifiable personal information obtained through healthcare

c. a federal law that makes it easier to obtain healthcare coverage and protects personal health information

d. an organized structure composed of many parts that work together and depend on each other to carry out a set of functions

e. a legally binding agreement between two or more people or agencies

f. a legal document prepared by a patient before a health crisis occurs to guide healthcare decisions in situations when the patient is unable to speak for himself or herself

g. an action that harms another person's body or property or takes away his or her freedom of action in some way

h. the branch of law that aims to protect individuals and society by defining certain actions as crimes, or offenses against society

i. a system that limits access to and use of healthcare to control costs

j. a condition that results in a person being unable to enter a contract, such as being under the age of consent, being ruled mentally incompetent, or having an altered mental state due to drugs or semi-consciousness

k. a term used to describe an action that fits with someone's personal morals or professional rules of conduct

l. placement on an official list, or registry, of qualified workers

13. **Term Charades.** Make term cards using the professional vocabulary terms in this chapter. You can use these cards to play term charades in groups of four or more students.

    - Use one deck of term cards for four or more players. Divide players into two teams.

    - The first team will draw a term card from the deck to act out for their team. They have one minute to nonverbally communicate the meaning of this term to their team through acting or drawing. They cannot use words or writing of any kind.

    - After one minute, if the team has not guessed the word, the other team can join in to guess the term.

    - The point goes to the team that correctly guesses the term and play alternates between the two teams. The team with the highest score at the end of the game is the winner. The game ends when class time runs out or you no longer have new term cards to choose.

REFLECT ON YOUR READING

14. Review the story about Mr. Stake at the beginning of the chapter. Using the notes you took in the *Map Your Reading* activity, identify the legal issues, ethical practices, systems, and safety issues that were encountered in Mr. Stake's story. What could have been done differently to prevent some of the legal, ethical, organizational, and safety problems? Try to use your new professional vocabulary in your explanation.

BUILD CORE SKILLS

15. **Reading.** Reread the section in this chapter that covers healthcare provider systems. Use a phone book or the Internet to search for providers in your community that fit the descriptions for five different types of healthcare provider systems.

16. **Critical Thinking.** Compare and contrast terms using a Venn diagram on a separate sheet of paper. What are the similarities and differences between *legal* and *ethical*? *independent living* and *home health care*? *HMO* and *PPO*? *CDC* and *NIH*? *Medicare* and *Medicaid*?

17. **Reading.** Go to the Department of Health and Human Services website to learn more about the agencies that protect our health. Write a brief summary of the duties and responsibilities of the Department of Health and Human Services.

18. **Writing.** If the government is responsible for healthcare, then should the government ensure that you take care of yourself and eat healthy foods? Should the government be able to regulate which foods people can eat? How do your state and local governments impact health services in your community? Write brief answers to each of these questions and then discuss with a partner.

19. **Critical Thinking.** Visit two different types of healthcare facilities. Use a Venn diagram to compare and contrast the two facilities you visited. How are they alike and different?

20. **Math.** Suppose a person who has health insurance has an 80/20 copay. How much would this person pay if billed for $300 worth of care? What would the cost to the insured person be if she had a $500 deductible and the copay didn't take effect until the deductible had been met?

21. **Math.** A family of four is trying to choose health insurance that will cost the least based on their typical care needs from the prior year. Compare the two plans listed here. Explain which plan you would choose for them and why.

Plan A has a monthly premium of $300 and charges a $10 copay per prescription, but all office visits and dental care are included.

Plan B has a monthly premium of $250 and charges a $15 copay per prescription and 10% copay per office visit. Two dental cleanings are included per person, but additional dental work requires a 20 percent copay.

The family visited the doctor's office 10 times last year at an actual cost before insurance averaging $120 per visit. They purchased a total of 20 prescriptions during the year. Each family member had two cleanings and there was one filling at an actual cost of $300.

22. **Listening.** Sit in a public area such as the lunchroom and listen to the conversations going on around you for 10 minutes. Did you hear an example of a tort? How did the conversation fit or not fit the definition of a tort?

23. **Speaking.** What is an appropriate response to a person who asks you to discuss someone's personal health information? Practice using that response so that you are prepared to say it when the situation really happens. Partner with a classmate and take turns role playing as the

healthcare worker and the person asking for information.

24. **Critical Thinking.** Use systems theory to consider how the following change in federal legislation might impact child welfare services. If federal laws require all adults (not just caregivers) to report suspected abuse, what effects might this have on the input, throughput, output, and feedback loops of child welfare services?

25. **Critical Thinking.** Suppose you are the medical assistant for Dr. Smith. Ms. Perez calls, complaining that she feels awful most of the time. You want to be sympathetic, so you say, "Don't worry, Dr. Smith will make you feel better in no time," and you help her to schedule an appointment for tomorrow. What are the terms of the contract you just created between Dr. Smith and Ms. Perez? On what basis can Dr. Smith be sued if the terms are not met?

ACTIVATE YOUR LEARNING

26. Evaluate the workspace of the healthcare worker pictured in Figure 4.19. What is wrong with this worker's ergonomics? What recommendations could you make to improve her ergonomics? Write a list of speaking points that she could use for discussing this issue with her supervisor.

27. Suppose you are a medical records technician. A parent is demanding a copy of his or her 18-year-old daughter's medical records from her recent visit to the doctor. The daughter is still in high school and her parent pays for the insurance. As a result, the parent feels that he or she has the right to know what is in the medical records. Role play how you will handle this situation.

28. Imagine that you are a public relations specialist for a local nonprofit organization. Search their website to gather information about the services they provide and the ways that youth could support their mission. Develop a brochure, public service announcement, or other promotional material to encourage people to support them.

THINK AND ACT LIKE A HEALTHCARE WORKER

29. Refer to the scenario in question 25. How should you have replied to Ms. Perez when she called? Would you have said something different? What is the best response according to professional standards? What are the legal and ethical issues involved in this situation?

30. Imagine that a patient who is preparing for surgery calls your healthcare facility with a question about the advance directives paperwork that was in her information packet. How will you explain her rights and choices based on the Patient Self-Determination Act?

31. Think of a healthcare provider system in your community, such as a hospital, nursing home, or mental health facility. Identify or describe each aspect of this system using the following prompts:

    * Input—who or what are the resources coming into the system?

    * Throughput—how does this facility's location connect with its purpose? How do people who use this facility pay for their care? How do people learn about this facility?

    * Output—what are the quantity, quality, or cost outcomes that result from this system's operation?

    * Feedback loop—how does the facility keep a flow of people, information, and resources coming back into the system?

    * Environmental constraints—identify a potential internal constraint (such as employee satisfaction or teamwork) and external constraint (such as changing cultural makeup of the community or closing the college that provides trained employees) that affect how this system functions.

32. You just observed your coworker sticking a note on her keyboard. She tells you that the note contains her new computer password. What comment or suggestion would be appropriate and helpful in this situation?

GO TO THE SOURCE

33. Review a summary of insurance benefits and coverage. You can find samples of this document for many health insurance plans online. Find an example of a limitation and an exclusion in a health insurance summary.

34. Find the Hippocratic Oath on the Internet. Compare the AHIMA Code of Ethics—listed in Figure 4.14—and the Hippocratic Oath. What are three ethical expectations they have in common?

Chapter 5
Academic Knowledge: Medical Terminology and Body Organization

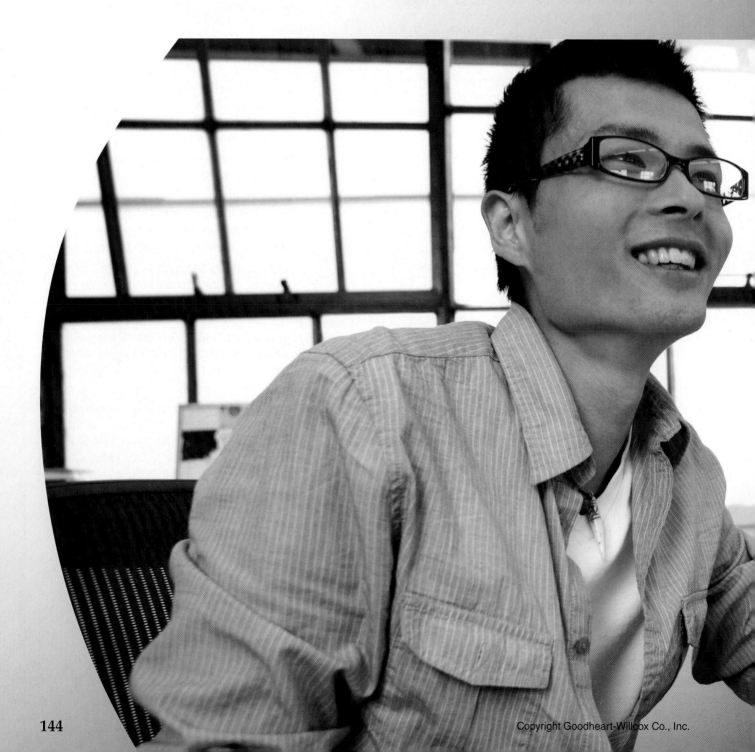

PROFESSIONAL VOCABULARY

E-flash
Cards

You will need to learn the essential terms listed below before you begin your reading. These terms will help you understand the main concepts of the chapter. These terms, which will be highlighted in yellow within the text, will become part of your professional vocabulary.

In addition to these essential terms, you will see bold terms throughout the chapter. The meanings of these terms are explained where the terms first appear. The bold terms, like the essential terms listed here, will become part of your professional vocabulary and deepen your understanding of the topics presented.

abdominal region one of nine equal areas of the abdomen that are named and used as reference points when discussing the body

anatomy the physical structures or parts of the body

body cavity a hollow space within the body that is lined by a membrane and contains bodily organs

body plane a flat or level surface seen by cutting away part of the body through surgery or medical imaging to serve as a point of reference when discussing anatomy

body region an area of the body with a specific name, which is used as a reference point when discussing anatomy

body system a group of organs working together to perform a vital function in the body

cell a small group of organelles that fulfill a specific purpose and are held together by a membrane

medical terminology special vocabulary that is used in healthcare and is often formed from Latin and Greek word parts

mnemonic device a learning tool that helps students memorize information

organ a distinct body structure made of different tissues working together for the same purpose

organelle a part of a cell that has a specific task

physiology the functions or inner workings of the body

standard anatomical position (SAP) the agreed-upon reference for body position when studying anatomy; standing erect on two legs, facing frontward, with the arms at the sides and palms facing forward

tissue a group of cells of the same type working together for the same purpose

CONNECT WITH YOUR READING

Before you read this chapter, organize the terms in the *Maximize Your Professional Vocabulary* list at the end of the chapter into logical categories based on your current knowledge. Use arrows or circles to show connections between related terms as needed. Share your newly organized list with a partner and discuss the differences in how you organized the terms.

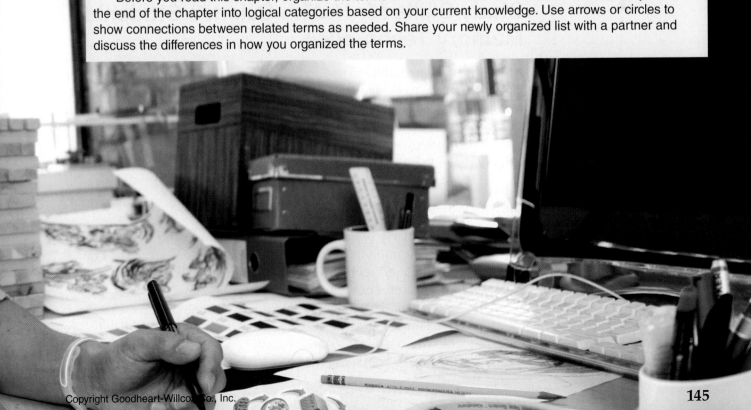

Understanding Body Organization
The Cell
Body Tissues
Organs
Body Systems
Body Directions
Body Regions & Quadrants
Body Cavities & Planes

MAP YOUR READING

Make a tablet organizer with four sheets of paper using the example shown at the left. Stack the sheets, keeping the sides even, but move each sheet of paper up so that its bottom edge is ½ inch to 1 inch above the bottom edge of the sheet below it. Holding the center of the stack, fold all the sheets down so the top edge of the top sheet is ½ inch to 1 inch above the bottom edge of the top sheet. Crease all the layers and staple at the folded edge. Write *Understanding Body Organization* on the outside flap and list what you know about the organization levels in the body. Label the edges of the flaps below the top one with the headings *The Cell*, *Body Tissues*, *Organs*, *Body Systems*, *Body Directions*, *Body Regions and Quadrants*, and *Body Cavities and Planes*. As you read, add visual cues, definitions of new terms, and notes on important concepts to each page of the booklet.

Knowledge of the body's anatomy and physiology is important for all healthcare workers. Information about how the body is organized is the foundation on which all other academic knowledge for healthcare workers is based. Learning the anatomy of the body means that you will be learning many new terms. This may seem overwhelming and you may need some new strategies for studying this new information.

In this chapter, you will be introduced to the language of medicine and techniques to help you learn new terminology and anatomy more quickly. Through these concepts, you will learn about the organization of the human body, including the directions and regions that are used to describe anatomy. You will also learn about the anatomy and physiology of the cell. After reading this chapter, you will be prepared to look at each body system in more depth in future chapters.

Study Skills for Health Science Students: Memory Techniques

It is nearly impossible to memorize all the medical terms you will hear in class or in the workplace, but learning some of the more common word parts will make it easier to understand the spoken and written terms used in patient care. It will also help you figure out the general meanings of body structures, diseases, and procedures. You will need to develop some ways to remember the large amount of information used in healthcare.

Memory Techniques for Learning Terms

People use a variety of methods to help them study and remember new terms. One common technique is to make and use flash cards. The time spent creating and reviewing the cards is what makes this technique work, so develop games or a schedule to use them often.

Some people play with the way a word looks to help remember its meaning. For example, *parallel* means *equal* and the *ll* in the middle of the word looks like a sideways equal sign. When studying a term, try creatively drawing or reshaping the letters.

Another technique is to look for familiar words that share the same word part, such as *ortho*dontists who straighten teeth and *ortho*pedists who straighten bones. This strategy may be used with everyday English words, too.

Some students like to investigate the origins of a new word. For example, *hypochondriac* [*hypo* = below, *chondr* = cartilage, *ac* = pertaining to] literally means *pertaining to the area below the cartilage*. However, in medical usage, it means *below the ribs* because some of the ribs are attached by cartilage. The term *hypochondriac* may also be used to mean a person who always thinks he or she is ill. Interestingly, many of us hold the area under our ribs when we complain that we don't feel well.

This book breaks medical terms down into their Latin and Greek origins to help you understand their meanings. All of the techniques described here can help you build a better vocabulary of new terms.

Mnemonic Devices

Mnemonic (nih-MAH-nihk) **devices** can be used to remember information. Sounds, colors, smells, tastes, touch, and emotions are all stored in different areas of the brain. By vividly connecting information with many senses, it is easier to recall the information later. The following are suggestions for basic techniques:

mnemonic device
a learning tool that helps students memorize information

- Make up acronyms to remember the parts of a concept or procedure. For example, the acronym *SOMBER* can remind you of the symptoms of depression—Sadness, Overwhelmed, Memory problems, Behavioral changes, Eating changes, and Restlessness.

- Use the spelling sequence of a word to remember the order of items in a list. For instance, *SOAP* tells you the steps in the system for recording narrative progress notes are Survey/Subjective, Observation/Objective, Assessment, and Planning.

- Use rhythm and rhyming to recall information. For example, "*i* before *e* except after *c*" reminds you of a basic spelling rule. You can also create lyrics from information and set them to a familiar tune or make up one of your own.

- Play the sound of the word you are learning off the sound of a word you already know. For instance, the word part *later*, which means *side*, sounds like *ladder*. To remember this term, you can imagine climbing up the side of a ladder.

- Use vivid or unusual images to recall new terms. Try imagining a deck of playing cards for the term *cardi*. This means *heart*, so you might see yourself holding a handful of pulsing, bloody hearts during your card game. The more vivid and unusual the image, the better.

- Exaggerate the size of important parts of an image. For example, a motor homunculus (hoh-MUHN-kyuh-luhs) [*homin* = human, *ule* = small, *us* = structure] is an exaggerated drawing used to help you recall how much area in the brain is required for muscle control of the different parts of the body (Figure 5.1). It has a very

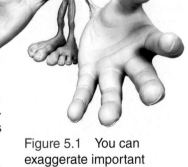

Figure 5.1   You can exaggerate important aspects of a term or image to better remember it. Which term in this chapter could you memorize by creating an exaggerated visual representation?

large tongue, lips, eyes, and hands to show that these parts use a larger area of the brain for motor control than the legs or nose. You can create an exaggerated image like the homunculus for whichever term you're trying to learn.

- Create a short scene with dramatic voices and actions to go with the information you are trying to remember, then practice acting it out. You will remember that the "brachial region" is on your arm if you hold your arm and say in a childish voice, "I breaky my arm!"

- Use humor, especially if it is shocking. This can make things very hard to forget. For example, you might think of the interesting contrast between *cleave*, which means *to cut or split apart*, and *cleavage*, which is created by pressing the breasts together.

The more strongly you can picture what you are trying to learn and associate it with something you already know, the more easily you will recall it later. Make your learning more memorable by using all of your senses as you study.

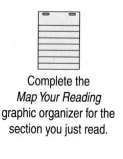

Complete the *Map Your Reading* graphic organizer for the section you just read.

RECALL YOUR READING

1. _____ devices can help students remember and organize new information.
2. Vividly connecting information with many _____ makes it easier to recall information later.
3. _____ use the first letters of each word to make a new word.
4. Use the _____ sequence of a word to remember the order of items in a list.

Medical Terminology

medical terminology
special vocabulary that is used in healthcare and is often formed from Latin and Greek word parts

Healthcare workers use a special language called **medical terminology** to communicate clearly about their patients. Understanding and using medical terminology is like speaking a foreign language. It takes effort and practice to speak another language, such as Spanish or French. You will find the same is true as you study medical terminology. Most medical terms come from Greek and Latin root words. Learning these origins may help you understand and remember terms.

All healthcare workers must be able to read, write, and understand medical terminology so they can communicate clearly with other professionals about their patients. Some healthcare workers, such as medical transcriptionists, will spend most of their day reading and writing medical terms. The ability to understand written and spoken medical terminology is essential to prevent errors at all stages of care and treatment.

Abbreviations

Abbreviations provide a shortened way to write or say medical words and phrases. You are already familiar with many abbreviations used in everyday language, such as *a.m.* and *p.m.* for morning and afternoon. Abbreviations are an important part of medical terminology. They can save time, space, and effort.

An abbreviation can be a shortened form of a word. For instance, *chemo* is a shortened way of saying *chemotherapy*. Some abbreviations are known as **acronyms**, meaning that each letter in the abbreviation stands for a word. For example, MRI is an acronym for *magnetic resonance imaging*. Sometimes each letter of an abbreviation represents a Greek or Latin word part, as in ECG, which is an abbreviation for *electrocardiography*. These abbreviations may not make sense until you understand their Latin and Greek origins.

Different medical facilities in different parts of the country may write abbreviations in different ways. Some use a period to separate lowercase letters, as in *b.i.d.* for *twice in a day*. Some use all capital letters, as in *BID*. Different facilities may or may not have lines over certain abbreviations. The abbreviation for *after* may be written as either $\overline{p}$ or *p*, depending on the facility in which you work.

Both writing messily and misreading letters and numbers that look alike can cause preventable medical errors (Figure 5.2 on the next page). Healthcare workers should be aware of and use only the abbreviations on the approved list for their facility. Never make up your own abbreviations. Use your best judgment about when abbreviations are helpful and when they should be avoided to prevent additional confusion. Always write neatly. Medical charts are a legal record and must be understandable for everyone who uses them.

Understanding Word Parts

Every language has rules that determine how it is properly written and spoken. The rules are different for each language. Medical terminology, like any other language, also follows specific rules for how words are formed, spelled, and pronounced.

A medical term is usually a combination of several word parts, like a train with many types of boxcars connected together (Figure 5.3 on the next page). Breaking down medical terms into their various parts will allow you to define many more terms than you could possibly memorize by studying them as whole words. Examples of all word parts are provided in Figure 5.4 on page 151.

A **root word** is the foundation of a medical term. It carries the term's main meaning, just as a train's boxcars hold the cargo to be delivered. It is usually a noun, such as a body part. For example, the root word *cardi* means *heart*, and the root word *pulmon* means *lung*.

Several root words may be combined in one word, like a compound word, but they need a **combining vowel** to connect them when the next root or suffix does not begin with a vowel. Think of combining vowels like couplers that hold a train's boxcars together. The most common combining vowel is *o*, but other vowels may sometimes be used. A combining vowel makes the complete term easier to pronounce. The word *cardiopulmonary* sounds smoother than *cardipulmonary* because of the letter *o* placed between the root words.

Figure 5.2 Error-Prone Abbreviations and Symbols			
Error-Prone Abbreviation or Symbol	**Intended Meaning**	**Misinterpretation**	**Solution**
l	lowercase *l*	numeral 1	Write in block letters and provide space between a word ending in *l* and a number following it.
1	numeral 1	lowercase *l*	When a quantity follows another word, place the number on the next line or provide enough space between words and numbers.
0	numeral 0	letter *o*	Use the word *zero*.
Z	letter *Z*	numeral 2	Use European-style letter (Ƶ).
7	numeral 7	numeral 1	Use European-style seven (7̶).
/	slash to separate items, meaning *per*	numeral 1	Use the word *per*.
cc	cubic centimeters (units)	numerals 00 *or* letters *oo*	Use *mL*.
HS or hs	half-strength *or* hour of sleep (bedtime)	hour of sleep (bedtime) *or* half-strength	Use the words *half-strength* or *bedtime*.
QOD	every other day	Q.D. (every day)	Use the words *every other day*.
no leading zero before a decimal point	.5 mg	5 mg (if the decimal is missed)	Write a zero to the left of the decimal when a number is less than a whole unit.
measurement abbreviations with a period following the abbreviation	mg. or mL.	period is unnecessary and could be interpreted as a number if writing is messy	Use *mg*, *mL*, or *etc*, without the period.

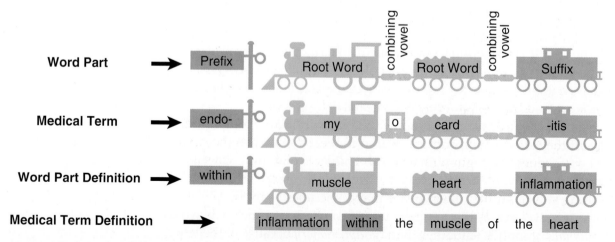

Figure 5.3   "Word trains" like these provide visuals to help you understand different parts of words.

Figure 5.4 Word Parts

Word Part	Purpose	Location	Use of Connecting Vowel	Example	Explanation
prefix	changes, adds to, or limits the meaning of the root; may tell you size, shape, color, position, or amount; is frequently a preposition or an adverb (not all words have a prefix)	beginning of the word	No connecting vowel is needed between the prefix and root word.	bi-	bi- = two bifocals = eyeglasses with two portions in each lens to adjust for both near and far vision
root word	main meaning of the word; usually a noun, such as a body part	middle of the word (or the beginning of the word if there isn't a prefix)	Drop the connecting vowel if the next word part begins with a vowel.	dent- or dento-	dent- = tooth dentist = a doctor who examines teeth and treats teeth-related health issues
suffix	changes the meaning of the root; makes the term a noun, an adjective, or a verb and tells what is being done to the root	end of the word	Use a connecting vowel if the suffix begins with a consonant.	-ology	-ology = the study of physiology = the study of nature
connecting vowel	makes it easier to pronounce the term	between word parts	When there is more than one root word, use a connecting vowel between the root words. When the suffix begins with a consonant, use a connecting vowel between the root and suffix.	-o-	musculoskeletal = muscul-**o**-skelet-al

A **prefix** [*pre* = before] appears at the beginning of a word, like a signal light in front of a train. The light tells the engineer whether to change the train's route or speed, just as the prefix can change, add to, or limit the meaning of the root word. The prefix may tell you the size, shape, color, position, or amount of the root. A combining vowel is not needed between a prefix and a root word. Not all words have a prefix.

A **suffix** appears at the end of a word, like the caboose of a train. It tells you what is being done to the root word, just as a brakeman used to ride in the train caboose to watch how the train and brakes were operating. The suffix can change the root into an adjective, a noun, or a verb. It can also add to the meaning of the root. It may identify size or describe a condition or procedure. If a suffix begins with a vowel (*a, e, i, o, u,* and sometimes *y*), it attaches directly to the root. If a suffix begins with a consonant (*b, c, d, f,* and so on), a connecting vowel is needed between the root and the suffix. All medical terms have at least one root and a suffix.

Creating a **plural** word in medical terminology does not follow the same rules as Standard English. In Standard English, the suffix *-s* or *-es* is added to show there is more than one. This is often not appropriate in medical terminology. Different plural endings are used with different Latin and Greek suffixes (Figure 5.5).

Defining medical terms is like solving a puzzle. To discover the meaning of a term, you will need to break it down into its individual parts and define each part. Define the suffix first, and then define the remaining word parts from left to right. Combine the definitions of the word parts to discover the meaning of the whole term. For example, *cardiopulmonary* can be broken into *cardi* (which means *heart*), *o* (the combining vowel), *pulmon* (which means *lung*), and *-ary* (which means *pertaining to*). Together they mean *pertaining to the heart and lung*.

Practice analyzing medical words that you see and hear. A medical dictionary will be an important tool when a term comes from a proper name, cannot be broken down, or has an unclear meaning. However, you will be able to understand the general meaning of most medical terms quickly by interpreting the word parts.

Pronunciation and Spelling

Healthcare workers also need to become comfortable reading and saying medical terms. These terms may seem hard to pronounce, especially if you haven't already heard them spoken. Many medical words have similar and sometimes confusing sounds. They may also look long

Figure 5.5 Plural Forms of Common Latin and Greek Suffixes

Ending	Singular Forms	Drop	Add	Plural Forms
-y	deformity, family	-y	-ies	deformities, families
-is	diagnosis, fibrosis	-is	-es	diagnoses, fibroses
-us	alveolus, stimulus	-us	-i	alveoli, stimuli
-um	ileum, bacterium	-um	-a	ilea, bacteria
-a	vertebra, ruga	-a	-ae	vertebrae, rugae
-ma	sarcoma, melanoma	-ma	-mata	sarcomata, melanomata
-ax	thorax, anthrax	-ax	-aces	thoraces, anthraces
-ex	cortex, index	-ex	-ices	cortices, indices
-ix	appendix, matrix	-ix	-ices	appendices, matrices
-on	spermatozoon, protozoon	-on	-a	spermatozoa, protozoa
-en	foramen, lumen	-en	-ina	foramina, lumina
-nx	larynx, pharynx	-x	-ges	larynges, pharynges
-yx	calyx	-yx	-yces	calyces

and difficult. These tips will help with pronunciation. First, break each term into its word parts. Then pronounce each word part separately. Figure 5.6 provides some basic pronunciation rules. The part of the word that appears in capital letters should be emphasized when you speak.

Although these rules will help you pronounce new terms, medical words should not be spelled by sounding them out. Some terms sound alike but are spelled differently. One letter can change the entire meaning of a body part or drug name. If you misspell a medical term, it can create confusion and may result in an incorrect diagnosis or procedure. You cannot rely on a computer to find your errors because spell-checkers may not recognize medical terminology. When you are unsure of a term's spelling or meaning, you should look up the term in a medical dictionary.

Figure 5.6 Pronunciation Rules	
Rule	**Examples**
• *c* and *g* have a soft sound (like *s* and *j*) when they appear before the letters *e, i,* and *y*	cycle (SI-kuhl) gender (JEHN-der) giant (JI-ant)
• *c* and *g* have a hard sound (like *k* and *guh*) when they appear before other letters	cranium (KRAY-nee-um) cut (KUHT) gonad (GOH-nad)
• *ch* sounds like *k* when it appears before consonants	chlorine (KLOHR-een) chronic (KRAHN-ik)
• *p* is silent at the beginning of a word when followed by the letters *s* and *n*	psychic (SI-kik) pneumonia (noo-MOH-nyuh)
• *i* sounds like *eye* when added to the end of a word to form a plural	stimuli (STIM-yoo-li) alveoli (al-VEE-oh-li)
• *ae* and *oe* sound like *ee*	coxae (kahk-SEE) amoeba (uh-MEE-buh)
• *es* is often pronounced as a separate syllable when found at the end of a word	nares (NAR-eez) stases (STAYS-eez)

RECALL YOUR READING

1. In all medical careers, it is important to understand, speak, spell, and use _____ correctly.

2. All medical terms have one or more _____ and a _____, but they may not have a _____.

3. It is important that you use only the _____ accepted by your facility.

4. _____ medical terms may not be formed by adding -*s* or -*es* to the end, as in common English words.

5. _____ rules can be used to sound out medical terms, but there may be more than one spelling for a particular sound.

Complete the *Map Your Reading* graphic organizer for the section you just read.

Body Organization and Related Medical Terms

anatomy
the physical structures or parts of the body

physiology
the functions or inner workings of the body

When healthcare workers discuss body systems, the parts of the body are its **anatomy** and how the body works is its **physiology** (fih-zee-AH-luh-jee) [*physi* = nature, *ology* = the study of]. Anatomy and physiology work together. The shape and location of a body part tells you a lot about what it does.

The anatomists who drew and studied the parts of the body hundreds of years ago spoke Greek and Latin, which explains the origins of our medical terms. Today, pathophysiologists (path-oh-fihz-ee-AHL-uh-jihsts) study *pathologies*, or diseases and disorders that occur when the body isn't functioning properly. All healthcare workers must understand anatomy and physiology so they can recognize what is normal and where a problem may exist. A medical coder's knowledge of anatomy will help them identify a code for a procedure that doesn't match the body part mentioned in the record. Many discoveries and treatments are developed by studying the body and its functions.

organelle
a part of a cell that has a specific task

Your body structures are put together in a very organized way. Each level of organization builds on the next to form a larger structure (Figure 5.7). At the smallest level are atoms, which bond together to form molecules (MAHL-uh-kyoolz). For example, hydrogen (H) and oxygen (O) atoms combine to form a molecule of water (H_2O). Groups of molecules form **organelles**, which are the structures within cells. Cells join together to form tissues. Different types of tissues work together as a body organ. A body system is a group of organs that perform a vital function in the body. All of these parts function together to form a living organism.

Molecular biologists study life at the cellular level. The information they discover about how genes, DNA, bacteria, and viruses work in a cell help healthcare professionals diagnose, prevent, and treat diseases. Biotechnology uses information about how microorganisms work to stay on the cutting edge of these types of discoveries.

The Cell and Its Organelles

cell
a small group of organelles that fulfill a specific purpose and are held together by a membrane

A **cell** is considered the smallest living thing. It is so small that it usually can't be seen without a microscope. Even though it is small, a cell is capable of performing all the activities that define life. Biologists say something is living if it can take care of its own structures, interact with its environment, grow, and reproduce. Cellular biologists study how the chemical reactions of cells can be supported or manipulated. Therefore, chemistry is very important in healthcare careers that require an understanding of how the body works. Some of the cellular structures will be covered in more detail in chapter 21.

The word *cell* comes from the Latin word *cellula*, which means "small room." You can think of each cell in your body as a room in a factory, creating a product or doing a job for that factory. Cells may have specialized roles as nerve, bone, blood, epithelial, or muscle cells. Although each room in your factory has the same basic structure and furniture, different rooms need special equipment for their specific jobs. Different types of cells also have the same basic parts, or *organelles*, but

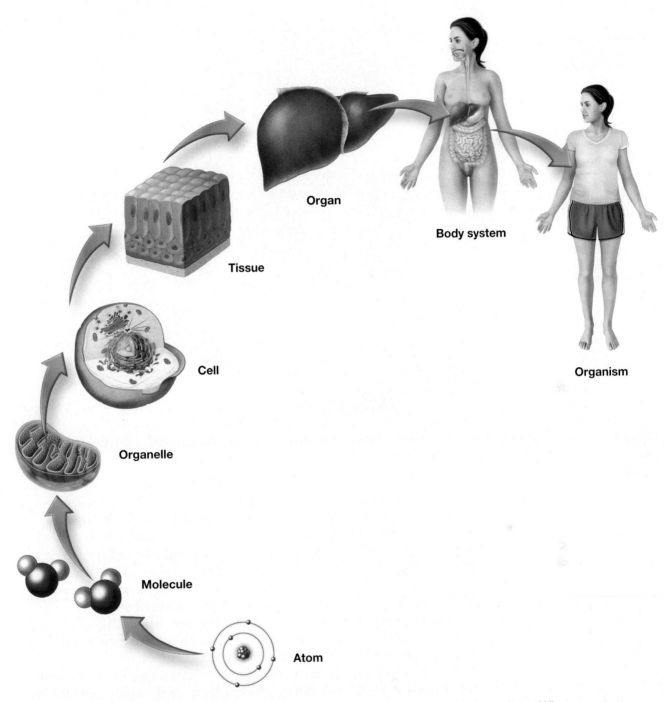

Figure 5.7 The organizational hierarchy of the body, from atom to organism, is shown here. What are some examples of organelles, organs, and body systems?

they contain different amounts and kinds of organelles depending on the cell's purpose. The anatomy or structure of a cell is closely related to its physiology, or function.

The cell's organelles can be seen as the furnishings and equipment in a factory (Figure 5.8). Every factory room needs walls for structure and protection from the environment outside, but also windows and doors to allow some things in and out. Similarly, the **cell membrane** is a semipermeable (sehm-ee-PER-mee-uh-buhl) [*semi* = half] outer covering with holes, or *pores*, that act as its doors and windows. Some

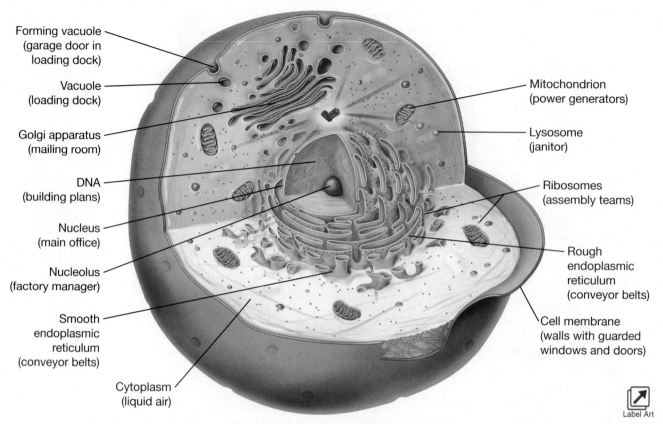

Forming vacuole
(garage door in
loading dock)

Vacuole
(loading dock)

Golgi apparatus
(mailing room)

DNA
(building plans)

Nucleus
(main office)

Nucleolus
(factory manager)

Smooth
endoplasmic
reticulum
(conveyor belts)

Cytoplasm
(liquid air)

Mitochondrion
(power generators)

Lysosome
(janitor)

Ribosomes
(assembly teams)

Rough
endoplasmic
reticulum
(conveyor belts)

Cell membrane
(walls with guarded
windows and doors)

Label Art

Figure 5.8   The parts of a cell can be compared to different parts of a factory. Choose one cell part and compare it to its corresponding factory component.

molecules can easily pass through the "security guards" at these pores; other molecules require cell energy to be carried actively through the membrane. **Vacuoles** (VAK-yu-wohlz) are like the doors of the loading dock. They allow larger enzymes and waste molecule packages to pass through the cell membrane. Fat cells have large vacuoles and not many other organelles. Cells use chemical messages to communicate about which materials need to be allowed through the membrane.

The cell membrane may have other structures that fulfill special needs. If a cell needs to be able to move, as with sperm, then it may have a flagellum (fluh-JEHL-uhm), or *tail*, as part of its cell membrane. This is like having a scooter to get around your factory. Some cells, like those of the intestines, need to absorb fluids or nutrients from the environment like a sponge. These cells have tiny hairs called cilia (SIHL-ee-ah) to increase the available surface area of their outer membrane. Just as air is contained within the walls of a factory, a semifluid **cytoplasm** (SI-toh-plaz-uhm) [*cyt* = cell, *plasm* = formation, structure] is contained within the walls of a cell. Chemical reactions take place in the cytoplasm as parts of the cell communicate and complete their work.

The **nucleus** is the factory's main office. It controls the cell's activity. The **nucleolus** (noo-KLEE-oh-luhs), located at the center of the nucleus, is the factory manager. It uses assembly teams called **ribosomes** (RI-buh-sohmz) to build proteins following the **DNA (deoxyribonucleic acid)** plans. The DNA are complete plans for items the cell builds. The nucleus interprets these directions and tells the cell what to build and when to build it. It also makes copies and produces its own new cells when needed.

Factories often use a conveyer belt to sort and transport materials for production. **Endoplasmic reticulum** (ehn-doh-PLAZ-mihk rih-TIHK-yuh-luhm) [*endo* = within, *plasm* = structure, *ic* = pertaining to, *reticulo* = network, *um* = structure], or *ER*, in the cell is like a conveyor belt on the production floor, moving construction materials (ribosomes) in and out of the nucleus as they are assembled. Rough ER is covered with ribosomes from the nucleus for building proteins. Smooth ER builds and stores fats and carbohydrates and detoxifies harmful substances. The **Golgi apparatus** (GOHL-jee ap-uh-RAT-uhs) is made up of layers of membranes in the cytoplasm that function like a mailing room. This organelle inspects, sorts, and packages proteins for use within or removal from the cell.

Cells and factories require energy to operate. Power stations provide energy to factories. **Mitochondria** (mI-toh-KAHN-dree-a) are power stations for cells. They produce adenosine triphosphate (ATP) from carbohydrates, fats, and proteins. Breaking the bonds of ATP creates energy for the cell. Muscle cells have more mitochondria than other cells because their work requires a lot of energy. After cells have used the available energy, digestive enzymes in the **lysosomes** (LI-suh-sohmz) [*lysis* = destruction] destroy used, dead, and foreign materials that are left behind, much like a factory janitor cleans up after workers.

Different types of cells have different functions, and each organelle has a different task within the cell. A cell may have more or fewer specific organelles, such as mitochondria, lysosomes, ribosomes, or cilia, depending on its job. Which organelles would you expect to find in a muscle cell? Which organelles would a liver's cells need to clean the blood, break down fat, and detoxify alcohol?

Body Tissues and Membranes

Tissue samples and analysis provide important information to healthcare professionals. If a doctor suspects a disease such as cancer, she may do a biopsy, obtaining a tissue sample to examine under a microscope. Histologists [*hist* = tissue, *ologist* = specialist in the study of] work with pathologists, studying these tissues to determine the cause and treatment of a disease.

tissue
a group of cells of the same type working together for the same purpose

There are four main types of tissues, and all four are found throughout the body:

- *Connective tissue* includes cartilage, bones, body fat, and blood. This tissue is important for providing support, absorbing shock, and storing and transporting nutrients.

- *Nervous tissue* conducts impulses to and from body organs.

- *Muscular tissue* is important for movement.

- *Epithelial tissue* forms the skin that covers the outside of the body, as well as the membranes that cover the organs and line body cavities. This tissue forms a protective covering, allows the absorption of nutrients, helps to filter harmful substances out of the blood, and forms secretions.

Body Organs and Systems

organ
a distinct body structure made of different tissues working together for the same purpose

body system
a group of organs working together to perform a vital function in the body

Groups of tissues working together form **organs**. Each organ performs specific bodily functions. For example, the heart pumps blood and the vessels carry blood to all parts of the body. Groups of organs work together as **body systems**, such as the circulatory system. Different medical professions may specialize in the study of specific organs and systems. A cardiologist studies the heart and cardiovascular system. An oncologist studies cancers of the blood and other tissues. Internal medicine doctors study multiple body systems and their interaction. In health informatics, a medical coder looks up surgical procedures by body system and subcategorizes them by the specific organ.

Body systems work together as part of a complete organism (the human body) to control, move, support, protect, and reproduce. The human body systems are listed with their major organs and functions in Figure 5.9. The table also tells you which future chapters contain detailed information for each system. The acronym *SLIC MEN R RED* will help you to remember the names of the systems.

The tasks of the body systems often overlap, and some organs belong to more than one system. For example, the pancreas is part of both the digestive and endocrine systems. Some systems, such as the musculoskeletal system (muscles and bones), combine body parts that depend on each other so they can be studied together. All cells, organs, and body systems work together to keep your body healthy and maintain

Figure 5.9 Body Systems			
Body System	**Major Organs**	**Major Functions**	**Chapter**
Skeletal	bones, ligaments	support, protection	9
Lymphatic (immune)	lymph nodes, tonsils, thymus, spleen	fluid return, immunity	13
Integumentary	skin, hair, nails	protection	9
Cardiovascular	heart, blood, vessels	transportation	13
Muscular	muscles, tendons	movement	9
Endocrine	glands, hormones	body communication and control	21
Nervous and special senses	brain, spinal cord, nerves, nose, mouth, ears, eyes, skin	body communication and control	21
Respiratory	pharynx, trachea, bronchi, lungs, alveoli, diaphragm	gas exchange	13
Reproductive	ovaries, uterus, fallopian tubes, testes, vas deferens, prostate	offspring production	17
Excretory (urinary)	kidneys, ureters, bladder, urethra	waste filtration	17
Digestive	stomach, liver, pancreas, intestines, colon	nutrient breakdown and absorption	17

a constant state of balance, or homeostasis (hoh-mee-oh-STAY-sihs) [*homeo* = same, *stasis* = stopping, controlling]. Diseases and disorders disturb this delicate balance.

Comparisons are a good learning tool because they help you organize and combine new information with ideas that are already familiar to you. The organizational structure of the human body, for example, can be compared to building a house (Figure 5.10 on the next page). When constructing a house, you need to begin with some basic building materials. The wood and nails you use to build the walls of a house are like the cells that make up body tissues. You need different types of body tissues to make body organs, just as the builder needs different kinds of wood, stone, and tile to make floors, counters, and walls. The fireplace, chimney, and vent of a house's heating system are like the lungs, bronchi, and trachea of your respiratory system. Just as the parts of the heating system work together for a common purpose, so do the organs of each body system.

The structural, plumbing, air conditioning, and electrical systems in a house can be compared to the skeletal, circulatory, respiratory, and nervous systems of the human body. Both a house and the human body need all of their systems to work together to provide a comfortable living environment. What other connections can you see between the organization of the body and the structures that form a house? Can you think of a different comparison?

Body Directions

Whether looking at a patient's body, writing about it in a medical chart, or coding patient information for the insurance company, all healthcare workers must use the same terms and points of reference. Medical examiners, surgeons, and medical illustrators all study the human body from the **standard anatomical position (SAP)**. When a cadaver (kuh-DAV-er)—a dead body—lies on the examination table for anatomical study, it is face up with the arms out to the side and palms facing up.

Directional terms are used to describe parts of the body or their position in reference to SAP. These terms usually occur in pairs with opposite meanings:

- **Anterior** [*ante* = front, before, *ior* = more toward] is the front side of the body; **posterior** [*poster/o* = back, behind, after] is the back. You can see the anterior view by looking in the mirror, but you need the reflection of another mirror to see the posterior.

- **Medial** [*med* = middle, *al* = pertaining to] refers to a point closer to the center of the body, while **lateral** [*later* = side] is toward the side. Men's clothing usually buttons and zips at the midline, but some women's clothing zips laterally at the hip.

- **Superior** [*super* = above, upon] means above or higher up on the body; **inferior** [*infer* = below] means lower down. The shoulders are superior to the hips but inferior to the ears.

- Sometimes we use more specific terms, such as **cranial** [*crani* = skull] to talk about a point closer to the head and **caudal** [*caud* = tail] for a point closer to the tailbone.

standard anatomical position (SAP)
the agreed-upon reference for body position when studying anatomy; standing erect on two legs, facing frontward, with the arms at the sides and palms facing forward

Figure 5.10 Comparing House Structure to Body Structure

House Diagram	House Structure Examples	Body Structure Examples	Body Diagram
	Building Materials	**Cells**	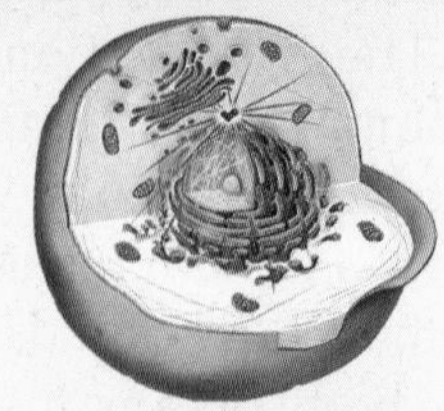
	nail	bone cell	
	wood stud	muscle cell	
	brick	skin cell	
	shingle		
	Groups of Materials	**Tissues**	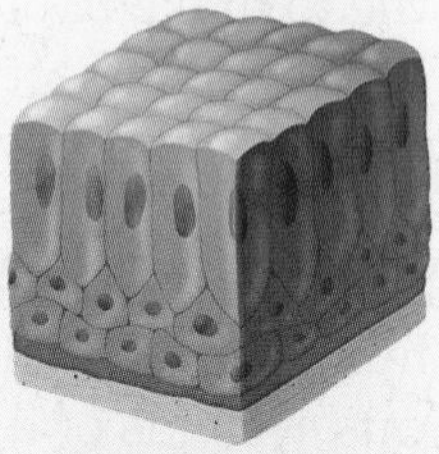
	wood rafters	connective tissue	
	wood flooring	muscular tissue	
	brick siding	epithelial tissue	
	roofing materials		
	Basic Structures	**Organs**	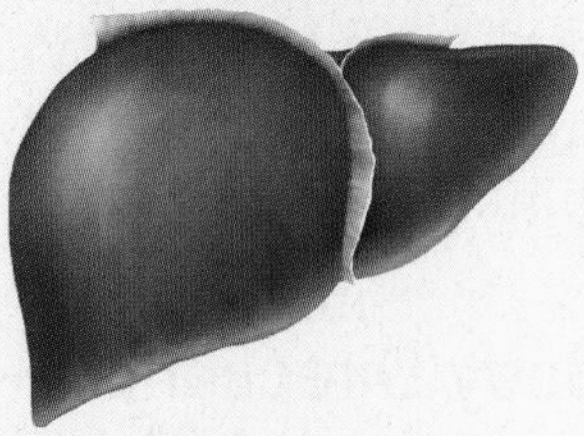
	walls	bones	
	floors	ligaments	
	counters	heart	
	air conditioner	blood vessels	
	fireplace	lungs	
	chimney vent	trachea	
		skin	
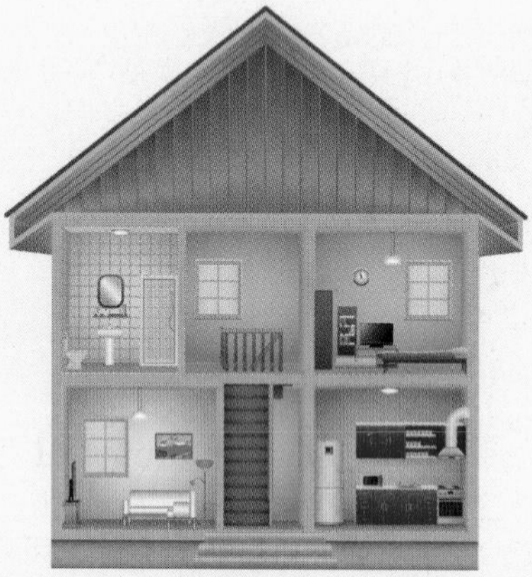	**Structural System**	**Body System**	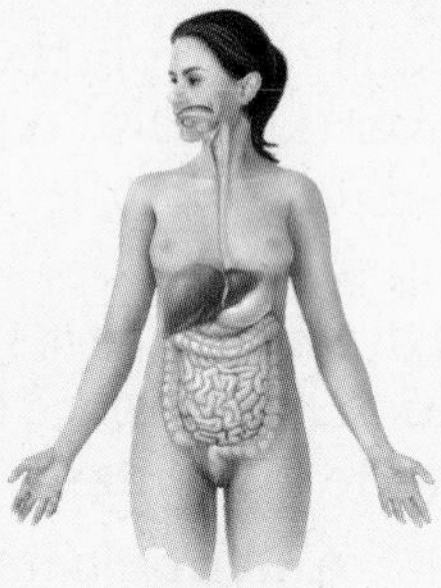
	plumbing system	skeletal system	
	air conditioning system	circulatory system	
	electrical system	respiratory system	
		nervous system	
	Structure	**Organism**	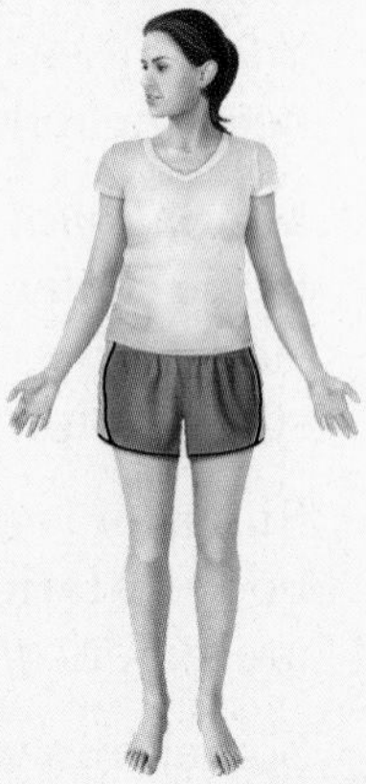
	house	human being	

- **Superficial** refers to the outside surface of the body, as opposed to **deep** tissues, which are farther below the surface. The heart is deep in the chest, and the ribs are more superficial.

- Left and right are labeled from the patient's perspective; the patient's right side is on your left.

Consider the differences and similarities of these directional terms for a two-legged creature compared to a four-legged creature (Figure 5.11). Which directional terms best describe the spine of a dog?

Descriptions of appendages (limbs) are based on their point of attachment to the body. For example, your arm is attached to your body at the shoulder, your hand is attached at the wrist, and your lower leg is attached at the knee. **Proximal** [*proxim* = near] indicates that the part being discussed is closer to the point of attachment, while **distal** [*dis* = apart] refers to a part that is farther away from the attachment site. As shown in Figure 5.12 on the next page, the proximal end of the humerus (a bone in your upper arm) is near the shoulder, and the distal end is at the elbow. The terms *proximal* and *distal* can also be used to describe internal organs. Like other terms based on SAP, these descriptions remain the same regardless of movement or repositioning of the body.

While the terms *anterior* and *ventral* as well as *posterior* and *dorsal* are frequently used interchangeably, there are specific differences in their meanings and uses. The terms *anterior* and *posterior* are used to describe the front and back of the body. The terms *ventral* [*ventr* = front] and *dorsal* [*dors* = back] describe body surfaces according to the way that joints flex.

Ventral (VEHN-truhl) surfaces move closer together when you bend a joint. They are generally lighter in color than dorsal surfaces and are often on the front side of the body. Try bending your arm at the elbow and you will see that the lighter-colored, ventral surfaces of your inner arm move toward each other. **Dorsal** (DOR-suhl) surfaces are located on the back of the body. They often receive the most sun, making them darker or hairier

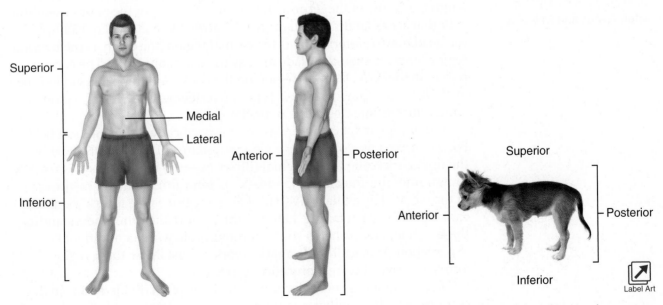

Figure 5.11   Directional terms usually come in pairs that have opposite meanings. What pairs of terms do you see in this figure? How are they opposite?

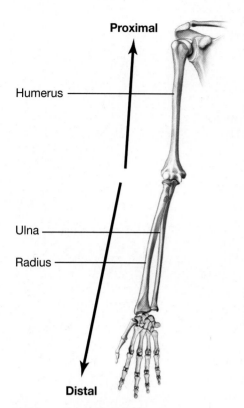

Proximal

Humerus

Ulna

Radius

Distal

Figure 5.12   Proximal means close to the site of attachment. Distal means farther away from the site of attachment.

body region
an area of the body with a specific name, which is used as a point of reference when discussing anatomy

than ventral surfaces. The backside of the upper and lower arm is dorsal. These surfaces move away from each other as the elbow is bent.

The legs on the human forms in Figure 5.13 illustrate the differences between the terms *ventral* and *dorsal* as opposed to *anterior* and *posterior*. When the knee is bent, the two lighter, ventral surfaces pulled toward each other are on the backside of the legs. The back of the legs are posterior by position, but they are ventral based on the way they move. The surfaces of the legs turned to the front in SAP are anterior by position, but they are dorsal based on the way they move. The hip joints of a human rotate the dorsal side of the legs toward the front to support us in a standing position.

You can see the difference between humans and four-legged animals in Figure 5.13. If you rub the belly of a dog, you will notice that the light coloring of its ventral underbelly carries over onto the ventral inside of its legs. If a person lies on his or her back like a dog and lets his or her legs relax and roll out to the sides, the lighter (ventral) surface of the person's legs will also rotate more toward the front side of their body. When they stand on two legs, these ventral surfaces will rotate in toward the back of the body.

Body Regions and Sections

When a patient complains of pain, healthcare workers need an easy way to communicate with each other about the different areas of the patient's body where the pain may be. This is why the medical community has given names to different **body regions**. These names provide a common language so you can easily refer to different areas on the surface of the body.

Some of these terms, such as *abdomen* and *calf*, are part of our everyday language. Many of the terms come from the names of the bones under the skin that act as landmarks and give the areas their shape. For example, the head may be referred to as the cranial region, the thigh as the femoral region, and the shoulder blade area as the scapular region. The cervical region in the neck, thoracic region on the chest, and lumbar region of the lower back are named for their types of vertebrae. The gluteal region is named for the muscles of the buttocks.

Other regional terms are used more specifically in the medical field. For example, a nurse wraps the blood pressure cuff around the part of the upper arm called the brachial (BRAY-kee-uhl) region. Blood is usually drawn from the antecubital (an-tee-KYU-bih-tuhl) region on the inside of the elbow. The axillary (AK-suh-lair-ee) region is the term a medical assistant uses when taking a temperature under the arm. Understanding these regional terms helps you to communicate without additional explanation. The health informatics worker must know these regional terms to arrive at correct procedural codes.

The abdomen is such a large area that it is often divided into smaller sections, which are either quadrants or regions (Figure 5.14). This helps healthcare professionals focus on which abdominal organs may be involved when a patient complains of abdominal pain. One method of

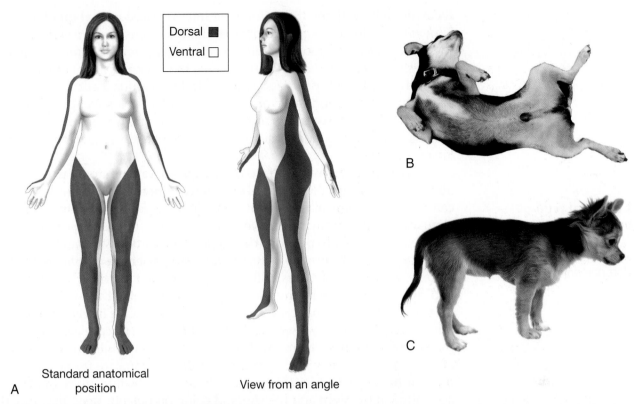

Dorsal ■
Ventral □

A   Standard anatomical position

View from an angle

B

C

Figure 5.13   Figure A shows that, in SAP, the fronts of the legs are anterior by position but dorsal based on how they move. The backs of the legs are posterior by position but ventral based on movement. The view from an angle shows the division between dorsal and ventral surfaces, which is hidden in the view from standard anatomical position. Figures B and C show the ventral and dorsal surfaces on a four-legged animal as opposed to a two-legged human.

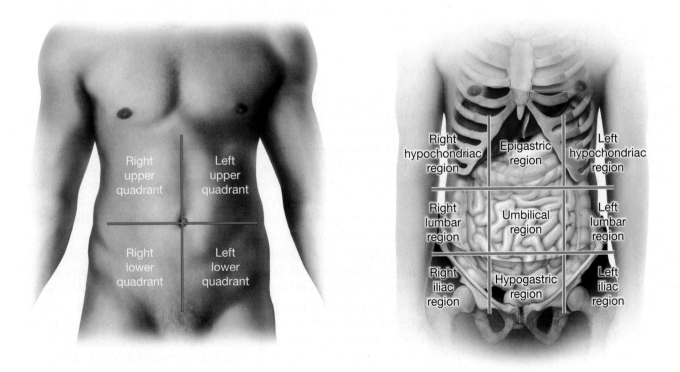

Right upper quadrant

Left upper quadrant

Right lower quadrant

Left lower quadrant

Right hypochondriac region

Epigastric region

Left hypochondriac region

Right lumbar region

Umbilical region

Left lumbar region

Right iliac region

Hypogastric region

Left iliac region

Figure 5.14   The abdomen can be divided into quadrants or regions. How might healthcare professionals use these quadrants and regions?

focusing in is to divide the abdomen it into four **abdominal quadrants** [*abdomin* = abdomen, *quad* = four] with the umbilicus, or *belly button*, at the center. Each of these quadrants contains just a few abdominal organs. The right upper quadrant (RUQ) contains the liver and gallbladder. The stomach, spleen, and pancreas lie in the left upper quadrant (LUQ). The appendix is a common cause of complaint in the right lower quadrant (RLQ), while the descending and sigmoid colon are in the lower left quadrant (LLQ). The small intestines are spread across the right and left lower quadrants.

A more detailed method is to divide the abdomen into nine **abdominal regions**, like a tic-tac-toe board, with the umbilicus at the center of the umbilical region. The epigastric region [*epi* = upon, *gastr* = stomach, *ic* = pertaining to] above it houses most of the stomach and pancreas. The right hypochondriac region [*hypo* = below, *chondr* = cartilage, *ac* = pertaining to] refers to the area under the cartilage of the ribcage, which contains the gallbladder and part of the liver, intestines, and right kidney. The left hypochondriac region holds the spleen and parts of the stomach, pancreas, colon, and left kidney. The right and left lumbar regions [*lumb* = lower back, loins] below the ribcage are named for the nearby lumbar vertebrae and contain parts of the intestines, kidneys, and colon. Below them, the right and left iliac regions are framed by the iliac bones of the hips. These regions contain the intestines and the appendix on the right and the sigmoid colon on the left. Keep in mind, the patient's right is your left! The hypogastric region [*hypo* = below, *gastr* = stomach, *ic* = pertaining to] is well below the stomach and includes the bladder, uterus (in females), and part of the small intestines.

These points of reference are helpful when a patient complains of abdominal pain. What organs would you expect to be coding treatments for if the progress notes indicated sharp pains in the patient's right iliac region?

Body Cavities

The interior of the body is divided into **body cavities** that contain the vital organs (Figure 5.15). Each body cavity is separated by a membrane that covers and protects the organs within. They are also protected by bones. The **ventral cavity** in the front is surrounded by the ribs and pelvic bones. The **dorsal cavity** in the back is protected by the bones of the skull and vertebrae. There are also smaller sinus, orbital, oral, and nasal cavities in the head.

The diaphragm muscle separates the ventral cavity into the **thoracic** [*thorac* = chest] **cavity** above and the **abdominopelvic** [*abdomino* = abdomen, *pelv* = pelvis, hip region] **cavity** below. This separation helps to prevent infections from moving from one part of the body to another. The thoracic cavity includes the pericardial [*peri* = around, *cardi* = heart] cavity for the heart, surrounded by two pleural (PLOOR-uhl) [*pleur* = side, rib] cavities for the lungs. The abdominopelvic cavity includes the abdominal cavity for the digestive organs and the pelvic cavity that houses the reproductive organs, bladder, and rectum. The peritoneum (pair-ih-toh-NEE-um) is a membrane that separates the abdominal and pelvic cavities along an imaginary line from the top of the iliac bones of the hips down to the pelvic bone.

abdominal region
one of nine equal areas of the abdomen that are named and used as reference points when discussing the body

body cavity
a hollow space within the body that is lined by a membrane and contains bodily organs

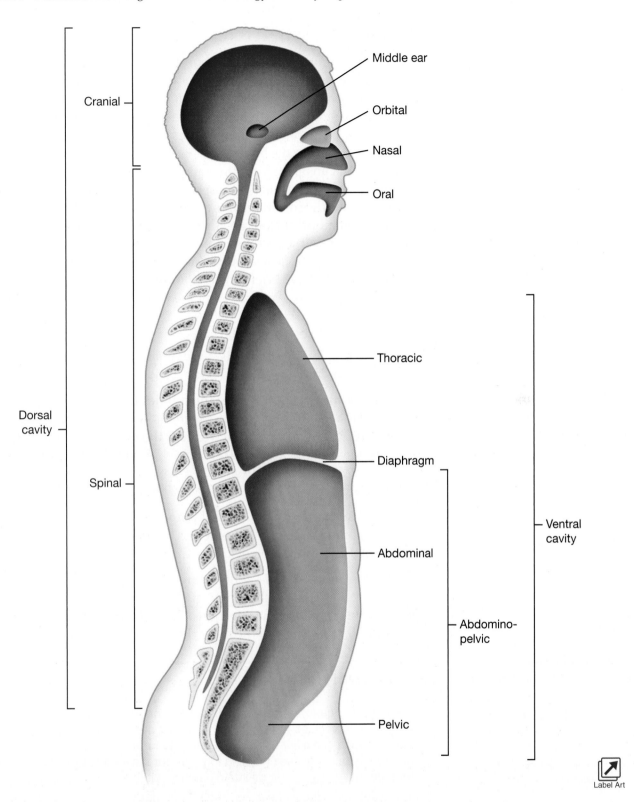

Figure 5.15   The interior of the body is divided into cavities that are separated by membranes. Which cavities are included in the head?

The dorsal cavity contains the **cranial cavity** for the brain and the **spinal cavity** for the spinal cord. In addition to the bony protection these cavities provide to the skull and vertebrae, they are lined by a membrane called the *meninges* (meh-NIHN-jeez).

Body Planes

Some medical professionals cut into the body with scalpels for surgery or dissection [*dis* = apart, *sect* = to cut, *ion* = action of]. Others use imaging technology to see inside the body without cutting it open. Body dissection and imaging technology both allow us to see the inside of the body in flat sections, or **body planes**. These planes help us refer more precisely to different points within the body.

If you look at an apple from the outside, you can only see the peel and overall shape. If you slice the apple from the top down through the core, you will see the inside, with the core down the middle and the seeds and flesh on each side of the core. If you had sliced the apple horizontally across the middle, you would have seen the core at the center, encircled by its seeds, and the apple flesh around that—a very different view.

Just as you can get a different view of the inside of an apple by cutting it in different directions, you can view the inside of a body along different planes, depending on what you are trying to see (Figure 5.16). The direction of the cut determines the name of the body plane:

- The **frontal plane**, also called the *coronal plane*, divides the body (or organ) into its front and back sections.

- The **sagittal** (SAJ-iht-uhl) **plane** divides the body, organ, or appendage into right and left sections. You can make a sagittal cut at various points along the width of the body. When the body is divided exactly down the midline, this is called the **midsagittal plane**. Zippers and buttons often appear on the midsagittal line. A midsagittal view of the head shows the different lobes of the brain.

- The **transverse** [*trans* = across] **plane** divides the body into top and bottom sections. It cuts across the body, perpendicular to the frontal and sagittal planes.

- Each section, or *plane*, shows different angles of different organs. Medical imaging technicians must be able to recognize the organs from different directions. These workers also know how superficial or deep in the body the organs are located.

body plane
a flat or level surface seen by cutting away part of the body through surgery or medical imaging to serve as a point of reference when discussing anatomy

Complete the *Map Your Reading* graphic organizer for the section you just read.

RECALL YOUR READING

1. Anatomy is organized in a hierarchy. Atoms bond to form molecules. Groups of molecules form _____, which are the basic structures of cells. Groups of similar cells join together to form _____. _____ are different types of tissues working together for the same purpose. They work together as _____ to maintain balance within the body.

2. Terms for body directions are based on standard _____ position, in which a person is standing erect, facing forward, with the arms at the sides and palms facing forward.

3. Abdominal _____ and _____ regions are two different ways of referring to areas of the belly.

4. Vital organs are protected inside _____ by membranes and bones.

5. Medical imaging views structures inside the body in flat _____.

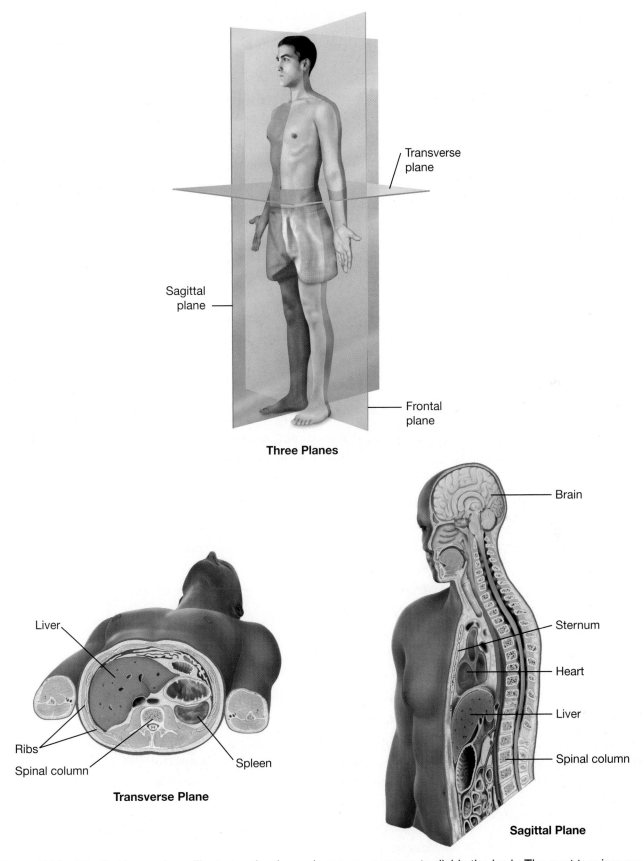

Three Planes

Transverse Plane

Sagittal Plane

Figure 5.16   The first image here illustrates the three planes you can use to divide the body. The next two images show cross-sections of two of those planes. Cutting along these planes allows you to view different organs and internal matter. What would you expect to see in the frontal cross-section of the figure above?

SUMMARY

Assess your understanding with chapter tests

- It is important to understand, speak, spell, and use medical terminology correctly in all medical careers.

- Medical terms are formed from Latin and Greek word parts.

- Abbreviations are a shortened way of writing medical terms. It is important that you only use the abbreviations approved by your facility.

- Plural forms of medical terms may not be formed in the same way as the plurals of common English words.

- Rules of pronunciation are helpful for sounding out medical terms, but you shouldn't spell medical terms based on how they sound.

- Mnemonic devices help you memorize new information.

- Anatomy refers to the parts of the body, while physiology refers to how the body works.

- Your body structures are built in an organized way, from atoms to a complete organism.

- Terms for body directions are based on standard anatomical position and are used to describe a body structure or its position.

- Body regions, such as abdominal quadrants and abdominal regions, provide a common set of terms for referring to areas of the body.

- Body cavities contain vital organs and are protected by membranes and bones.

- Body planes divide the body into sections to show structures inside the body.

MAXIMIZE YOUR PROFESSIONAL VOCABULARY

 Build vocabulary with e-flash cards, games, and audio glossary

Listed below are the essential, yellow-highlighted terms and the additional professional vocabulary terms that you encountered in this chapter. Complete the activities that follow the list to make all of these terms part of your everyday professional vocabulary.

abdominal quadrant	distal	plural
abdominal region	dorsal	posterior
abdominopelvic cavity	dorsal cavity	prefix
acronyms	endoplasmic reticulum (ER)	proximal
anatomy	frontal plane	ribosomes
anterior	Golgi apparatus	root word
body cavity	inferior	sagittal plane
body plane	lateral	spinal cavity
body region	lysosomes	standard anatomical position (SAP)
body system	medial	
caudal	medical terminology	suffix
cell	midsagittal plane	superficial
cell membrane	mitochondria	superior
combining vowel	mnemonic device	thoracic cavity
cranial	nucleolus	tissue
cranial cavity	nucleus	transverse plane
cytoplasm	organ	vacuole
deep	organelle	ventral
deoxyribonucleic acid (DNA)	physiology	ventral cavity

Matching. Match each essential term from this chapter with the correct definition below by writing the letter of the definition next to the number of the essential term on a separate sheet of paper.

1. body plane
2. medical terminology
3. abdominal region
4. body system
5. anatomy
6. cell
7. tissue
8. standard anatomical position
9. organelle
10. body region
11. physiology
12. mnemonic device
13. organ
14. body cavity

a. a group of similar cells working together for the same purpose

b. special vocabulary that is used in healthcare and is often formed from Latin and Greek word parts

c. a hollow space within the body that is lined by a membrane and contains bodily organs

d. a distinct body structure made of different tissues working together for the same purpose

e. an area of the body with a specific name, which is used as a reference point when discussing anatomy

f. one of nine equal areas of the abdomen

g. a small group of organelles that fulfill a specific purpose and are held together by a membrane

h. the functions or inner workings of the body

i. a learning tool that helps students memorize information

j. the agreed-upon reference for body position when studying anatomy

k. a part of a cell that has a specific task

l. the physical structures or parts of the body

m. a flat or level surface seen by cutting away part of the body through surgery or medical imaging

n. a group of organs working together to perform a vital function in the body

15. Make flash cards for each of the medical word parts listed in this table, placing the word part on one side of the card and its definition and a visual aid on the other side. When you have your completed set of flash cards, follow the directions listed on the next page to play the Word Train Game.

Word Parts				
Prefix	**Root Word**		**Suffix**	
ante-	abdomin/o	lumb/o	-ac	-ologist
dis-	cardi/o	med/o	-al	-ology
endo-	caud/o	pelv/o	-cyte	-plasm
epi-	chondr/o	physi/o	-ic	-stasis
hypo-	crani/o	plasm/o	-ion	-ule
infer-	cyt/o	pleur/o	-ior	-um
peri-	dors/o	poster/o	-lysis	-us
pre-	gastr/o	proxim/o		
quad-	hist/o	reticul/o		
semi-	home/o	sect/o		
super-	homin/o	thorac/o		
trans-	infer/o	ventr/o		
	later/o			

- The first player chooses a root word and a suffix and/or prefix card from his or her deck to form a medical term. The player lays the cards down with the word parts facing up, says the medical term that was created, and defines it.

- The next player must place a word part card on top of a word part that is already showing, then read the new term and define it.

- If a definition is challenged by other players, the cards are turned over and a definition is formed. If the definition was wrong, all of the cards on the table go to the hand of the person who defined the term incorrectly. If the definition is correct, all cards go to the challenger's hand.

- Play begins again with the next player placing a root word, suffix, and/or prefix card on the table and defining the new term. Players may not place an identical card on top of a card that is already displayed.

- The object of the game is to get rid of as many cards as possible. Players may only "pass" if they are unable to make a word with their current cards, or if they only have cards identical to those on the table. The game ends when no more words can be made. The player with the fewest cards left at the end of the game is the winner.

16. Choose a term from the list on page 168 to study. Create a poster for the term that includes its definition, a synonym, an antonym, another term with the same root, a sentence using the term, and a picture that helps you understand the term. If there is not a true antonym for the term, substitute a term that might be confused with the term you chose.

REFLECT ON YOUR READING

17. Review your sorted word list from the *Connect with Your Reading* activity at the beginning of the chapter. Make changes to your organization based on what you learned and remember from your reading of the chapter.

BUILD CORE SKILLS

18. **Critical Thinking.** Explain how nonstandard abbreviations could have a negative effect on the patient, the workers in your healthcare facility, and the workers in other healthcare facilities who receive your records.

19. **Critical Thinking.** Review the requirements a biologist uses to define a living thing. What evidence did you find in the chapter section on the cell to support the fact that a cell is alive?

20. **Writing.** Type the following paragraph into a word processor. Correct any errors found by the spell-check feature.

All patience complained of stomach pane. The gastrenterologist noted stomach distention in every patient examined. The CNA reported that the patients complained of nawzea. Lab tests were ordered to confirm a diagnosis.

a. What problems were corrected?

b. What problems were missed?

c. What problems were created?

21. **Reading.** Research the work of three of the following people who made important discoveries about the human cell. What were their roles in forming our current understanding of the cell? Be prepared to share your information with the class.

a. Robert Hooke

b. Anton Van Leeuwenhoek

c. Rudolf Virchow

d. Theodor Schwann

e. Camillo Golgi

f. James Watson and Francis Crick

ACTIVATE YOUR LEARNING

22. Build the following "edible cell" model or create a model using different edible materials. Then answer the questions below.

- cell membrane—slice of bread with the crust left on

- cytoplasm—honey

- nucleus and nucleolus—sucker or lollipop with the stick cut off

- vacuoles—small pretzel twists

- lysosomes—black jelly beans

- mitochondria—gummy bears

- endoplasmic reticulum—fruit leather cut and unrolled into long, thin strips

- ribosomes—sprinkles

- Golgi apparatus—gummy worms

a. Explain how each of the edible cell parts looks like or represents the organelles of a cell.

b. If you add a few more gummy bears, what type of cell would this be?

c. If you add a few more black jellybeans, how does the cell's function change?

23. Create a model of a person using a pickle or snack cake for the body, a marshmallow for the head, and toothpicks for arms and legs. Perform the following steps of an autopsy. Use the professional vocabulary you learned in this chapter to describe the body regions, directions, and planes as you write up the death report.

a. For the gross assessment, examine the body surface. Note the location, size, shape, and color of any unusual markings. Draw an anterior and posterior view of the victim and mark the location of your findings.

b. Weigh and measure the victim.

c. Open the ventral body cavity with a deep, Y-shaped incision (see below). The arms of the Y should start at the anterior surface of the shoulders (A) and join at the inferior point of the sternum (B) to form a single cut that extends to the pubic area (C). Perform medial to lateral incisions from the umbilical area and down both sides (D) to open the abdominal cavity.

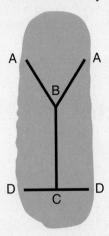

d. Open the thoracic cavity to examine the "internal organs." Weigh and measure them. Describe your findings, noting any abnormalities.

e. Decide on a cause of death and describe how your findings support that conclusion.

24. Trace a gingerbread man cookie cutter or draw the outline of a person with the arms and legs out to the sides. Draw a face and hair to show the front side and back side. Cut out the shape. Color the ventral surfaces on the front and back in green. Color the dorsal surfaces on the front and back in red. Add labels for ventral and dorsal on both the front and back sides.

THINK AND ACT LIKE A HEALTHCARE WORKER

25. Suppose that you are an internal medicine doctor. Your patient is complaining of a stomachache. What locations would you examine based on your patient's complaint? Use professional vocabulary from this chapter in your description.

26. Suppose you hear or see a new term at work. List three different steps you can take to increase your understanding of this term.

GO TO THE SOURCE

27. Search the Internet for "stem cell research articles for high school students." Find an article that interests you and print it out. Then follow the steps listed here.

a. Prepare for your reading by checking the source—who wrote the article? Why would this person be a qualified source on this topic? Who is the intended audience for this article?

b. After reading the article title and subheadings, predict what you anticipate to learn from the article.

c. Read the article. Then reread the article and underline any words that relate to or describe cells. Finally, read the article again and highlight main ideas about stem cell research.

d. Review the underlined and highlighted material, looking for common themes or ideas. Use the template below to write a paragraph summarizing the article.

In the article _____ (title), _____ (author) discusses _____ (main topic of the article). This information will be used in the future to _____.

Unit 2
Therapeutic

Chapter 6
Career Skills in Therapeutic Services

Chapter 7
Fundamental Skills in Therapeutic Services

Chapter 8
Professional Knowledge in Therapeutic Services

Chapter 9
Academic Knowledge: Body Systems for Support and Movement

While studying, look for the online icon to:
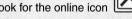

Companion
G-W Learning

- **Listen** to the audio Glossary and review e-flash cards
- **Assess** learning with quizzes and online exercises
- **Expand** knowledge with animations and activities
- **Simulate** healthcare tasks and employability skills

www.g-wlearning.com/healthsciences

Mobile
G-W Learning

Study on the Go
Use your mobile device to practice vocabulary and assess learning

www.m.g-wlearning.com

Career Pathway

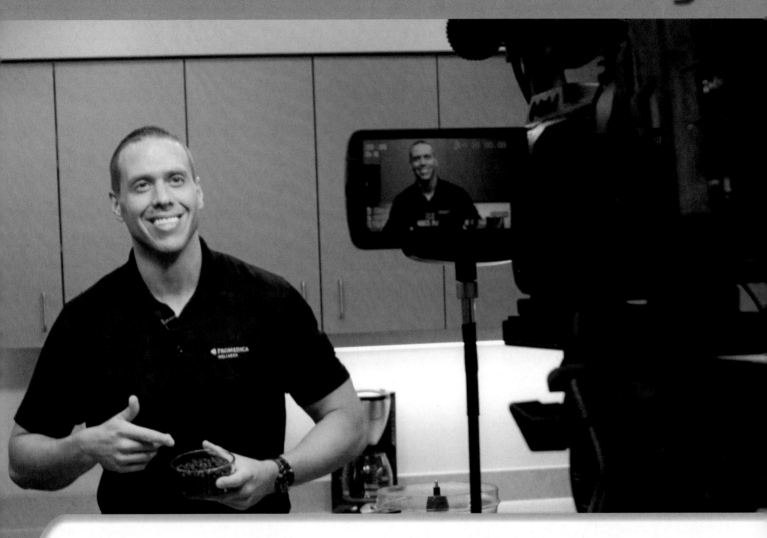

Healthcare Insider:

Nathan Drendel, M.S., R.D., L.D.
ProMedica's Wellness Dietitian

"When people hear I'm a dietitian, they always think I'm in the hospital telling people what to eat. In reality, I have such an amazingly unique job that it's hard to explain. Being a Wellness Dietitian means I get to test recipes and try to improve them, but also film cooking and educational videos and provide educational lectures. I'm able to counsel individuals to help them achieve their nutritional and wellness goals. My work days are never the same, which is just another perk of my job. Being in the role of a "proactive dietitian" rather than a "reactive dietitian" means I get to help people prevent nutritional issues before they progress to serious health issues."

Chapter 6
Career Skills in Therapeutic Services

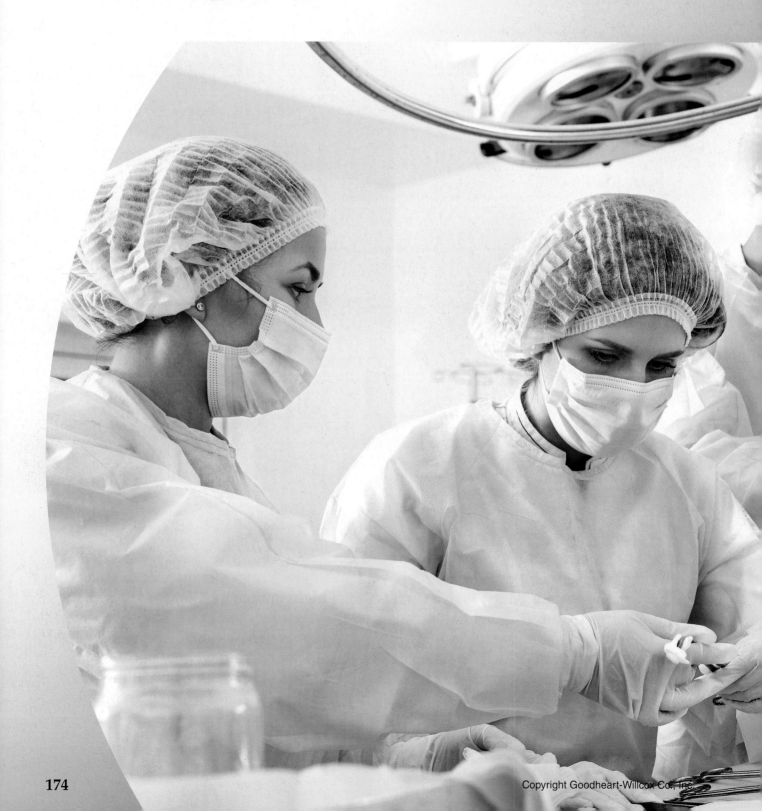

PROFESSIONAL VOCABULARY

 E-flash Cards

You will need to learn the essential terms listed below before you begin your reading. These terms will help you understand the main concepts of the chapter. These terms, which will be highlighted in yellow within the text, will become part of your professional vocabulary.

In addition to these essential terms, you will see bold terms throughout the chapter. The meanings of these terms are explained where the terms first appear. The bold terms, like the essential terms listed here, will also become part of your professional vocabulary and deepen your understanding of the topics presented.

clinical training term that describes hands-on work with patients that students do under the supervision of a licensed healthcare provider

collaborate to work together; to consult with each other

cover letter a message sent with a résumé to introduce the job applicant and give the reasons he or she is applying for a particular job

delegate to direct another healthcare worker to perform a care task that is within that worker's training and experience and within the scope of practice of the licensed provider giving the direction

empathy the ability to identify with another person's feelings and thoughts

interview etiquette accepted appearance and behavior for the interview process

multidisciplinary healthcare team a group of healthcare workers from different healthcare specialties, each providing specific services to the patient

personal protective equipment (PPE) equipment such as gloves, masks, gowns, respirators, and eyewear worn to protect skin, clothing, and the respiratory tract from infectious agents

postgraduate term that describes education and training completed after receiving a bachelor's degree

range of motion (ROM) the full extent of movement for a joint

residents (1) individuals living in long-term care facilities; (2) medical school graduates who are completing the last portion of their medical training before becoming licensed physicians

standard precautions steps that a healthcare worker takes with all patients to prevent the spread of infection

tact the ability to communicate difficult or embarrassing information without giving offense

technical training education lasting two years or less and leading to an industry certificate, a technical diploma, or an associate's degree

therapeutic term that describes treatment given to maintain or restore health

CONNECT WITH YOUR READING

Make a list of the first 10 healthcare occupations that come to mind. As you read this chapter, take note of how many jobs on your list are therapeutic services careers. The therapeutic services pathway includes the largest number of healthcare careers. Since these workers focus on treating patients, they are the people you most often meet when you receive care.

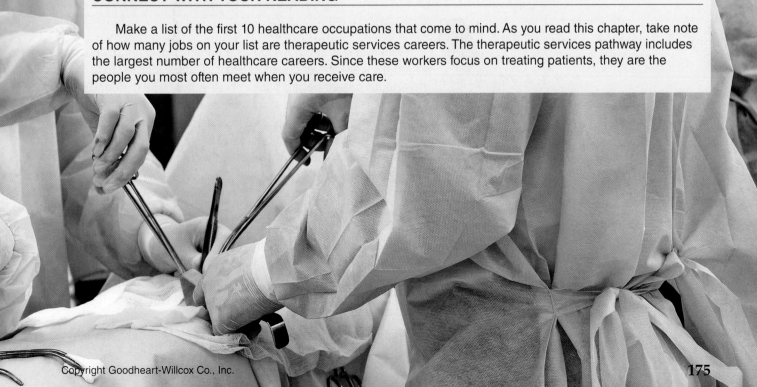

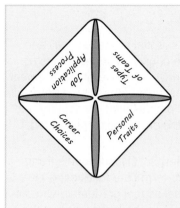

MAP YOUR READING

Create a visual summary of this chapter, just as you did in chapter 2. Begin with a square sheet of paper—an 8½-inch square works well. Fold each of the four points of the square to the center. Label each of the four resulting flaps with one of these topics: *Personal Traits*, *Career Choices*, *Types of Teams*, and *Job Application Process*. When you finish reading each of these sections in the chapter, open the corresponding flap and draw a picture or symbol to illustrate what you have read. Ask yourself what each topic looks like, how you could draw it, and what graphic or symbol best represents it. Finally, for each of the four topics, write two words that explain how the topic relates to you personally in the center square of your visual summary.

In difficult situations, do you find yourself taking care of others? If a family member gets sick, are you the one who cares for them? A desire to help and take care of people is important for those in the therapeutic services career pathway. You have likely encountered therapeutic workers at the dentist's office, in hospitals, and at doctors' offices. Therapeutic services workers are dedicated to helping others through direct contact with patients.

If you want to help patients by providing care and treatment to improve their health, consider a therapeutic services career. This chapter will introduce you to several broad categories of these careers and explain the different levels of training for occupations in each category. You will see how special types of teams deliver patient care in various healthcare settings. As you practice basic therapeutic skills, you can begin to evaluate your personal interest in providing hands-on care. Completing job application forms and practicing job interview skills will prepare you for HOSA competitions and for future healthcare employment.

The Therapeutic Worker: Darius

When asked about his job as a nursing assistant, Darius smiled his slow grin and said, "I like it." Darius' journey to a therapeutic career began back in high school. His girlfriend's mom was a nurse, and she talked to him about healthcare job opportunities. He decided to take the *Introduction to Healthcare Careers* class offered at his high school. He liked the idea of a diagnostics job and thought he might like to become an X-ray technician.

Around that same time, Darius' friend from football practice, who was interested in nursing, convinced him to sign up for the nursing assistant class. There were some things that Darius was unsure of as he studied the duties of a nursing assistant. He wasn't sure of his ability to give a bed bath, but training at a nursing home helped him master certain tasks. His clinical instructor at the nursing home gave him some good insights into caring for another person.

After passing his state certification test, Darius got a part-time job at the nursing home where he had completed his training. Within a few months, he realized that he really enjoyed caring for people and his employer had already taken notice of his skills. His calm demeanor, his patience with people, and his slow, easy grin made him a favorite with the residents. As a result of his education, training, and experience in the field, Darius chose the therapeutic pathway and a career as a registered nurse.

Personal Traits

Are you a "people person?" Are you the one who listens to your friends' problems? Do you enjoy showing another person how to do a task? Do you get satisfaction from helping someone who is sick? Careers in the **therapeutic** services pathway focus on interacting with patients. Because these are the careers that require close contact with patients, you need a strong interest in people to find job satisfaction in therapeutic careers. Many therapeutic workers have social or "helper" personalities according to their John Holland career personality assessments.

therapeutic
term that describes treatment given to maintain or restore health

The Therapeutic Worker: Tina

Tina always loved children, so she took a child development class in high school and became an assistant teacher at a local childcare center. During her senior year, she also took a nursing assistant class to gain more skills and experience. She would have to live on her own and support herself after graduation, so she would need a full-time job. She knew that the more job skills she had, the better her chances would be for getting that full-time job.

After graduation, Tina worked at an assisted living facility for one year and then moved on to work at a university hospital. Several years later, she is still in that hospital position. She is the person with the most experience on her floor. In addition to her nursing assistant duties, she teaches the orientation class for all newly hired nurses and the university student nurses who complete clinical training on her floor. Notice that all of Tina's jobs—teaching children, caring for residents and patients, and teaching her fellow employees—involve working with people.

Can you remain calm and patient under stress? Therapeutic workers must handle patient emergencies, sometimes on a daily basis. Even when you are helping a person who could bleed to death in a few minutes, you must respond calmly.

When you work with sick people, you can't expect them to be polite and concerned about your feelings. You have to be the patient one when a difficult client keeps complaining about his food. You have to be the patient one when a resident with **dementia** (dih-MEHN-chuh), a condition that causes memory loss, repeatedly asks you what day it is. You have to be the patient one when a coworker takes his frustration out on you. Caring for sick people is stressful work.

empathy
the ability to identify with another person's feelings and thoughts

Therapeutic workers must have **empathy** for their patients. Understanding the emotions of your patient will help you deliver compassionate care. Successful therapeutic workers know that a patient's mental, social, and spiritual needs are just as important to wellness as the physical needs for which he or she is receiving medical treatment.

The Therapeutic Worker: Selena

Selena is a therapeutic worker. One Friday evening, Selena is preparing to leave work when she is called on to help a patient. The patient, an older woman, requires surgery to **amputate** (AM-pyoo-tayt), or surgically remove her leg due to spreading cancer. The patient asks Selena if she can talk to the pastor at her church. Even though Selena's shift has ended, she takes the time to look in the patient's medical record and call the religious contact listed there. Selena arranges for a visit and lets the patient know when she will see her pastor. After she has helped the patient, Selena heads home.

tact
the ability to communicate difficult or embarrassing information without giving offense

Successful healthcare workers use **tact** when communicating with patients. Could you respond without embarrassment to a patient who wants to know if he will be able to have sex after his surgery? Could you politely ask a patient with digestive problems to describe her bowel movements? Could you find the right words to convince a visitor not to feed her special homemade brownies to her diabetic grandmother? All of these situations require an honest but tactful approach.

Accepting criticism can be a difficult experience for anyone. It is human nature to feel hurt and angry when criticized; we want to "defend" our position. Even when we know we have made a mistake, we have a strong urge to fight back by blaming something or someone else. Too often, we retaliate with our own criticism and create a hostile work environment.

Criticism is, however, part of working in healthcare. For therapeutic workers, criticism can be undeserved when it comes from a client who is in pain or is frustrated by the physical limitations caused by illness. These are the situations in which patience is required. It helps to remember that the criticism isn't really about you, but is instead about the emotions of your patient. Sometimes you are just the convenient target of those emotions. Learning how to accept criticism is a valuable skill that will improve your work performance.

The Therapeutic Worker: Lynn

Fatou and Lynn both work as personal care attendants. Fatou notices that Lynn is always wearing gloves. She even wears them from one resident's room to the next. Fatou mentions to Lynn that she needs to change her gloves when she moves to a new resident, even if she didn't provide direct care to the previous resident. Fatou is surprised by Lynn's angry reaction, "You're not my boss! I don't have to listen to what you say!"

Actually, Lynn was embarrassed and felt stupid for not knowing the standard precautions guidelines. Instead of becoming defensive, she should have taken a deep breath and waited until she calmed down. Then she could really think about Fatou's advice. When she realized that Fatou was helping her protect residents from the risk of infection, she apologized for her outburst and thanked Fatou for her help. The next day she registered to retake the infection control training class so she could feel confident about following the guidelines correctly.

During a performance evaluation, the boss is looking not only at what workers do well, but also at how they can improve. Successful workers take time to think about possible areas for improvement in their job performance before an evaluation. They also ask the boss questions during the evaluation to clarify any suggestions that do not seem accurate or are confusing. Finally, they actually create a plan to improve their job performance and stick to that plan.

When it's time for their next evaluation, these workers can show the boss exactly what they have done to improve job performance. Would you value a worker who takes your suggestions and implements them without arguing, complaining, or becoming defensive? You can be sure that healthcare managers do. Showing improvement on the job is an important skill for receiving promotions and pay raises at work.

Dependability seems an obvious trait of a successful healthcare worker, but for therapeutic workers it is essential. Since patients rely on you, regular work attendance and prompt responses to patient needs are crucial to providing quality patient care. Suppose that a healthcare worker named Matt heard the call buzzer for one of his patients but was in the middle of charting. He quickly finished the charting but forgot about the buzzer. When he remembered and checked on his patient, he found the man unconscious on the floor of his hospital room. The patient had to use the bathroom and was embarrassed that he might wet the bed. Even though he was at risk of falling, he tried to get to the bathroom on his own. Matt's failure to respond promptly to a patient's call led to that patient being injured.

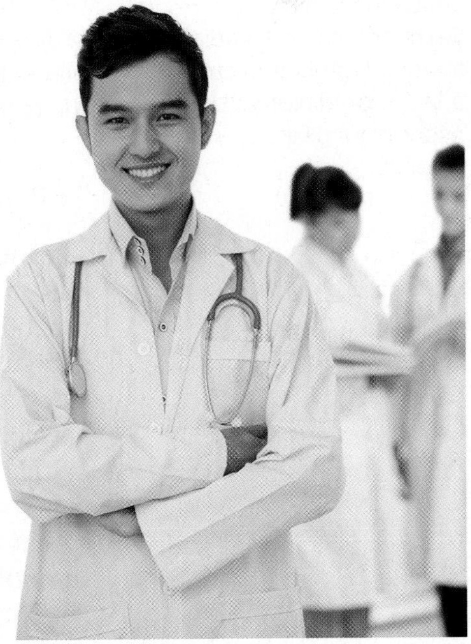

Your fellow workers also depend on you (Figure 6.1). When you are absent from work, another trained employee must take your place. Paperwork can sometimes wait, but patient care never can. Frequent absences place a burden on fellow workers and create resentment.

For therapeutic workers, being dependable requires a commitment to maintaining personal health. Because you are working with sick people who may have weakened immune systems, you must be healthy when you are providing care. Without good health, you can't be a dependable worker. Are you willing to eat a healthy diet, get regular exercise, and take the time to get adequate sleep so your team and patients can rely on you?

Figure 6.1   One of your responsibilities as a healthcare worker is to be dependable. What does it mean to be a dependable therapeutic worker?

Therapeutic Career Choices

Therapeutic occupations are primarily involved in changing the health status of a patient over time. Therapy means treatment, and workers in therapeutic services use a variety of treatments to improve patient health. These treatments may improve physical, mental, or emotional health. The therapeutic services pathway includes the largest number of healthcare careers. Since therapeutic services require the most worker-to-patient interaction, facilities cannot easily **outsource** these jobs to a foreign country—a frequent practice in information technology services. However, many hospitals, behavioral health facilities, and long-term care organizations outsource medical, nursing, therapy, support, and other services through local agencies to save money. In this type of outsourcing, outside staff members provide care or treatment within the healthcare organization or under its name.

The job outlook for therapeutic workers is changing because of the rising costs of healthcare. Therapeutic work is increasingly being assigned to lower paid workers to cut costs. For example, physician assistants, medical assistants, dental hygienists (hI-JEHN-ists), and physical therapy aides are performing tasks that were previously performed by doctors, nurses, dentists, or physical therapists. This trend has created a new **tier**, or level of careers for workers with **technical training**. While the professionals still complete the patient evaluation and create treatment plans, technical workers often deliver part of the treatment. As a result, the technical worker may actually have more contact with the patient.

technical training
education lasting two years or less and leading to an industry certificate, a technical diploma, or an associate's degree

Therapy Careers

There is a wide variety of therapy careers, but all therapists use a special set of knowledge and skills to assist people with impaired functions in becoming as self-sufficient and productive as possible. A patient's limited functions may be caused by physical illness or injury, emotional disorder, **congenital** (kahn-JEHN-ih-tuhl) birth disorder, developmental disability, or the aging process.

Therapists evaluate the needs of each patient and develop a treatment plan to improve the person's health status. Therapists specialize in specific types of treatments, and the result is a large number of different specialties (Figure 6.2).

Therapists work in many different settings, including hospitals, clinics, schools, private offices, clients' homes, gyms, outdoors, and at private swimming pools. Therapy work can be both physically demanding and emotionally challenging. A therapist must remain patient when clients make slow progress. A lack of progress can be frustrating for the therapist as well as for the client, but seeing eventual improvement is very satisfying.

While you may be acquainted with the work of physical and occupational therapists, the field of therapy is expanding. For example, the field of massage therapy is growing as more people learn about its health benefits. Trained and licensed therapists have the best opportunity for employment. However, many massage therapists work part-time until they build a client base large enough to support full-time employment.

Figure 6.2 Types of Therapists

Specialist	Services Provided
athletic trainer	prevents and treats muscle and bone injuries
audiologist	assesses and treats hearing, balance, and related ear problems
exercise physiologist/ kinesiotherapist	plans and implements fitness programs
massage therapist	performs therapeutic massage of soft tissues and joints
mental health therapist	counsels individuals and groups to promote mental and emotional health
occupational therapist	plans rehabilitative programs to restore vocational and daily living skills
physical therapist	plans rehabilitative programs to relieve pain, improve mobility, and increase strength
radiation therapist	administers radiation to treat cancer
recreational therapist (art/music/dance therapist)	provides treatment services and recreational activities for people with disabilities or illnesses
rehabilitation counselor	designs rehabilitation programs that include personal and vocational counseling, training, and job placement
respiratory therapist	treats and cares for patients with breathing disorders
speech-language pathologist	assesses and treats people with speech, language, voice, and fluency disorders
vision rehabilitation therapist	provides instruction for adaptive living skills to adults who are blind or visually impaired

Recreational therapy includes many distinct types of treatment. These therapists use sports, games, arts, crafts, and music to help patients build confidence and restore physical and social function. Recreational therapists are not the same as the recreational workers who conduct games for fun at parks and other locations. Therapists use patient medical records and interviews with the healthcare team to design specific treatment activities. For example, a treatment plan might include helping a right-handed girl who can't use her right arm anymore learn to throw a ball with her left arm.

Currently, hospitals and nursing homes provide the most jobs for therapists. However, as healthcare is delivered increasingly in alternative settings, adult day care, assisted living facilities, and physical rehabilitation sites will also provide many job opportunities. Be aware that activity aides, rather than certified therapists, are more frequently involved in recreational therapy programs as a cost-control measure.

Patients sometimes use alternative therapies such as Reiki (RAY-kee), acupuncture, and traditional Chinese medicine to complement Western treatments. Patients feel that their clinical treatment plans benefit from complementary therapies, and demand for such therapies is growing. If you want to provide alternative therapies, look for an accredited training program that leads to certification. The National Certification Commission

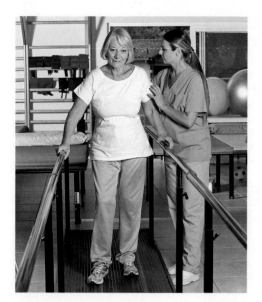

Figure 6.3   Residents in long-term care facilities might receive physical therapy as part of their treatment.

residents
(1) individuals living in long-term care facilities;
(2) medical school graduates who are completing the last portion of their medical training before becoming licensed physicians

clinical training
term that describes hands-on work with patients that students do under the supervision of a licensed healthcare provider

for Acupuncture and Oriental Medicine (NCCAOM) is a national organization whose certification process will show employers that you are competent. In most states, NCCAOM certification is a requirement for licensure.

Therapeutic workers use different terms to identify the people they treat based on the care setting where treatment is given. Patients receive treatment in hospitals and clinics. **Clients** receive treatment in privately owned offices and treatment facilities, as well as in their own homes. **Residents** live in long-term care facilities such as group homes, assisted living facilities, and nursing homes (Figure 6.3).

Most but not all therapists require a bachelor's or a graduate degree to practice. Therapy assistants often require an associate's degree. Therapy aides may require a specialized training course of one year or less. Regardless of the type of degree, therapeutic workers develop their skills during **clinical training**. This volunteer work is part of their educational program. Although clinical training is required for all therapeutic workers, each worker experiences a unique path through education and training. Note the differences in training and work responsibilities for the physical therapy and occupational therapy career ladders shown in Figure 6.4.

Workers can specialize within their chosen field of therapy as they learn new treatments or work with a specific patient population. For example, some occupational therapists train to treat patients who have swollen limbs due to excess fluid in the tissues. They are lymphedema (limf-uh-DEE-muh) therapists. Physical therapists may specialize in working with patients who have spinal cord injuries or with infants who have birth disorders, birth injuries, or delays in motor development.

The need for therapists is increasing due to the aging population of the United States. Older adults have an increased incidence of heart attack and stroke, both of which require therapy in the recovery process. Those who are 75 years of age and older suffer from high incidences of disabling conditions, which means an increased demand for therapeutic services. In addition, more patients with critical conditions or injuries are surviving because of medical advancements. These patients may need extensive therapy. However, growth in therapy careers may be slowed by the impact of federal legislation that limits reimbursement for therapy services.

Dental Careers

Why do you think job opportunities in dental careers are increasing rapidly? If you recognize that we have an aging population and that older adults are keeping their natural teeth rather than getting dentures these days, you have identified a major reason for growth in the dental field.

General dentists complete a bachelor's degree with an emphasis on science. They take the dental admissions test, which is very competitive, before entering dental school. During their four years of dental school, students continue their study of science and learn lab techniques for patient treatment. During the final two years of dental school, students treat patients in special clinics, working under the supervision of a licensed dentist. Graduates must pass a licensing exam before beginning to practice dentistry.

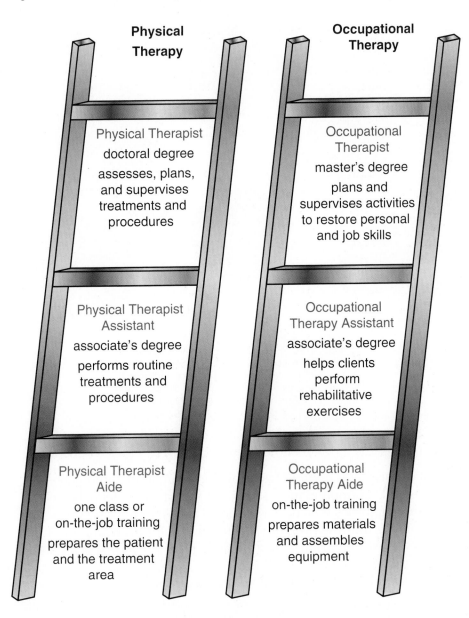

Physical Therapy

Physical Therapist
doctoral degree
assesses, plans, and supervises treatments and procedures

Physical Therapist Assistant
associate's degree
performs routine treatments and procedures

Physical Therapist Aide
one class or on-the-job training
prepares the patient and the treatment area

Occupational Therapy

Occupational Therapist
master's degree
plans and supervises activities to restore personal and job skills

Occupational Therapy Assistant
associate's degree
helps clients perform rehabilitative exercises

Occupational Therapy Aide
on-the-job training
prepares materials and assembles equipment

Figure 6.4   Jobs at the top of the career ladder require more training and education, which generally means more responsibilities at work. In addition to their patient responsibilities, physical and occupational therapists supervise the work of their assistants and aides.

Dentists can specialize in treating specific dental conditions by completing two to four years of additional **postgraduate** education. For some specialties, a two-year postgraduate residency is required, during which the dentist practices the specialty under the supervision of an experienced specialist (Figure 6.5 on the next page).

Dentistry requires skill both in diagnosing dental problems and in working with your hands. Many dentists work in private practice. This means they also need good business sense, self-discipline, and communication skills to succeed in running their own businesses.

While there will be jobs for dentists as older dentists retire, much of the growth in dental careers is currently focused on dental hygienists and dental assistants. Hygienists complete an associate's degree. They work directly with patients to clean teeth, take and develop oral X-rays, assess the health of patients' gums, and teach patients how to practice good oral care. Dental hygiene is one of the fastest growing healthcare occupations in the Unites States. However, about half of all hygienists work part-time, so dental hygiene is ideal for someone interested in a flexible work schedule.

postgraduate
term that describes education and training completed after receiving a bachelor's degree

Figure 6.5   Within the field of dentistry, there are specialties that you can pursue. Can you identify some advantages and disadvantages of career specialization?

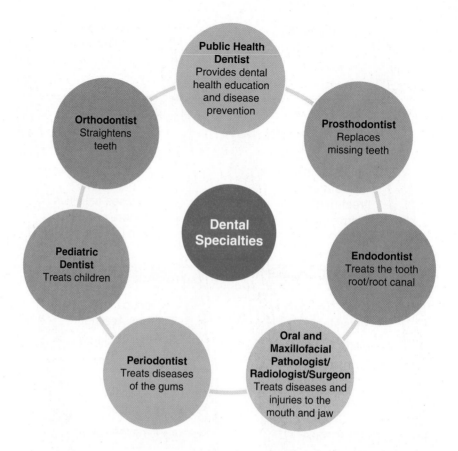

Dental assisting is another fast-growing occupation. On-the-job training is still common in most states, but increasingly dentists are looking for employees who have completed a six-month or one-year dental assisting training program. Requirements for licensure of dental assistants vary widely from state to state, so research your specific state regulations when preparing for this career.

Like medical assistants, dental assistants can perform a wide range of duties:

- Chairside assistants work directly with the dentist in the treatment area by setting up instrument trays, preparing the patient, and handing materials and instruments to the dentist.

- Laboratory assistants make casts of the teeth and mouth from impressions, clean and polish removable appliances, and make temporary crowns.

- Office assistants schedule and confirm appointments, receive patients, keep treatment records, send bills, receive payments, and order dental supplies and materials.

With additional education and work experience, dental assistants may work as claims approvers for insurance companies, as dental office managers, or as dental sales representatives.

Medical Careers

So, you want to become a doctor. To many students, the life of a physician seems glamorous. Physicians work in a highly respected profession and they earn a high rate of pay. While this is true, you should consider every aspect of the profession before pursuing medicine.

There are two types of physicians—the medical doctor (MD) and the doctor of osteopathic (ahs-tee-oh-PA-thihk) medicine (DO). Both MDs and DOs may use all accepted methods of treatment, including drugs and surgery. However, DOs place special emphasis on the body's musculoskeletal system, preventive medicine, and holistic patient care. They are most likely to be primary care physicians, whereas medical doctors can work in one or more specialties (Figure 6.6).

Figure 6.6 Medical Specialties

Specialty	Treatment Areas	Specialty	Treatment Areas
allergy and immunology	immune system disorders such as asthma and AIDS	oncology	diagnosis of and treatment for cancerous tumors
anesthesiology	pain relief for surgery	ophthalmology	disorders of the eye
cardiology	disorders of the heart and blood vessels	orthopedics	disorders of muscles and bones
dermatology	disorders of the skin, hair, and nails	otolaryngology	diseases of the ear, nose, and throat
emergency medicine	quick evaluation and action to prevent death	pathology	examination of tissue to diagnose disease
family medicine	comprehensive healthcare for the individual and family	pediatrics	diseases and disorders in children
gastroenterology	diagnosis of and treatment for diseases of the digestive organs	plastic surgery	reconstruction of malformed body parts
general surgery	disorders of the abdomen, digestive tract, etc.	preventive medicine	health promotion and disease prevention
internal medicine	comprehensive care for adults and the elderly	proctology	diseases of the colon and rectum
medical genetics	treatment for genetically linked diseases	psychiatry	diseases and disorders of the mind
neurological surgery	treatment for disorders of the nerves and brain	radiology	use of radiation to diagnose and treat disease
neurology	diagnosis of brain and nervous system disorders	rehabilitation medicine	treatment of patients with physical disabilities
nuclear medicine	anatomic and molecular imaging for diagnosis	thoracic surgery	surgery of the lungs, heart, or chest cavity
obstetrics and gynecology	care of pregnant women; evaluation and treatment of women's reproductive health	urology	diseases of the kidney or bladder

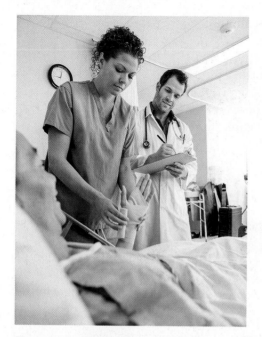

Figure 6.7   Medical students receive hands-on training with physician supervision. How does experience working in several different specialty areas benefit medical students?

The education and training requirements for physicians are among the most demanding of any occupation. Preparation begins with an undergraduate degree in a field of the student's choice. Science coursework is important, but a well-rounded education is an asset for anyone entering the field of medicine. Some students volunteer at local hospitals or clinics to gain practical experience in the health professions.

Application to medical school is highly competitive. Students must score well on the Medical College Admissions Test (MCAT). College transcripts and letters of recommendation are important. Schools also consider an applicant's character, personality, and leadership qualities, which can be demonstrated through extracurricular activities, including healthcare experiences. Most schools require candidates to participate in an interview with members of the admissions committee.

The first two years of medical school are mostly classroom work, but the last two years include clinical or hands-on patient work under the supervision of a physician (Figure 6.7). During this time, students rotate through different specialties such as surgery, pediatrics, and neurology to learn about each field so they can decide which one is of most interest to them. You may see these medical students in hospitals, but they haven't finished their training and are not yet licensed doctors. Upon graduating from medical school, students add the MD or DO to their names and become residents.

After School. As they are finishing medical school, students apply for a residency program and hope they will be matched with the program of their choice. The term *resident* comes from the time when most residents actually lived on the hospital grounds to be on call at all times.

The term **intern** describes a student doctor when he or she is completing rotations through various specialties in the first year of residency. To become licensed as specialists, these new doctors still have many more years of study to go, depending on their chosen field. For example, an internal medicine doctor will study for three more years, and a neurologist will study for six or seven more years. Some highly specialized programs and subspecialties, such as endocrinology or pediatric cardiology, can require even more training. These types of programs are known as **fellowships**.

Have you added up the years of education and training? A physician completes 11 to 14 years of training after high school before being licensed to practice medicine. This is a huge investment of time and money. Doctors do receive a small salary during residency, but most physicians have large school loans to repay when they begin to earn an income.

Finding a Job. Job prospects are best for physicians who are willing to practice in rural and low-income areas because these medically underserved areas typically have difficulty attracting medical professionals. Physicians in specialties that treat the rapidly growing elderly population will also have better opportunities for employment. Cardiologists and radiologists will particularly be needed because the risks for heart disease and cancer increase as people age.

While the job prospects for physicians are good, the job prospects for **physician assistants (PAs)** are even better. These workers practice medicine under the supervision of a physician (Figure 6.8). They can diagnose, treat, and prescribe medication for patients. Each state determines the duties that may be performed by a PA. Many PAs work in primary care areas such as internal medicine, pediatrics, or family medicine. They may also train to work in medical specialties.

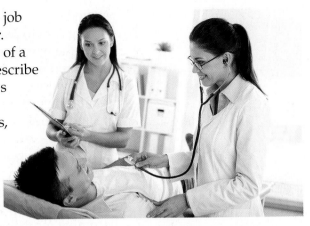

Figure 6.8   A physician assistant works under the supervision of a physician. What duties can a physician assistant perform?

Physician assistants begin their training with an undergraduate degree. Many PAs have prior experience as registered nurses, emergency medical technicians, and paramedics. Physician assistant schooling includes two years of classroom and lab training along with clinical rotations in several areas. Graduates earn a master's degree and pass a national examination to become certified.

Physician assistants work an average of 40 hours a week. They may work nights and weekends if they are employed in a hospital setting. Physicians, however, work long and irregular hours averaging more than 50 hours a week.

Whether you choose a physician or a physician assistant career, you must have a strong desire to serve patients, a good bedside manner, emotional stability, and the ability to make decisions in an emergency. Do you enjoy learning? As a physician or a PA, you will need to study medical advancements constantly to provide quality care for your patients.

When you hear the word *doctor*, you probably think of an MD. However, many other therapeutic healthcare professionals also hold doctoral degrees. Optometrists, chiropractors, veterinarians, and pharmacists are required to obtain doctoral degrees. The Doctor of Optometry (OD), Doctor of Chiropractic (DC), and Doctor of Veterinary Medicine (DVM) use the word *doctor* in their title, but the Doctor of Pharmacy (PharmD) does not. Advanced practice nurses and physical therapists may also obtain doctoral degrees. Each of these professionals completes several years of education and training beyond their bachelor's degree to prepare for their chosen healthcare profession or to advance their professional skills.

Nursing Careers

You may plan to become a pediatric nurse, but why limit yourself? The nursing field has an incredible variety of job opportunities. Nursing has the largest number of job openings and employs more workers than any other healthcare occupation (Figure 6.9).

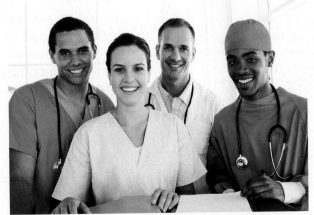

Figure 6.9   The field of nursing offers many healthcare job opportunities. What are some job titles that appear on nursing's career ladder?

Nursing also has a well-developed career ladder. At the entry level, home health aides work to assist their clients with daily activities. After completing a nursing assisting class and passing a certification test, a person becomes a **certified nursing assistant (CNA)** and can work in assisted living facilities, nursing homes, and hospitals providing basic nursing care to patients and residents.

At the next level, a **licensed practical nurse (LPN)** or **licensed vocational nurse (LVN)** completes a one-year technical training program and can perform additional nursing tasks such as giving injections, monitoring catheters, and dressing wounds. Each state determines the specific care skills an LPN may perform.

A **registered nurse (RN)** has either an associate's degree in nursing (ADN) or a bachelor's of science in nursing (BSN). The ADN and the BSN take the same examination and have the same license to practice. Individuals who complete a BSN receive more training in areas such as communication, leadership, and critical thinking. These skills are becoming more important as nursing practice becomes more complex. A bachelor's degree or higher is often necessary for administrative, research, consulting, and teaching positions.

Advanced practice nurses—which include the clinical nurse specialist (CNS), nurse practitioner (NP), registered nurse anesthetist (a-NEHS-theh-tist) (RNA), and certified nurse midwife (CNM)—need at least a master's degree. Many programs are now offering a doctor of nursing practice (DNP) degree as well. Nurses who are already working can often take advantage of tuition reimbursement from their employers to advance their education and earn a bachelor's, master's, or doctoral degree.

Using orders from the physician and input from other team members, nurses establish a care plan for the patient and make sure the plan is carried out. They perform a variety of tasks, including but certainly not limited to the following:

- administering medications, carefully checking dosages and avoiding interactions between certain types of medication

- starting, maintaining, and discontinuing intravenous (IV) lines

- administering therapies and treatments

- observing the patient and recording those observations

- consulting with physicians and other healthcare clinicians

delegate
to direct another healthcare worker to perform a care task that is within that worker's training and experience and within the scope of practice of the licensed provider giving the direction

Registered nurses also **delegate** nursing tasks and supervise the work of the LPNs and CNAs on their care team.

Today's nurses are assuming more technically challenging roles than at any other point in history. As a result, nurses are becoming more and more specialized in the work they perform (Figure 6.10). The duties of RNs vary widely and are often determined by their work setting or the patient population they serve. Registered nurses can specialize by

- working in a particular setting or with a particular type of treatment;

- specializing in a specific health condition;

- working with a specific body system; and

- working with a specific patient population.

Some nurses have jobs that require an RN license but include little or no direct patient care. For example, a forensic (fuh-REHN-zihk) nurse provides care to victims of crimes, collects evidence after crimes occur, and provides care to patients within the prison system. Infection control

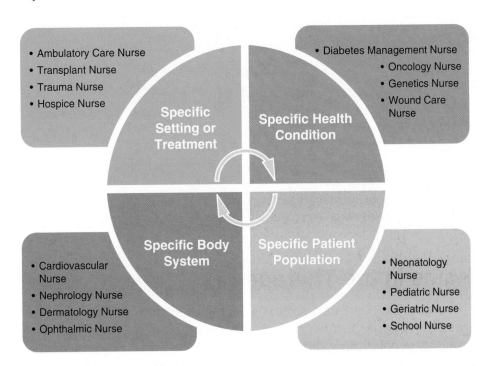

- Ambulatory Care Nurse
- Transplant Nurse
- Trauma Nurse
- Hospice Nurse

Specific Setting or Treatment

- Diabetes Management Nurse
- Oncology Nurse
- Genetics Nurse
- Wound Care Nurse

Specific Health Condition

Specific Body System

- Cardiovascular Nurse
- Nephrology Nurse
- Dermatology Nurse
- Ophthalmic Nurse

Specific Patient Population

- Neonatology Nurse
- Pediatric Nurse
- Geriatric Nurse
- School Nurse

Figure 6.10   Nurses are becoming increasingly specialized, meaning their duties can vary widely according to their work setting and the patients they serve. This diagram shows four areas of specialization in the field of nursing.

nurses track and work to control infectious outbreaks in healthcare facilities. Nurse informaticists manage and communicate nursing data to improve healthcare decisions.

If you have an interest in caring for people, take the time to research a career in nursing. Because there are so many opportunities in this field, you are almost certain to find one that fits your skills and interests.

Technical Workers in Therapeutic Services

As stated earlier, more tasks are being delegated to workers with technical training rather than those with a professional degree in an effort to reduce costs. According to the Bureau of Labor Statistics, the following therapeutic healthcare careers require an associate's degree or less training:

- dental hygienist and dental assistant
- home health aide
- occupational therapy aide and assistant
- pharmacy technician (Figure 6.11)
- physical therapy aide and assistant
- veterinary technician

These careers offer good opportunities for students who do not wish to pursue a professional degree. Typically, the job prospects for these careers will be good.

Therapeutic services offer a multitude of job choices. Review the listing of job titles in the therapeutic section of the health science careers chart found in chapter 1. Whether you want on-the-job training or are ready to study for several years, you can find a career in therapeutic services.

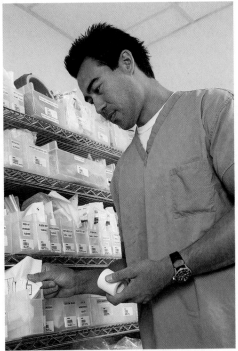

Figure 6.11   Pharmacy technician is one example of a technical position in the therapeutic pathway.

Complete the
Map Your Reading
graphic organizer for the
section you just read.

RECALL YOUR READING

1. Therapeutic healthcare services focus on changing a patient's _____.
2. Because therapeutic workers interact directly with patients, they must remain _____ in emergencies and feel _____ for their patients.
3. Dental careers are experiencing rapid _____, in part because many aging baby boomers are not getting dentures.
4. _____ has the largest number of job openings and employs more workers than any other healthcare occupation.
5. To reduce costs, healthcare facilities are using more _____ workers and fewer professional employees.

Teams in the Therapeutic Pathway

Teams deliver patient care in all kinds of healthcare settings. Working in teams allows healthcare professionals to provide better care to a larger number of people. Using the combined skills of many health professionals reduces medical costs for patients and helps bring healthcare to underserved areas of the country.

As physician specialties were developed during the past 50 years, many different doctors could work with a single patient. A single patient might see a podiatrist, dermatologist, cardiologist, obstetrician, and so on. These doctors could be located at several different offices. Each office maintained its own set of records and did not share patient records with other offices. Unless the patient talked about his or her other doctors, many physicians remained unaware that a patient was receiving any other treatment. The patient was being treated by a **multidisciplinary healthcare team**, but care was not coordinated, especially because patient records were not shared. If a general practice physician referred a patient to a specialist, he or she would receive a consult report, but could not access complete patient records.

In healthcare today, the interdisciplinary healthcare team approach is becoming more common. The change to interdisciplinary teams focuses on coordination of care to improve patient outcomes by preventing conflicting treatments and avoiding duplication of services. It also saves money. As interoperability of patient records expands, communication between interdisciplinary team members becomes less difficult.

In this section you will learn how interdisciplinary teams function and what kinds of interdisciplinary teams are used in healthcare. In addition, you will learn about the types of teams used by nurses to provide continuous patient care.

multidisciplinary healthcare team
a group of healthcare workers from different healthcare specialties, each providing specific services to the patient

Interdisciplinary Teams

Interdisciplinary teams consist of different types of healthcare professionals just like multidisciplinary teams. However, interdisciplinary team members **collaborate** to provide a coordinated plan of treatment for the patient. Interdisciplinary teams can be described as *primary* or *secondary*. Primary care teams function in clinical and community settings, while secondary care teams provide hospital services.

collaborate
to work together; to consult with each other

Primary care teams include the primary care physician along with physician assistants and nurse practitioners who see the patient in the clinic setting. Depending on the needs of its patient, the team may also include nutritionists, pharmacists, social workers, or others. The team decides which additional healthcare practitioners will be most beneficial in promoting health and wellness for its patient population. For example, a community-based health team may add dentists, health educators, or mental health professionals, while a rehabilitation team would include physical, occupational, and speech therapists.

Secondary care teams deliver services to hospital patients. Surgical teams include surgeons, surgical technicians, nurse anesthetists, and operating room nurses. Cardiovascular teams are made up of cardiologists, dietitians, and exercise therapists. An infection control team might consist of infectious disease specialists, a pharmacologist, a social worker, and so on.

Collaboration is a key element in the interdisciplinary team model (Figure 6.12). Regardless of the type of healthcare team or setting involved, team members communicate on a regular basis. Hospital-based teams go on rounds together or hold conferences to communicate about patients in their care. A team working with outpatients in an office or a clinic meets frequently to keep team members up-to-date on which patients have been seen and which treatments they've received. Team members work together to plan and carry out patient treatments. The physician diagnoses and prescribes medications, the nurse practitioner educates the patient about the illness and treatment, and the social worker counsels the patient on community resources available to him or her.

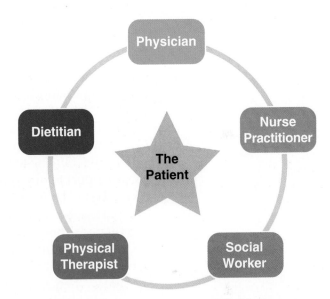

Figure 6.12 Healthcare team members collaborate by communicating with each other and with the patient as they coordinate the plan of treatment for the patient.

The development of computers and **teleconferencing** allows healthcare professionals to interact and collaborate over long distances. As a result, healthcare team members can be spread out over a wide geographic area. This has been important when providing care to patients in rural areas. Telemedicine allows a primary physician to seek the opinion of a specialist without having to send the patient hundreds of miles to see that specialist. Similarly, an anesthesiologist (an-ehs-thee-zee-AH-luh-jihst) working at a major medical center in another city can use telemedicine to supervise a nurse anesthetist in a small community hospital.

Nursing Teams

While nurses function as members of the healthcare team, they also have their own system of teamwork to provide the round-the-clock care required in hospitals and long-term care facilities. The most basic nursing team includes the nurse (RN, LPN, or LVN) and the nursing assistant (CNA). The nurse carries out the doctor's orders, and the nursing assistant completes the care tasks assigned by the nurse. The nurse has the authority to delegate tasks that are within the nursing assistant's scope of practice.

Additional nursing team members may include the charge nurse who supervises all the nurses for a specific shift, the head nurse who oversees a department, and the director of nursing (DON) who supervises all of the nursing care within a facility.

Nurses provide care using a variety of nursing care models. Each healthcare facility determines which model its nurses will use. A **case manager** model is often used in home health care. The RN serving as the case manager develops a care plan along with the client and his or her family. The nursing assistant follows this plan when visiting the client, and the case manager supervises the care being provided.

In a **primary nursing** model, one RN, LPN, or LVN is assigned several patients or residents and is responsible for planning and carrying out all aspects of care for as long as the patients are in the care unit. Other nurses will follow this care plan when the primary nurse is not working, but the primary nurse has 24-hour responsibility for planning patient care. Patients report higher levels of satisfaction with this model.

A **functional nursing** model assigns tasks. Each nurse is responsible for completing a set of assigned tasks for every patient or resident. So one nurse may administer medications, while another nurse delivers special treatments, and the nursing assistant takes all vital signs and assists with meals. Patient care becomes fragmented with this system, and patients don't like this model as much as they like others.

An RN functions as the team leader in the **team nursing** model (Figure 6.13). The team leader has a group of nursing staff members who report to him or her, and together the group divides the nursing care tasks. Team members complete tasks based on their training and expertise, but the team leader is still accountable for all of the care provided. The input and expertise of all team members (RN, LPN, and CNA) is used in planning patient care. In this model, the team leader not only needs clinical nursing skills but must also be an effective group leader. When a nursing team communicates effectively, patient needs are met quickly. Patients are very satisfied with this model, especially when an effort is made to keep the members of the nursing team consistent for each patient.

Figure 6.13   In the team nursing model, tasks are divided up according to each member's training and expertise.

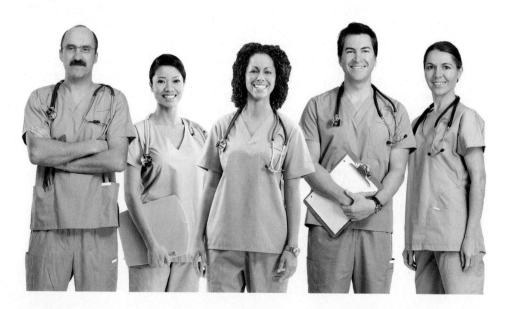

Complete the *Map Your Reading* graphic organizer for the section you just read.

RECALL YOUR READING

1. Healthcare teams rely on effective _____ to function successfully.

2. Through _____, a patient can be "seen" by a specialist without leaving his or her primary physician's office.

3. While nursing teams use a variety of models, patients like the _____ model the least.

4. A cardiovascular team is an example of a _____ healthcare team.

Technical Skills for Therapeutic Workers

In this section, you will learn basic skills used by healthcare workers to promote patient safety. You will also practice a common therapeutic task from the fields of nursing, therapy, and pharmacy. As you practice these new skills, think about your preferences. Do any of these career fields appeal to you?

Standard Precautions

Therapeutic workers perform many career-specific care tasks, but all healthcare workers practice **standard precautions**. Healthcare workers in traditional hospital settings as well as outpatient surgery centers, long-term care facilities, rehabilitation centers, and community clinics all routinely use standard precautions.

The Centers for Disease Control and Prevention developed standard precautions to prevent the spread of infections in healthcare settings. Proper use of these steps protects the healthcare worker from infections carried by patients and protects the patient from infections present in the healthcare facility. One in every twenty hospital patients in the United States gets an infection, and these infections can be life threatening and hard to treat. Hospital-acquired infections are called **nosocomial** (nahs-uh-KOH-mee-uhl) **infections**.

Infections acquired in any healthcare facility are called *healthcare-associated infections (HAIs)*. These infections are caused by a wide variety of both common and unusual bacteria, fungi, and viruses to which the patient is exposed while receiving medical care. Following infection control guidelines ensures that all care is safe care.

Standard precautions are the basic level of infection control that should be used in the care of *all* patients, *all* the time. Using standard precautions prevents the transmission of diseases that can be acquired by contact with blood, body fluids, **non-intact skin** (broken skin, including rashes), and mucous membranes. The term *body fluids* refers to all secretions and excretions, excluding sweat, even if they don't contain visible blood. Standard precautions include guidelines for each of the following:

- hand hygiene

- personal protective equipment (Figure 6.14)

standard precautions steps that a healthcare worker takes with all patients to prevent the spread of infection

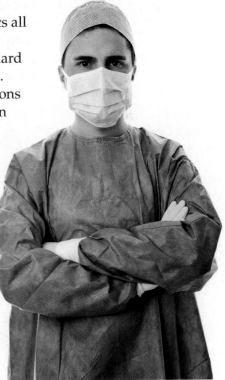

Figure 6.14   Personal protective equipment (PPE) is part of standard precautions. What does PPE include?

- respiratory hygiene (cough etiquette)

- needlestick and sharps injury prevention

- cleaning and disinfection

- waste disposal

- safe injection practices

Hand Hygiene. Hand hygiene is an extremely important part of reducing the spread of infection. Since you can't disinfect or sterilize skin, frequent hand washing removes pathogens that cause disease. In addition to all healthcare workers, patients and their loved ones also play an important role in preventing infections. When people practice hand hygiene and remind their healthcare providers to wash their hands, they reduce their own as well as others' risk. Hand hygiene includes regular hand washing using plain or antibacterial soap and the use of alcohol-based gels. Alcohol-based hand gels are the preferred method of hand hygiene when hands are not visibly soiled. Hand hygiene should be practiced before and after care is given in healthcare settings, as well as in all other situations (Figure 6.15).

The goal of the hand washing procedure is to clean your hands without recontaminating them by touching a dirty surface in the process. Pay close attention to the length of time you are supposed to wash and to what you should *not* touch with your clean hands. Figure 6.16 shows the steps to follow when washing your hands.

Alcohol-based hand gels act quickly to kill microorganisms and reduce the amount of bacteria on your hands. A dime-sized amount of gel is all you need, but remember to rub all hand surfaces. Figure 6.17 on page 196 shows steps to follow when using alcohol-based hand gels.

Figure 6.15   Hand hygiene controls the spread of infection in daily life as well as in healthcare settings. *Always* wash hands that are visibly dirty or contaminated with body fluids. If your hands are not visibly soiled, what other hand hygiene method can you use?

IN ALL SETTINGS

Before...
preparing food
eating
touching animals
putting contacts in eyes
treating any injury
giving medicine
caring for a sick person

After...
handling raw foods
eating
using the restroom
changing a diaper
caring for animals
blowing your nose
coughing or sneezing
caring for a sick person
handling garbage or chemicals

IN HEALTHCARE SETTINGS

Before...
touching a patient
putting on gloves
performing clean/aseptic care
moving from a contaminated
   body site to a clean body site
using a restroom

After...
touching a patient
touching objects in the care
   environment
being exposed to body fluids

How to Handwash?

WASH HANDS WHEN VISIBLY SOILED! OTHERWISE, USE HANDRUB

🕐 **Duration of the entire procedure:** 40–60 seconds

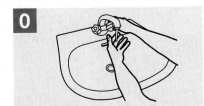

0 Wet hands with water;

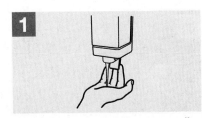

1 Apply enough soap to cover all hand surfaces;

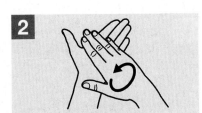

2 Rub hands palm to palm;

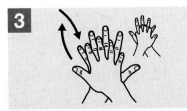

3 Right palm over left hand with interlaced fingers and vice versa;

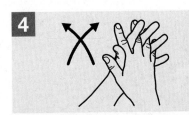

4 Palm to palm with fingers interlaced;

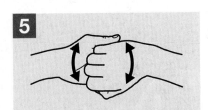

5 Backs of fingers to opposing palms with fingers interlocked;

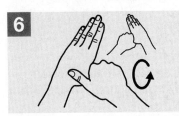

6 Rotational rubbing of left thumb clasped in right palm and vice versa;

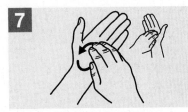

7 Rotational rubbing backward and forward with clasped fingers of right hand in left palm and vice versa;

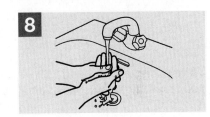

8 Rinse hands with water;

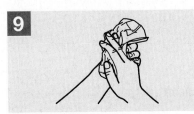

9 Dry hands thoroughly with a single use towel;

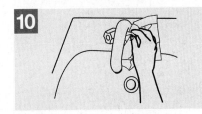

10 Use towel to turn off faucet;

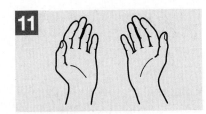

11 Your hands are now safe.

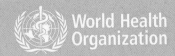 **World Health Organization** | **Patient Safety** A World Alliance for Safer Health Care | **SAVE LIVES** Clean **Your** Hands

Figure 6.16   This instructional poster shows how to properly wash your hands.

How to Handrub?

RUB HANDS FOR HAND HYGIENE! WASH HANDS WHEN VISIBLY SOILED

🕐 **Duration of the entire procedure:** 20–30 seconds

1a 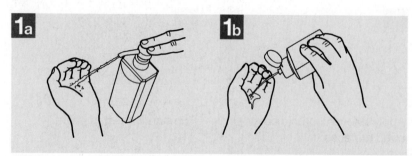 **1b**

Apply a palmful of the product in a cupped hand, covering all surfaces

2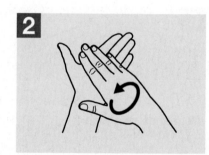

Rub hands palm to palm;

3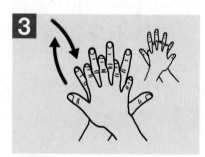

Right palm over left hand with interlaced fingers and vice versa;

4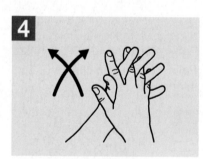

Palm to palm with fingers interlaced;

5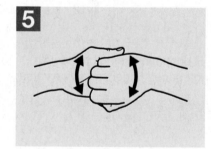

Backs of fingers to opposing palms with fingers interlocked;

6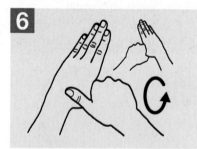

Rotational rubbing of left thumb clasped in right palm and vice versa;

7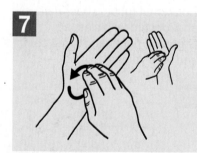

Rotations rubbing, backward and forward with clasped fingers of right hand in left palm and vice versa;

8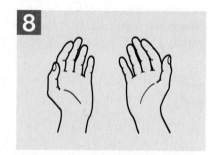

Once dry, your hands are safe.

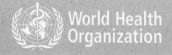 **World Health Organization** | **Patient Safety** A World Alliance for Safer Health Care | **SAVE LIVES** Clean **Your** Hands

Figure 6.17   The correct method of using alcohol-based hand gel is shown here.

Personal Protective Equipment. **Personal protective equipment (PPE)** creates a barrier to protect the skin, clothing, mucous membranes, and respiratory tract from infectious agents. PPE is used whenever the possibility of exposure exists. Here are a few guidelines for the use of PPE:

- Wear *gloves* when touching blood, body fluids, non-intact skin, mucous membranes, and contaminated objects.

- Wear a *mask, face shield,* or *goggles* when there is a risk of body fluid or blood splashing into the eyes, mouth, or nose.

- Wear a *gown* if skin or clothing will be exposed to blood or body fluids.

Remove PPE immediately after use and always wash your hands. Follow your facility's guidelines for disposing of PPE. In some instances, when the PPE is saturated with blood or body fluid, a special biohazard bag is needed for safe disposal. Following the correct steps for removing PPE helps you to avoid contaminating your skin or clothing (Figure 6.18 on the next page).

personal protective equipment (PPE) equipment such as gloves, masks, gowns, respirators, and eyewear worn to protect skin, clothing, and the respiratory tract from infectious agents

Respiratory Hygiene. Patients in waiting rooms can easily spread infection, so healthcare workers must practice **respiratory hygiene**, or *cough etiquette*, and teach these practices to their patients. Respiratory hygiene practices seek to protect people from airborne infectious particles. Healthcare facilities as a whole must take steps to reduce the spread of infection in common areas such as waiting rooms and cafeterias. The following are basic elements of respiratory hygiene:

- Cover your nose and mouth with a tissue or the crook of your elbow when coughing or sneezing.

- Discard tissues after one use and perform hand hygiene.

- Ask patients with signs of respiratory illness to wear a mask in common areas, or provide them with a private waiting area.

- Place seats in waiting areas at least three feet apart to reduce close contact.

- Provide tissues, hand gel, masks, and waste receptacles in waiting areas.

- Post respiratory hygiene guidelines in common areas.

Additional Precautions. Guidelines for the use and disposal of needles and other sharp objects protect healthcare workers from bloodborne pathogens. Specially designed safety syringes may be used, and sharps are discarded in specially designed, clearly labeled containers. Facilities follow special guidelines for disposing of sharps containers.

Housekeeping staff members clean and disinfect healthcare facilities. They are specially trained to use the correct cleaning agents to prevent the spread of infection without damaging expensive equipment. Central supply workers in hospitals use special equipment and procedures to produce the sterile environment required for surgical procedures.

Medical waste disposal requires extra care and caution. Disposal records for medical waste show how much contaminated material was transported and where it was taken. Medical facilities must maintain

SEQUENCE FOR DONNING PERSONAL PROTECTIVE EQUIPMENT (PPE)

The type of PPE used will vary based on the level of precautions required; e.g., Standard and Contact, Droplet or Airborne Infection Isolation.

1. GOWN
- Fully cover torso from neck to knees, arms to end of wrists, and wrap around the back
- Fasten in back of neck and waist

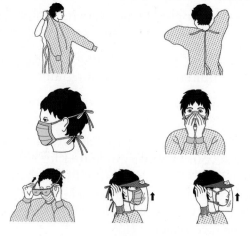

2. MASK OR RESPIRATOR
- Secure ties or elastic bands at middle of head and neck
- Fit flexible band to nose bridge
- Fit snug to face and below chin
- Fit-check respirator

3. GOGGLES OR FACE SHIELD
- Place over face and eyes and adjust to fit

4. GLOVES
- Extend to cover wrist of isolation gown

USE SAFE WORK PRACTICES TO PROTECT YOURSELF AND LIMIT THE SPREAD OF CONTAMINATION

- Keep hands away from face
- Limit surfaces touched
- Change gloves when torn or heavily contaminated
- Perform hand hygiene

SEQUENCE FOR REMOVING PERSONAL PROTECTIVE EQUIPMENT (PPE)

Except for respirator, remove PPE at doorway or in anteroom. Remove respirator after leaving patient room and closing door.

1. GLOVES
- Outside of gloves is contaminated!
- Grasp outside of glove with opposite gloved hand; peel off
- Hold removed glove in gloved hand
- Slide fingers of ungloved hand under remaining glove at wrist
- Peel glove off over first glove
- Discard gloves in waste container

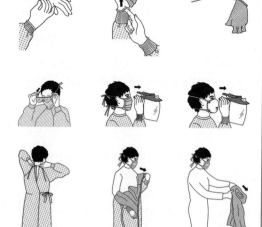

2. GOGGLES OR FACE SHIELD
- Outside of goggles or face shield is contaminated!
- To remove, handle by head band or ear pieces
- Place in designated receptacle for reprocessing or in waste container

3. GOWN
- Gown front and sleeves are contaminated!
- Unfasten ties
- Pull away from neck and shoulders, touching inside of gown only
- Turn gown inside out
- Fold or roll into a bundle and discard

4. MASK OR RESPIRATOR
- Front of mask/respirator is contaminated — DO NOT TOUCH!
- Grasp bottom, then top ties or elastics and remove
- Discard in waste container

PERFORM HAND HYGIENE ¡MMEDIATELY AFTER REMOVING ALL PPE

Courtesy of the Centers for Disease Control and Prevention

Figure 6.18 It is important to carefully follow the steps for putting on and taking off personal protective equipment.

sanitary procedures by using biohazard bags and sharps containers for disposal. They must also be careful to keep waste materials away from clean items and to disinfect vehicles after hauling contaminated waste items.

Safe injection practices protect patients from the spread of bloodborne diseases such as hepatitis. Healthcare workers should use a new needle and syringe each time they access an IV line or a medicine vial. They should also use a new needle and syringe for each patient when giving injections.

Hand Care

Many therapeutic workers provide close personal care for their patients. As a nurse or therapist, you need to feel comfortable with providing a caring touch to another person. Practicing the steps for giving hand care will help you develop this skill.

The first step is getting authorization from your supervisor. Sometimes, normal care tasks are **contraindicated** (kahn-truh-IHN-duh-kay-ted). This means that the patient has a particular condition that makes normal care tasks uncomfortable or dangerous for him or her. For example, a patient with an open sore on his hand would not be able to soak the hand in water because bacteria in the water could enter his body through the open sore. A patient with heart disease might not receive certain types of massage because massage can affect her circulation.

Once you have authorization, you can prepare for providing hand care. Assemble your supplies and knock on the patient's door before entering his room. Always introduce yourself and make sure you have the correct patient by saying her name and checking her ID band or record. Explain your care task and provide an appropriate level of privacy. Finally, wash your hands. Now you can begin providing hand care.

Fill a basin with warm water (about 105°F). Place the basin at a comfortable level for your patient and soak her hands for 5 to 10 minutes. This is a good opportunity to make some observations. Tell your supervisor if you see any of these signs:

- reddened skin that feels hot to the touch

- very dry or cracked skin

- areas of skin that are painful or tender

- nail beds that are blue or bruised

- nails that are unusually thick or yellow

- nails that are ingrown

- cuticles that are torn, red, or swollen

- any skin rash, cuts, scrapes, or bruises

If you will be cleaning the patient's nails, you should wear gloves. The following description does not include the steps for nail care.

Remove the patient's hands from the basin and pat them dry using a clean towel. Apply oil or lotion to soften the skin and begin these simple steps for hand massage (Figure 6.19). If the patient reports any pain, stop massaging immediately and report the patient's pain to your supervisor.

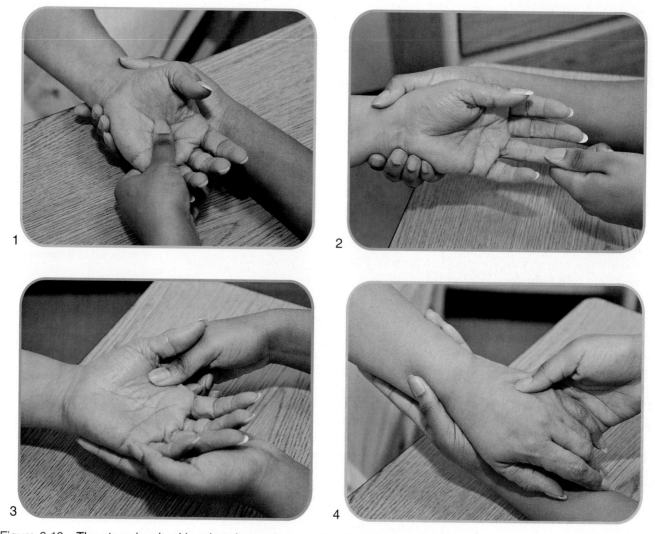

Figure 6.19   The steps involved in a hand massage are detailed in these photos.

1. Place the back of the patient's hand in your palm and use the thumb of your free hand to apply pressure in a circular motion all around her palm. Use firm pressure so as not to tickle or irritate the skin. Continue to support the hand and wrist as you complete the massage movements.

2. Gently pull and stretch each finger. Do not pull hard enough to cause pain or crack the joint at the knuckle.

3. Squeeze and gently knead the webbing between the patient's thumb and index finger with your thumb and index finger. Gently open her fingers to stretch the area between them.

4. Support the patient's wrist with the palm of your hand and gently massage the muscles and tendons between the bones of the hand and wrist.

Once you have completed the hand care procedure, make sure your patient is in a safe and comfortable position. Place the call signal within reach. Clean and store all of your equipment. Wash your hands. Report and record the completion of your care task.

You already know that you are practicing hand massage to become comfortable with touching patients. However, do you know the benefits of massage? We all use our hands daily. Think of the texting and computer use that is common in everyday life, not to mention doing and undoing buttons and zippers, driving a car, and even opening a bag of chips. Hand massage relieves muscle tension, reduces stress, and promotes relaxation.

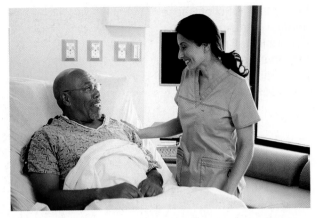

Figure 6.20   Preprocedure and postprocedure actions are intended to improve a patient's care. What pre- or postprocedure actions are shown in this image?

Patient Interaction Guidelines

As you followed the hand care skills steps, did you notice that you were learning additional requirements associated with patient care, such as identifying your patient and providing privacy? Specific steps are followed before and after providing any care procedure. Preprocedure actions promote safety and courtesy while protecting the patient's or resident's rights. Postprocedure actions provide for patient comfort and safety and for communication among healthcare team members. Caregivers learn the following steps to perform before and after every care procedure (Figure 6.20).

Preprocedure Actions

- Gather your supplies.
- Knock and identify yourself by name and title.
- Identify and greet the patient.
- Explain the procedure.
- Provide privacy.
- Wash your hands and follow standard precautions.
- Follow safety precautions for the use of equipment.

Postprocedure Actions

- Provide for the patient's comfort and good body alignment.
- Leave the call button within the patient's reach.
- Lower the bed, lock the wheels, and position the side rails as required.
- Open the curtain or door according to the patient's preference.
- Wash your hands.
- Report and record your care actions.

Range-of-Motion Exercises

Range-of-motion (ROM) exercises—movements that put each joint through its full range of motion—are performed to preserve joint and muscle function for a patient whose movement is limited (Figure 6.21 on the next page). When they are not used, muscles become weak and joints become stiff. Eventually, a contracture may occur (Figure 6.22). In this condition, the muscle is permanently shortened and use of the joint is lost.

In some cases, patients do their own exercises. This is called *active ROM*. Sometimes patients can do the exercises but need assistance to achieve full range. This is called *active ROM* or *active assistive ROM*. When

range of motion (ROM)
the full extent of movement for a joint

Figure 6.21 Follow these general guidelines for performing all range-of-motion exercises. When might range-of-motion exercises be used?

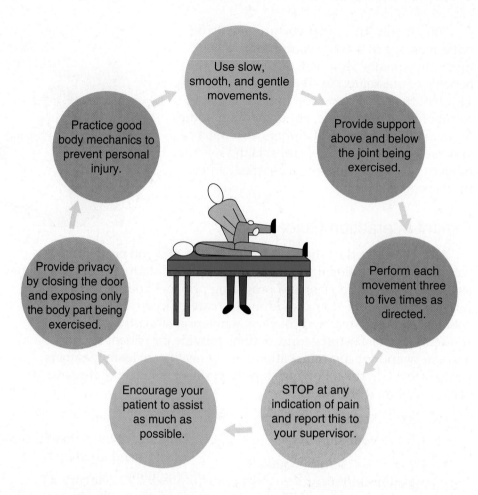

Use slow, smooth, and gentle movements.

Provide support above and below the joint being exercised.

Perform each movement three to five times as directed.

STOP at any indication of pain and report this to your supervisor.

Encourage your patient to assist as much as possible.

Provide privacy by closing the door and exposing only the body part being exercised.

Practice good body mechanics to prevent personal injury.

Figure 6.22 In the condition known as a *contracture*, an unused muscle is permanently shortened and use of the joint is lost. The type of contracture pictured here, in which the bent fingers cannot be straightened, usually affects the pinkie and ring fingers and occurs most frequently among older men.

the patient needs another person to move each joint, the procedure is called *passive ROM*.

Before they begin to work with a patient, healthcare workers must check with their supervisor to find out which range-of-motion exercises will be performed and if there are any limitations to the exercises. For example, after a hip or knee replacement, certain exercises are restricted.

A healthcare worker must also be aware of his or her scope of practice regarding ROM exercises. For example, in some states and some facilities, nursing assistants are not allowed to perform range-of-motion exercises for the neck.

Practice performing passive ROM for the hand by following these steps (Figure 6.23):

1. Complete the preprocedure actions you learned in the previous section.

2. Position the patient comfortably.

3. Support the patient's wrist with one hand. Use your other hand to bend the patient's fingers, making a fist (A). Tuck the thumb under the fingers. Then straighten each finger and the thumb individually (B).

4. Hold the patient's fingers together with one hand. With your other hand, move the thumb and each finger apart and back again (C).

5. Finally, touch the thumb to the tip of each finger (D).

6. Complete your postprocedure actions.

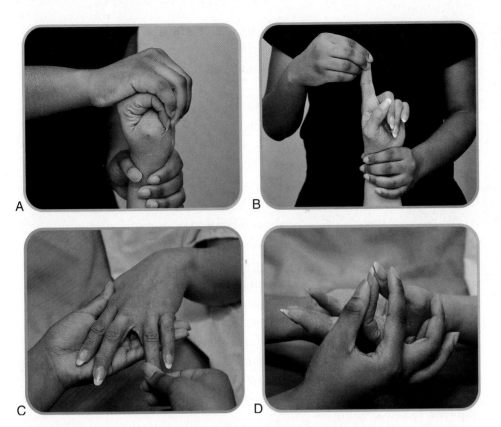

Figure 6.23 Range-of-motion exercises, which are shown here, help to preserve joint and muscle functions for patients who have limited movement due to various conditions.

Preparing a Medication

The position of a pharmacy technician falls under the category of therapeutic services careers. Filling a prescription is one of the most important and most common duties a pharmacy technician performs. With the increased use of electronic medical records, many prescriptions are automatically sent to the pharmacy. Other prescriptions are brought to the pharmacy by patients. There are specific steps involved with filling a prescription. Note that each step followed by an asterisk (*) is a point at which the technician rechecks the prescription to avoid medication errors. Attention to detail is very important in the work of a pharmacy technician.

The technician's first task is to make sure the correct information is listed on the prescription.* It must list the patient's full name, the medication name and dosage, directions for taking the medication, the physician's signature, and refill information.

Next, the technician translates the physician's written prescription. During this step, the technician consults with the pharmacist to interpret any prescriptions that are difficult to read. Computerized systems have greatly reduced the problem of reading a physician's poor handwriting. Finally, the technician enters the prescription into the computer program.

The computer prints a prescription label, which the pharmacist checks for accuracy. The pharmacist also checks which other medications the patient is taking. If drug interactions are possible, the pharmacist contacts the physician.

The technician then follows these steps to fill the prescription:

1. Select the correct medication from the stock shelf area. Check the bottle label and the national drug code number in the computer to make sure it matches the prescription.*

Simulate
EHR

2. Count out the necessary amount of the medication and fill the vial, taking care not to touch the medication. Select and attach the correct lid based on size and the patient's preference for a childproof or easy-open lid.

3. Attach the label to the vial,* and initial the bottom right-hand side of the printed label.

4. Attach auxiliary labels. These give additional information, such as whether the medication needs to be taken with water or on an empty stomach.

5. Put the medication on top of the original prescription.*

6. Present the medication to the pharmacist for final approval (Figure 6.24).

When the patient picks up the prescription, the pharmacist is required to check it one more time. The pharmacist consults with each patient to answer questions and explain information about the medication. When the pharmacist has finished, the technician can ring up the sale. The technician also gets the signature of the person picking up the prescription as part of required record keeping.

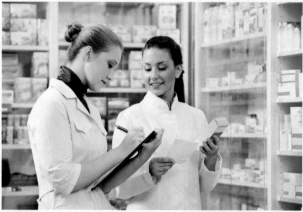

Figure 6.24   A pharmacy technician must get final approval on prescriptions from his or her supervising pharmacist.

Complete the
Map Your Reading
graphic organizer for the section you just read.

RECALL YOUR READING

1. All therapeutic workers practice _____ to protect their patients and _____ from the spread of infection.

2. Since hands are the main pathways of germ transmission in healthcare settings, _____ is the most important measure to prevent healthcare-associated infections.

3. Because many therapeutic workers provide close personal care for their patients, they must become _____ with giving a caring touch to another person.

4. The purpose of performing range-of-motion exercises is to preserve _____ and _____ function.

5. The pharmacy technician may prepare a medication, but a _____ answers patient questions.

Employability Skills for Healthcare Workers

Perhaps you've completed a couple of health science classes, or you've passed your nursing assistant certification test, and you're ready to find a job. You will need to think creatively to locate an entry-level opportunity in the healthcare field because most healthcare jobs require a degree and a license or certification. However difficult finding that first job might be, work experience in healthcare is an asset when you apply for future professional positions. Entry-level work experience also helps you make a decision about your future career goals.

The Therapeutic Worker: Brittany

Brittany completed a nursing assistant class during high school and worked at a nearby nursing home all through college. In her sophomore year, she changed her mind about majoring in nursing and pursued a business degree instead. After graduation, she looked for a sales job in the medical field. The employer who hired her said that her previous CNA job set her apart from all the other applicants. That job gave her work experience in the field and proved that she could be a successful healthcare employee.

The Job Search

Your first job doesn't have to be directly related to your future career. It should, however, provide opportunities to learn skills that you can use in your professional life. For example, becoming a dietary aide may not teach you physical therapy skills, but it will teach you how to interact with residents, and you will be able to observe how physical limitations affect their lives. Likewise, a dental receptionist learns the scheduling process and skills for communicating with patients, and a pharmacy assistant learns a great deal about pharmacology and medical record keeping. The skills learned in these entry-level positions are also important skills for higher-level careers such as professional therapist, dentist, and pharmacist.

Begin your job search by creating a list of all the settings where healthcare is delivered. Then make a list of the businesses in your area. Search their websites to find available jobs for which you are qualified. Job search websites can help you to identify healthcare businesses in your area and alert you to those that are currently hiring. However, be aware that creating an account with a site could bring unwanted advertising, and it may take a lot of searching on a national site to locate healthcare jobs in your specific area.

Ask your health science teacher and guidance counselor for names of businesses that hire entry-level workers. Check the jobs board at your school. A few jobs are still advertised in local papers, so you should look there as well. Stop by the chiropractor's, dentist's, or veterinarian's office on your way home. Ask if they are hiring and if you can fill out an application. Most important, use your personal network. Many times, jobs are filled based on "who you know" before they are ever posted.

A **network** is the group of people you know who work in healthcare. Is your friend's mom a dentist? Ask her about a job. Have you asked your own optometrist about job openings? The best job opportunity is the one that involves someone you know telling you that his or her company is hiring and offering to recommend you. Make a list of all the people you know who already work in healthcare. Take the time to connect with them. These contacts can lead to a job.

The Job Application Process

Applying for a job includes different steps for each employer. Searching the job listings on a company website and applying online is common today. You may be asked to attach your résumé at the end of the application, so have a current copy ready. Many companies hire a firm to operate their online job application process. Be cautious about the personal information you supply. Check for a secure website before providing any identifying information.

Smaller companies may require a paper application form. Some job advertisements will ask you to send your résumé along with a letter expressing your interest in a particular job (Figure 6.25). This letter is called a **cover letter**, or a *letter of application*.

cover letter
a message sent with a résumé to introduce the job applicant and give the reasons he or she is applying for a particular job

Figure 6.25   Job advertisements tell you how to apply for the position being advertised. What different application methods do you see in these ads?

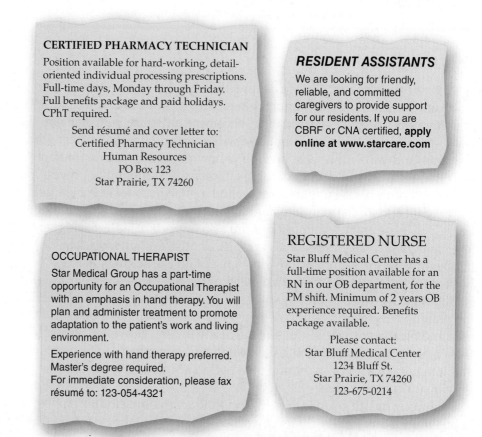

CERTIFIED PHARMACY TECHNICIAN

Position available for hard-working, detail-oriented individual processing prescriptions. Full-time days, Monday through Friday. Full benefits package and paid holidays. CPhT required.

Send résumé and cover letter to:
Certified Pharmacy Technician
Human Resources
PO Box 123
Star Prairie, TX 74260

RESIDENT ASSISTANTS

We are looking for friendly, reliable, and committed caregivers to provide support for our residents. If you are CBRF or CNA certified, **apply online at www.starcare.com**

OCCUPATIONAL THERAPIST

Star Medical Group has a part-time opportunity for an Occupational Therapist with an emphasis in hand therapy. You will plan and administer treatment to promote adaptation to the patient's work and living environment.

Experience with hand therapy preferred. Master's degree required.
For immediate consideration, please fax résumé to: 123-054-4321

REGISTERED NURSE

Star Bluff Medical Center has a full-time position available for an RN in our OB department, for the PM shift. Minimum of 2 years OB experience required. Benefits package available.

Please contact:
Star Bluff Medical Center
1234 Bluff St.
Star Prairie, TX 74260
123-675-0214

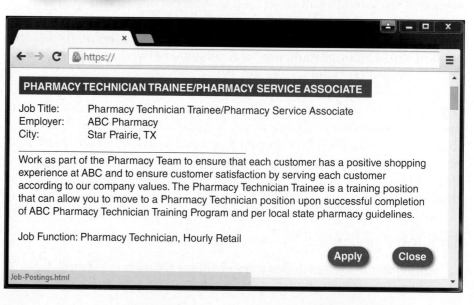

PHARMACY TECHNICIAN TRAINEE/PHARMACY SERVICE ASSOCIATE

Job Title: Pharmacy Technician Trainee/Pharmacy Service Associate
Employer: ABC Pharmacy
City: Star Prairie, TX

Work as part of the Pharmacy Team to ensure that each customer has a positive shopping experience at ABC and to ensure customer satisfaction by serving each customer according to our company values. The Pharmacy Technician Trainee is a training position that can allow you to move to a Pharmacy Technician position upon successful completion of ABC Pharmacy Technician Training Program and per local state pharmacy guidelines.

Job Function: Pharmacy Technician, Hourly Retail

Apply   Close

Job-Postings.html

Personal Data Page. Whether you complete an application form at the beginning of your job search or after you have been interviewed, you will need to access your personal data. The easiest way to do this is to prepare a **personal data page** for your career portfolio and use it as you complete job applications. Include the following information in your personal data page:

- **Contact information.** Your name, address, phone number, and e-mail; you will also need to know your Social Security number but may submit that after you are hired.

- **Education.** List the names and locations of all the schools you have attended along with the years you attended. List any diplomas or degrees you were awarded and your grade point average. Many applications don't request all of this information, but this will prepare you for the ones that do.

- **Work experience.** List all of your work experience, including volunteer work. Write the name, address, and phone number of each employer, and include the years you worked there. Record your job title, duties, the name of your supervisor, and your beginning and ending wage.

- **Skills.** List whatever skills you have that apply to the jobs you are seeking. For example, fast and accurate keyboard skills are important in a medical office.

- **References.** Create a list of three or four **references**. These are people who know you well and are willing to discuss your skills and job qualifications with potential employers. Former employers, teachers, club advisors, or coaches make good references. Your relatives and friends do not make good references because they are considered biased; they should not be listed. Write the name, title, address, and phone number for each reference. You must ask permission from all of these individuals before listing them as references.

Application Form. Whether you complete your application online or on paper, you will follow the same guidelines. Neatness, accuracy, and correct spelling are all very important. Sloppy applications are discarded—even if you're well qualified for the job, you won't be considered if your application is sloppy. Employers think sloppy applications indicate that people will be sloppy in their work. Complete paper applications by printing in ink but use cursive handwriting for your signature. Have your personal data page nearby to use as a reference.

Build Portfolio

Complete every question on the job application form. If some questions don't apply to you, write "does not apply" or "N/A" in the space so the employer knows that you didn't skip the question. For questions related to salary, write "negotiable." If you write a higher wage than what the job pays, you may be eliminated from consideration. Remain positive when stating your reasons for leaving previous jobs. Examples might include "reduction of workforce" or "return to school." Negative comments about former employers will not help your employment prospects.

For privacy reasons, you may choose not to list your Social Security number on a job application form. In this case, you can write "available upon job offer." If you are hired, the business will need your Social Security number before you can be paid. If you are applying online, make sure you are accessing a legitimate website and a secure page before entering your Social Security number.

In the field of healthcare, you may need to complete a **caregiver background form** or **Background Information Disclosure (BID) form**. This process eliminates workers who have a history of harming others. The background check is designed to protect clients, patients, and residents. A Social Security number is required for completing a background check.

Make positive choices about your behavior now! Students who are involved in fights can be **barred**, or prevented from working in healthcare if the charges result in a criminal record. Many companies also do an Internet search. Be very careful about posting personal information on social networking sites (Figure 6.26). People have been eliminated from hiring processes and have lost current jobs because of information or photos they posted on the Internet.

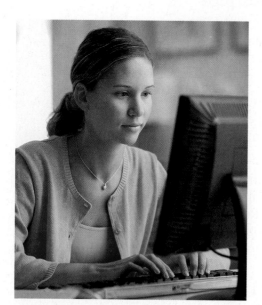

Figure 6.26   Other people can see what you post online—even potential employers. Use good judgment about what you post to social media and elsewhere.

Cover Letter/Letter of Application. When you mail a résumé or post it online, you should include a cover letter to introduce yourself and explain why you are applying for the job. This letter summarizes your main qualifications and expresses positive interest in the job. Just like your résumé and your application form, your cover letter must be error-free.

Your cover letter should be typed using a business letter format and should contain three sections (Figure 6.27):

- **Introduction.** The introduction tells the employer how you learned about the job or company and why you are interested in the position.

- **Body.** The body of the message explains to the employer how your skills will meet the organization's needs. Do not repeat all the facts on your résumé but include enough information to get the employer interested in reading it.

- **Conclusion.** In your conclusion, you should request an interview and provide the contact information needed for the employer to reach you easily.

The Job Interview

The job interview is a conversation between you and a possible future employer. The employer wants to know if you will be a good fit for the healthcare facility, and you want to know if you will enjoy working at this facility. You should prepare for your interview by learning as much as you can about the business. Search online and talk with someone who works there. Read the job description carefully.

Consider your knowledge and experience. Then prepare examples that you can talk about to illustrate your job qualifications. The employer will want to know that you have the technical skill for the job but will also be looking for examples of your communication, teamwork, and problem-solving skills. Don't be afraid to talk about school classes, clubs, or athletic team experiences that demonstrate these skills.

Sam Sanchez
4035 Starlight Ct.
Star Prairie, TX 74260

November 3, 2015

Human Resources
PO Box 123
Star Prairie, TX 74260

Greeting ——————| Dear Hiring Manager:

Introduction ——— I am writing in response to your advertisement in the Star Prairie News for a certified pharmacy technician. After reading your job description, I am confident that my skills and aptitudes are a perfect match for this position.

I began working in a pharmacy during my senior year of high school through the health youth apprenticeship program. During my senior year, I completed a full year of pharmacy technician coursework. Upon graduation, I took the state certification exam and became a certified pharmacy technician last June.

Body ———

My youth apprenticeship mentor ranked my attention to detail and responsible work attitude as outstanding on my work program evaluations. In addition to my pharmacy coursework, I have completed courses in medical terminology, body structure and function, and computer concepts. I was an active member of HOSA, attending state conferences and competing in pharmacology and prepared speaking.

Conclusion ——— I would welcome the opportunity to discuss this position with you. If you have questions or would like to schedule an interview, please contact me by phone at 123-217-2130 or by e-mail at SSanchez@gmail.com. I have enclosed my résumé for your review, and I look forward to hearing from you.

Sincerely,

Sam Sanchez

Sam Sanchez

Enclosure

Figure 6.27   This cover message is in letter format because it will be mailed. When responding to an online job ad, your cover message will begin with the greeting. You will list your contact information after your name at the end of the message. Attach your résumé to the e-mail.

Next, prepare a few questions to ask about the healthcare facility and the position for which you're applying. Avoid asking questions about pay and benefits before you have been offered the job. Be prepared to answer typical interview questions by practicing your answers at home. Know that some personal questions are considered illegal in the interview process (Figure 6.28).

Practicing proper **interview etiquette** includes choosing business-like attire (Figure 6.29). You are not dressing for a party or for school. Avoid jeans, T-shirts, tank tops, tennis shoes, hats, and sunglasses. Limit jewelry, wear only light makeup, and avoid fake nails and colored nail polish. Remove all visible piercings and cover tattoos.

We expect healthcare facilities to be clean, so make sure that you are as well. Your hair, clothing, nails, hands, and shoes should all look clean and neat. Know that strong fragrances can be irritating and unpleasant when you are ill or have allergies and demonstrate that knowledge by limiting your use of scented products.

Bring your career portfolio with you. Have extra copies of your résumé to leave with the employer. Arrive a few minutes early and alone. Do not bring a friend or family member with you because that person may make a bad impression. Turn off your cell phone or just don't bring it if you are tempted to check messages. Greet the interviewer with a smile and a firm, but not gripping, handshake.

interview etiquette
accepted appearance and behavior for the interview process

Questions you might ask

What are the specific duties of this position?
What skills are most important in this position?
What are the working hours?
What do you consider your facility's most important assets?
How is your facility organized, and how does your department fit into the organization?
What types of services are provided at your facility?
What is the next step in your hiring process?

Questions to avoid asking until you have a job offer

How much does this job pay?
How much vacation time do I get each year?
Will I have to work overtime?
Do you pay bonuses?

NEVER ask:
Can I use your phone to call my ride?
I hated my last boss. How does management work here?
This job sounds pretty neat. How come the last person left?

Questions they might ask

What are your strengths/weaknesses?
What makes you a good employee?
Describe your work experiences.
Why do you want to work for this organization?
Tell me something about yourself.
What subjects did you enjoy in school and why?
How do you manage your time?
What does success mean to you?

Questions they can't legally ask

Do you have children?
Are you single or married?
How old are you?
How tall are you? or How much do you weigh?
Do you have any disabilities?
How's your family's health?
Have you ever been arrested?
Do you go to church?
ANY question about nationality/color/religion

Figure 6.28   Reviewing these four categories of questions will help you prepare for the question-and-answer format used in job interviews.

Your goal is to convince the employer that you are the right person to hire. Let your appearance say that you take work seriously and think this interview is important. Let your behavior say that you will be easy to talk with, easy to work with, and a positive addition to the staff. Thank the interviewer for taking the time to speak with you.

Send a thank-you e-mail the next day (Figure 6.30). If you want the job, express your interest again in the thank-you e-mail. Add any information you forgot to provide during the interview.

Primary Work Tasks

As you continue to search for a satisfying health science career, consider the primary tasks of an occupation. Look for jobs that include tasks you enjoy performing. Knowing your likes and dislikes in your hobbies and activities will help you plan for a career that is a good match for you. All job tasks focus primarily on people, data, things, or ideas:

- People-oriented jobs provide care and services to people, lead or guide people, or sell products to people. These jobs may be a good choice if you enjoy helping someone who is sick, running for an office, listening to a friend's problems, or showing a child how to do a new task.

- Data-oriented jobs deal with facts, numbers, and files of information, and involve business procedures. Do you like to complete science experiments? serve as a club treasurer? write a computer program? research an interesting topic?

- Ideas-oriented jobs work with knowledge, insights, theories, and new ways of doing or saying something. Are you interested in

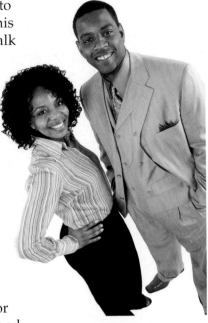

Figure 6.29 Professional, business-like attire is required for a job interview.

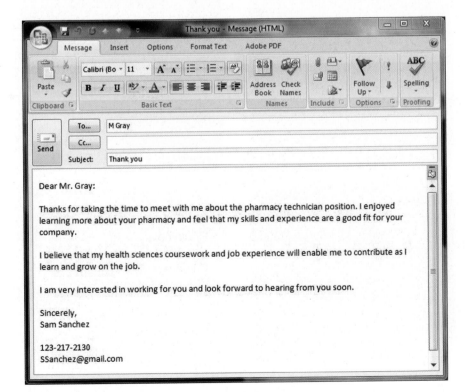

Figure 6.30 Send a thank-you note within a day of your interview. An e-mail is generally acceptable now, but you can send a written note if you think that would be preferred. This sample shows a thank-you note in an e-mail format.

decorating a room? writing stories or music? performing in a play or a concert? inventing a new product?

- Things-oriented jobs involve working with equipment and machines; living things; and materials such as food, metal, or plastic. Do you find satisfaction in repairing a car; building something out of wood; gardening and lawn care; making craft projects; preparing food; or operating computers, cameras, and other electronic equipment?

While all jobs involve a combination of people-, data-, ideas-, and things-related tasks, you will be most satisfied when your preference for one or two of these areas matches the primary tasks of your job (Figure 6.31).

Do you remember Brittany, the nursing student who became a medical sales representative, whom we mentioned earlier in the chapter? She knew that she was a people person. She pursued nursing because she wanted to work with people but learned that she also had a strong entrepreneurial personality. She enjoyed the tasks of guiding people and helping them choose appropriate products more than the tasks of caring for them directly.

When you research specific careers, read about the nature of the work to learn about the actual tasks performed by workers in your chosen career. Ask yourself if a job's tasks match your own preferences for working with people, data, ideas, or things.

HOSA Connections

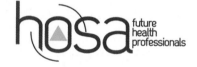

HOSA provides many opportunities to build your therapeutic skills as well as your employability skills. Attend HOSA conferences to practice

Figure 6.31   Based on your interests, you may want to pursue jobs that specifically include people-, data-, ideas-, or things-related tasks. Choose the category that best fits with your interests and research which jobs include that type of task.

DATA
Medical Coder
Biostatistician
Admitting Clerk
Clinical Data Specialist
Unit Coordinator
Patient Account Technician
Quality Control Technician

PEOPLE
Nurse
Paramedic
Pharmaceutical Sales
  Representative
Rehabilitation Counselor
Dietary Manager
Healthcare Administrator
Social Worker

THINGS
Central Service Technician
Hospital Maintenance Engineer
Medical Lab Technologist
Product Safety Scientist
Dental Lab Technician
Optician
Nurse Anesthetist

IDEAS
Radiologist
Geneticist
Epidemiologist
Forensic Scientist
Speech-Language Pathologist
Molecular Biologist
Exercise Physiologist

wearing business-like attire and to interact with other members in a professional development setting. Several HOSA competitive events can strengthen your career skills. Read about all of these in the *competitive events* section of the HOSA website (Figure 6.32).

Figure 6.32 HOSA Events	
Event Name	**Event Description**
Dental Terminology	written test
Pharmacology	written test
Medical Math	written test
Human Growth and Development	written test
Transcultural Healthcare	written test
Medical Reading	written test
Job Seeking Skills/ Interviewing Skills	cover letter, résumé, job application, and interview
Clinical Nursing	written test and skills demonstration
Dental Science	written test and skills demonstration
Home Health Aide	written test and skills demonstration
Medical Assisting	written test and skills demonstration
Nursing Assistant/ Personal Care	written test and skills demonstration
Physical Therapy	written test and skills demonstration
Sports Medicine	written test and skills demonstration
Veterinary Science	written test and skills demonstration

RECALL YOUR READING

1. Connecting with your healthcare _____ can contribute to success in acquiring a job.
2. Today, many job applications are completed _____.
3. Submitting the _____ form eliminates healthcare workers who have a history of harming others.
4. A career portfolio that has all of your information in one place and is easily available will streamline the _____ process.
5. HOSA provides opportunities to imiprove your _____ skills and _____ skills.

Complete the
Map Your Reading
graphic organizer for the
section you just read.

Chapter 6 Review

SUMMARY

 Assess your understanding with chapter tests

- Therapeutic occupations are primarily involved in changing the health status of the patient over time.

- Therapeutic workers must be skilled at showing empathy and using tact when communicating with patients.

- The education and training requirements for physicians are among the most demanding of any occupation.

- Nursing has the largest number of job openings and employs more workers than any other healthcare occupation.

- As a cost-saving measure, therapeutic tasks are increasingly being delegated to workers with technical training.

- Collaboration is a key element in the interdisciplinary team model.

- Nurses provide care using a variety of nursing care models that include the case manager model, primary nursing, functional nursing, and the team nursing model.

- All therapeutic workers practice standard precautions to prevent the spread of infection in healthcare settings.

- Since many therapeutic workers provide close personal care for their patients, they must become comfortable with giving caring touch to another person.

- A well-developed career portfolio is an important asset in your job search.

- Attending HOSA conferences provides valuable experiences in modeling professional career etiquette.

MAXIMIZE YOUR PROFESSIONAL VOCABULARY

Build vocabulary with e-flash cards, games, and audio glossary

Listed below are the essential, yellow-highlighted terms and the additional professional vocabulary terms that you encountered in this chapter. Complete the activities that follow the list to make all of these terms part of your everyday professional vocabulary.

amputate
Background Information
    Disclosure (BID) form
barred
caregiver background form
case manager
certified nursing assistant
    (CNA)
clients
clinical training
collaborate
congenital
contraindicated
cover letter
delegate
dementia
empathy

fellowship
functional nursing
hand hygiene
intern
interview etiquette
licensed practical nurse (LPN)
licensed vocational nurse
    (LVN)
multidisciplinary healthcare
    team
network
non-intact skin
nosocomial infections
outsource
personal data page
personal protective equipment
    (PPE)

physician assistant (PA)
postgraduate
primary care teams
primary nursing
range of motion (ROM)
references
registered nurse (RN)
residents
respiratory hygiene
secondary care teams
standard precautions
tact
team nursing
technical training
teleconferencing
therapeutic
tier

Matching. Match each essential term from this chapter with the correct definition below by writing the letter of the definition next to the number of the essential term on a separate sheet of paper.

1. clinical training
2. collaborate
3. cover letter
4. delegate
5. empathy
6. interview etiquette
7. multidisciplinary healthcare team
8. personal protective equipment (PPE)
9. postgraduate
10. range of motion (ROM)
11. residents
12. standard precautions
13. tact
14. technical training
15. therapeutic

a. the ability to identify with another person's feelings and thoughts

b. the ability to communicate difficult or embarrassing information without giving offense

c. accepted appearance and behavior for the interview process

d. a message sent with a résumé to introduce the job applicant and give the reasons he or she is applying for a particular job

e. term that describes "hands-on" work with patients that students do under the supervision of a licensed healthcare provider

f. the full extent of movement for a joint

g. education lasting two years or less and leading to an industry certificate, a technical diploma, or an associate's degree

h. a group of healthcare workers from different healthcare specialties, each providing specific services to the patient

i. to work together; to consult with each other

j. (1) individuals living in long-term care facilities; (2) medical school graduates who are completing the last portion of their medical training before becoming licensed physicians

k. term that describes education and training completed after receiving a bachelor's degree

l. to direct another healthcare worker to perform a care task that is within that worker's training and experience and within the scope of practice of the licensed provider giving the direction

m. steps that a healthcare worker takes with all patients to prevent the spread of infection

n. term that describes treatment given to maintain or restore health

o. equipment such as gloves, masks, gowns, respirators, and eyewear worn to protect skin, clothing, and the respiratory tract from infectious agents

16. **Hollywood Squares Terms Review.** The teacher will select nine students to be the "celebrities" and then divide the remaining students into two teams. Each celebrity holds a large card marked with an O on one side and an X on the other. Three students sit on chairs placed at the front of the classroom, three sit on the floor in front of the chairs, and three stand behind to simulate the tic-tac-toe board.

Contestants from each team take turns selecting a celebrity to answer a question for them. The contestants must then agree or disagree with their celebrity's answer. Each team tries to create a row of Xs or Os to win. Rotate contestants after each vocabulary question and rotate celebrities after each game to allow all students to participate.

REFLECT ON YOUR READING

17. Review the list of 10 occupations you created for the *Connect with Your Reading* activity. How many of those occupations are in the therapeutic pathway? You can use the career chart in chapter 1 to check this. For each therapeutic occupation on your list, indicate whether it requires technical training (two years or less) or professional training (four years or more). Mark the occupations on your list that you believe will provide good job opportunities in the future. Be prepared to discuss your list with your classmates.

BUILD CORE SKILLS

18. **Writing.** Review the section in this chapter that discusses personal traits for therapeutic workers. Think about your own life and write a paragraph about a personal experience that shows you are empathetic, dependable, or have the ability to accept criticism.

19. **Problem Solving.** Which type of therapist would each of these people see?

    - Jim, a three-year-old, has a high fever.
    - Mr. Jones is experiencing symptoms of depression following his divorce.
    - Mr. Rogers needs to learn what a particular shadow on his X-ray means.
    - Kim's eyes are not focusing, and they are red and itchy.
    - Grandpa has a bad heart and his circulation is poor.

20. **Critical Thinking.** Create a five-point chart to compare two occupations—physician and physician assistant. As you prepare your chart, consider the following topics: education and training, work environment, job outlook, job tasks and responsibilities, and earnings. Based on your comparison, which occupation would you like to pursue? Why?

21. **Critical Thinking.** Review the section in this chapter on nursing careers to identify the scope of practice for a certified nursing assistant, licensed practical nurse/licensed vocational nurse, registered nurse, and nurse practitioner. Then list all nurses qualified to complete each of the following tasks:

    - making a hospital bed
    - diagnosing a patient condition
    - giving a vaccination
    - writing a prescription
    - providing wound care
    - assisting with ambulation
    - feeding a patient
    - training nursing students

22. **Critical Thinking.** Review Figure 6.12, which shows healthcare team collaboration. Then answer the following questions about healthcare teamwork.

    a. What do the lines between each of the healthcare workers listed in this diagram tell us about the functioning of healthcare teams?

    b. Why is the patient in the middle of the diagram?

    c. Each point of the star (the patient) points to a healthcare worker. Why is that significant? What does that indicate about healthcare team communication?

23. **Critical Thinking.** Choose one of the job ads from Figure 6.25 and pretend you are interviewing for the job. Show your knowledge of etiquette as you answer the following questions:

    - What will you wear to the interview?
    - What will you take with you to the interview? What will you not take with you?
    - How do you greet the interviewer?
    - How do you end the interview, and what do you do after the interview?

24. **Speaking and Listening.** Refer to Figure 6.28 in your text. Select any three questions that an interviewer might ask, prepare your responses, and practice answering the questions aloud. Be prepared to give your answers during a classroom interview simulation.

25. **Reading.** Read the following statements taken from a job application form.

Please Read Before Signing:

The information that you provide on this application is subject to verification. Falsifications or misrepresentations may disqualify you from consideration for employment or, if you are hired, may be grounds for termination later.

With my signature below, I certify that all information on this application is true, correct, and complete to the best of my knowledge and contains no willful falsifications or misrepresentations. I authorize all former employers to release job-related information they may have about me, and I release all persons or companies from any liability or responsibility for providing such information.

Signature _____
Date _____

You may be required to sign a job application form that looks like this. Will you know what are you signing? Define the following terms: *verification*, *falsification*, *misrepresentation*, *grounds for termination*, *certify*, *willful*, *authorize*, *liability*. With these definitions in mind, rewrite the passage in your own words. Do you understand what you're signing?

ACTIVATE YOUR LEARNING

26. Review the principles of standard precautions. Then assemble supplies and follow the steps described in your text to practice hand hygiene and putting on and removing personal protective equipment.

27. Review the steps for filling a prescription on page 204. Then copy the sample label shown here and practice filling the following prescription for Jane Doe.

Star Prairie Clinic
Dr. John Smith
333 Clinic Street
Star Prairie, TX 74260
123-701-3000
Medication: 500mg M&M tablets
Three times each day for three days
to treat fungal infection
NO REFILLS
Signature: *Dr. John Smith*

Prescription

Star Prairie Pharmacy   Date _____
123 Clinic St.
Star Prairie, TX 74260
123-701-5000
Patient's Name _____
Medication _____
Direction _____
_____
# of tablets _____
NO REFILLS   Rx# 345678

Label

THINK AND ACT LIKE A HEALTHCARE WORKER

28. Sasha was excited to get a part-time job in a dental office. She had always wanted to become a dental hygienist and knew this would be the perfect opportunity to expand her knowledge and skills while still in high school. Two months later, she was having doubts about her career choice. She didn't think she

could perform the same tasks every day as part of her job. According to the John Holland chart in chapter 2, which personality type finds satisfaction in dental careers? What are the primary work tasks of the dental hygienist? What would you suggest that Sasha do next to prepare for a satisfying healthcare career?

GO TO THE SOURCE

29. Use the Internet to learn more about careers in therapeutic services. Select two careers of interest to you and complete a career profile page for each career. Use at least one site that ends in .gov and one site that ends in .org. Record the following information for each career:

- name of the career
- tasks involved in this career
- personal traits and abilities needed
- educational requirements
- type of credential needed and how it is obtained
- work conditions
- wages and benefits
- job outlook for the future
- the websites you accessed

How do the two careers compare? Why might you prefer one to the other?

DEVELOP YOUR HEALTH SCIENCE CAREER PORTFOLIO

30. Create your personal data page. Include all the information listed in the text. Place your completed page in your career portfolio.

31. Locate an advertisement for a health science job that interests you. Create a cover letter using the sample in the text as a guideline. Place the completed letter in your career portfolio.

32. Complete a sample job application form for practice. Follow the guidelines described on pages 207 and 208. Place the completed form in your career portfolio.

33. Research the HOSA competitive events listed in this chapter on the HOSA website. Select and note which event is your top choice and list reasons for your choice.

Chapter 7
Fundamental Skills in Therapeutic Services

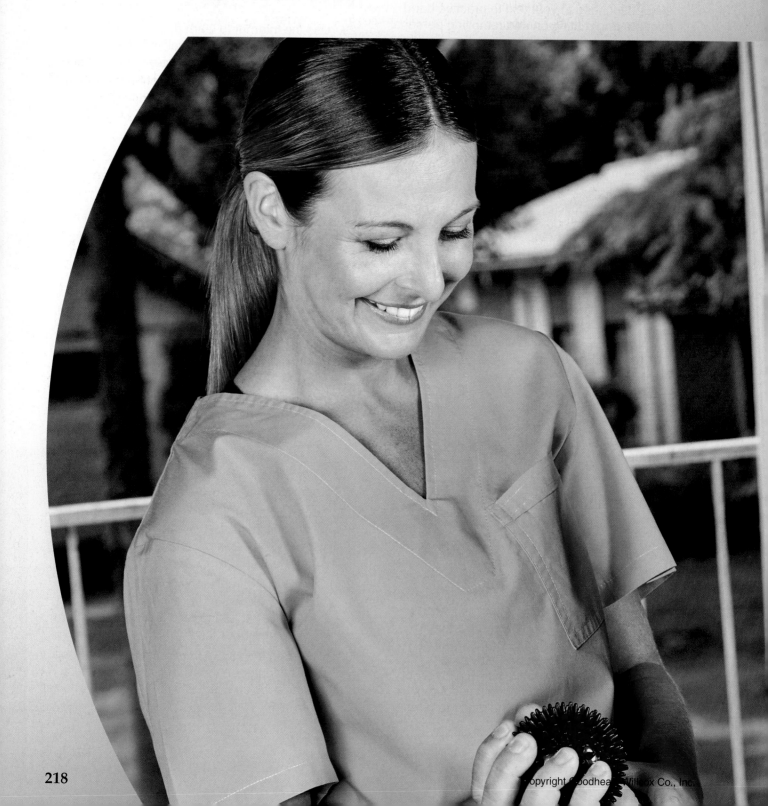

PROFESSIONAL VOCABULARY

E-flash Cards

You will need to learn the essential terms listed below before you begin your reading. These terms will help you understand the main concepts of the chapter. These terms, which will be highlighted in yellow within the text, will become part of your professional vocabulary.

In addition to the essential terms, you will see bold terms throughout the chapter. The meanings of these terms are explained where the terms first appear. The bold terms, like the essential terms listed here, will also become part of your professional vocabulary and deepen your understanding of the topics presented.

24-hour clock a method of telling time that assigns a number to each hour of the day; also known as *military time*

apps applications; software that is accessed through the Internet and runs on a computer, smartphone, tablet, or other mobile device

assertive communication a communication style characterized by confidence and consideration for others

communication barrier anything that blocks or interferes with the exchange of information

communication style a person's preferred method for exchanging information, which includes words, tone of voice, and nonverbal signals

cultural diversity term that describes differences in age, gender, physical and intellectual abilities, sexual orientation, race, or ethnicity that influence what we believe, the way we think, and what we do

e-prescribing electronic generation, transmission, and filling of a medical prescription

goniometer an instrument for measuring angles

medication a substance or mixture of substances that have been proven through research to have a clear value in the prevention, diagnosis, or treatment of diseases

metric system the decimal measurement system based on the meter, liter, and gram as its primary units of length, volume, and weight or mass respectively

open-ended question a question that requires more than a one- or two-word response

patient interview a structured communication between a patient and a healthcare worker for the purpose of collecting subjective data such as a medical history

social media a group of online communication tools that allow people to share information and resources via the Internet

US customary units the main system of weights and measures used in the United States based on the yard, pound, and gallon as units of length, weight, and liquid volume respectively; also known as *household measurements*

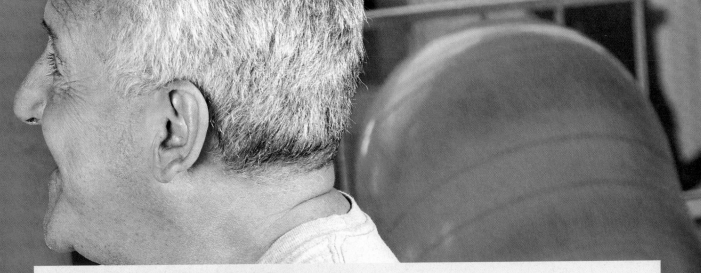

CONNECT WITH YOUR READING

Because of the increasing diversity of the general population, the US healthcare system needs a culturally competent workforce. How do you define culture? How does a person's culture influence healthcare practices? What skills or characteristics does a culturally competent healthcare worker possess? Consider these questions and share your thoughts with a classmate.

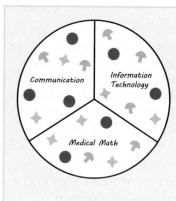

MAP YOUR READING

Create a visual summary by drawing a large circle on a blank sheet of paper. Divide the circle into three pizza slices. Label one slice *Communication*, another *Information Technology*, and the third *Medical Math*. As you finish reading each section of the chapter, place the following "toppings" on your pizza:

- Draw "pepperoni" circles containing the main ideas, or the "meat" of the information.
- Draw "mushroom" shapes containing bits of information that are new or interesting for you and kept you from "vegging out" as you read.
- Draw "mystery" toppings (you create the shapes) that contain questions you still have about your reading.

In this chapter, you will examine common communication styles and consider your own preferred style. You will also learn techniques for communicating clearly with coworkers and patients and for recognizing and overcoming barriers to clear communication. As you consider the expanding use of electronic health records and information systems, you will recognize the advantages of this technology. You will also become aware of concerns regarding the use of computers, social media, and mobile technologies in the field of healthcare.

You will study how to record time using the 24-hour clock and how to work accurately within and convert between the metric system of measurement used in healthcare and the household system used by US citizens. An introduction to math and medications highlights the critical role that accuracy plays in the preparation and administration of medication. Practice in using a goniometer to measure range of motion will acquaint you with a technique used by therapists to evaluate patient progress.

Communicating with Patients and Coworkers

Communication is especially important in healthcare settings because it is a vital factor in patient care (Figure 7.1). In fact, studies of

Figure 7.1 Improving communication between caregivers improves patient outcomes.

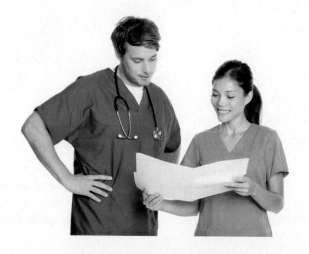

medical errors show that communication difficulties cause the majority of preventable problems in healthcare. According to The Joint Commission, an organization that accredits and certifies US healthcare programs, improving communication between caregivers can prevent negative patient outcomes and strengthen a teamwork approach to patient care.

The Therapeutic Worker: Karen

Karen, a registered nurse at the hospital, was worried about her patient, Mr. Benning. Instead of feeling better after his surgery, his pain was increasing. He didn't look quite right, either. Karen believed that something was seriously wrong with her patient. She decided to call the doctor.

"Hello, Doctor Black," she said. "This is Karen, one of the nurses. Mr. Benning is in pain that he says is at 10. I just don't feel right about him."

The doctor replied that Karen should increase the dose of Tylenol for Mr. Benning.

Now Karen was frustrated. She really wanted the doctor to examine her patient, but what could she do?

Communication Styles

While communication is certainly about the words we choose, our tone of voice and nonverbal signals are just as important. Our **communication style** is a combination of all three of these aspects (Figure 7.2). Every person has a preferred communication style based on

communication style
a person's preferred method for exchanging information, which includes words, tone of voice, and nonverbal signals

Figure 7.2 Communication Style Self-Assessment				
	Passive	**Aggressive**	**Passive/Aggressive**	**Assertive**
How it sounds	apologetic; soft/tentative tone of voice	loud, demanding tone of voice; uses "you" statements to accuse or humiliate others	sarcastic tone of voice; says *yes* but means *no*	firm tone of voice; uses "I" statements to express feelings and opinions clearly
How it looks	no eye contact; stooped posture	tense and rigid posture; points fingers at others	appears satisfied with decision, but will complain about it later	direct eye contact; relaxed posture
How it feels	I'm shy; I'll go with the flow; my feelings aren't important.	My feelings are most important; I think I'm superior.	I'm uncomfortable saying what I think.	I think we are equal; we are both important.
How it turns out	I feel angry and resentful.	No one trusts me; they just avoid me.	I don't have real friends anymore.	I expressed my opinion even if it didn't go my way this time.

personality and environment, including individual experiences. Do you recognize your style in any of the following descriptions?

- **Passive.** You may be shy or very easygoing. You usually say, "I'll just go with whatever the group decides." You want to avoid conflict. This attitude creates problems because you're sending the message that your thoughts and feelings aren't as important as those of other people. When you are too passive, you allow other people to disregard your wants and needs. That can make you feel angry and resentful, increasing your stress level.

- **Aggressive.** You may act like a bully by disregarding the feelings and opinions of others. You may even humiliate and intimidate others. While you appear to get what you want, your aggression may be destroying trust. Others may avoid you or oppose your ideas because they don't trust you.

- **Passive-Aggressive.** You may say *yes* when you want to say *no*. You may be sarcastic or complain about others behind their backs. Feeling uncomfortable about stating your needs and feelings can lead to passive-aggressive behavior. This communication style damages relationships and makes it harder to meet goals.

- **Assertive.** You state your opinions and feelings clearly. You stick up for your rights and needs but respect the rights of others in the process. This style tells people your needs and opinions are important. Assertiveness is a healthy communication style because it is effective, diplomatic, and can help you manage stress levels.

How can you recognize **assertive communication**? Assertive people make eye contact. They stand up straight and look like they are ready to talk and to listen. Assertive people give their opinions, but they don't try to argue and they don't become mean or sarcastic. They listen to criticism and consider it carefully, but they don't let it make them feel inferior or inadequate. They understand that being assertive includes respecting the opinions of others and not always getting what you want.

assertive communication
a communication style characterized by confidence and consideration for others

Communicating with Coworkers

Reconsider the story about Karen, the nurse who had trouble communicating with the physician. Do you recognize her style? Because she used a passive style, Karen was unable to communicate her concerns and opinions about her patient's needs. She didn't even tell the doctor that she wanted her patient to be evaluated for a serious complication. Communicating assertively in a healthcare environment increases the level of patient care. Several healthcare facilities have developed training programs to teach assertive communication skills to employees.

The **SBAR system** is a method that helps healthcare workers communicate with each other more clearly (Figure 7.3). The system creates a standardized communication format that is very useful for reporting changes in a patient's status. SBAR is an acronym that stands for *Situation, Background, Assessment,* and *Recommendation.* Each of these terms means something specific in a healthcare setting:

- **Situation.** What is currently happening? Begin by identifying yourself, your occupation, and your location. Then identify your patient by name and date of birth. Describe the patient's current status and your reason for communicating.

- **Background.** What are the circumstances leading to this situation? Give a brief summary of relevant past medical history. Provide details of the patient's status, including vital signs, pain scale, and level of consciousness.

- **Assessment.** What is the problem? Note any signs that are outside the normal ranges, your impressions, and any additional concerns.

- **Recommendation.** What should be done to correct the problem? Explain what you want to happen and how soon you think it should happen. Suggest possible actions and then clarify your expectations.

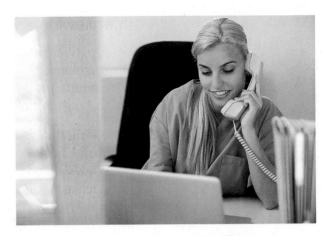

Figure 7.3 This nurse might be using the SBAR system to talk to a colleague. According to SBAR, what is one thing she should include in her communication?

The Therapeutic Worker: Karen

The SBAR system helps healthcare workers communicate with each other. If Karen, the nurse mentioned earlier in the chapter, used SBAR to communicate with the physician, she might communicate her concerns more clearly:

- **Situation.** Dr. Black, my name is Karen. I'm the RN on 6 west caring for your patient, Mr. Benning, DOB 12/06/51. He is here for a GI bleed. He is currently complaining of chest pain, looks pale, and is sweating profusely.

- **Background.** Mr. Benning received two units of red blood cells this morning. At 3 p.m., he had blood drawn, and his hematocrit (hih-MA-tuh-krit) is 31. His vital signs are BP, 88/52; pulse, 120; respiration, 24. His pain is a 10 on a scale of 10. I just administered 2 L/min oxygen by nasal cannula (KAN-yoo-luh).

- **Assessment.** It looks like he may have internal bleeding or an MI, but I think additional tests are needed to know for sure.

- **Recommendation.** I would like an order for an EKG, a blood test to check hemoglobin and hematocrit, medication for increased pain, and I need you to evaluate him without delay. What questions do you have for me?

Learning to communicate assertively has many benefits. It reduces anxiety and increases self-esteem. It helps you achieve your goals and allows you to make decisions more easily. More important, learning to communicate assertively in a healthcare setting by using a system such as SBAR can improve patient outcomes.

Interviewing a Patient

patient interview
a structured communication
between a patient and
a healthcare worker for
the purpose of collecting
subjective data such as a
medical history

A **patient interview** is useful when taking a patient's medical history. During interviews, you want patients to feel comfortable about explaining their symptoms. When healthcare workers conduct a patient interview, they follow a set of guidelines, or *protocols*.

Following Professional Protocols. Successful interviews begin with courtesy. Knock before entering the exam room. Remember that patient interviews are conducted in private. Greet your patient using a formal title such as *Mr. Benning*, and introduce yourself by giving your name and job title. Use first names only when requested. Limit interruptions and be prepared with your forms and questions. Avoid going straight to the computer and barely looking at the patient.

The next steps in the interview process are meant to build trust. Use your positive nonverbal communication skills. Sit so you are facing the patient at eye level and making eye contact as the patient speaks. The patient needs to feel that you understand his or her symptoms. If you're not looking at the patient as he or she is talking, you will be perceived as not listening, even if you have heard every word. Maintain a distance of two to four feet to avoid invading the patient's personal space.

Show respect by keeping an open mind about what the patient tells you. Differences in culture or experience can impair effective communication with your patient. Examine your own values and beliefs to minimize any personal biases that could interfere with the interview. Healthcare workers apply a "therapeutic use of self." This means they remain nonjudgmental as they use their interpersonal skills to help their patients (Figure 7.4). Avoid talking about your own problems. Professional healthcare workers set aside their own difficulties when they care for others.

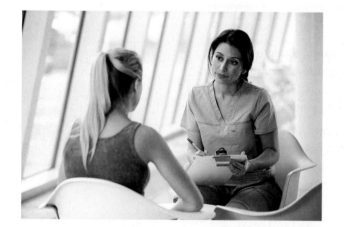

Figure 7.4 Use positive body language and remain nonjudgmental during a patient interview.

open-ended question
a question that requires
more than a one- or two-
word response

Asking Open-Ended Questions. Communicating with patients requires the use of techniques that encourage a patient to share information. Always begin by asking **open-ended questions**. Of course, if a patient has trouble breathing or speaking, you will want to receive a short response, but more information is beneficial in most patient interactions. For example, if you ask, "Would you say you are in good health?" the patient will reply *yes* or *no*, and the conversation will be over. If you say, "Tell me about your health," the patient is more likely to name a problem or give a description.

Avoid asking questions that begin with the word *why*. Perhaps you are caring for a patient who finds it difficult to communicate. While discussing how he feels about his illness, he stops talking mid-sentence. If you ask, "Why did you stop?" he is likely to reply, "I don't know," and your conversation will be over. If instead you acknowledge his feelings by saying, "You seem uncomfortable," he will see that you are empathetic and may be willing to talk further about his feelings.

Rephrasing what the patient has said is another method for encouraging conversation. If a patient says, "I don't know how I'll be able to pay for this hospitalization," try rephrasing this in the form of a question such as, "You're worried about finances?" This shows that you are listening and encourages further communication.

Address sensitive topics at the end of the patient interview, after you've had a chance to build a connection with the patient. Practice asking sensitive questions before the interview so you can ask them calmly when you're with a patient. You will become more comfortable with practice, and this will make your patients more willing to voice problems and concerns (Figure 7.5).

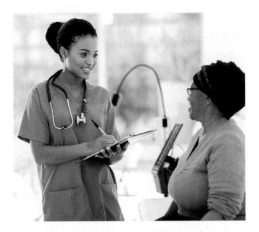

Figure 7.5   You can learn more about a patient's health concerns by asking open-ended questions and showing sensitivity.

The Patient Interview Process. Follow these steps as you complete a patient interview:

1. Gather your tools. These may include forms, a computer tablet, a pen, and equipment for measuring vital signs.

2. Introduce yourself and state your role at the healthcare facility. For example: "Hi, Mr. Benning. I'm Amy, Dr. Black's medical assistant. I would like to ask you a few questions to update your medical history, and I want to take your vital signs before the doctor sees you."

3. Verify the patient's name and birth date. Then update the patient's medical history. Note any surgeries or family medical history that might mean a patient is more at risk for a particular medical condition.

4. Record a list of medications the patient is currently taking, including vitamins and herbal supplements. This allows the physician to check for drug-related symptoms or drug interactions. For each medication, list the amount, dosage, frequency, and time of day the medication is taken. Spell out each medication to make sure you have the correct one. A patient may give you a list of his or her medications, but you should verify each item on the list to make sure it is current.

5. Measure and record vital signs.

6. Ask the reason for the patient's visit. This is the time to use your open-ended questions. Don't rush. If you give your patient time to think, you will receive answers that are more reliable. Record the patient's responses in detail. If your computerized record uses a drop-down menu, make sure the correct symptoms have been checked. Then add details in the comment section.

7. Review the patient's information and reason for seeing the doctor. This will verify your data and act as a polite ending to the interview. Let the patient know how soon to expect the doctor and excuse yourself, closing the door as you exit.

Communication Barriers

Now that you've studied the communication process and are working to develop assertive communication skills, your communication should be effective. That sounds logical, but in reality, our communication can be interrupted by a multitude of barriers. Recognizing possible

communication barrier
anything that blocks or
interferes with the exchange
of information

communication barriers and using techniques to overcome these barriers goes a long way toward making your communication truly effective.

Environmental barriers are distractions in the surrounding area that cause our attention to wander. Healthcare workers learn to ignore many of these barriers, but they can distract patients. These barriers can be created by people talking in the hallway, an overhead speaker announcement, the radio or TV playing in a patient's room, checking your pager, or answering a phone call during a patient interview (Figure 7.6). Check your environment and eliminate or reduce as many distractions as possible before you begin to communicate with someone.

Sensory impairments such as hearing loss, vision loss, or speech difficulties also create communication barriers. Learn to recognize these barriers and adjust your communication style accordingly. The elderly hospital patient who directs the TV remote at you and presses the volume button while you are talking might strike you as humorous. However, she is sending a clear message that you need to talk louder. Does your patient turn one ear toward you, ask you to repeat things, or just smile and nod? Do you check for understanding or just assume that she has heard you? Figure 7.7 shows a variety of techniques to improve communication when sensory impairments create barriers.

Cognitive impairments occur when a patient's ability to think is affected by pain or medication, when the patient is confused or disoriented, and when the patient suffers from dementia. All of these conditions create barriers to effective communication. Sometimes common sense will guide your methods. Consider the physician who caught himself asking the patient to consider the pros and cons of a caesarean delivery while she was in the middle of a strong labor contraction. Of course, he waited and resumed the conversation when she wasn't in as much pain.

The following techniques will improve communication with patients who have cognitive impairments:

- Identify yourself and greet your patient by name.

- Use simple language and short sentences.

- Speak slowly and clearly but not loudly. Hearing is not the problem.

Figure 7.6   Interruptions distract you and your patient and create barriers to effective healthcare communication. How can the interruption shown here be avoided? Who is causing this interruption?

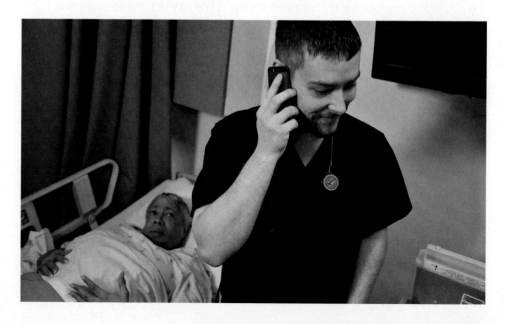

Figure 7.7 Techniques for Improving Communication with Patients Who Have Sensory Impairments

hearing loss or deafness	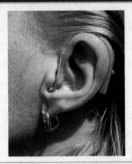	• Check hearing aids: Are the batteries working? Is the hearing aid inserted correctly? • Face the person as you speak to improve lip reading. • Use gestures and signs or write your message. • Use the help of a sign language interpreter.
impaired vision or blindness	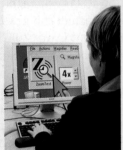	• Use a soft tone of voice. • Announce your presence and identify yourself. • Explain sounds and describe equipment and its location. • Explain each care step as you do it. Let the patient know when and where you will touch. • Provide more detailed instructions since you can't demonstrate actions for the patient. • Let the patient know when you leave the room.
speech impairment	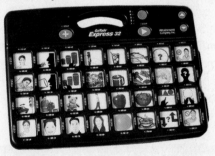	• Encourage speech as appropriate. • Ask questions that require a short answer and allow time for the patient to respond. • Encourage the use of gestures, pointing to objects, or writing requests if appropriate. • Use communication boards and computer tablet applications to provide verbal responses.

- Provide plenty of time for the patient to respond.

- If you repeat the message, use the same words both times.

- Check for understanding and provide additional written information if appropriate.

- Use pictures and objects or demonstrate actions when patients do not understand verbal instructions.

Cultural differences can create communication barriers, and the most obvious of these is speaking a different language. When you and your patient speak different languages, you might enlist the help of a family member or friend of the patient. With the patient's permission, that individual can interpret, but be aware that culture may also limit what a family member is willing to communicate. One nurse assumed that her patient's daughter would communicate care instructions to her father because the daughter spoke fluent English as well as Korean. When her father continued to risk a fall by getting out of bed, the nurse found a Korean nurse to speak with him. He was unaware of his diagnosis or the risk of falling. The daughter

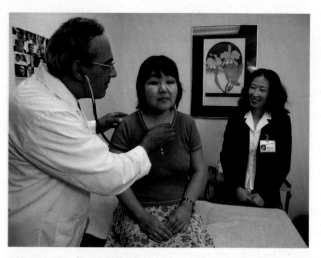

Figure 7.8   Request the help of a medical interpreter when necessary to ensure that your patient's needs are met. In addition to language, what other cultural differences must a medical interpreter recognize?

cultural diversity
term that describes differences in age, gender, physical and intellectual abilities, sexual orientation, race, or ethnicity that influence what we believe, the way we think, and what we do

explained that her brother would arrive the next day and talk to her father. Culture dictated that it was not her place to tell her father what he should do.

When there is no one to interpret, greet your patient with a smile. Use gestures and pictures, or demonstrate your message, but don't speak loudly. Increasing your volume does nothing to improve a patient's understanding if you do not speak the same language. If necessary, request help from a **medical interpreter** to ensure that your patient's needs are met (Figure 7.8).

In addition to language, cultural differences in communication affect the use of gestures, touch, and sense of time (Figure 7.9). To you, a thumbs up may be a sign that everything is OK, but it's a rude sexual gesture in Islamic culture. You may hug a coworker as a sign of encouragement and empathy, but be aware that hugging could make an Asian coworker very uncomfortable. Some patients stop taking their medication after a few days because they feel better. You may need to explain the long-term outcomes by using the patient's interpretation of time. For example, you can tell a grandmother that taking the medicine every day will keep her feeling strong enough to hold her new grandchild.

Cultural diversity, however, is much larger than communication differences. It influences what people believe, think, and do. Do men and women see the world in the same way? Do young and old people make the same choices? Do you expect people of differing racial and ethnic backgrounds to share your views on healthcare issues? If so, then your expectations will create barriers in communication.

Figure 7.9 Cultural Issues That May Affect Healthcare Communication	
language	The same language can vary—words have different meanings. Do you drink from a *water fountain* or a *bubbler*? When you pass out, do you *graduate* or *become unconscious*?
names	Using first names can be seen either as friendliness or as inappropriate and discourteous.
pain	Some patients are expressive, while others are stoic. How do you know who needs pain relief?
eye contact	Lack of eye contact can indicate disinterest or respect for the speaker.
visitors and family	A large number of demanding family members shows respect for an ailing parent.
gender and authority	The patient may not have the authority to speak. A relative may control communication between the patient and the healthcare worker.

Cultural background influences both conscious and unconscious choices. Does your cultural background influence the way you dress, where you live, or your choice of friends? How has your culture influenced your level of education, your career, your hobbies, and your interests? Does it affect your marital status, parental status, or religious views? These choices provide visible clues to your culture, but they don't tell the whole story. Do you assume that people who live near you, go to school with you, and have the same career interests as you will have the same beliefs about the practice of healthcare? If so, these assumptions will create barriers in communication.

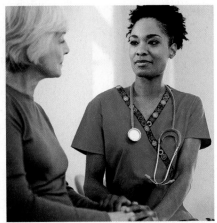

To meet the demands of increasing cultural diversity, our country needs a culturally competent workforce (Figure 7.10). Cultural competence includes being knowledgeable about possible cultural differences that might occur in the healthcare setting. However, it also means learning not to make assumptions about the viewpoints and beliefs of others. Most important, culturally competent healthcare workers are motivated to overcome cultural communication barriers to serve their patients.

Figure 7.10 Cultural competence is an important skill for healthcare workers.

Cultural competence begins with learning about possible cultural differences. You become culturally sensitive when you develop awareness about how the thoughts of patients and coworkers may differ from your own. For instance, when a patient refuses to look at you while you provide care instructions, do you assume he is not interested? If he is Asian, he may be showing respect for your position. In his culture, looking you in the eye is rude. One employer refused to hire any nursing assistants who wouldn't look her in the eye during the interview. She believed these applicants could not be trusted. Two excellent caregivers of Nigerian descent failed the test because they looked down as a sign of respect. A culturally competent healthcare worker would be aware of and account for these differences.

RECALL YOUR READING

1. Because it is direct, but still tactful, _____ is considered the healthiest style of communication.

2. The SBAR system can help workers communicate more effectively. SBAR stands for _____, _____, _____, and _____.

3. Use _____ questions when interviewing patients to encourage them to share more information about their symptoms.

4. Noise in the environment, problems with vision or hearing, and cognitive impairments create _____ to effective communication.

5. Healthcare workers who recognize cultural differences, but don't make assumptions about differences exhibit _____.

Complete the *Map Your Reading* graphic organizer for the section you just read.

Information Technology

Advances in information technology are causing rapid changes in the methods for storing patient information and performing patient treatments. Therapeutic workers need to consider implementing these changes carefully so that patient privacy and safety is preserved.

Government Influences on Electronic Health Records

In 2009, the **Health Information Technology for Economic and Clinical Health (HITECH) Act** was signed into law. HITECH made significant changes to the HIPAA privacy and security regulations. For example, the new law specifies the penalties that the US Department of Health and Human Services (HHS) can impose for violations of the HIPAA rules. HITECH also requires that business associates of healthcare providers maintain the same level of security whenever health information is accessed or exchanged between organizations. This means that an independent medical transcriptionist or an accounting firm must have the same level of security as the healthcare provider when they are working with protected health information.

HITECH provides the funding to address concerns about the security and privacy of protected health information as records of that information move toward electronic rather than paper media. The new privacy and security requirements support the federal government's plans to increase the use of health information technology (HIT) and health information exchange (HIE). The ultimate goals of nationwide use of electronic health records (EHRs) are to reduce healthcare costs by avoiding duplication of tests and to improve patient outcomes through point-of-care access to a patient's complete medical history (Figure 7.11).

To support this goal, the HITECH law offers financial incentives to healthcare providers who demonstrate **meaningful use** of EHRs. The requirements for demonstrating a meaningful use of electronic health records follow a series of stages with sets of objectives to meet in each stage. In stage one, for example, providers must use electronic prescribing software, maintain current medication and allergy lists for patients, and provide summaries for patients following each clinic visit. These examples represent 3 of the 15 core objectives for this stage. Each stage has its own list of core objectives for developing meaningful use of EHRs. The financial incentives for meaningful use are provided by HITECH through 2015. In subsequent years, however, the government may penalize facilities that fail to use effective EHR systems.

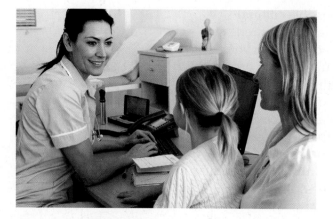

Figure 7.11   Electronic health records provide easy access to a patient's medical history.

Therapeutic Applications

Therapeutic workers will recognize many advantages to working with EHRs, including the speed of accessing patient information and the clarity of typewritten rather than handwritten entries. However, electronic health records systems do not eliminate the need for chart entries that are timely, complete, and accurate.

Electronic Charting and e-Prescribing. Electronic records contain all of the information found in a paper chart, but EHR software combines many additional medical office functions (Figure 7.12). For example, the EHR system can

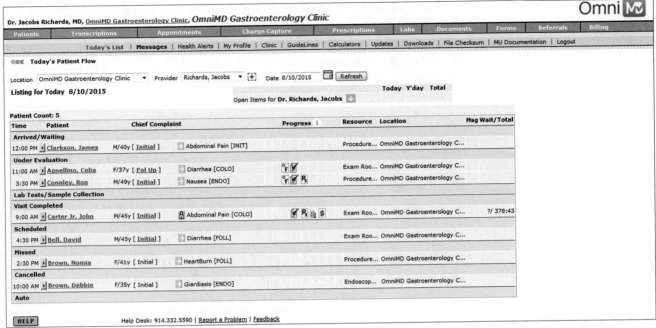

Figure 7.12   Electronic health records contain all the information of a paper record, but can also provide drug information, recommended codes for medical services, and much more.

Simulate EHR

- link to sites that show drug formularies and dosages;
- print patient education instructions;
- recommend codes for medical services;
- search charts to find patients who are due for routine health screenings;
- alert providers to a patient's drug and allergy interactions;
- streamline medical office communication using e-mail, messaging, and templates for letters; and
- provide immediate access to a patient record from multiple facility locations.

In a paper record system, all of these functions require the use of separate resources for looking up information, manually searching patient records, and repeatedly entering the same information for every new document.

The Therapeutic Worker: Maricela

Maricela, who works as an LPN at a medical clinic, compares electronic records to paper records by asking if you would prefer a car (the electronic record) to a horse and buggy (the paper record). She says that disadvantages of paper records include

- trying to read handwriting;
- struggling to locate the exact information desired;
- damaging paper with a spill or tear;
- misplacing records; and
- being unable to keep records completely secure.

She also says that when records are kept behind a desk or in a patient's room, private information in those records can easily fall into the wrong hands.

Maricela also recalls the difficulty of sharing a patient's paper record with another facility. The record, which could contain as many as 100 pages, had to be located and photocopied by taking each page out and copying it individually. If a clinic called to request all records on a patient for the past year, you would need to flip through each section of the chart—including subcategories such as *Labs*, *Images*, and *Progress Notes*—look at the dates, pull out the correct pages, and photocopy them.

By comparison, reading the text in a computerized record is far simpler. The requested record can be found with the click of a mouse and shared with another clinic through a secure electronic data transfer. When you need to find a specific record—for instance, lab results for the past month—the computer finds exactly what you want.

Maricela believes that computerized records are more secure. As long as each person accessing the information remembers to lock the computer after use, no one should be able to gain unauthorized access to protected information.

e-prescribing
electronic generation, transmission, and filling of a medical prescription

The system of electronic prescribing, or **e-prescribing**, replaces handwritten prescriptions, faxed notes, or prescriptions called in by phone (Figure 7.13). An e-prescription is automatically sent to the patient's preferred pharmacy over the Internet. This process improves patient safety by automatically checking for drug and allergy interactions and eliminating medication errors due to poor handwriting.

With all of the improvements that come with electronic health records, you might think that a healthcare professional can quickly go into the record, check a few boxes, and be done with charting. However, a healthcare worker may need to access several charts, click on multiple tabs, and complete several entries. Using a computerized chart is like turning pages in a book—you don't see everything at once. When you chart tasks in a computer, you access different screens and follow assigned tasks. There is a screen for pain management, another for vital signs, a third for intake and output, and so on.

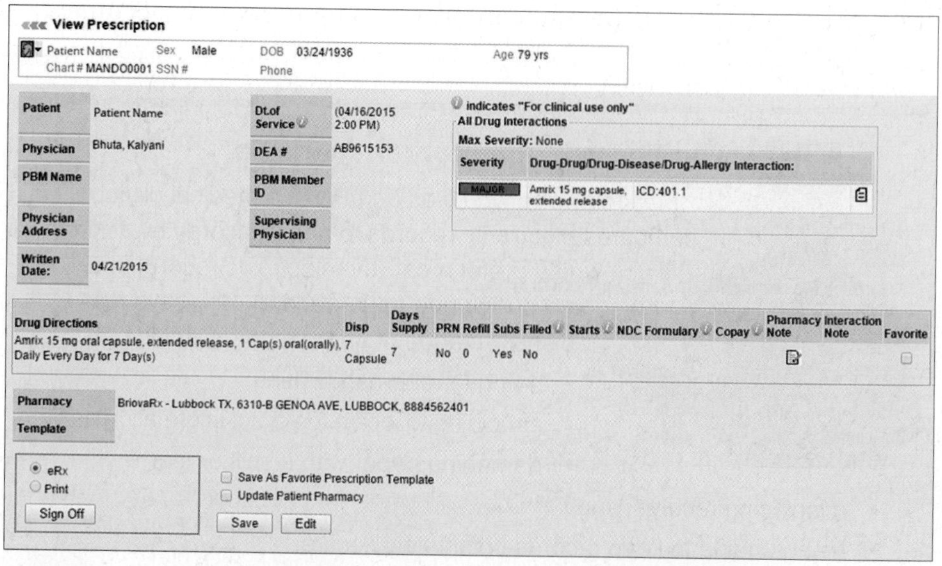

Figure 7.13 E-prescribing software helps reduce the adverse effects of drug and allergy interactions.

The **face page**, or *summary screen*, on a patient's chart shows contact information, insurance information, and medical history. Healthcare workers edit the face page to record changes and additions such as a new insurance provider (Figure 7.14). Each office visit, or *encounter*, has a separate file showing progress notes for that visit. Information can be extracted or collected from different encounters to track specific services such as immunizations.

Completing a thorough charting of patient assessments, medications, treatments, education, changes in condition, care plans, and other patient information can take a long time. Even though electronic records have dramatically improved the process of charting, it remains complex and can still be a time-consuming part of patient care.

Correcting Errors in the Electronic Record. Correcting errors in an electronic record can be a simple process, but it is important to remember never to delete errors. Because the patient record is a legal document, you must be able to retrieve the original chart. This means that you cannot remove parts of an active patient's medical record. If a change is made to

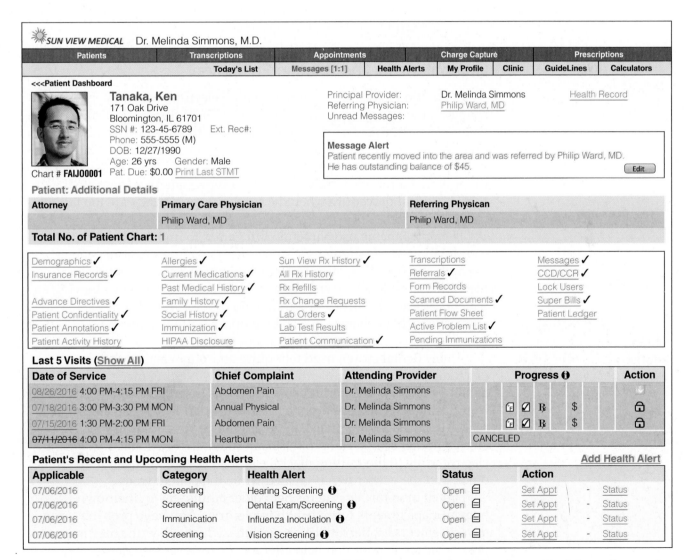

Figure 7.14   The face page in an electronic health record shows contact information, insurance information, and medical history. What else do you see here that might improve the healthcare experience?

correct an error, the original electronic document—including the error—must be stored and accessible. Keep these guidelines in mind as you correct errors in an electronic chart:

Simulate
EHR

- If you find an error recorded by another healthcare worker, talk to that worker to verify that it truly is an error and ask that person to correct it. Remember that you are responsible for charting only the care that you provide. Never allow another worker to chart care under your username.

- To correct an error, note an **addendum** (uh-DEHN-duhm) on the electronic chart. This means that new or corrected information is being added. Then type the reason for the addendum as well as the corrected information.

- Label information that has been forgotten as *late entry*.

- **Authenticate** (aw-THEHN-tih-kayt), or give legal authority to, all addendums and late entries with your digital signature and healthcare credentials. Include the date and time with your signature.

- Follow your healthcare facility's specific protocols when correcting errors in electronic charts.

Computerized Therapeutic Equipment

In addition to health records becoming electronic, technology is changing therapeutic procedures (Figure 7.15). In the surgical suite, a physician can rotate a 3-D image to practice the steps in a surgical procedure before performing the surgery. Medical students actually play video games to learn how to use joystick technology for future surgeries. Computerized robotic hands guided by a physician may complete the actual surgical procedure when the surgeon's own hands are too large for the surgical site.

Therapy patients use Nintendo Wii games to improve balance and coordination. Work simulators and exercise machines restore patients' strength and mobility following injuries or joint replacement surgery. Electronic stimulation strengthens muscles and improves swallowing for patients affected by stroke or Parkinson's disease. Tablet computers with applications that generate speech by tapping buttons with symbols restore communication for patients who cannot speak.

A new dental crown used to require an initial visit for the placement of a temporary crown while the new crown was being made in an offsite dental laboratory. The permanent crown was installed a couple weeks later during a second appointment. Now the dentist uses an electronic sensor to take a digital image of the original tooth and draws the crown on a computer screen right in the exam room. Dimensional data is sent electronically to the milling machine or a 3-D printer located in the same office, and the new crown is created while the patient waits.

Patient monitoring systems help older adults stay in their own homes or apartments when health issues arise. You have probably seen advertisements for personal alert systems, which allow the user to press a button to summon help after a fall. However, a wide variety of sensors has increased the scope of patient monitoring. These sensors can monitor how often a person gets out of bed, flushes the toilet, or opens the

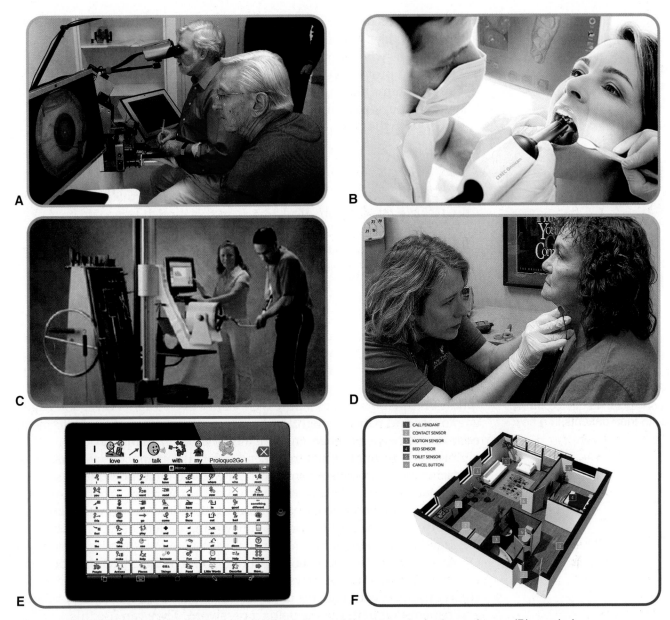

Figure 7.15   New technology such as surgery simulators (A), crown-designing software (B), workplace simulators (C), electric stimulation (D), speech simulator apps (E), and sensor systems (F) contribute to and change therapeutic procedures. Proloquo2Go® is an AssistiveWare® product. Used with permission.

refrigerator. No cameras or microphones are used, but family members and healthcare providers can be alerted if typical patterns change. For example, an increase in toilet flushing could signal a urinary tract infection. These sensor-based monitoring systems are far less expensive than full-time assisted living or nursing home care. Combined with home health services, a sensor system allows elderly individuals to continue living in their own homes or apartments.

Social Media

Social media networks such as Facebook and Twitter have changed the way people interact and communicate with each other. Should they also change the interactions and communication between healthcare providers

social media
a group of online communication tools that allow people to share information and resources via the Internet

and patients? As the worlds of social media and healthcare intersect, people are experiencing positive results but also finding areas of concern.

Physicians who embrace the use of social media emphasize that personal and professional communication must remain separate. One doctor maintains both a professional Facebook page, which anyone can view, and a personal page limited to friends and family. In this way, he complies with the American Medical Association guidelines that advise physicians to protect privacy and maintain appropriate boundaries when communicating with patients through social media.

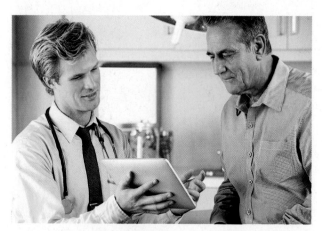

Figure 7.16 Doctors can use social media to connect with their patients in a new way.

Since anyone can post information online, medical advice on social media sites can be inaccurate. For this reason, patients are advised to only use links provided by physicians. Because social media allows physicians to reach a much wider audience, tech-savvy physicians often post links to updated medical guidelines and patient education resources (Figure 7.16). With patient permission, a cosmetic surgery center might post success stories along with a description of treatment options, and an obstetrician might post photos of newborns. When an orthopedist (or-thuh-PEE-dihst) promotes a fitness challenge event on his Facebook page, employees and patients might post photos of themselves working to meet each week's new challenge, creating a motivational competition.

"Tweets" from physicians can send helpful alerts and reminders. One physician alerts patients when he is running late for appointments so they don't have to sit for a long time in the waiting room. Another sends a reminder about an upcoming immunization clinic. However, Twitter messages aren't the best method for answering patient questions. The messages' limited length may require a physician to oversimplify a response.

Answering patient questions through social media also raises privacy concerns. For this reason, physicians use secure web portals for e-mail communication with patients to better answer their questions. Physicians and patients log in to the site using a password. They can use this same site to download their lab test results or schedule appointments. Physicians are learning that communicating with patients by e-mail throughout the day can reduce the time needed to make phone calls to patients at the end of the day.

Healthcare workers must use common sense when posting information online. While violating patient confidentiality and making derogatory (dih-RAH-guh-tor-ee) remarks about patients are obvious errors in online communication, the details of a diagnosis and treatment can be enough to identify a patient even if the information is posted without other identifiers. One physician posted the details of a patient injury on Facebook. Even though no name was given, readers figured out the identity of the patient, and the physician was fined for unprofessional conduct.

While social media can enhance provider and patient communication, it can't replace office visits. The **Affordable Care Act (ACA)**, however, which encourages the use of electronic health records and the electronic exchange of health information, is expected to increase the use of social media and virtual communication for patient care. Even in this new, tech-savvy environment, healthcare workers must recognize that using social media does not remove their obligation to protect patient privacy and to maintain professional relationships with patients.

Mobile Apps and Electronic Resources

The mobile technology of smartphones and tablet computers has already changed our personal lives. It provides entertainment through music, games, and videos. We use it for online shopping, photos, and personal banking. It has also largely replaced GPS devices as well as paper maps and phone books.

Apps, short for *applications*, have fueled growth in mobile technology. The wide range of available apps has expanded to include healthcare. Thousands of health-related apps are now available. How are they making healthcare more mobile?

Healthcare apps, which are sometimes called **mHealth** (mobile health) programs, can be divided into categories according to their purpose (Figure 7.17):

apps
applications; software that is accessed through the Internet and runs on a computer, smartphone, tablet, or other mobile device

- **Electronic health records.** Healthcare professionals can access patient records and check lab results. With full access, physicians can dictate into the record, monitor a patient's vital signs, and e-prescribe from a smartphone.

- **Point of care.** Providers can communicate with patients using images and videos to explain disorders and treatments. Some programs break down language barriers by providing medical phrases in languages other than English.

- **Medical reference and education.** These programs provide interactive images of human anatomy and disorders, drug interactions, procedure references, medical news updates, professional journal articles, and research case studies that can enhance diagnosis.

- **Consumer health.** As you might expect, food and exercise diaries, calorie trackers, and pedometer programs are widely available. Mobile pharmacy apps let you place a refill request by scanning the barcode on your prescription. Practical apps for travelers can track medication schedules across time zones, send medication alerts, or locate the nearest emergency room.

Newer programs use devices that plug into the phone or tablet to measure and track health data. With these devices, you can monitor your blood pressure or blood glucose levels and send the data to your physician through your smartphone or tablet.

Older adults and their caregivers are expected to be big users of mobile health apps. Patients with chronic health conditions will use apps to improve at-home monitoring. This will reduce costs and improve patient outcomes as it decreases the number of patients who are readmitted to hospitals.

Regulations from the US Food and Drug Administration (FDA) may slow the development of innovative mHealth programs, but they will also remove apps that make false medical claims. Linking large information technology systems such as an EHR with apps for mobile devices is technologically challenging.

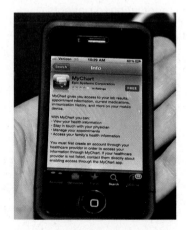

Figure 7.17   Mobile health (mHealth) programs provide health information on mobile devices such as tablets and smartphones. Name two resources that mHealth programs offer.

Security and privacy remain a concern. Healthcare workers who carry a smartphone for mHealth purposes must discipline themselves not to check personal messages or use a camera to record patient images. Some workers have been suspended or fired for posting patient images. This violates patient privacy and can cause unanticipated problems. Remember, once you make something public online, you have no control over the number of people who will view your post and forward the information to others.

Complete the *Map Your Reading* graphic organizer for the section you just read.

RECALL YOUR READING

1. More healthcare facilities are implementing electronic health records to meet the standards of the _____ Act.
2. Electronic charting is more efficient, but it is still a _____ process.
3. Errors in electronic records must never be _____ because the original record must be stored for legal reasons.
4. When using _____, personal communication must never contain references to work-related information.
5. The development of new _____ is improving access to electronic records and medical education resources.

Medical Math

Therapeutic workers use math on a daily basis as they record care given to patients and prepare or administer medications (Figure 7.18). Whether they are using metric units or US customary units, they always recognize that accuracy is vital to patient health and safety.

Figure 7.18 Therapeutic workers often administer medication to patients. What might be the result of a healthcare worker failing to be accurate in a medication dose?

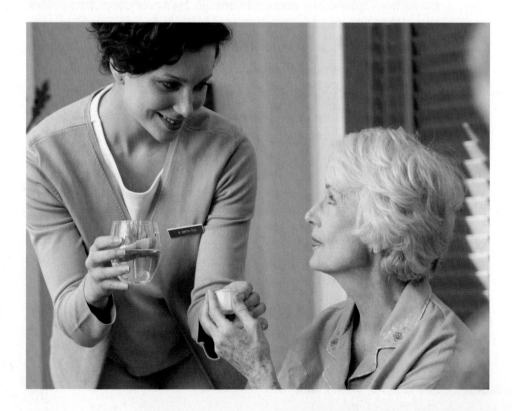

The 24-Hour Clock

Although we usually use Greenwich (GREHN-itch) Mean Time (GMT) in our day-to-day lives, many healthcare facilities use the **24-hour clock**, also called *military time* (Figure 7.19). Rather than twelve hours with an a.m. or p.m. designation, the 24-hour clock uses the numbers 1 through 24. Each hour of the day has its own number. This avoids confusion between a.m. and p.m. and prevents medication or chart documentation errors when the a.m. or p.m. designation is omitted or misread.

Guidelines for using the 24-hour clock include the following:

- Always write the time using four digits with no colons to separate hours and minutes. For example, 9:00 a.m. is 0900, and 12:00 noon is 1200.

- Always state time in hundreds when speaking. For example, 2:00 a.m. is 0200 and is stated as "zero two hundred hours" or "oh two hundred hours;" 7:00 p.m. is 1900 and is stated as "nineteen hundred hours."

- The last two numbers at the end of each time represent minutes after the hour. For example, 11:15 a.m. is 1115. This means it is fifteen minutes past eleven o'clock.

- If the time is between whole hours, drop the word *hundred* when speaking. Thus, 1115 is spoken as "eleven fifteen hours."

- Midnight (12:00 a.m.) is presented as 0000 or 2400 in military time, whereas 1200 is 12:00 noon.

- From midnight to noon, you can use the numbers on a standard clock (1 through 12) to tell military time. For example, 1:00 a.m. is 0100, and 10:00 a.m. is 1000.

- Convert p.m. hours to military time by adding 1200 to the time. For example, 1:00 p.m. plus 1200 is 1300, and 4:30 p.m. plus 1200 is 1630. Reverse the process and subtract 1200 when converting from military to Greenwich Time. Figure 7.20 on the next page shows how you can convert from Greenwich Mean Time to military time.

24-hour clock
a method of telling time that assigns a number to each hour of the day; also known as *military time*

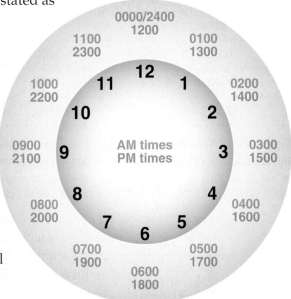

Figure 7.19   Using the 24-hour clock helps healthcare workers avoid confusion between a.m. and p.m. times.

Systems of Measurement

Knowing which system of measurement you are working with is very important in a healthcare setting. When communicating with fellow healthcare workers, or with patients, be sure that you are both using the same system of measurement. Otherwise, mistakes can easily be made. In healthcare settings, you are likely to encounter two different systems of measurement—the metric system and the US system. To avoid errors, pay careful attention to the system of measurement being used.

Consider the story of a British family whose dream vacation to the United States took a frightening turn. The family's young son had an

Figure 7.20 Conversion of the 12-Hour Clock to the 24-Hour Clock

Greenwich Mean Time	Military Time	Greenwich Mean Time	Military Time
1:00 a.m.	0100	1:00 p.m.	1300
2:00 a.m.	0200	2:00 p.m.	1400
3:00 a.m.	0300	3:00 p.m.	1500
4:00 a.m.	0400	4:00 p.m.	1600
5:00 a.m.	0500	5:00 p.m.	1700
6:00 a.m.	0600	6:00 p.m.	1800
7:00 a.m.	0700	7:00 p.m.	1900
8:00 a.m.	0800	8:00 p.m.	2000
9:00 a.m.	0900	9:00 p.m.	2100
10:00 a.m.	1000	10:00 p.m.	2200
11:00 a.m.	1100	11:00 p.m.	2300
12:00 p.m.	1200	12:00 a.m.	0000/2400

Figure 7.20   This chart shows how to convert times between Greenwich Mean Time and military time. When using the 24-hour clock, you must remember to insert the leading 0 or 00 for a.m. hours. 12:01 a.m. is written as *0001*, while 12:01 p.m. is written as *1201*. 2400 is the highest number that can be used since there are only 24 hours in each day. What time do you start work or begin school each day? Convert those times into military time.

asthma attack, so his mother took him to the emergency room to get a prescription for asthma medication. She gave her son the prescribed asthma medication, but there was no improvement in his breathing, so she took him back to the emergency room. As the physician reviewed the medication label, he asked the woman to confirm her son's weight. She said 40, meaning kilograms, but the label listed dosage amounts for a child weighing 40 pounds. Because 40 kilograms is closer to 88 pounds, her son was receiving only half the medication needed to alleviate his symptoms.

Since the United States is the only industrialized country that does not use the **metric system** as its official system of measurement, the mother's assumption that weight measurements would be in kilograms is understandable. The scientific community, and increasingly the healthcare community, both use metric measurement. Therefore, healthcare workers must know how to use this system. Yet most healthcare workers—and their patients—still think in pounds, ounces, inches, and feet.

Healthcare workers must be comfortable with converting between US customary measurements and metric measurements. They will likely measure in the metric system, but must present information to patients in the most commonly used terms. A nurse in America might measure and record a newborn's weight as 3000 grams but will tell the parents that the baby weighs 6 pounds, 10 ounces.

metric system
the decimal measurement system based on the meter, liter, and gram as its primary units of length, volume, and weight or mass respectively

At the same time, there is an attempt in the healthcare field to teach patients about metric measurements for medication. Some companies are providing cups and syringes with measurements marked in metric along with the medication. This is being done for educational purposes, but also for the sake of increased accuracy of doses. Some patients use kitchen silverware to measure out their medication, which can result in inaccurate doses. The size of household teaspoons can vary significantly, and it's easy to misread *tbsp* (tablespoon) as *tsp* (teaspoon). Using kitchen silverware instead of an actual measuring spoon or other device that comes with a medicine can result in the wrong dosing—too much or too little of the medicine.

Metric System Basics. The metric system, or *International System of Units*, uses four basic units of measurement: the meter, gram, liter, and Celsius. The meter (m) is used to measure length, the gram (g) measures weight, the liter (L) measures volume, and Celsius (C°) identifies temperature. The L for liter is capitalized to avoid confusion with the numeral 1. Working within the metric system is mathematically easy because all of the units are based on multiples of ten. All conversions are calculated by multiplying by 10, 100, 1000, and so on (Figure 7.21).

Moving a decimal point easily converts units within the metric system. Suppose that an order for 1000 milligrams of medication needs to be converted to 1-gram tablets. Since *milli* represents 0.001 of a gram, it is three places to the right of *gram*, as pictured in Figure 7.21. This means you will move the decimal point three spaces to the left to convert the measurement to grams. Thus, 1000 milligrams becomes 1 gram. The dose is 1 gram or one tablet.

Follow these guidelines to reduce errors when recording metric measurements:

- Avoid using a comma as a thousands separator (write 1000 mg rather than 1,000 mg).

- Avoid unnecessarily large numbers or trailing zeros (simplify 1000 mg to 1 gram).

- If possible, use whole numbers rather than decimals (write 25 mm rather than 2.5 cm).

United States Customary Units. The **US customary units**, more commonly known as the *household system* of measurement, are familiar to students educated in the United States. The terms *inch* (in) and *foot* (ft) for length, *cup* (c) and *quart* (qt) for volume, and *ounce* (oz) or *pound* (lb) for

US customary units
the main system of weights and measures used in the United States, based on the yard, pound, and gallon as units of length, weight, and liquid volume respectively; also known as *household measurement*

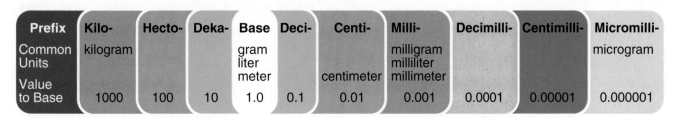

Prefix	Kilo-	Hecto-	Deka-	Base	Deci-	Centi-	Milli-	Decimilli-	Centimilli-	Micromilli-
Common Units	kilogram			gram liter meter		centimeter	milligram milliliter millimeter			microgram
Value to Base	1000	100	10	1.0	0.1	0.01	0.001	0.0001	0.00001	0.000001

Figure 7.21   Working within the metric system is mathematically easy since all of the units are based on multiples of ten.

weight are common. Converting between the units, however, may not be as familiar and requires knowledge of several *equivalents* (Figure 7.22).

When you know the basic equivalents, you can convert to other units by using a proportion. For example, you need to measure 4 tablespoons (T) of a liquid but have a measuring cup marked in ounces. You know the equivalent that states 2 tablespoons equal 1 ounce. If 2 tablespoons are equal to 1 ounce, then how many ounces does 4 tablespoons equal? Your proportion problem should look like this:

$$\frac{2T}{4T} \diagup\!\!\!\!\diagdown \frac{1\,oz}{x\,oz}$$

Solve the problem using the following steps:

1. Cross multiply to get $2x = 4$ oz
2. Divide each side of the equation by the number in front of x.
    $2x \div 2 = 1x$
    $4 \div 2 = 2$
    $x = 2$ oz

Thus, measuring 2 ounces will be equal to 4 tablespoons.

Other Systems of Measurement. While the metric system is becoming the standard for healthcare measurement, you may see a prescription that looks like this: *aspirin gr xv.* Seeing the unit—grains, in this case—listed first and the amount listed second using lowercase Roman numerals tells you it is an **apothecary** (uh-PAH-thuh-kair-ee) **system** prescription. The apothecary system is an older system used by early pharmacists, or *apothecaries,* as they were called. The system may still be used for herbal

Figure 7.22 Common Household Measurements and Equivalents		
Type	**Name and Abbreviation**	**Equivalents**
distance/length	inch (″ or in)	12 in = 1 ft
	foot (′ or ft)	3 ft = 1 yd
	yard (yd)	1760 yds = 1 mi
	mile (mi)	
capacity/volume	drop (gtt)	60 gtts = 1 t
	teaspoon (t or tsp)	3 t = 1 T
	tablespoon (T or tbsp)	2 T = 1 oz
	ounce (oz)	8 oz = 1 c
	cup (c)	2 c = 1 pt
	pint (pt)	2 pts = 1 qt
	quart (qt)	4 qts = 1 gal
	gallon (gal)	
mass/weight	ounce (oz)*	16 oz = 1 lb
	pound (lb)	

* Ounce is used for measures of volume and weight in household measurement

medicines but has largely been replaced by the metric system. When you see measurements listed as drams, grains, and minims, you are working with the apothecary system. These measurements will use lowercase Roman numerals and fractions rather than decimals.

While the numbering of the Super Bowl might be your only exposure to Roman numerals, this ancient numbering system is quite easy to interpret (Figure 7.23). Roman numerals use letters to express numeric values:

I or *i* stands for 1
V or *v* stands for 5
X or *x* stands for 10
L or *l* stands for 50
C or *c* stands for 100
D or *d* stands for 500
M or *m* stands for 1,000

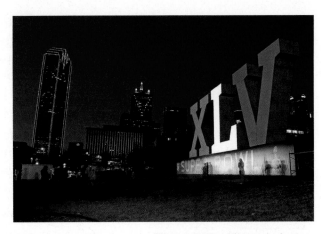

Figure 7.23   You may have seen Roman numerals while watching the Superbowl. What do the Roman numerals here mean?

The following are guidelines for reading and writing Roman numerals:

- The letters should be arranged from largest to smallest.

  1,510 is written *MDX*, largest to smallest

- When the same letter is repeated twice in a row, the two are added together. However, don't repeat a letter more than three times in a row.

  100 is written *LL*, not *XXXXXXXXXX*

- When a letter with a smaller value precedes one with a larger value, the smaller number is subtracted from the larger number.

  4 is written *IV*, which literally means *5 minus 1*

- When a letter with a smaller value follows one with a larger value, the smaller number is added to the larger number.

  6 is written *VI*, which literally means *5 plus 1*

When you see *aspirin gr xv*, it means the prescription calls for aspirin at a strength of 15 grains. You will have to calculate how many tablets the patient must take to equal 15 grains of medication.

The word *units* commonly indicates a measure of insulin or heparin. These **International Units (IU)** are also used for measuring the biological effect of manufactured medicinal drugs and vitamins. For every substance to which an IU is assigned, there is an internationally accepted biological effect expected with a dose of 1 IU.

Because each substance is tested individually, there is no standard conversion from international units to metric equivalents. For example, 1 International Unit is equivalent to 0.0455 milligrams of insulin. However, one International Unit is equivalent to just 0.0003 milligrams of vitamin A and just 0.000025 milligrams of vitamin D.

Converting Between Systems of Measurement. Remember the nurse who measured the infant at 3000 grams but told the new parents that the baby weighed 6 pounds, 10 ounces? It's common for US healthcare workers to convert measurements like this from one system to another, such as from metric to household measurement. Therefore, workers must know equivalents between the units of each system (Figure 7.24). There are often no exact equivalents, so close approximations must be used. Memorizing the following equivalents will provide a foundation to help you evaluate conversions from system to system:

1 fluid oz = 30 cc or mL = 6 teaspoons (t) or 2 T = 8 fluid drams

Using approximate equivalents, you can set up a proportion to convert measurements. For example, if you are the nurse weighing the newborn baby, you know the baby weighs 3000 grams, and you know that 30 grams = 1 ounce. So how many ounces is 3000 grams?

$$\frac{30 \text{ g}}{3000 \text{ g}} = \frac{1 \text{ oz}}{x \text{ oz}}$$

1. Cross multiply to get $30x = 3000$
2. Divide each side of the equation by the number in front of x

$$30x \div 30 = 1x$$

$$3000 \div 30 = 100 \text{ oz}$$

The correct answer is $x = 100$ ounces, but that isn't a typical measurement. Now you will have to convert these ounces into pounds. You know that 16 ounces = 1 pound, so how many pounds is 100 ounces?

$$\frac{16 \text{ oz}}{100 \text{ oz}} = \frac{1 \text{ lb}}{x \text{ lb}}$$

1. Cross multiply to get $16x = 100$
2. Divide each side of the equation by the number in front of x

$$16x \div 16 = 1x$$

$$100 \div 16 = 6.25 \text{ lbs}$$

You know the baby weighs 6.25 pounds, but now you need to determine how many ounces are in 0.25 pounds. We know that 16 ounces = 1 pound, so how many ounces are in 0.25 pounds?

$$\frac{1 \text{ lb}}{0.25 \text{ lb}} = \frac{16 \text{ oz}}{x \text{ oz}}$$

Figure 7.24 Conversion Table: Apothecary to Metric to Household				
Apothecary Volume	**Apothecary Weight**	**Metric Volume**	**Metric Weight**	**Common Household**
1 ounce	1 ounce	30 mL	30 g	2 tbsp
4 drams	4 drams	15 mL	15 g	1 tbsp
2 drams	2 drams	7.5 mL	7.5 g	½ tbsp
1 dram	60 grains	4 mL	4 g	1 tsp
½ dram	30 grains	2 mL	2 g	½ tsp

1. Cross multiply to get $1x = 4$
2. Divide each side of the equation by the number in front of x

   $1x \div 1 = 1x$

   $4 \div 1 = 4\ oz$

So the answer is 6 pounds, 4 ounces. However, the nurse said the baby weighed 6 pounds, 10 ounces! This illustrates a problem with using equivalents—they are only approximately equal. In large numbers such as 3000 grams, the resulting conversion will be less accurate. A difference of 5 ounces may not be critical when recording your child's weight in a baby book, but it would be very important when calculating the amount of medicine needed by a newborn infant. A more exact equivalent, such as 1 ounce = 28.34 grams, is needed. This equivalent will convert 3000 grams to 6 pounds, 10 ounces.

The more equivalents you know, the more accurate your converted measurements will be. You can also increase the speed at which you convert measurements. You can convert 3000 grams to kilograms by simply moving the decimal point three spaces to the left, giving you 3 kilograms.

To convert kilograms to pounds, remember that 2.2 kilograms = 1 pound, so you simply multiply 3 kilograms by 2.2 (3 kg × 2.2 = 6.6 lb). To convert 0.6 to ounces, multiply by the number of ounces in one pound (0.6 lb × 16 oz = 9.6 oz). Your answer is 6 pounds, 10 ounces (rounded to the nearest whole number). Using kilograms instead of grams was both faster and more accurate. Of course, the easiest conversions use equipment labeled with both metric and household measurements. Figure 7.25 shows mathematical operations that will help you perform faster conversions.

Visualizing Metric Measurements. If you are familiar with the household system, you are able to visualize its units of measurement. For

Figure 7.25 Conversion Table: Metric to Household and Household to Metric				
Metric		**US Customary (Household)**	**Convert from metric to household**	**Convert household to metric**
2.5 centimeters	length	1 inch	divide by 2.5 (100 cm ÷ 2.5 = 40 in)	multiply by 2.54
30 centimeters	length	1 foot	divide by 30 (100 cm ÷ 30 = 3.3 ft = 3 ft 4 in)	multiply by 30.48
30 grams	weight	1 ounce	divide by 30 (1000 g ÷ 30 = 33 oz)	multiply by 30
0.45 kilograms	weight	1 pound	multiply by 2.2 (50 kg × 2.2 = 110 lb)	multiply by .45
30 milliliters	volume	1 ounce	divide by 30 (30 mL ÷ 30 = 1 oz)	multiply by 30

example, you know what a pound of butter looks like and how heavy it feels when you hold it. So, if you read that a truck weighed 10 pounds, you would know that was obviously an error. As you work with the metric system, you should try to develop a visual sense for basic units of metric measurement. This will improve your accuracy because it helps you spot obvious errors (Figure 7.26).

Math and Medications

Suppose a prescription label gives instructions for a young child to receive 3.5 teaspoons of antibiotic liquid a day instead of the 3.5 milliliters the doctor ordered. Since 3.5 teaspoons equals 17.25 milliliters, the child will be receiving five times the amount of medicine prescribed if the label's instructions are followed. Because of this error, the child may experience severe diarrhea, a yeast infection, and a fungal infection.

Clearly, accuracy is critical when administering medications to patients. For this reason, only authorized persons who have received specialized training can prepare or administer medication. While some **medications** cure a disease, others assist the body to overcome a disease. The following information will introduce you to the knowledge and skills needed to work with medications.

medication
a substance or mixture of substances that have been proven through research to have a clear value in the prevention, diagnosis, or treatment of diseases

First, medications come in different forms—liquid, solid, and semisolid. Liquid medications can come in several different forms as well. These include an *aqueous suspension* (a mixture of water and undissolved particles of medicine), a *suspension* (a liquid into which particles of medicine have been mixed but not dissolved), a syrup, and a *tincture* (an alcoholic base in which medicine has been dissolved).

Solid medications may come in the form of a capsule, caplet, tablet, or lozenge (LAH-zehnj), which is a small, flat pill that dissolves in

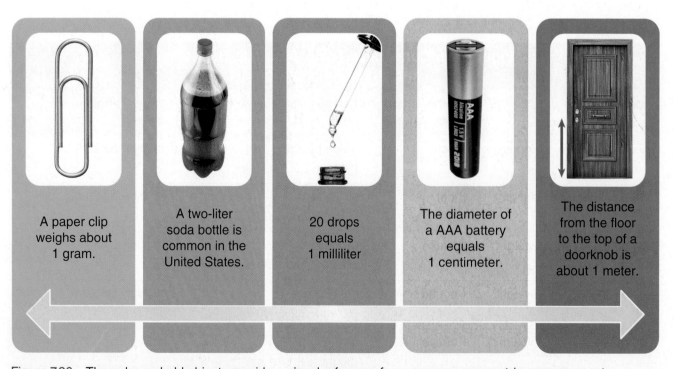

A paper clip weighs about 1 gram.

A two-liter soda bottle is common in the United States.

20 drops equals 1 milliliter

The diameter of a AAA battery equals 1 centimeter.

The distance from the floor to the top of a doorknob is about 1 meter.

Figure 7.26   These household objects provide a visual reference for some common metric measurements.

the mouth. Semisolid medications may come as an ointment, or as a *suppository* (suh-PAH-zuh-tor-ee), which is a small, firm mass of medicine that dissolves when inserted into a body cavity other than the mouth.

Medications can be administered in several ways or by different routes such as:

- oral: given by mouth; used for liquid and solid forms of medicine

- rectal: given in the rectum; used for liquids and suppositories

- topical: applied directly to the skin; used for ointments, liquids, and adhesive patches

- sublingual: given under the tongue; used for tablets, lozenges, or suspensions

- injection: given with a needle and syringe; used for liquids

- inhalation: medication that is inhaled or breathed in; used with sprays, inhalers, or other special machines

When calculating amounts of medication, you will hear the terms **dose** and **dosage** (Figure 7.27). A dose is the portion of medicine to be administered at one time. The dosage is the total quantity of medicine that is to be administered. Dosage depends on the weight, sex, and age of the patient; the disease being treated; how the drug is to be administered; and the patient's tolerance of the drug. The following terms describe different types of doses:

- initial dose: the first dose

- average dose: the amount of medication that has proven most effective with minimal toxic effects

- maximum dose: the largest amount of medication that can safely be administered at one time

- lethal dose: the amount that could cause death

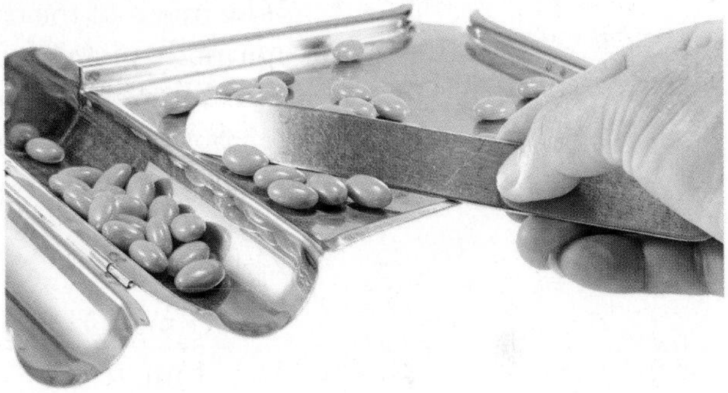

Figure 7.27   Medications must be calculated carefully to ensure the correct dose and dosage.

Oral administration of medications is the safest and most common route. Oral medications are produced at different strengths to meet individual patient needs. Therefore, you may have to calculate the amount of medication needed based on the strength you have available. For example, if the prescription calls for 200 mg, but your pharmacy only carries 100-mg tablets, you will have to double the number of tablets and adjust the prescription instructions accordingly.

Make sure that your medication label and the prescribed medication are in the same measurement system or have been converted to the same system. Then follow this formula for calculating oral medication dosages:

$$\frac{\text{DA (dosage available)}}{\text{DF (dosage form)}} = \frac{\text{DO (dose ordered)}}{\text{DG (dose to be given)}}$$

For example, suppose you are a pharmacist and a patient prescription calls for 500 mg of amoxicillin to be taken three times each day for three days. Your pharmacy has 250-mg amoxicillin tablets. You will use a proportion to determine the dose.

$$\frac{250 \text{ mg (DA)}}{1 \text{ tablet (DF)}} = \frac{500 \text{ mg (DO)}}{x \text{ (DG)}}$$

1. Cross multiply to get $250x = 500$
2. Divide each side by the number in front of x

$$250 \div 250 = 1x$$

$$500 \div 250 = 2 \text{ tablets}$$

Each dose will require two tablets, which means 2 tablets × 3 doses/day = 6 tablets × 3 days = 18 tablets in the entire dosage. Therefore, you will fill the pill bottle with 18 amoxicillin tablets. The prescription's label should direct the patient to take two tablets three times each day for three days.

Liquid medications are measured with a dosing syringe, dosing cup, or specially-marked dosing spoon (Figure 7.28). For accuracy, use the measuring device provided with the medicine instead of kitchen silverware. Medication dosages depend on the weight of the patient, so accuracy is especially important when giving liquid medicine to children. A small difference in the amount of medicine can have a serious negative effect on a young child. Be sure to measure liquid medicine at eye level, and never guess at the dose. Use the dose shown on the medication label.

When preparing liquid medications, you must calculate how many milliliters of medicine a patient should receive. For this calculation, you must know the **concentration** of the drug. The concentration describes how much of the drug is in a specific volume of liquid. Concentrations are normally given as a fraction, such as 20 mg/mL, which means there are 20 milligrams of medication in every milliliter of liquid.

Suppose the dose ordered (DO) from the physician is 30 mg of ketorolac liquid every six hours for 24 hours. The dose available (DA) is 15 mg/mL. How many milliliters of ketorolac liquid are needed in the 24-hour period?

$$\frac{15 \text{ mg (DA)}}{1 \text{ mL (DF)}} = \frac{30 \text{ mg (DO)}}{x \text{ mL (DG)}}$$

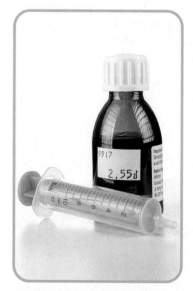
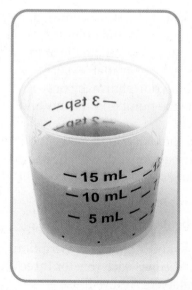
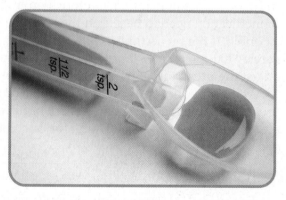

Figure 7.28   Dosing devices include the dosing syringe, dosing cup, and dosing spoon.

1. Cross multiply to get $15x = 30$, and then divide each side of the equation by 15. This means that $x = 2$ mL, which tells us the patient needs 2 mL of ketorolac per dose.

2. We know the patient receives a dose every six hours. In a 24-hour period, the patient will receive four doses of medication ($24 \div 6 = 4$).

3. Finally, multiply the total number of doses in a 24-hour period by the total number of milliliters per dose (4 doses/24 hr × 2mL/dose = 8 mL/24 hr).

Physicians commonly use abbreviations to indicate the route and times for administering medication. For example, *240 mg of aspirin, qd in am* means the patient will take 240 mg of aspirin every day in the morning. Technicians interpret the abbreviations and clarify the time and frequency for taking each medication. They print instructions on the medication label that are easy for the patient to understand. For the prescription example above, the label instructions might read, "Take one tablet by mouth each day in the morning" (Figure 7.29).

Figure 7.29 Prescription Abbreviations

Question	Abbreviation and Meaning	
How often should you take your medication?	ad lib—freely, as needed bid—twice a day prn—as needed q—every q3h—every 3 hours	q4h—every 4 hours qd—every day qid—four times a day qod—every other day tid—three times a day
When should you take your medication?	ac—before meals hs—at bedtime	int—between meals pc—after meals
Where should you get your medication?	Rx—prescription OTC—over the counter	
How much medication should you take?	caps—capsule gtt—drops i, ii, iii, or iiii—the number of doses (1, 2, 3, or 4) mg—milligrams mL—milliliters	ss—one half T, TT, TTT—the number of tabs/caps (1, 2, 3) tabs—tablets tbsp—tablespoon (15 mL) tsp—teaspoon (5 mL)
Where should you administer your medication?	ad—right ear al—left ear c̄ —with od—right eye os—left eye ou—both eyes	po—by mouth s or ø—without sl—sublingual top—apply topically IV—intravenously

Some long-term care facilities receive residents' medications in prepackaged doses ready to be administered at timed intervals (Figure 7.30). This type of packaging can also be helpful when patients are away from home for long periods, such as children who go to summer

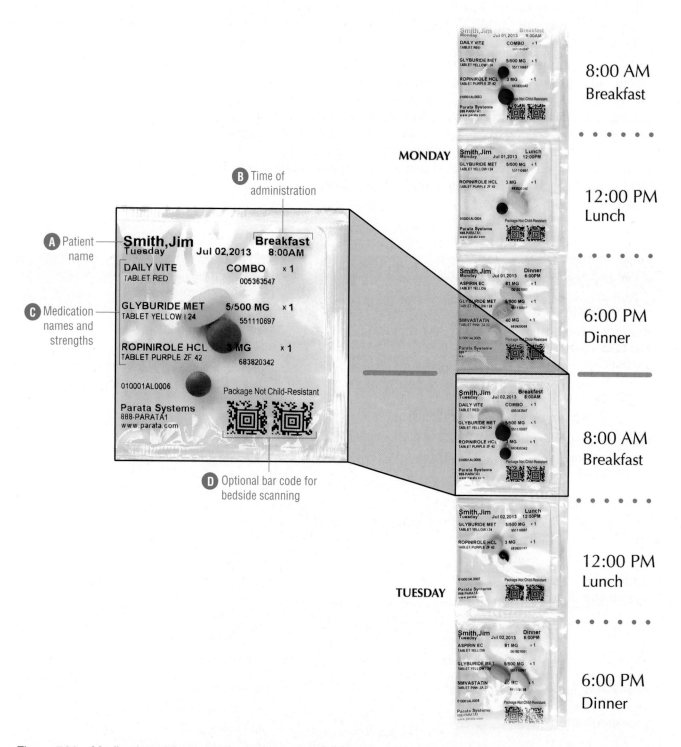

Figure 7.30   Medications can be prepackaged in pouches labeled with the following information: (A) patient name, (B) time of administration, (C) medication names and strengths, and (D) an optional bar code for bedside scanning. In addition, any special instructions—such as the need to take a medication with food—will be listed below the name of that medication.

camp or businesspeople who travel to several cities or countries in a row. For patients who take several medications each day, this packaging can save time and prevent dosing errors. According to a 2006 report by the Institute of Medicine, medication errors harm an estimated 1.5 million people in the United States each year, resulting in more than $3.5 billion in extra medical costs.

The more medications a patient takes, the easier it is to make an error. For example, a patient taking five different medications three times each day must open and select a correct dose from a medication container fifteen times each day. Figure 7.31 shows the medication orders for a patient named Adrian Hartman, who lives in a long-term care facility. The pharmacy technician who receives these orders sees that the resident takes six different medications each day and a seventh only when needed. The technician interprets the routes and times for each medication and groups the medicines that are taken at the same time into one package. Each package lists the date, time to administer, and the name and dosage of each medication in the package. So the pouch for 0800 (8:00 a.m.) will contain Furosemide, Plavix, Lipitor, aspirin, and Toprol; the pouch for 1130 (11:30 a.m.) will contain Furosemide; and the pouch for 2200 (10:00 p.m.) will contain Tylenol. Nitrostat is delivered in a separate pouch to be administered as needed.

Of course, technicians follow medication safety practices that promote giving the right medication at the right time and in the right dose. Pharmacists check each package to ensure that medications, amounts, and times are correct. They pay attention to possible drug interactions and special instructions such as taking medicines before, with, or after meals.

Measuring Angles

Healthcare workers use angles to measure and describe joint movement, to inject medications correctly, and to position patients in bed.

Figure 7.31 Medication Orders for Adrian Hartman		
Medication Orders	**Dosing Times**	**Interpretation of Medication Orders**
20 mg Furosemide	bid in am hours	twice each day, in the morning
75 mg Plavix	qd in am	every day in the morning
10 mg Lipitor	qd in am	every day in the morning
240 mg Aspirin	qd in am	every day in the morning
25 mg Toprol XL	qd in am	every day in the morning
650 mg Tylenol	qd hs OTC	every day at bedtime; not a prescription; purchase over the counter
0.4 mg Nitrostat	prn sbl	use as needed for chest pain; place under the tongue

Angles are measured in degrees from a *reference plane*. For example, when you are lying flat on your back in bed, your body is the reference plane at 0 degrees. When you raise your arm straight toward the ceiling, you have created a 90-degree angle between your body and your arm. Raising your arm above your head and moving it all the way back down to the bed surface creates a 180-degree angle (Figure 7.32).

When injecting medications, healthcare workers vary the angle of the needle based on the type of medication they are administering or the procedure they are performing. The surface of the patient's skin is the reference plane at 0 degrees (Figure 7.33).

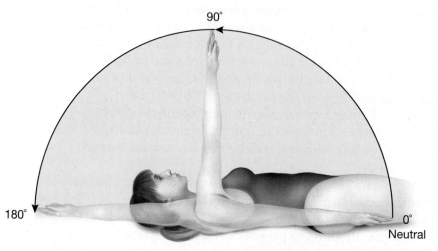

Figure 7.32   Healthcare workers use angles to measure and describe joint movement. If a patient can raise his or her arm straight up, what degree of movement would you record in the patient's chart?

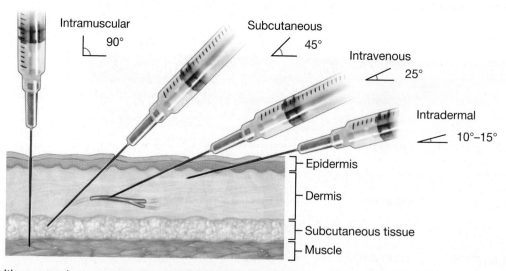

Figure 7.33   Healthcare workers use specific angles for different types of injections. Intramuscular injections are given through the skin and into the muscle at a 90-degree angle. Subcutaneous injections go into the tissue layer between the skin and the muscle at a 45-degree angle. Intravenous injections are given into a vein at 25-degree angle. Intradermal injections are given into the dermis layer of the skin at a 10- to 15-degree angle.

Angles are also important for determining how to position patients. Physicians may order the head of a patient's bed to be elevated 30 to 45 degrees. The purpose of this position is to help the patient breathe more easily or to prevent aspiration of fluids into the lungs. Nurses will raise the bed from 60 to 90 degrees when feeding a patient to help them swallow more easily. These are called *Fowler's positions* and include **semi-Fowler's** (30 degrees), **Fowler's** (45 degrees), and **high Fowler's** (90 degrees). These terms indicate the number of degrees the patient is elevated from the 0-degree plane, which is lying flat on the bed in supine position (Figure 7.34).

Angles are also used during patient rehabilitation, when the physical therapist measures the range of motion for an injured joint. As therapy progresses, the measurements will document the improvements in range of motion. The therapist uses a tool called the **goniometer** (goh-nee-AH-meh-ter) to measure joint angles and records range of motion in degrees (Figure 7.35). While the most accurate measurements are taken from radiographs (X-ray images), the goniometer is a less expensive tool that works like a protractor to measure joint angles on the human body.

goniometer
an instrument for measuring angles

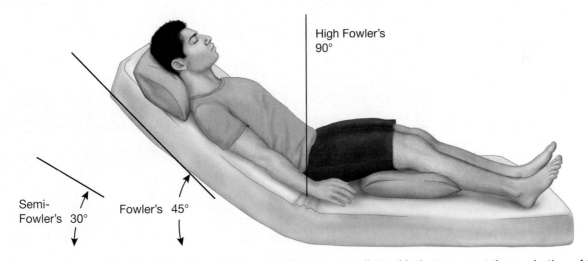

Figure 7.34   Fowler's positions allow the patient to breathe more easily and help to prevent the aspiration of fluids.

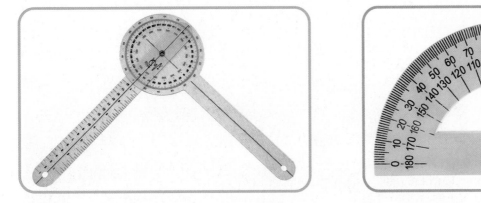

Figure 7.35   A goniometer and a protractor both measure angles.

When taking a joint measurement with a goniometer, always stabilize the stationary part of the body (the part that does not move), which is proximal to the joint you are testing (Figure 7.36). This isolates the joint movement and results in a more accurate measurement. Follow these steps to measure the angle of a joint:

1. Align the fulcrum or pin of the goniometer with the fulcrum of the joint to be measured. Since the location of the fulcrum can vary, you will need to check the location for each specific joint. In the knee and elbow joints for example, the pin of the goniometer is placed over the lateral epicondyle (ehp-ih-KAHN-dihl).

2. Align one arm of the goniometer with the stationary limb.

3. Align the other arm of the goniometer with the limb that moves.

4. Read the goniometer by noting the degree measurement from the 0 point to the endpoint at the arrow or line before removing it from

Figure 7.36   The arms of the goniometer must be positioned correctly for an accurate measurement. The range of motion measurement is 180 degrees.

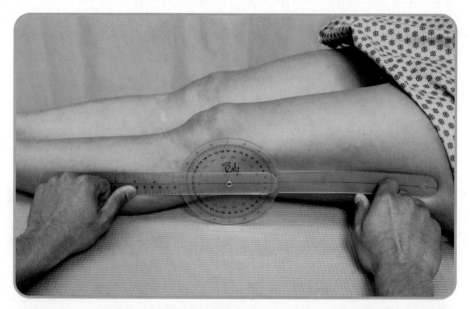

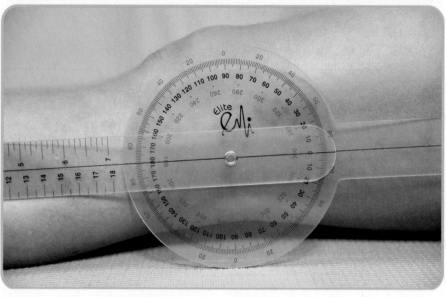

the patient's body. The degrees between the zero point and the endpoint represent the entire range of motion.

5. Record the range of motion for the joint.

A therapist will compare the patient's range of motion with previous records and the average range of motion to determine his or her progress and to develop therapy plans for continued improvement (Figure 7.37).

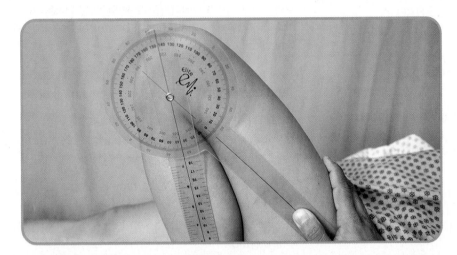

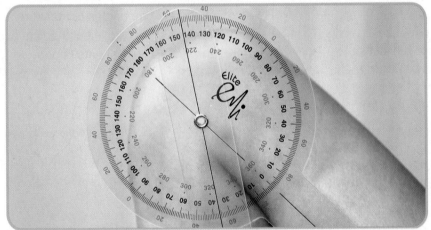

Figure 7.37   This angle shows that the patient has full range of motion. Read the measurement shown on the goniometer here. What is the patient's range of motion for knee flexion?

RECALL YOUR READING

1. You can avoid confusion between _____ and _____ times by using the 24-hour clock.

2. US healthcare workers must be able to make accurate conversions between _____ and _____ systems of measurement.

3. You can make conversions within the household system by understanding _____.

4. Special _____ and authorization are required for healthcare workers who administer medications.

5. To assess range of motion, a healthcare worker measures the _____ of a joint and records the range of motion in degrees.

Complete the *Map Your Reading* graphic organizer for the section you just read.

SUMMARY

Assess your understanding with chapter tests

- While each person has a preferred communication style, assertive communication is considered the healthiest style because it is both effective and diplomatic.

- Healthcare workers use standardized communication formats such as SBAR to communicate more clearly and improve patient outcomes.

- Open-ended questions encourage patients to share information.

- Environmental barriers, sensory impairments, and cognitive impairments require healthcare workers to use special techniques for maintaining effective communication.

- Culturally competent healthcare workers are aware of possible cultural differences, but do not make assumptions about the viewpoints or beliefs of others.

- Electronic health records systems contain all of the same information found in a paper chart along with many additional medical office functions.

- Errors in an EHR should not be deleted. The original document—including errors—must be stored and accessible.

- The use of mobile technologies is increasing as apps are developed to improve access to EHR, patient monitoring, consumer health, and medical education resources.

- Using the 24-hour clock prevents chart errors and confusion between a.m. and p.m. times.

- US healthcare workers must be proficient in both metric and household measurement systems.

- Since mathematical accuracy is a critical element in working with medications, only trained and authorized workers can administer medication.

- Healthcare workers use angles to measure and describe joint movement, to inject medications correctly, and to position patients in bed.

MAXIMIZE YOUR PROFESSIONAL VOCABULARY

Build vocabulary with e-flash cards, games, and audio glossary

Listed below are the essential, yellow-highlighted terms and the additional professional vocabulary terms that you encountered in this chapter. Complete the activities that follow the list to make all of these terms part of your everyday professional vocabulary.

24-hour clock
addendum
Affordable Care Act (ACA)
apothecary system
apps
assertive communication
authenticate
cognitive impairments
communication barrier
communication style
concentration
cultural differences

cultural diversity
dosage
dose
environmental barriers
e-prescribing
face page
Fowler's
goniometer
Health Information Technology for Economic and Clinical Health (HITECH) Act
high Fowler's
International Units (IU)

meaningful use
medical interpreter
medication
metric system
mHealth
open-ended question
patient interview
SBAR system
semi-Fowler's
sensory impairments
social media
US customary units

VOCABULARY DEVELOPMENT

Matching. Match each essential term from this chapter with the correct definition below by writing the letter of the definition next to the number of the essential term on a separate sheet of paper.

1. 24-hour clock
2. apps
3. assertive communication
4. communication barrier
5. communication style
6. cultural diversity
7. e-prescribing
8. goniometer
9. medication
10. metric system
11. open-ended question
12. patient interview
13. social media
14. US customary units

a. a group of online communication tools that allow people to share information and resources via the Internet

b. a person's preferred method for exchanging information, which includes words, tone of voice, and nonverbal signs

c. a question that requires more than a one- or two-word response

d. a communication style characterized by confidence and consideration for others

e. a method of telling time that assigns a number to each hour of the day; also known as *military time*

f. an instrument for measuring angles

g. applications; software that is accessed through the Internet and runs on a computer, smartphone, tablet, or other mobile device

h. a structured communication between a patient and a healthcare worker for the purpose of collecting subjective data such as a medical history

i. electronic generation, transmission, and filling of a medical prescription

j. the main system of weights and measures used in the United States, based on the yard, pound, and gallon as units of length, weight, and liquid volume respectively; also known as the *household measurements*

k. the decimal measurement system based on the meter, liter, and gram as its primary units of length, volume, and weight or mass respectively

l. anything that blocks or interferes with the exchange of information

m. a substance or mixture of substances that have been proven through research to have a clear value in the prevention, diagnosis, or treatment of diseases

n. term that describes differences in age, gender, physical and intellectual abilities, sexual orientation, race, or ethnicity that influence what we believe, the way we think, and what we do

15. **Draw A Visual.** Draw a visual that will help you remember each of the following terms: *environmental barriers*, *sensory impairment*, *cognitive impairments*, *cultural differences*. Reread the section of the chapter that introduces the vocabulary term to refresh your memory, if necessary. All visuals should be appropriate and respectful. Compare your visuals with your classmates' visuals to see their ideas.

16. **Name Your Terms.** For each letter in your name, select a term from the vocabulary list that begins with that letter. Skip letters that do not appear in the terms list. Write each term and define it in your own words. Then share your terms with a classmate and compare different definitions.

REFLECT ON YOUR READING

17. What characteristics other than language differences create diversity? Name at least five of these characteristics and describe yourself based on each characteristic. For example, gender is a diversifying characteristic. What is your gender? Consider each description and explain ways that each characteristic shapes your beliefs, thoughts, and actions. For example, how has your gender influenced your choice of hobby or career?

BUILD CORE SKILLS

18. **Critical Thinking.** Think about a disagreement you've recently experienced

and consider how you communicated with the other person involved in your disagreement. Then review the self-assessment in Figure 7.2. Which style of communication did you use? Provide examples to explain your choice.

19. **Critical Thinking.** Which of the following questions are open-ended? Rewrite any of the questions that can be answered with a one- or two-word response so that they are open-ended.

   a. What symptoms bring you to the emergency room today, Mr. Wright?

   b. Do you have pain?

   c. Are you taking any medications, Pablo?

   d. When are you most likely to feel faint?

   e. When are supposed to take you medication(s)?

   f. What foods do you eat in a typical day?

   g. Will there be someone to help you after the surgery?

20. **Speaking and Listening.** To learn more about your own cultural healthcare background, ask a parent or grandparent these questions about childhood experience:

   a. What was your religion? What are your healthcare-related religious beliefs?

   b. What did you believe caused illness?

   c. What did you do to treat and prevent illness?

Now consider these questions about your own childhood experiences:

   a. How were you told to stay healthy?

   b. When you got a common illness like a cold, how was your condition treated? Did you use special foods or other remedies?

What has changed and what has stayed the same from your parents' or grandparents' childhood to your own childhood? What is unique about your healthcare identity?

21. **Writing.** Create a five-point chart to compare and contrast the features of electronic and paper medical records.

22. **Problem Solving.** Develop a set of guidelines for healthcare workers to follow when they use social media to communicate with patients.

23. **Math.** Convert the Greenwich times below to military time.

   a. 2:30 p.m.

   b. 1:15 a.m.

   c. 4:50 a.m.

   d. 12:00 a.m.

   e. 5:30 a.m.

24. **Math.** Convert the following military times into Greenwich time.

   a. 1415

   b. 0300

   c. 1230

   d. 0645

   e. 1130

25. **Math.** Move the decimal point to convert these metric measurements.

   a. 70,263 g = _____ kg

   b. 24,100 g = _____ kg

   c. 12.7 cm = _____ mm

   d. 1,450 cm = _____ m

   e. 23.27 L = _____ mL

   f. 76.25 L = _____ mL

26. **Math.** Refer to Figure 7.22 and use equivalents to convert these household measurements.

   a. 67 oz = _____ lbs

   b. 6½ lbs = _____ oz

   c. 63 in = _____ ft, _____ in

   d. 12 ft = _____ yd

   e. 500 yd = _____ mi

   f. 120 gtt = _____ tsp

   g. 6 T = _____ oz

   h. 18 oz = _____ c

   i. 6 c = _____ pt

   j. 3 gal = _____ qt

27. **Math.** Refer to the conversion tables in Figures 7.24 and 7.25 to convert these measurements into units in a different measurement system.

   a. Mrs. Jergens' newborn baby weighs 7.5 lbs and is 20½ in long. How will you record this information in metric measurements for the baby's medical record?

   b. Mr. Castillo drank 6 oz of orange juice, 12 oz of lemonade, and 4 oz of water during your work shift. How many total ounces of liquid intake is this? How will you record this in metric measurements on his chart?

   c. Stacy Judd's physician advised her to take 30 mL of cold medication. How can she measure that amount accurately using her household measuring spoons?

28. **Critical Thinking.** For each of the descriptions below, identify the specific form of medication that will be used.

a. used on the skin to help heal sunburn

b. dissolved in the mouth to ease throat pain

c. swallowed to calm a cough

d. this medicine is shaken to mix the drug with the liquid before measuring the dose

29. **Reading.** Refer to Figure 7.29 to translate these prescriptions. Then write easy-to-understand instructions for patients to follow when taking each prescription. Label the dose and the dosage listed in each prescription.

Example: Toradol 10 mg #20

$\dot{T}$ tab q6h for inflammation

Answer: Take one 10 milligram Toradol tablet (dose) every 6 hours for inflammation. Dispense 20 tablets (dosage).

a. Amoxicillin 500 mg #30

$\dot{T}$ cap po tid x 10 days

b. Motrin 800 mg #90

$\dot{T}$ tab po tid $\bar{c}$ food

c. Colace 100 mg #30

$\dot{T}$ tab po qhs

d. Zofran 4 mg IV

q4h prn nausea

30. **Math.** For each example listed here, calculate the dose, or amount to administer.

Example:

Ordered: Thorazine 20 mg po tid

On hand: Thorazine 10 mg tablets

Dose = 2 tablets

a. Ordered: Ceclor 0.375 g po bid

On hand: Ceclor Oral Suspension 187 mg per 5 mL

b. Ordered: Ketoconazole 100 mg po qd

On hand: Ketoconazole 200-mg scored tablets

c. Ordered: Tranxene 30 mg po qhs

On hand: Tranxene 15 mg tablets

d. Ordered: Keflex 500 mg po q12h

On hand: Keflex 250 mg per 5mL

ACTIVATE YOUR LEARNING

31. Use a doll provided by your instructor to take the following measurements. Measure the doll's weight, length, head circumference, and abdominal circumference in metric units. Use equivalents to convert these measurements into household units.

32. Use the goniometer provided by your instructor for this exercise. With a partner, practice measuring joint angles for flexion and extension of the knee and elbow. Record your measurements.

THINK AND ACT LIKE A HEALTHCARE WORKER

33. Suppose you are caring for an elderly woman in a long-term care facility. You have cared for Mrs. Skylar for three years and are very familiar with her routines and interests. She has not been acting like herself all day. This morning she decided not to get dressed or go to breakfast. She usually likes to dress up and chat with other residents at mealtime. When you brought her medications, she seemed distracted and even dropped a couple of her tablets. She decided not to watch TV because it was too blurry. You think she needs to see a doctor. Use the SBAR system to organize your communication and write out what you would say to convey your concerns to your supervisor.

GO TO THE SOURCE

34. Search the Internet for an article on robotic surgery and make a printout. Make sure the source is reliable and reputable. Highlight the key ideas presented in the article. Look for possible responses to the following questions:

- What types of surgeries are typically done with robotics?
- What are the advantages of robotic surgery vs. manual surgery?
- What is the success rate of robotic surgeries or a particular type of robotic surgery?
- What skills does the person controlling the robot need?
- What questions might a patient ask when considering robotic surgery?
- What other questions need to be asked about robotic surgery?

35. Share your article about robotic surgery with the rest of the class. Mention five key things that you learned about robotic surgery. Do your findings agree or disagree with those of other students?

Chapter 8
Professional Knowledge in Therapeutic Services

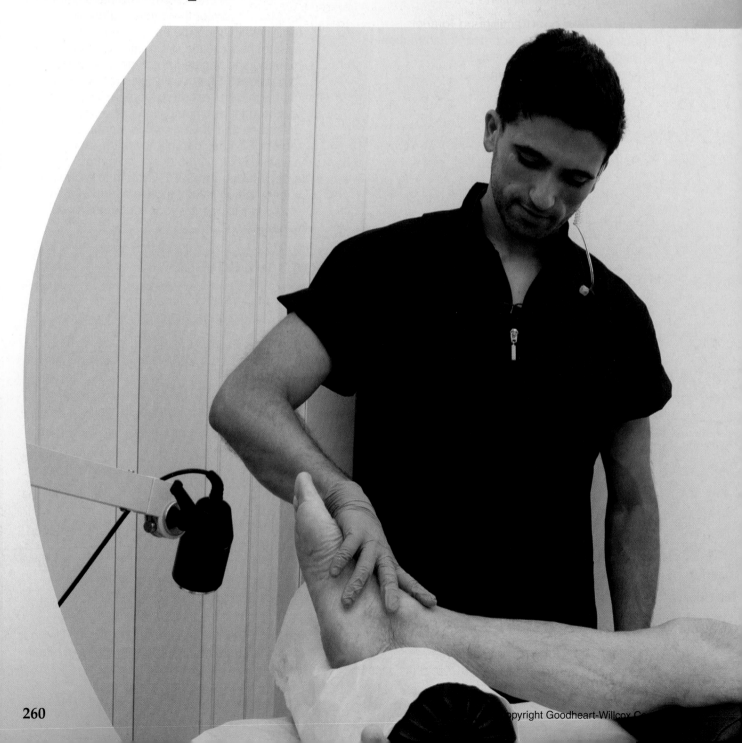

PROFESSIONAL VOCABULARY

E-flash Cards

You will need to learn the essential terms listed below before you begin your reading. These terms will help you understand the main concepts of the chapter. These terms, which will be highlighted in yellow within the text, will become part of your professional vocabulary.

In addition to these essential terms, you will see bold terms throughout the chapter. The meanings of these terms are explained where the terms first appear. The bold terms, like the essential terms listed here, will also become part of your professional vocabulary and deepen your understanding of the topics presented.

body mechanics specific positions for muscles and joints that help a person avoid injury during a physical task

informed consent a patient's choice to accept or reject a procedure after receiving information on available options and possible consequences

malpractice term for actions that violate a professional's scope of practice or standard of care and result in injury to a patient that could reasonably have been expected

mandatory reporting the legal requirement for certain health issues to be reported to authorities

medical errors preventable mistakes that can occur at any point in the healthcare process and may potentially cause harm to the patient

organizational chart a diagram that shows how departments in an organization are related to one another

safety check the process of looking for and removing potential hazards that could cause injury or harm

safety precautions information about the safe operation of a piece of equipment, which is usually found in the instruction manual or on equipment labels

scope of practice tasks that an employee is legally allowed to perform based on his or her training and certification

standard of care the level of service that a healthcare professional is expected to provide to a patient based on that professional's position and the patient's condition

workplace violence acts of verbal abuse, threats, physical assault, or homicide that occur at work

CONNECT WITH YOUR READING

How do patient expectations affect healthcare? Consider that question as you read the following scenario.

Jai Vang was visiting an oncologist for the first time. She usually saw the healer in her community when she was ill, but she had felt a lump in her breast, and a cousin said she'd be more likely to survive an illness like this if she saw the American doctors at her neighborhood clinic. The clinic didn't have an interpreter available, but Jai thought she could manage without one because she'd been speaking English for several years. Her insurance plan said it would pay for the doctor's visits and prescriptions. She had never needed more than a few herbal treatments in the past, so she felt sure that would be fine.

Language turned out not to be a problem, but Jai had other difficulties at the clinic. She wasn't sure how to respond to all of the items in the registration form she was given, and she didn't feel comfortable answering confusing and personal questions from people she didn't know. She was embarrassed when she was asked to take her clothes off in the examination room. When the doctor attempted to touch her breasts, she was startled and slapped his hands away. He was equally surprised by her reaction. How did things go so wrong?

After reading Jai Vang's story, look for connections you can make to her experience. Is her story similar to something you've experienced? When have you felt like this? Why do you think that Jai reacted in this way?

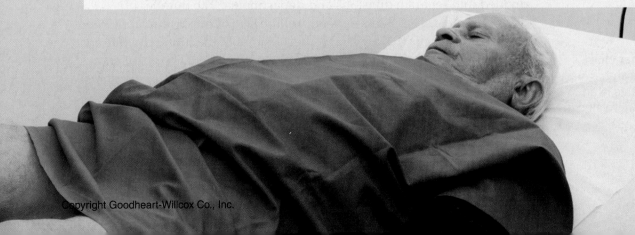

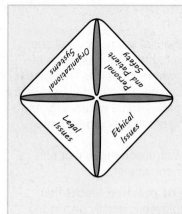

MAP YOUR READING

Can you figure out what went wrong in Jai Vang's situation? Create a visual summary to record your ideas. Begin with a square sheet of paper—an 8½-inch square works well. Fold each of the four points of the square to the center. Label each of the four resulting flaps with one of these topics: *Organizational Systems*, *Legal Issues*, *Ethical Issues*, and *Personal and Patient Safety*. Open each flap and draw a picture or symbol to illustrate something related to that topic that you believe caused Jai Vang's reaction. When you finish reading each of these sections in the chapter, open the corresponding flap and draw a picture or symbol to illustrate what you have read. Ask yourself how therapeutic workers are affected by organizational, legal, ethical, and safety issues. Finally, for each of the four topics, write three or four words that highlight important issues related to the topic.

As you have already learned, there are many legal and ethical issues in the field of healthcare. Therapeutic workers often work closely with patients, ensuring the quality of their care. This makes the therapeutic pathway a great option for those who enjoy helping people. But it can also mean that therapeutic workers encounter many legal and ethical issues in their day-to-day work.

In this chapter, you will consider how therapeutic workers are affected by organizational, legal, ethical, and safety issues. You will be introduced to common organizational structures and learn to follow the chain of command. You will also learn about legal and ethical issues that therapeutic workers encounter, such as scope of practice and abuse.

Organizational Systems

Healthcare workers need to understand the organization within which they work. They may even find themselves trying to explain it to their patients as they help them obtain care services. The healthcare system is a whole network of interconnected agencies, facilities, insurers, and providers working together to provide and finance healthcare services.

The Structure of Organizations

Within healthcare organizations, care providers and services are divided into separate divisions and departments. The number of divisions and departments depends on the size of the organization. The **organizational chart** is a visual representation of the **hierarchy** (HI-er-ahr-kee), or levels of authority, within an organization. Figure 8.1 shows an organizational chart for a large medical clinic. This chart represents the levels of responsibility and flow of information vertically within a department and horizontally between different departments. This structure helps the organization achieve its goals. It also helps workers understand who is responsible for different jobs and to whom they should report when they have questions about their job.

organizational chart
a diagram that shows how departments in an organization are related to one another

Medical Center Organizational Chart

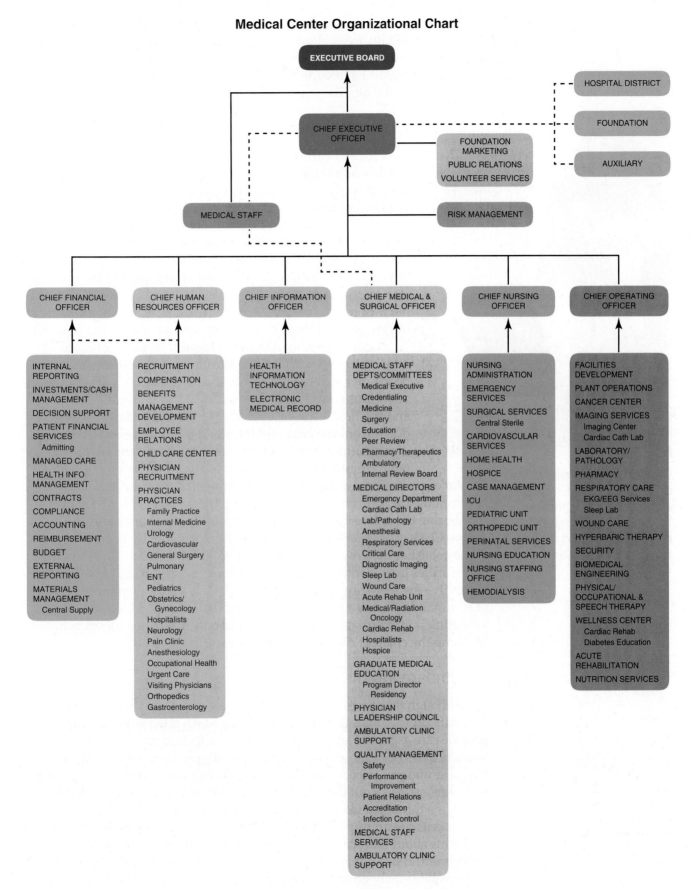

Figure 8.1   An organizational chart shows the levels of authority in an organization—in this case, a hospital. According to this chart, who would be your immediate supervisor if you worked in the emergency services department?

Within the organizational chart, therapeutic medical services are usually divided by areas of medical specialty. For example, the emergency department, anesthesiology, and respiratory services would each have their own director. Each department serves a different role in the overall functioning of the facility.

Lines of Authority

Lines of authority are the hierarchy of command from the top down through all the different ranks of employees. These lines show who is in charge and who reports to whom. Workers with more training and experience have more authority than workers with fewer credentials. For instance, in the medical department, medical assistants work under the direction of a physician (Figure 8.2). Residents have more authority than interns but less than a fellow or attending physician. On the nursing staff, certified nursing assistants report to a licensed practical nurse or registered nurse, and the director of nursing oversees all nurses. Some of these lines of authority are shown in Figure 8.1.

A governing board has the highest level of decision-making power within large healthcare organizations. The board includes the chief executive officer (CEO) and the heads of various committees. They address both administrative and medical issues. Decisions from the board are passed down from the administrator to department heads. Smaller organizations have a smaller management structure and may not have many of these upper levels of management.

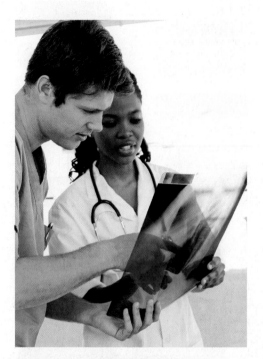

Figure 8.2   According to the chain of command, medical assistants must report to their supervising physician if they are concerned about a test result such as an X-ray.

An organizational structure creates a smooth flow of information between the decision makers at the top and the workers below. It shows the sharing of responsibilities and provides a **chain of command** to follow. *Chain of command* is another name for the hierarchy of authority that establishes the flow of decision making and directives. This structure also clarifies how workers should bring problems up through the lines of authority—by reporting issues to the individuals above them in the chain of command. When you raise concerns but they are not addressed in a way you think is appropriate, you must seek support from your supervisor. Move up the chain of command until the issue is resolved.

Healthcare Teams

Although the organizational chart appears to separate departments and staff, professionals from different departments often work together to provide care as part of an interdisciplinary healthcare team. A primary care team includes doctors, nurses, and allied health professionals. The doctors diagnose and prescribe treatments. Nurses, therapists, and pharmacists help to design and carry out the treatment plan. Secondary care is provided by specialists through a referral from the primary care provider when needed.

Patients are an important part of the care team. They make the final decisions about their care. In some states, if a patient is unable to make decisions and has not appointed a power of attorney for healthcare, this responsibility may go to the highest-ranking member of the healthcare team. Each member of the team has a separate role in providing care, but they all share the common goal of wellness for the patient.

Reporting

Care teams share information through both written records and oral reports. Therapeutic workers use **handoff care reports** with each new shift or change in the level of patient care to explain a patient's current situation. These reports are needed during *handoffs*, which are times when one healthcare worker is transferring the care of a patient to another healthcare worker. A transfer between units, a change in services, and a discharge all create the need for handoff care reports. The Joint Commission, which reviews the quality of care provided by healthcare organizations, identified handoffs as a key time when medical errors may occur. You can help prevent such errors by compiling complete information and organizing it logically in your report.

You will be responsible for recording and reporting the care you give. As you perform care tasks, it will be your job to keep accurate notes to use in your reports. You will need to use critical thinking skills to determine what information must be reported immediately and what can be charted or shared during handoff. Changes in the patient's condition are usually reported immediately. Whether you write these changes in the patient's chart or report to someone else who does the charting will depend on your level of responsibility and the rules in your facility.

Reporting and recording usually follow a standard format. You identify the patient, diagnosis, current condition, recent events, and anticipated changes. Your reports need to be clear and concise. Follow the IDEAL format shown in Figure 8.3 when making verbal or written reports and allow for questions from the person who is receiving the handoff of care.

Figure 8.3 IDEAL Method for Handoff Communication	
Identify	Identify patient by name, patient record number, date of birth, and physician name
Diagnosis	Diagnosis and current condition
Events	Recent events or changes in condition or treatment
Anticipated	Anticipate changes and what to watch for
Leave	Leave time for questions and clarification

RECALL YOUR READING

1. The _____ shows the connections between departments and the hierarchy within a department.
2. The hierarchy established by lines of _____ tells you to whom you report and from whom you take orders.
3. Members of a(n) _____ team share a common goal of wellness for the patient.
4. Changes in a patient's condition must be _____ and recorded in a clear and concise manner.

Complete the *Map Your Reading* graphic organizer for the section you just read.

Legal and Ethical Issues for Therapeutic Workers

Common legal and ethical issues for therapeutic workers cover a broad range of topics. Professionals who work in therapeutic careers are always aware of the limits placed on their actions by their credentials and **scope of practice**. They understand the consequences of exceeding those limits. They also need to be aware of the consequences of errors made in the course of providing healthcare. In addition, therapeutic workers need to understand how alternative medicine can affect patient care. Because these workers are hands-on caregivers, they are more likely to be exposed to issues of patient rights, informed consent, and mandatory reporting.

scope of practice
tasks that an employee is legally allowed to perform based on their training and certification

Credentials

As discussed in chapter 1, credentials provide evidence that you have the legal and professional requirements to practice your career. Credentials are represented by a license, certificate, or similar document you have earned and the initials placed after your name, such as "Mary Johnson, CST" (certified surgical technologist). Figure 8.4 provides a list of common credential abbreviations for therapeutic workers. The credentialing process is designed to make sure providers are qualified to handle their patients' healthcare needs. Licensing boards and professional associations grant credentials.

Licensure is required by law for some professions to protect public health, safety, and welfare. Medical doctors, nurses, pharmacists, and therapists are among the professionals who must have a license to

Figure 8.4 Common Credential Abbreviations

Abbreviation	Credential	Abbreviation	Credential
CFNP	Certified Family Nurse Practitioner	LPN	Licensed Practical Nurse
CNA	Certified Nursing Assistant	MA	Medical Assistant
CNM	Certified Nurse Midwife	MD	Medical Doctor
COTA	Certified Occupational Therapy Assistant	MSN	Master of Science–Nursing
CRNA	Certified Registered Nurse Anesthetist	NP	Nurse Practitioner
CRNP	Certified Registered Nurse Practitioner	OD	Doctor of Optometry
DC	Doctor of Chiropractic	PA-C	Physician Assistant–Certified
DDS; DMD	Dentist	PNP	Pediatric Nurse Practitioner
DO	Doctor of Osteopathic Medicine	PT	Physical Therapist
DPM	Podiatrist	RD	Registered Dietitian
EMT	Emergency Medical Technician	RN	Registered Nurse
FNP	Family Nurse Practitioner	WHCNP	Women's Health Care Nurse Practitioner

practice. Licensing is usually managed by each state's department of health. These state agencies make sure the applicant has the education and experience required to practice the profession in question.

Individuals who want a license must supply proof of their education and pass a licensing examination. These examinations may include multiple sections addressing different aspects of the field. For example, becoming licensed as a physical therapy assistant in California requires passing the National Physical Therapy Examination (NPTE), which assesses knowledge of the field, and the California Law Examination (CLE), which covers state legal issues.

Licenses are only valid for a certain period of time, and then they must be renewed. Renewing a license typically means completing a certain number of **continuing education units (CEUs)**. This coursework ensures that the individual remains up-to-date on knowledge and skills in the field. Practicing with an expired license is illegal.

State and federal laws **regulate**, or *control*, the training and practice of many healthcare careers to protect public safety. Most federal laws are very broad, while state laws provide requirements that are more specific for practice and which may vary from state to state. For instance, the federal **Omnibus Budget Reconciliation Act (OBRA)** requires certified nursing assistants (CNAs) to have at least 75 hours of training and to pass written and skill tests. Individual state requirements range from 75 to 200 hours of training for CNAs. Similarly, a psychologist in Alaska must have 1,500 hours of supervised experience for licensure, but Florida requires 4,000 hours.

Some healthcare careers are less regulated than others. For example, veterinary assistants, physical therapy aides, and cardiovascular technicians do not require either licensure or certification. **Certification** is typically a voluntary credential created by a professional association, not a mandatory one required by law. Even if the law does not require certification for a particular career, employers may look for this qualification as a sign of job applicants' knowledge and skills. In turn, certified healthcare workers usually earn more money and are more employable. Federally funded facilities generally require their employees to be licensed or certified.

Employers must check a **registry** to make sure employee credentials are up to date. They also verify work history with past employers. For example, before they can work at a hospital, physicians must apply to the hospital board for medical staff membership and hospital privileges. Doctors currently on the medical staff at that hospital review the applicants' credentials and recommend whether or not the board should accept them (Figure 8.5). This review includes providing evidence of past training and experience and demonstrating competence. The review also considers applicants' character and judgment shown in their past practice. If a doctor is accepted, the hospital will list which procedures he or she is allowed to perform there. A hospital doesn't want staff members who aren't well-qualified because they would jeopardize the facility's accreditation and reputation.

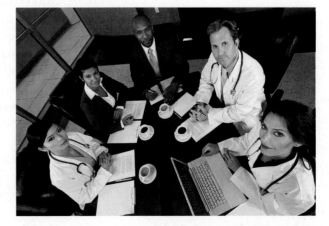

Figure 8.5 A hospital board must approve a physician's application for membership in the hospital staff. What kind of information does the hospital board review in these situations?

Scope of Practice

Your scope of practice includes all the skills you are trained in and allowed to use. Most healthcare careers require you to take classes to learn the necessary skills, but some skills are learned on the job. Scope of practice is different for each career. The higher you climb up your career ladder, the more skills you will learn, the broader your scope of practice will be, and the more responsibilities you will have. Healthcare workers should never provide care that is outside their scope of practice.

Healthcare Workers: Scope of Practice

As a physical therapy assistant, Debbie was trained to provide range-of-motion exercises to those needing rehabilitation under the supervision of a physical therapist. She knows she must notify her supervisor if a patient is not responding well, but she is also aware that she is not authorized to change the prescribed exercises herself. That authority lies outside her scope of practice.

Sarah learned her job as a pharmacy technician through on-the-job training at a local pharmacy. She prepares prescriptions that are written by a doctor, but they must always be checked by a pharmacist who also answers any questions that customers have about the medications.

As a nursing assistant, Claudio is trained to carry out the nursing plan set by a registered nurse. Although he may recognize and report common symptoms, he cannot tell the patient what diagnosis he suspects or recommend a treatment.

Scope of practice is a legal concept. A healthcare worker can be held **liable**—legally responsible—for not performing tasks within his or her scope of practice. Consider Patel, a radiation therapist who delivers radiation treatments to cancer patients. If he fails to deliver the doses of radiation ordered by an oncologist, Patel could be liable for negative effects on a patient's health. If he provides the required amount of radiation and the patient shows no visible signs of distress *during* treatment, Patel is not responsible for any ill effects the patient experiences *after* treatment.

Remember that scope of practice places limits on what healthcare workers are allowed to do. Liability also arises if a worker goes beyond those limits. If Patel decides on his own that a particular patient should receive radiation for a longer period than ordered, he has exceeded his scope of practice. Working outside your scope of practice could be considered as operating without a license, which is illegal.

standard of care
the level of service that a healthcare professional is expected to provide to a patient based on that professional's position and the patient's condition

Malpractice

Within a healthcare professional's scope of practice, he or she is expected to provide a certain **standard of care**. For example, physicians are expected to respond to patients with particular illnesses and conditions with generally accepted treatments. When a trained professional knowingly provides care that is below this standard and the patient suffers harm that could reasonably have been anticipated, that professional is guilty of **malpractice**.

Malpractice is most often the result of negligence. **Negligence** is the failure to do something a person with training should have known enough to do. In cases of negligence, however, the error is not intentional. For example, dental hygienists know that their dental tools must be sterilized between uses. If Sue is in a hurry and just rinses the instruments off, she is *knowingly* taking the chance of transmitting a serious disease. This is malpractice. If Sue removes the tools from the autoclave and doesn't realize they have not yet been sterilized, this is negligence (Figure 8.6).

Malpractice is generally a matter of civil law rather than criminal law. A patient who believes he or she has suffered injury can bring a malpractice suit. The patient bringing the suit—the plaintiff—must prove that the practitioner had a duty to provide care, that the practitioner did not meet that duty, and that the plaintiff suffered injury as a result of that failure. Failure to cure a disease or condition is not grounds for malpractice as long as the physician treating the patient followed standards of care for that disease or condition. Treatments are not guaranteed to succeed.

Malpractice suits are typically brought against physicians, but other healthcare professionals can also face these charges. Healthcare professionals who face the possibility of malpractice charges usually purchase insurance to protect themselves from the cost of losing a malpractice suit.

Mistreatment of Patients

Caregiver laws govern people who provide direct care, supervision, and protection to children, the elderly, and people with disabilities. These laws vary by state. They cover topics such as neglect, abuse, and misappropriation of property. Violations of these laws can affect your ability to work.

Abuse is an act that inflicts physical or emotional harm. There are many types of abuse. Slapping or pinching a patient are examples of physical abuse. Verbal abuse uses words to damage a patient's self-esteem. Sexual abuse includes any unwanted sexual contact. Physical and emotional neglect are passive forms of abuse in which the caregiver fails to provide the care needed. Some families have charged elder-care facilities with another form of abuse called **involuntary seclusion**. This is the practice of isolating a person and preventing him or her from interacting with others.

Charges of abuse look at the degree of harm to determine if the crime is a misdemeanor or felony. A felony is a serious crime that is punished by imprisonment or large fines. Misdemeanors, which are less serious than felonies, entail shorter jail sentences and smaller fines. In some states, people with felony abuse or neglect convictions are permanently barred from caregiver jobs and facilities.

False imprisonment is holding people against their will or limiting their movement without the right to do so. This includes the wrongful use of restraints or not allowing a patient to leave the hospital. Patients with

malpractice
term for actions that violate a professional's scope of practice or standard of care and result in injury to a patient that could reasonably have been expected

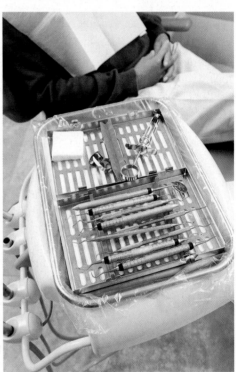

Figure 8.6   Failing to properly sterilize medical instruments, such as these dental tools, is considered malpractice. What could happen if unsterilized tools were used on a patient?

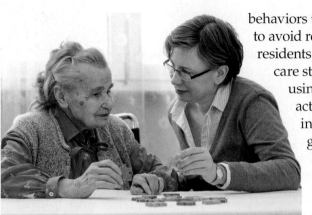

Figure 8.7   Elderly residents are at risk for falling, but don't necessarily need to be restrained. What kinds of activities might distract a person and avoid the use of restraints?

behaviors that are difficult to manage will require a care plan to avoid restraints by adapting to their needs. For instance, residents with dementia are at high risk for falling. Long-term care staff can avoid restraining them in a wheelchair by using interventions such as distracting them with an activity or a snack (Figure 8.7). Environmental safeguards include monitors to draw staff attention when residents get out of their chair or open a door. Patients may be asked to sign a waiver form if they wish to leave their care facility against medical advice.

Words or actions that lead a person to fear that you intend to harm him or her are considered **assault**. Assault is often charged along with **battery**, which is touching a person without his or her consent. Both assault and battery are crimes. Be sure to let your patient know what you are doing, and get his or her permission for the action before proceeding. Be careful in your choice of words and actions so that your patients don't feel threatened. Failing to get permission before removing a patient's clothing is battery. Telling a patient that if he doesn't go to the bathroom on the toilet you'll hang his soiled clothes out for everyone to see is considered assault. If you become frustrated with a patient, get help from a coworker rather than taking it out on the patient. An incident report must be filed whenever a patient, an employee, or a visitor reports an injury.

Patient Rights

The first Patient's Bill of Rights was developed in 1973 by the American Hospital Association. Created to help improve patient care, this Bill of Rights reminded healthcare workers of their responsibilities to the patient and encouraged patients to be more active in their own care.

In 1997, President Bill Clinton appointed an advisory committee on consumer protection and quality in healthcare. In 1998, that committee recommended a national set of consumer rights and responsibilities based on the following ideas:

1. **Information disclosure.** Consumers have the right to receive accurate and understandable information about their diagnosis, prognosis, treatment options, costs, and the facility rules to make informed healthcare decisions.

2. **Choice of providers and plans.** Consumers have the right to a variety of high-quality healthcare providers and insurance options from which to choose.

3. **Access to services.** Another consumer right guarantees access to medically necessary healthcare services and a reasonable continuity of care from one healthcare facility to another. Consumers have a right to be informed of business, educational, or other partnerships between providers that may influence their treatment or care.

4. **Participation in treatment decisions.** Consumers, or their designated representatives, have the right to participate fully in all decisions related to their healthcare. This includes the consumer's right to refuse treatment and to choose whether or not to participate in experimental research.

5. **Respect and nondiscrimination.** Consumers have the right to receive considerate, respectful care from all members of the healthcare team (Figure 8.8).

6. **Confidentiality of health information.** Consumers have the right to privacy regarding their information. Consumers also have the right to review, request corrections to, and make a copy of their own medical records.

7. **Complaints and appeals.** Consumers have the right to a fair and efficient process for resolving differences with their healthcare plans, providers, and facilities.

8. **Consumer responsibilities.** Consumers are encouraged to be more involved in their care and to support a cost-conscious environment. They are expected to share information about their health with the care provider, follow instructions for their treatment, and make arrangements to pay their bills.

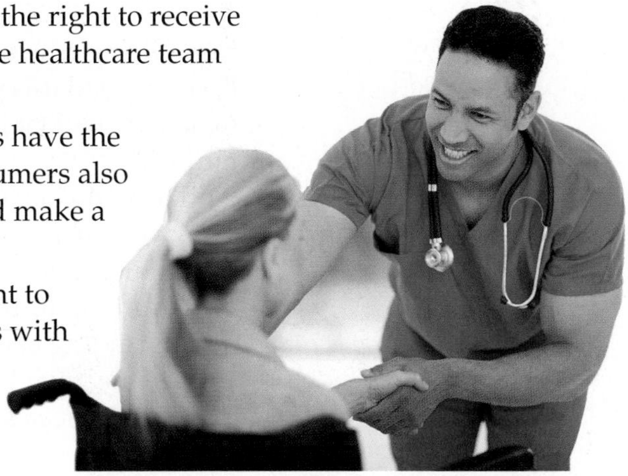

Figure 8.8 Consumers have the right to considerate, respectful care from healthcare workers. What are some simple ways you can show respect for patients?

The Patient Protection and Affordable Care Act (ACA) of 2010 also specifies certain rights for all Americans. These rights tend to focus on health insurance plans, but they can also affect the healthcare that people receive:

1. **Reducing limits on care.** The ACA bans the use of preexisting condition limitations and prevents insurers from denying treatments due to unintentional errors on insurance applications. This blocks health insurance providers from preventing consumers from receiving care. The act also limits insurers' use of annual coverage limits and bans lifetime coverage limits.

2. **Ensuring access to care.** The ACA guarantees that individuals with insurance can choose a healthcare provider from their insurer's network of providers. It also allows women to see an OB-GYN without a referral and allows emergency care without prior insurer approval.

The Older Americans Act initially required every state to have an **ombudsman** (ahm-BUDZ-muhn) program to address complaints and advocate for improvements in the long-term care system. Changes in 2006 authorized the addition of mental health and elder abuse prevention and services staff at the federal level. Funding and services to help promote training, community involvement, and prevention of elder abuse were also expanded.

Informed Consent. Patient rights are the underlying idea of **informed consent**. It relies on healthcare workers giving patients clear descriptions of the following elements of healthcare:

- the patient's condition (the diagnosis)
- the purpose and nature of the treatment
- benefits and risks of the treatment
- possible alternative treatments
- potential risks of not receiving the treatment

informed consent
a patient's choice to accept or reject a procedure after receiving information on available options and possible consequences

Informed consent applies to all medical or surgical procedures, from taking a prescribed medication to undergoing open-heart surgery. Exceptions to this policy include emergency situations, situations in which the patient is incapable of making a decision, and treatment of minors.

The main element of informed consent is receiving a clear decision about treatment from the patient. It is your job to make sure the patient has enough information to make informed decisions. Always explain procedures in terms that the patient can understand. Check his or her understanding and answer questions before you begin. Try asking, "Can you tell me what you are expecting will be done today?" If the patient's response indicates a lack of complete understanding of the procedure or includes incorrect information, explain what is missing or incorrect. Do not perform a procedure if the patient refuses or asks for more information.

Remember that illness affects each patient and his or her family differently (Figure 8.9). Some react better to pain and disease than others. Each patient has his or her own fears and concerns. One patient may be reacting to a negative healthcare experience from the past. Another may be worrying about how her family will manage without her. The family of still another may be stressed about paying his or her medical bills. Treat each person as an individual. Use your listening skills and be sympathetic to patients' needs.

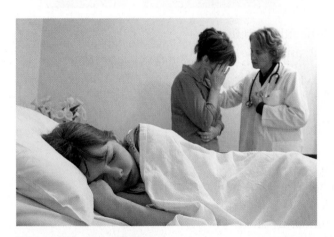

Figure 8.9 The stress of illness affects everyone differently. Some patients may be optimistic and focused on recovery, while others are focused on fears and concerns. What concerns might this family be experiencing?

Privileged Communication. Healthcare providers have a special duty to maintain privacy. This duty goes beyond the rules of confidentiality that restrict the sharing of patient information outside of the care team without patient consent. A patient must feel free to communicate openly with his or her care provider. Therefore, private conversations between a healthcare professional and a patient cannot be disclosed in court. A care provider cannot be required to testify about these conversations, which are known as **privileged communication**. The patient would have to give permission for this information to be shared.

This privilege is granted by state statutes, so the extent of protection may vary from one state to another. Generally, the only exception to this policy is when a patient threatens to harm himself or others and has a plan and means to do it. In all situations that place a person in imminent danger, care providers are obligated to warn authorities and the person who is at risk.

Privacy. An important focus of HIPAA laws is protecting patient privacy. As described in chapter 4, HIPAA restricts the sharing of protected health information with anyone who is not involved in a patient's care. HIPAA allows the patient to control how much information is shared and with whom it is shared. Strict guidelines must be followed to ensure the safety of patient information.

Demonstrating respect for patients' privacy helps them feel free to discuss their health issues openly. In turn, open communication helps care providers make the proper diagnosis, design the best treatment, and ensure the treatment is followed. For instance, a patient with HIV needs to feel comfortable discussing his or her health status with care providers. Patients with cancer need to talk about their views on quality of life and end of life without feeling pressured to receive excess treatment.

Physical privacy is also important to patients during their care. If a patient is in a public area, ask to move him or her to a more private area before discussing specific care issues or beginning personal care. Always knock on the door before entering a patient's room, even if the door is ajar. Be sure to use the privacy curtain before providing care, even when the door is closed. This helps the patient feel protected and prevents unintended exposure of his or her body if someone else enters the room during the procedure (Figure 8.10). Announce yourself and pause before going behind a privacy curtain that is already closed. If visitors are in the patient's room, ask them to step into the waiting room until you are done. Most people don't want others watching when they are receiving personal care.

Different cultures may have different requirements in the area of privacy. For example, Muslims may prefer receiving care from a caregiver of the same gender to follow their rules of modesty with the opposite sex. In addition to being an important patient right, showing concern for your patient's dignity and privacy helps build trust with the patient.

Ethical Dilemmas

We all face ethical **dilemmas** at various points in our lives. These are problems that require us to choose between two conflicting obligations. When you must make a difficult decision, you can use a decision-making process as a guide. First, determine what the problem is and which people are involved or affected. It is important to differentiate between assumptions and facts. Next, explore all of the possible actions, including inaction. What are the effects or potential outcomes of each option? Establish what is most important in this situation. Look at the issue from different points of view. Finally, choose the best action for all those involved.

Ethical decision making has become more difficult as new advances are made in healthcare. New techniques, medications, and technology have extended life and redefined death. Healthcare providers and families are left with difficult decisions that didn't exist a generation ago. Today, healthcare providers must ask what "quality of life" is and how they can preserve or improve it for patients.

Imagine that a child is left paralyzed and in a persistent vegetative state after an accident. How far should healthcare workers go to save that child's life? Suppose a patient has hepatitis, a communicable disease, and doesn't want his or her life partner to know. How far does the right to privacy extend when another person's health may be at risk?

As mentioned in chapter 4, many occupations have professional codes of ethics to set out the standards of conduct expected of members in that profession. One of the most famous codes of ethics is the Hippocratic Oath, which doctors take when they graduate from medical school (Figure 8.11 on the next page). The oath dates back to the time of Hippocrates, an ancient Greek philosopher who is called the "father of medicine." The words have

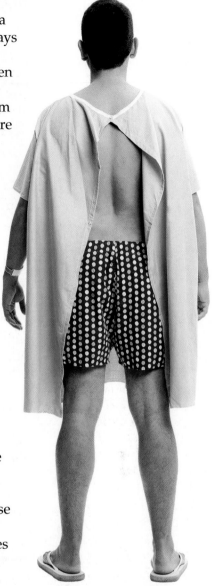

Figure 8.10   Healthcare workers must always preserve the privacy of their patients. If you saw a patient standing in the hallway with a loose hospital gown, how would you handle the situation?

Figure 8.11   These medical students at Wayne State University are swearing the Hippocratic Oath as part of their graduation ceremony. What questions or concerns would you have about swearing a professional oath?

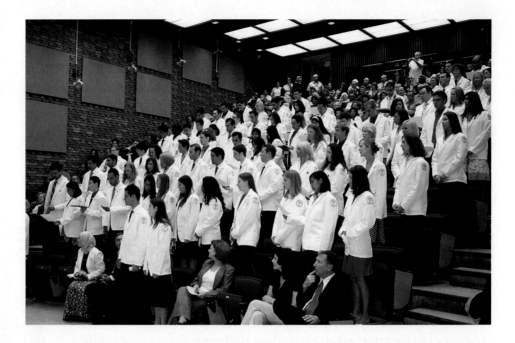

changed many times over the years, reflecting more modern language and avoiding the more controversial ethical topics discussed in the original version.

Many healthcare institutions have **ethics boards** that meet to discuss unusual or controversial cases. These boards advise professionals on ethical dilemmas but do not make final decisions. The opinion of the ethics board can help to clarify ethical issues.

While providing hands-on care, therapeutic workers may observe cases of suspicious injuries or suspected abuse. An emergency medical technician may see that the bleeding wounds she's treating were made by a knife or bullets. An emergency room nurse may smell alcohol on the breath of a car accident victim he is treating. A school nurse may hear stories that suggest a child has been sexually abused. Sharing this information is not a violation of confidentiality. These are incidents and conditions that involve people's safety, so they must be reported.

The Therapeutic Worker: Dyna

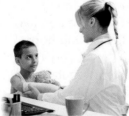

As a physician assistant (PA) in a hospital emergency room, Dyna often places casts on broken bones. As she wrapped one young boy's arm, Dyna was shocked to see round scars that looked like cigarette burns on his arm. The boy's mother said he had poked himself by accident.

Dyna knew this needed to be reported as a possible case of child abuse. But she thought the mother seemed nice, and she could see the woman's close bond with the child. She knew the process of investigating child abuse would probably involve removing the boy from his home until the situation could be investigated. Dyna didn't want to cause the boy further distress. She also knew that abuse victims often know and protect their abusers. What would you do in Dyna's position?

Mandatory reporting laws are written to protect people from abuse. Protecting people from harm is more important than protecting the doctor-patient relationship or the parent-child relationship. Under the federal Child Abuse Prevention and Treatment Act (CAPTA), healthcare workers are required to report suspected physical, sexual, or emotional neglect or abuse to the state's child protective services (CPS). Reportable issues include apparent failure to provide for the basic needs of food, clothing, shelter, and medical care. Rules vary from state to state. It is your responsibility to know the rules at the facility and in the state where you work. Failure to report suspected abuse is typically classified as a misdemeanor. Knowingly making a false report of abuse is also punishable by law. Persons reporting "suspicions of abuse in good faith" cannot be held liable for a report that is unsubstantiated.

mandatory reporting
the legal requirement for certain health issues to be reported to authorities

Alternative Therapies

The use of **complementary and alternative medicine (CAM)** has been increasing in the United States. These practices sometimes fall outside of the system for medical regulation. The National Certification Commission for Acupuncture and Oriental Medicine provides credentialing and licensing standards for some CAM professions in some, but not all, states. Some states regulate chiropractors, osteopaths, and massage therapists. Without a licensing or credentialing system, patients often find it difficult to judge which providers are qualified and which are fraudulent.

Dietary supplements and medical devices are regulated by the Food and Drug Administration or the Public Health Service Act. Biofeedback machines and acupuncture needles are considered medical devices, and their production and use must follow federal law. Herbal supplements, however, are less regulated than medications and are not held to the same rigorous testing and quality control standards (Figure 8.12). Some people argue that this creates unsafe conditions for consumers. Others feel that less expense and regulation in Western medicine would encourage development of more potentially useful therapies.

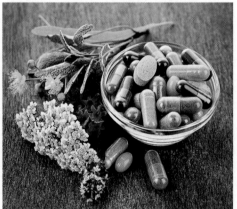

Patients need information to judge which practices are safe or effective, and which are not. Research funded by the National Center for Complementary and Alternative Medicine (NCCAM) aims to increase the amount of reliable information in this area. Keep in mind that being labeled "natural" does not automatically mean that a product is safe. Herbal supplements can have an effect on a person's body as well as on the other medications he or she takes. It is important that patients discuss all alternative treatments and practices with their care provider.

At the same time, doctors need to be sensitive to the cultural beliefs of their patients. Alternative medicine is an important part of cultural practices for some ethnic groups (Figure 8.13 on the next page). Fear and lack of understanding are common barriers to providing culturally sensitive care. Some patients feel their alternative healthcare practices are seen as inferior and that mainstream medicine is forced upon them. This cultural bias weakens the trust of the patient and the patient's cultural community in healthcare providers. If a doctor forces blood products on

Figure 8.12   A lack of regulation on herbal supplements and alternative treatments means a patient needs to communicate with his or her healthcare provider about their use and what is safe or effective.

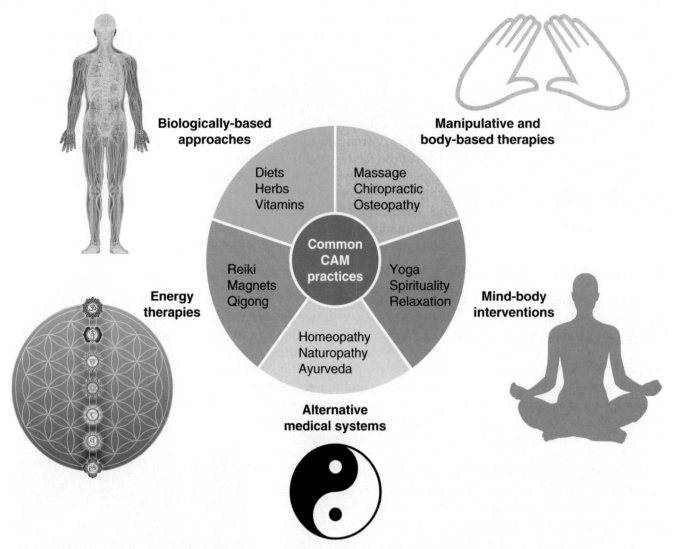

Biologically-based approaches

Manipulative and body-based therapies

Diets
Herbs
Vitamins

Massage
Chiropractic
Osteopathy

Common CAM practices

Reiki
Magnets
Qigong

Yoga
Spirituality
Relaxation

Energy therapies

Mind-body interventions

Homeopathy
Naturopathy
Ayurveda

Alternative medical systems

Figure 8.13   Complementary and alternative medicine (CAM) practices involve concepts different from those in Western medicine. For example, most traditional Chinese medicine practices are based in complementary or opposing forces, as represented by the black-and-white "yin and yang" symbol. Energy therapies are based on different types of energy that can be focused on an area of the body, as represented by the image here.

the sick child of a Jehovah's Witness or breathing machines on an Amish person, others who hold similar beliefs in prayer healing may stay away from the doctor's office altogether.

How do we balance a patient's right to his or her cultural beliefs and a doctor's obligation to preserve life? When should a judge intervene over parents' rights to make decisions about their child? Remember not to impose your own goals and assumptions on patients. Use your listening skills. Consider the whole patient, including differences in gender roles, beliefs about illness, opinions on foods that heal, and the decision of whether or not to show pain. All cultures have something important to teach us.

Another issue concerning CAM is insurance coverage. Some insurers provide coverage for massage therapy and chiropractic manipulations to treat certain conditions. Wellness rebates from insurance companies may cover massage, acupuncture, tai chi, Pilates, or yoga. Even practices that are not covered by insurance must be openly discussed in a healthy doctor-patient relationship.

RECALL YOUR READING

1. Healthcare workers are responsible for operating within their _____ and providing the expected _____.
2. The Patient's Bill of Rights provides patients with _____ in their treatment decisions, _____ of their health information, and the right to a _____ of healthcare providers.
3. Lack of licensing or credentialing makes it difficult to judge if _____ providers are qualified.
4. Therapeutic workers must check for understanding and obtain _____ before beginning a procedure.

Complete the *Map Your Reading* graphic organizer for the section you just read.

Personal and Patient Safety

Many laws are in place to make healthcare safe for both patients and employees. Patient safety is protected by licensure laws, standards of practice, and the patient's bill of rights. Employment laws exist to protect healthcare workers.

Worker Safety

Certain laws are in place to protect the safety of employees. State and federal employment laws define minimum wage and safe working conditions. The Fair Labor Standards Act specifies age requirements for various jobs to help prevent injuries. Although minors are generally able to work at 16 years of age, jobs that are considered **hazardous** may require workers to be 18 years of age or older. For example, healthcare workers who must lift patients, such as home health aides, are at risk of hurting themselves or their patients. Working with physically violent patients in a mental health facility can be dangerous. Both of these situations require workers to be older and have specific training to maintain a safe work and care environment.

Under the Occupational Safety and Health Act (OSHA), employers must provide a work environment free from recognized hazards. Inspectors look for cleanliness, attention to safety procedures, and safety of the physical environment in a workplace. Health codes and fire codes must be obeyed. Employees should be trained in ways to prevent the spread of infection and ways to avoid injury (Figure 8.14). The Occupational Health and Safety Administration (OSHA), the federal agency responsible for workplace safety, has specific guidelines for preventing the transmission of bloodborne pathogens and handling hazardous materials. Employees who report unsafe conditions are also protected by law from employer retaliation. This means they cannot be disciplined by their employer for making the report.

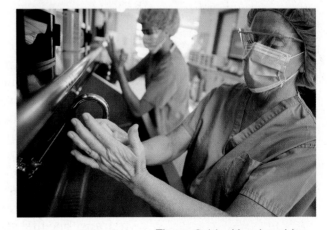

Figure 8.14   Handwashing is a simple but important way to prevent the spread of infection. When are healthcare workers required to wash their hands?

Nurse aides, orderlies, and attendants have the third highest injury rate among American healthcare workers, with more than 40,000 cases reported each year. Back strain is the most common type of injury in healthcare. Needlesticks are a concern but account for less than 1 percent of the healthcare injuries reported to OSHA.

Healthcare workers involved in direct patient care may be required to work mandatory overtime. This extends workers' shifts beyond an eight-hour day, usually when there is a staffing emergency. Mandatory overtime ensures that patients are not abandoned, but it creates problems for both workers and employers. Longer shifts may mean that workers are not getting enough sleep. Workers who are sleep deprived have twice the risk of being injured on the job as those who are well rested. Employees who work long hours are also more likely to make errors in judgment, have difficulty concentrating, and work at a slower pace.

Workplace Violence. Threats of physical violence, harassment, and intimidation are a major concern for both employers and employees. **Workplace violence** may come from patients, their families, or coworkers. Healthcare and social services workers who are in direct contact with the public or work in high-crime areas are at the greatest risk for workplace violence.

workplace violence
acts of verbal abuse, threats, physical assault, or homicide that occur at work

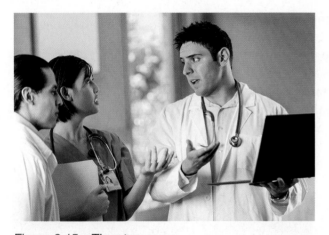

Figure 8.15   The stress involved in a healthcare job may cause tempers to flare among coworkers. How can you avoid conflicts with fellow healthcare workers?

Working with volatile or unstable people increases workers' chances of being injured on the job. Patients and family members dealing with difficult choices and bad news are more likely to become emotional. This can be difficult for hands-on care providers, who are likely to be the bearers of bad news. Approximately ¼ of all healthcare worker injuries are caused by patients. Healthcare workers also face great stress in their jobs and may react inappropriately toward their peers (Figure 8.15).

Healthcare workers are trained to recognize signs of abuse in their patients but often fail to look out for their own needs. You may be embarrassed or feel uncomfortable reporting a coworker who threatens or harasses you. This is a situation in which a strong administration is important. A **zero-tolerance policy** sends a message to all employees that no one will be allowed to harass or intimidate another employee, no matter what their rank in the organization. When a patient or coworker, even a person in a position of power, treats others inappropriately, his or her behavior should be corrected.

Many incidents can be avoided by creating a prevention program that includes an evaluation process, preventive measures, and employee training. The first step is for organizations to assess the environment in which their workers practice and identify where risks of violence occur. For example, emergency room staff may be at risk when treating wounded gang members or women with abusive spouses. Home health aides may be called upon to visit clients in violent neighborhoods or abusive households.

Next, employers need to notify workers of potential hazards and train them to recognize and report workplace violence. Workers need to learn how to evaluate situations, what preventive measures they can take to protect themselves, how to respond to violent situations, and how and when to ask for help. For instance, if a floor nurse is preparing to give an injection to a patient who is known to react violently to anyone touching him, hospital protocol may require the nurse to have one or two orderlies or other staff members with her when she approaches the patient. The system for reporting workplace violence needs to be easy and provide for response at any time of day.

Constantly providing direct care to patients—especially those in difficult situations such as hospice, trauma units, and children's cancer wards—can be very stressful (Figure 8.16). Workers may experience discrimination or bias from coworkers based on age, gender, race, religion, or other factors. Personal problems can add to on-the-job worries and cause some workers to lash out at both patients and colleagues. Most organizations provide free employee assistance programs to help with problems that are causing emotional distress. Many organizations also suggest or require that staff receive training in cultural sensitivity and sexual harassment issues. Simply stated, if a person finds your behavior offensive and asks you to stop, then you should stop. All healthcare workers and patients should be treated with respect.

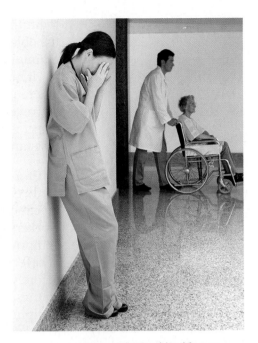

Figure 8.16   Healthcare workers may witness traumatic events and experience secondhand stress from their patients. How can you reduce work-related stress?

Preventing Injury with Good Body Mechanics. Healthcare workers are more prone to injury than workers in many other careers. Approximately 5 in every 100 healthcare workers are injured on the job each year. Forty percent of those injuries are due to strains and sprains. Back, shoulder, or neck injuries can result from improperly lifting and transferring patients. Standing in an incorrect position and carrying an off-balance load can cause workers to fall. The number of workplace injuries can be reduced by following some basic rules for body mechanics and lifting.

Body mechanics describe the correct positions for muscles and joints that allow healthcare workers to complete tasks safely and efficiently, without unnecessary strain or injury. Using good body mechanics is important to prevent injury to both you and your patient. Muscles are most efficient and avoid unnecessary strain when they are used properly. Paying attention to proper body mechanics reduces fatigue and makes the job of lifting, pulling, or pushing safer and easier.

Good **posture** is an important part of body mechanics. When lifting, you should keep your head, back, and hips in a straight line. Tighten your abdominal muscles to protect your back. Creating a broad base of support gives you the most stability, so place your feet shoulder-width apart. Put one foot slightly in front of the other to increase your balance. Point your feet in the direction you are about to move. If you need to turn, pivot on the balls of your feet. Turn your whole body rather than just twisting at the waist; this will protect the small muscles in your back.

When lifting heavy objects, use your leg muscles to lift the weight rather than relying on your back muscles. Your legs are stronger than your back. To make use of your leg muscles, bend at the knees and hips

body mechanics
specific positions for muscles and joints that help a person avoid injury during a physical task

to lift the object rather than reaching down by curling your spine. Bring the object close to your body before lifting, and keep your chin up to help maintain a straight back (Figure 8.17).

It may be easier to push a heavy object instead of lifting it. This allows you to use the weight of your entire body. Avoid pulling a heavy object to prevent injury to your wrist, arm, or shoulder muscles and joints. If an object is too heavy to lift or push by yourself, get help. You may need the assistance of coworkers or a lift device.

Lifting Patients with Lift Equipment. The task of lifting patients can be made easier and safer with the use of lift equipment, as long as proper precautions are observed. Proper use of equipment can protect both workers and patients from injury. It is important to be trained on new equipment before you use it. Each piece of equipment has its own set of **safety precautions**. These contain information you need to know before you begin using the equipment. You can refresh your memory on these precautions by reading the operating instructions found on the equipment labels or in the manual (Figure 8.18). If you are unsure of how to use a piece of equipment, stop and ask for help. Using equipment the wrong way can be very dangerous.

Inspect all equipment before each session. Check for frayed cords or straps. Make sure the equipment is functioning properly. Remove damaged or malfunctioning equipment, if possible, or report it immediately. If protective pads are used for your procedure, be sure they are in place before beginning. If additional staff are needed to safely use the equipment, be sure they are available and prepared before starting a procedure.

When using equipment to lift a patient, you should plan out where you are going, how the equipment will fit, and what each person's role in the lift procedure is. You may need to clear a path for the lift. Will you be able to maneuver in the space available? If you are transferring the patient from a bed to a chair, is the chair prepared? Does each person involved understand what is expected of him or her?

Providing instructions for your patient is one of the most important steps in safe equipment use. Let the patient know what will happen to him or her and ask for cooperation during the procedure. Communicate clearly with your coworkers as well. Be sure that each person knows

safety precautions
information about the safe operation of a piece of equipment, which is usually found in the instruction manual or on equipment labels

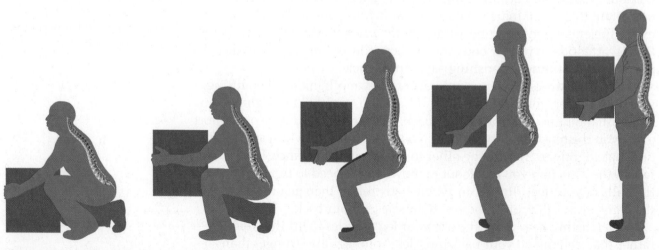

Figure 8.17   When lifting heavy objects, always bend at the knees and keep your chin up to maintain a straight back.

his or her role. Agree on a signal, such as "One, two, three, lift," so that everyone's actions are coordinated. Remember that an informed team is able to anticipate needs and avoid problems.

Perform a **safety check** as part of your ending procedures. Be sure to remove lift equipment and return furniture to its place before you leave a patient's room. Can the patient reach everything he or she may need while avoiding unnecessary movements that may cause pain or injury?

safety check
the process of looking for and removing potential hazards that could cause injury or harm

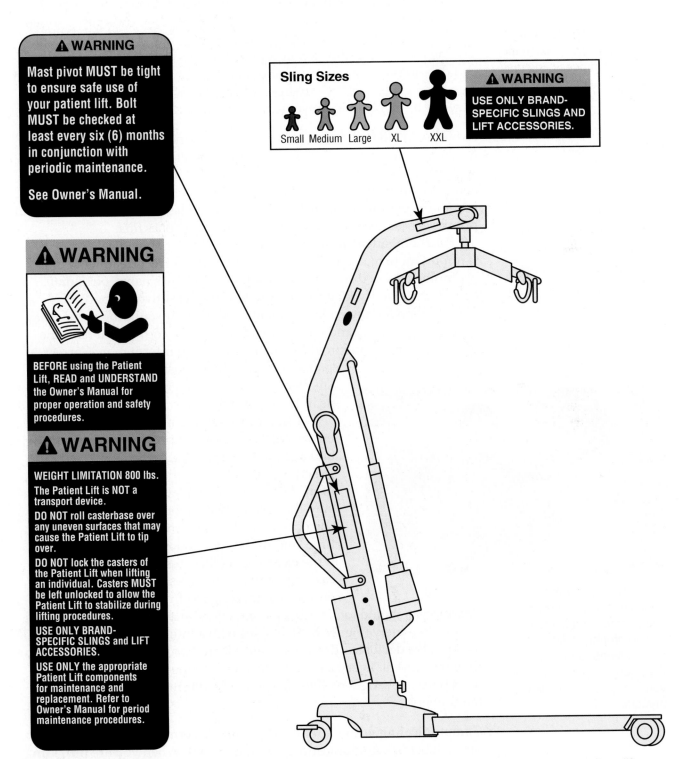

⚠ WARNING

Mast pivot MUST be tight to ensure safe use of your patient lift. Bolt MUST be checked at least every six (6) months in conjunction with periodic maintenance.

See Owner's Manual.

⚠ WARNING

BEFORE using the Patient Lift, READ and UNDERSTAND the Owner's Manual for proper operation and safety procedures.

⚠ WARNING

WEIGHT LIMITATION 800 lbs.
The Patient Lift is NOT a transport device.

DO NOT roll casterbase over any uneven surfaces that may cause the Patient Lift to tip over.

DO NOT lock the casters of the Patient Lift when lifting an individual. Casters MUST be left unlocked to allow the Patient Lift to stabilize during lifting procedures.

USE ONLY BRAND-SPECIFIC SLINGS and LIFT ACCESSORIES.

USE ONLY the appropriate Patient Lift components for maintenance and replacement. Refer to Owner's Manual for period maintenance procedures.

Sling Sizes

Small   Medium   Large   XL   XXL

⚠ WARNING

USE ONLY BRAND-SPECIFIC SLINGS AND LIFT ACCESSORIES.

Figure 8.18   Healthcare workers must follow the operating instructions on equipment such as this patient lift.

Is the call button within reach? Is the bed in the lowest position? Can the patient reach a cane, crutches, or walker if needed?

Ensuring Patient Safety

Every healthcare worker must take an active role in creating a safe healthcare system. The healthcare system is so complex that errors can happen anywhere. **Medical errors** cost billions of dollars, drive up the price of malpractice insurance for healthcare workers, and cause serious problems for patients and their families. Errors may occur when people use the wrong procedures or equipment. Errors can also be the result of bad decisions or miscommunication. Because of their role in direct patient care, therapeutic workers are more likely than workers in other pathways to see or be involved in preventable errors that cause patients harm.

medical errors
preventable mistakes that can occur at any point in the healthcare process and may potentially cause harm to the patient

Avoiding Misidentification. When you are assigned a list of patients to care for during your shift, you are required to be familiar with their needs. To do so, you can check patient charts, care orders, and handoff reports to find out about your patients before coming to the floor. At the beginning of your shift, introduce yourself to each patient and ask about his or her needs. You should prioritize these needs and care for the most urgent ones first.

Patient **misidentification** is a significant cause of medical errors. It is important to match the correct patient to the correct treatment before beginning a procedure. You can ask for the patient's name, birth date, or address to verify identity. Be sure to use at least two methods of identification for any patient. Patients with similar sounding names may have a "name alert" and require extra caution. Be certain you have the correct patient before providing care or charting information. Correct patient identification is just as important in smaller healthcare settings, like a dentist's office, as in large hospitals.

Misidentification can also lead to medication errors. Mistakes made in prescribing, dispensing, and administering medications can all result in serious harm to the patient. Every member of the healthcare team plays a role in making sure the correct medications are given to the correct patient, by the correct route, at the correct time, and in the correct dosage. Doctors must write clear and legible prescriptions, which is easier now that many prescriptions are written on computers using electronic signatures.

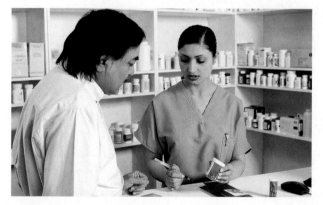

Figure 8.19 Pharmacists educate their patients on safety precautions and how to properly take their prescriptions. Can you recall the pharmacist instructions you received for your last prescription?

Pharmacists should look for drug interactions and educate the patient on medication safety (Figure 8.19). Nurses who administer medications need to check the doctor's order, the patient's identity, and the medication each time they give it. Everyone who interacts with the patient is responsible for reporting changes or side effects that result from treatments and medications.

Communicating with Patients. Some medical errors can be avoided through better communication with the patient. When you are providing care, listen to your patients. Getting a complete medical history from them can help prevent misdiagnosis. Patients can often tell you what is wrong and what they need. They may also tell you what they don't need or want. They do not always communicate these messages verbally, so healthcare workers must be aware of nonverbal signals from patients. For example, what do clenched fists, gritted teeth, and favoring one leg over the other indicate? Does a patient claim to have no pain but flinch every time you touch him or her? It is your job to look for subtle signs of discomfort and depression. Missing important symptoms can lead to misdiagnosis and improper treatment.

Patients can help to reduce adverse, or *harmful*, reactions by telling you what medications they currently take and which cause allergic reactions for them. Surgeons avoid cutting into the wrong body part by having patients mark the correct location themselves. Letting a patient know what you are doing will allow him or her to ask questions and participate more effectively in the care they are receiving. Patient communication and involvement in treatment is an important part of creating a safer healthcare system.

Promoting Health Literacy. In a therapeutic health career, part of your role is to educate your patients about their treatment. Physical therapists need to teach patients how to do recommended exercises (Figure 8.20). Pharmacists explain side effects to watch for and make sure the customer knows how to take medication. Nurses may have to teach patients how to change a wound's dressing after being discharged from the hospital. This education plays a big role in the patient's well-being.

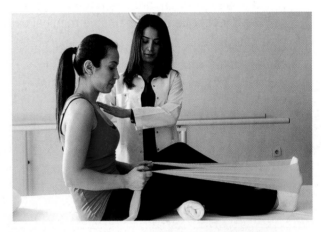

As explained in chapter 3, health literacy is how well people are able to find, understand, and use basic health information and services to make good decisions about their care. Health literacy is affected by a person's education, age, background knowledge, culture, and access to resources. Older adults, minorities, people with limited English skills, and people with less than a college education are most likely to have low health literacy skills. For instance, a person who speaks English as a second language may not understand your directions for taking medication. Poor eyesight or arthritis may keep someone from reading brochures about an upcoming surgery. It is your job to provide health information in a way that your patient can understand.

Figure 8.20 Physical therapists can help improve patients' health literacy by teaching them how to do recommended exercises. How can physical therapists check for understanding?

RECALL YOUR READING

1. Employees are protected from unsafe work conditions by a federal agency known as _____.
2. Workplace _____, such as harassment and physical injuries, can be caused by either patients or coworkers.
3. Good _____ use proper positioning to protect the muscles.
4. _____ with your patient prevents errors such as _____ and increases patient satisfaction and cooperation by involving them in their care.
5. Health _____ varies depending on factors such as age, education, culture, and background knowledge.

Complete the
Map Your Reading
graphic organizer for the
section you just read.

SUMMARY

 Assess your understanding with chapter tests

- An organizational chart shows the vertical and horizontal relationships between people in an organization.

- The lines of authority in an organizational chart show who is in charge.

- Care teams may be interdisciplinary, with staff from different departments sharing the goal of wellness for the patient.

- Care teams communicate about changes in a patient's condition through charting and handoff care reports.

- State and federal laws protect patients and healthcare employees. Licensure laws, standards of practice, and the patient's bill of rights protect patients from unsafe medical care.

- Some healthcare careers require a license or certificate, which are regulated by state and federal laws or issued by professional organizations.

- A healthcare worker is legally liable for care provided and should always take care to remain within his or her scope of practice.

- Showing respect for a patient's rights encourages patients to participate in their care.

- Most patient information is privileged, but some types of patient information must be reported by law in certain situations.

- Professional codes of ethics set the standards of conduct expected of healthcare workers.

- Complementary and alternative medicine is less regulated than western medical practices, which makes it difficult to judge which providers are well qualified and which practices are effective.

- Employment laws protect employees from unsafe work conditions.

- Workplace violence is more common in high-stress jobs, such as healthcare.

- Using good body mechanics can help healthcare workers avoid injuries.

- Healthcare workers should always identify patients before beginning treatment, verify medications before giving them, listen to their patients, and check for understanding.

MAXIMIZE YOUR PROFESSIONAL VOCABULARY

 Build vocabulary with e-flash cards, games, and audio glossary

Listed below are the essential, yellow-highlighted terms and the additional professional vocabulary that you encountered in this chapter. Complete the activities that follow the list to make all of these terms part of your everyday professional vocabulary.

abuse	hazardous	Omnibus Budget Reconciliation Act (OBRA)
assault	hierarchy	
battery	informed consent	organizational chart
body mechanics	involuntary seclusion	posture
certification	liable	privileged communication
chain of command	licensure	registry
complementary and alternative medicine (CAM)	lines of authority	regulate
continuing education units (CEUs)	malpractice	safety check
	mandatory reporting	safety precautions
dilemma	medical errors	scope of practice
ethics board	misidentification	standard of care
false imprisonment	negligence	workplace violence
handoff care report	ombudsman	zero-tolerance policy

VOCABULARY DEVELOPMENT

Matching. Match each essential term from this chapter with the correct definition below by writing the letter of the description next to the number of the essential term on a separate sheet of paper.

1. body mechanics
2. informed consent
3. malpractice
4. mandatory reporting
5. medical errors
6. organizational chart
7. safety check
8. safety precautions
9. scope of practice
10. standard of care
11. workplace violence

a. the process of looking for and removing potential hazards that could cause injury or harm

b. term for actions that violate a professional's scope of practice or standard of care and result in injury to a patient that could reasonably have been expected

c. a patient's choice to accept or reject a procedure after receiving information on available options and possible consequences

d. a diagram that shows how departments in an organization are related to one another

e. acts of verbal abuse, threats, physical assault, or homicide that occur at work

f. specific positions for muscles and joints that help a person avoid injury during a physical task

g. the legal requirement for certain health issues to be reported to authorities

h. the level of service that a healthcare professional is expected to provide to a patient based on that professional's position and the patient's condition

i. tasks that an employee is legally allowed to perform based on their training and certification

j. information about the safe operation of a piece of equipment, which is usually found in the instruction manual or on equipment labels

k. preventable mistakes that can occur at any point in the healthcare process and may potentially cause harm to the patient

12. **Scrambled Vocab Terms.** Unscramble the following professional terms from the chapter. Then use them appropriately in a new sentence to show your understanding.
    a. cidmlea rsorer
    b. tfeays nitpecauosr
    c. dyob csmaechin
    d. taogzianlrioan rathc
    e. medfirno tensnoc
    f. daytaonmr gneprtior
    g. kpcaoelwr nceoilve

13. **Remembering Terms.** Select the vocabulary words from this chapter that you are least likely to remember. Without using the term itself, develop a simple two- to five-word phrase or sentence to help you remember the term. For example, "hazardous—a dangerous situation or item," or "abuse—inappropriate, hurtful treatment to someone by another."

REFLECT ON YOUR READING

14. Review the story about Jai Vang at the beginning of the chapter. Use your notes from the *Map Your Reading* activity to identify what should have been done differently to prevent the liability, ethical, organizational, and safety errors made in this situation. Try to use your new professional vocabulary as you support your points.

BUILD CORE SKILLS

15. **Problem Solving.** Where would you place the following information on a handoff care report? Prepare an IDEAL chart and insert the following information into the correct category:

    • potential for redness to occur at site of injection

- ran a low-grade fever of 101°F last evening at 3:00 a.m.
- 12/15/1978
- Dr. Smith
- feeling lethargic with cold extremities within the last 12 hours
- Martin Olsen
- What should happen if the fever spikes higher? What medications is Martin allergic to?
- #6945

Which of the IDEAL categories is missing in the information presented here?

16. **Critical Thinking.** What is the difference between an interdisciplinary team and a primary care team? What is the value for the patient and healthcare workers to have each of these teams in place? What situations would warrant the addition of an interdisciplinary team? What is the common goal for all involved?

17. **Writing.** Write out the healthcare credential that corresponds to each of the following abbreviations. Refer to Figure 8.4.

OD	DO
PA-C	CRNA
WHCNP	DC
DPM	DMD

18. **Writing.** Write the corresponding abbreviation for each of the following therapeutic workers. Refer to Figure 8.4.

Pediatric Nurse Practitioner

Registered Dietitian

Master of Science–Nursing

Certified Nurse Midwife

Emergency Medical Technician

Certified Occupational Therapy Assistant

19. **Critical Thinking.** Review the ethical dilemmas presented near the bottom of page 273. Choose one and discuss both sides of the issue. Who are the people affected by this dilemma? What are the possible consequences for each of these people? If you sat on the board of ethics for this case, what recommendations would you make?

20. **Critical Thinking.** Use a real world example to explain your understanding of how the standard of care relates to malpractice and negligence.

21. **Reading.** Review the section in this chapter that covers patient rights. Why is it so important that healthcare professionals understand and honor patient rights?

22. **Writing.** Using information from the section on patient rights, write a five-sentence paragraph demonstrating your understanding of patient rights. Use terms and concepts from the chapter to demonstrate your understanding.

23. **Problem Solving.** What problems are solved or prevented by the HIPAA laws? What steps would you take to ensure a patient's privacy while providing care with visitors in the room? How would you handle the situation?

24. **Writing.** Review the scenario on page 274, which features Dyna, the therapeutic worker. Would you do what is considered safe and ethical in her situation? Explain your answer.

25. **Critical Thinking.** Do some research on the use of complementary and alternative medicine (CAM). Then write a two-paragraph essay on two of the following questions: How or why do these practices sometimes fall outside the medical regulation system? How do herbal supplements and medications differ in terms of regulation? How does CAM enter into healthcare for certain patients? Why should insurance questions and certain treatments be discussed between the doctor and the patient? What guidelines need to be considered during discussions related to CAM?

26. **Speaking and Listening.** Why do medical personnel ask the same questions over and over? Why is communicating with patients so important? Act out a scenario with a partner in which one student is the healthcare worker and the other is the patient. The student acting as the healthcare worker should not listen to what the patient is saying. When the scenario has finished, imagine what problems could arise as a result of the healthcare worker not listening to the patient's needs and requests.

27. **Math.** A study of 780 Medicare patients discharged from hospitals in October 2008 revealed the following statistics related to medical errors:

- 1.5% of these patients died due to medical error.
- 14.3% experienced permanent medical harm.
- 14.3% suffered temporary harm that was caught and reversed.

Using these statistics, answer the following questions. How many patients died? How many experienced permanent harm? Now put these statistics in perspective. What is the ratio of your school population to this group of Medicare patients? If your school were that group of patients, how many students in your school would die and how many would be personally affected by medical errors?

ACTIVATE YOUR LEARNING

28. Mario is a patient of yours who has come in with chest pains, difficulty breathing, and pain down his left arm. Considering what you learned in this chapter about informed consent, what are you obligated to tell Mario?

29. Charles works in a residential care facility as a COTA. He was asked to present a brief demonstration on proper body mechanics for lifting and transporting patients. What are the key points that Charles needs to make and demonstrate for the safety of both healthcare workers and patients? What are the legal and practical advantages to knowing proper body mechanics on the job for employees and patients? What constitutes good posture and how is it a vital aspect of body mechanics? Create a basic outline or a PowerPoint presentation that Charles could use with his demonstration.

30. Contact a local healthcare facility. Ask for a copy of the professional code of ethics given to their employees. Which items did you expect to see in this code? Which items were new or different from what you expected? Compare your findings with classmates who found codes from different healthcare facilities.

THINK AND ACT LIKE A HEALTHCARE WORKER

31. Suppose you have been transferring patients in the nursing home from their beds to their wheelchairs. You begin to feel muscle strain in your back and neck. You realize that you have not been using proper body mechanics for transfers. Describe or demonstrate how you can prevent personal injury through good body mechanics.

32. Suppose you work in a hospital as a nursing assistant and have been concerned that a fellow CNA is treating patients inappropriately. The CNA became irritated when an elderly patient forgot where he put his glasses. Handoff reports from this CNA are often missing information, such as the patient's current condition and changes that occurred during his shift. You actually heard him swear at a patient who didn't make it to the bathroom on time. The CNA then left the soiled laundry on the patient's floor. You are concerned for patient treatment and safety. To whom would you report these incidents? Would you worry about retaliation? Why or why not? If the nurse supervisor was a good friend of the CNA in question, to whom would you consider reporting the incidents? How would you resolve these safety and care issues?

GO TO THE SOURCE

33. Use the Internet to find a career site that has information about a health career that you are interested in. Find out what certifications, licensing, CEUs, or additional requirements are needed once you have the initial degree.

34. On the NCCAM website, follow the "Be Informed" link on the left. Find and print a fact sheet that interests you from one of these three categories: *Issues to Consider*, *Consumer Tips*, or *Safety Information*. After reading the information on your fact sheet, share three key ideas with the class.

35. Use the Internet to research an actual healthcare malpractice or negligence suit. What details are provided? What was the claim? Was the case settled in or out of court? Was there monetary compensation? If so, what was the amount? Do you agree or disagree with the results? Why or why not? Considering the context of the situation, do you think the settlement was fair? Why or why not? What might you learn from the case that could help you avoid a malpractice suit in your professional career?

Chapter 9
Academic Knowledge: Body Systems for Support and Movement

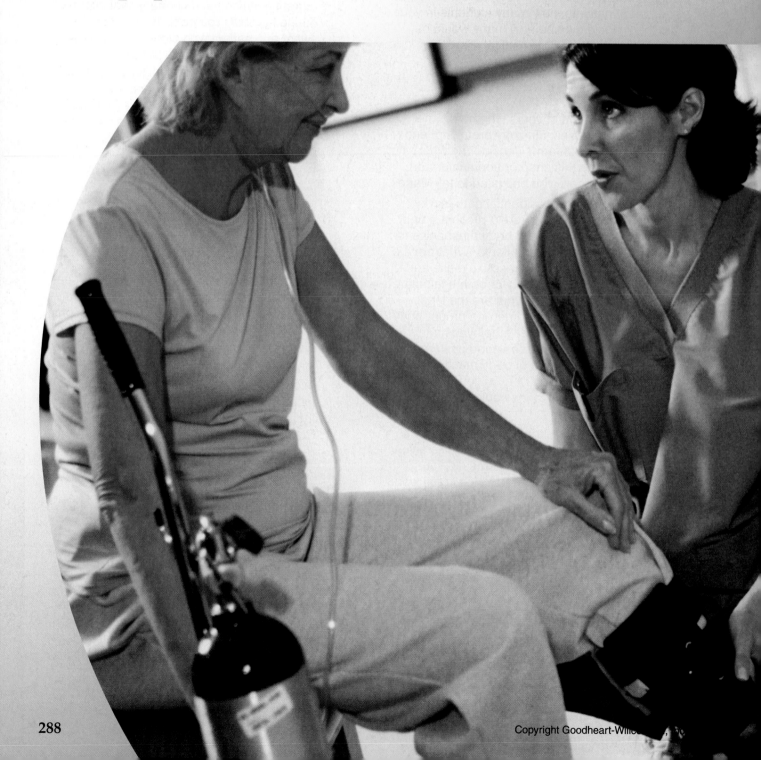

PROFESSIONAL VOCABULARY

E-flash
Cards

You will need to learn the essential terms listed below before you begin your reading. These terms will help you understand the main concepts of the chapter. These terms, which will be highlighted in yellow within the text, will become part of your professional vocabulary.

In addition to these essential terms, you will see bold terms throughout the chapter. The meanings of these terms are explained where the terms first appear. These bold terms, like the essential terms listed here, will also become part of your professional vocabulary and deepen your understanding of the topics presented.

appendicular skeleton term that describes the bones of the arms and legs, including the shoulder and hip bones where they are attached

axial skeleton term that applies to the skull, spine, and rib cage, which rotate around an imaginary center line of the body

cardiac muscle an involuntary, striated muscle tissue located in the walls of the heart

collagen a protein fiber that connects, supports, and gives strength to body tissues such as the skin, muscle tendons, and bone ligaments

dermis the middle layer of the skin, which contains most of the skin's structures

epidermis the thin, outer layer of the skin

hypodermis the innermost layer of the skin, which stores fat

integumentary related to the skin

ligament a tough, fibrous tissue that connects bones to other bones and holds organs in place

skeletal muscle a voluntary, striated muscle that connects to bones and is responsible for movement

smooth muscle an involuntary muscle located in the body's visceral organs and blood vessels; also known as *visceral muscle*

tendon a tough, fibrous tissue that connects muscles to bones

CONNECT WITH YOUR READING

Connecting what you read to what you already know is an important part of learning. As you read this chapter, use sticky notes to mark information in the chapter that makes you think of things you've observed before or already know. When the chapter reminds you of something you've read somewhere else, such as a book or newspaper, label the sticky note *T→T* for *text to text*. If something in the chapter connects to something you've experienced in your own life, label it *T→S* for *text to self*. If information in the chapter sounds like something you've seen or heard about happening somewhere in the world, such as on the news, label it *T→W* for *text to world*. Be prepared to share at least one of your connections with the class.

MAP YOUR READING

Systems for Support and Movement

Collagen adds strength, structure, and elasticity to the skin, bones, and muscles...

INTEGUMENTARY SYSTEM (the skin)

SKELETAL SYSTEM

MUSCULAR SYSTEM

Make a tablet organizer with two sheets of paper using the example shown here. Stack the sheets, keeping the sides even, but move the top sheet up so its bottom edge is ½ inch to 1 inch above the bottom edge of the sheet below it. Holding both sheets of paper, fold both sheets down so the top edge of the top sheet is ½ inch to 1 inch above the bottom edge of the top sheet. Crease both layers and staple at the folded edge. Write the title *Systems for Support and Movement* on the top flap. Label the edges of the flaps below it with the headings *Integumentary System*, *Skeletal System*, and *Muscular System*. On the top flap, summarize what you know about the role of collagen in these systems. As you read, add a picture, the main functions, a related career, and a related disease to each system's page.

Did you know there are entire systems in your body that support you and help you to move? The muscles and bones that make up the frame of your body also help you walk from class to class and even take notes while reading this textbook. Of course, being able to move your hands is not the only technique you need for taking notes in class.

This chapter will give you a step-by-step process for taking effective notes as you read. A better note-taking technique will help you review topics and recall information more easily. You will be able to apply your note-taking skills as you study the rest of the chapter, which describes the major systems that support and move the body. These systems include the skin and its layers; the skeleton and different types of bone; and the various muscles, ligaments, and tendons in the body.

Study Skills for Health Science Students: Note Taking

One of the most challenging aspects of studying the health sciences, especially the therapeutic fields, is the large amount of information you have to learn. You need to find ways to identify the most important material and take notes that will help you remember that material more easily.

Identifying Main Ideas

Because there is a limit to how much new information you can remember, your first task will be selecting what is most important for your purpose. What should you highlight or write in your notes?

When you are taking notes from a textbook or a lecture, you will need to ask yourself what the main idea is, or what you are supposed to be learning. Your teacher may tell you the topic before you begin. You can also find clues to the main idea of a textbook by previewing the headings. Notice topics that occur in both the text and your teacher's lecture. Listen for the ideas your teacher emphasizes or spends the most time on in class. Pay attention to what he or she writes on the board or hands out in class. These are the main ideas to highlight or write in your notes.

As you read, set a purpose for each section of your reading. You can do this by turning the chapter title and each main heading into a question. For example, if a section is titled *Study Skills for Health Science Students*, you should begin by asking yourself, "What are some study skills I will need?" If the subtitle is *Identifying Main Ideas*, you should ask yourself, "How can I identify main ideas?" Ask yourself who, what, when, where, why, or how for each heading before you begin to read. Once you've set the purpose by developing a question, you will be prepared to read and find the answer.

It may be helpful to mark your text as you read (Figure 9.1). Write in the margins of the book (if allowed) or use sticky notes that can be removed. E-books generally have a note-taking feature that allows you to virtually mark up the text. Write down the question you created as you set your purpose for reading. Stop to ask yourself what you already know about this topic. Look ahead at the subtitles in the section to organize your thinking. Check for any pictures or figures that will support the text. As you read, allow yourself to ask more questions about the material and look for connections to things you already know. Make short notes of these questions and connections. Many e-books have a feature that lets you highlight or bookmark text that you find helpful or important.

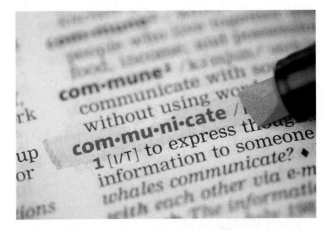

Figure 9.1   If it is allowed, highlighting important terms in your textbook can help you better remember them. Use sticky notes if you are not supposed to write in your book.

All of these strategies are only useful if they point out important information. Focus on information that answers the question you created for the chapter or section. Highlight or circle the main idea or key terms. Use a different color highlighter or underlining for supporting details. If you stayed focused on the most important points, less than one-third of your page should be marked up when you're done.

Methods for Taking Notes

Next, you should organize your information in a meaningful way. There are many styles to use for organizing your thoughts (Figure 9.2 on the next page). Notes taken in an outline format are easy to do if you use the headings and subtitles from the chapter. However, you may end up with a list of details you don't understand if you aren't reading the information as you outline. Stop after reading each section and restate the main idea aloud before adding it to your notes.

The two-column, or *Cornell*, style is good for merging notes from more than one source and reviewing information. In this style, you list the main ideas and supporting details from the lecture or textbook on the right side of a notebook page and use the left side to note prior knowledge, additional information from the lecture, remaining questions, or memory cues. Leave a blank line between topics.

Mind maps, or *web notes*, use color, symbols, arrows, size, and other visual connections to show how ideas are connected. They do not use many words. If a visual image for your mind map doesn't exist, create one! Your mind map should group information into manageable chunks and relate the categories of information to each other.

OUTLINE NOTES

1. Organized
   A. Hierarchy
      i. Big ideas to left
      ii. Smaller ideas indented
         a. dash/bullet
         b. number/letter
   B. Follows textbook format well
      i. Use heading size as clue
      ii. Follows in order
      iii. Details from reading
   C. Teacher may provide outline format for lecture
      i. Copy format from board or overhead
      ii. Add details by listening
         a. Word signals—"there are two ways..."
         b. Examples
      iii. Need to keep up
   D. Easy to share/Get notes from a friend
2. Use
   A. Phrases—not complete sentences
   B. Own words
   C. Key words and facts
3. Leave space between topics
   A. Review in text/lecture/study time and add more info
   B. May come back to ideas again in lecture

Outline Style Notes

Class Notes/Textbook Notes

Name: _____
Class: _____
Period/Block: _____
Date: _____

Topic:

Questions/Main Ideas	Notes

Summary, Reflection, Analysis

Cornell Style Notes

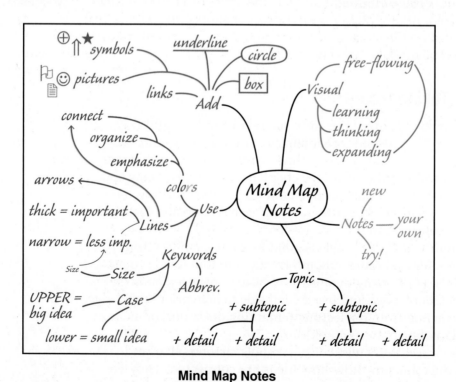

Mind Map Notes

Figure 9.2   Depending on how you learn best, one of these styles of note taking might help you learn and study. Which of these styles would you be most likely to use?

This style of note taking helps to organize information so you can make meaningful connections.

No matter what style of note taking you use, your brain needs review time to process and absorb the new information. If you took notes during a lecture, go back to your textbook and compare the information. If you took notes from your textbook, notice how the teacher's lecture and activities organize and connect the same ideas in a new way. It may be helpful to guess potential test questions from the main headings of your text, then attempt to answer the questions from memory and check against your notes. Put the information into your own words or explain it to someone else to help you sort through it and build your own understanding. Add notes about connections you see between this topic and other classes, your personal life, the news, and other reading material.

Review your notes in small chunks on a regular basis. A few short review sessions are better for learning than one long cram session. Walking into a test (or doing a medical procedure) when you are tired and your brain is overloaded will not lead to long-term memory or success. Review notes or practice with flash cards or a smartphone app for a few minutes several times a day—on the bus, waiting in line, or during TV commercials. The more times you reread the information, the more easily you will recall it later. Put the information in your own words and repeat it aloud before you put the notes away. These short practice sessions will build both understanding and memory.

RECALL YOUR READING

1. Before you begin to take notes, identify the _____ idea.
2. Make _____ as you read your text, either in the margins of your textbook or on sticky notes.
3. Cornell notes, mind maps, and outlining each provide a different way to _____ your notes.
4. _____ chunks of your notes in short, frequent sessions to build understanding and memory.

Complete the *Map Your Reading* graphic organizer for the section you just read.

Body Systems for Support and Movement

The **integumentary** (ihn-tehg-yoo-MEHN-tuh-ree) [*integument* = skin, *ary* = pertaining to], muscular, and skeletal systems work together to support and move the body (Figure 9.3 on the next page). Connective tissue gives these systems support and structure, while muscular tissue provides movement. Muscular tissue uses connective tissue to attach to both skin and bones.

Most types of connective tissue contain **collagen** (KAH-luh-jehn) [*colla* = glue, *gen* = origin, formation, producing] fibers to add strength. Collagen is found in the skin and hair of the integumentary system, tendons and muscle coverings of the muscular system, and bones and ligaments of the skeletal system. Collagen is the "glue" that keeps the skin firm, muscles flexible, and bones strong.

integumentary
related to the skin

collagen
a protein fiber that connects, supports, and gives strength to body tissues such as the skin, muscle tendons, and bone ligaments

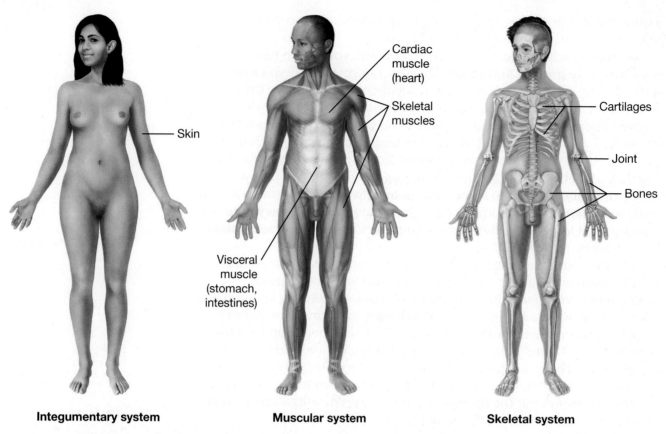

Skin

Cardiac muscle (heart)

Skeletal muscles

Visceral muscle (stomach, intestines)

Cartilages

Joint

Bones

Integumentary system

Muscular system

Skeletal system

Figure 9.3   Support and movement are provided by the integumentary, muscular, and skeletal systems. How is collagen important to each of these systems?

Vitamin C is very important for the production of collagen. Sailors used to develop a disease called *scurvy* because they didn't have access to fresh fruits and vegetables—a good source of vitamin C—on long voyages. Sailors with scurvy experienced bleeding gums, weakness, bone pain, and tooth loss. Their bodies were not able to build the collagen needed for healthy skin, muscles, and bones because they didn't have the correct nutrients. In the 1700s, James Lind proved that citrus fruits, such as oranges and limes, were an effective treatment for scurvy.

Different types of collagen serve different purposes. In tendons and muscle coverings, collagen fibers are lined up to provide strength for muscles pulling in one direction. In the skin and bones, collagen fibers run in different directions; they are not organized. This gives the body's structures extra protection.

The Integumentary System

If you have an interest in diseases and disorders of the skin, you might want to become a dermatologist [*dermat* = skin, *ologist* = specialist in the study of]. To do so, you must earn a medical degree, then complete another year of medical or surgical internship and three years of residency in dermatology. Once you've finished this training, you may decide to specialize in immune disorders, laser medicine, cosmetic surgery, or diseases of the skin. Dermatology appeals to people who are both social and investigative but who want work that provides independence and a sense of accomplishment.

Many other healthcare workers also observe the skin, hair, and nails for early signs of serious medical conditions. For instance, emergency medical technicians look for color changes in the nails and skin that show a problem with breathing or blood flow. Hematologists (hee-muh-TAH-luh-jihsts) know that unusual bruises on the skin can mean a problem with the body's ability to stop bleeding. Very dry skin or excess sweating could be reasons to consult an endocrinologist (ehn-doh-krih-NAH-luh-jihst) about a hormone imbalance. A rash can indicate the need to see an allergist. Pathologists [*path* = disease] know that hair loss may result from both hereditary conditions and poisoning. Any change in the condition of the skin, hair, or nails could be important. Healthcare professionals must understand what is normal for skin structures so they can recognize an abnormal change.

The integumentary system, or *skin*, forms the outside surface of the body. Skin protects and supports the bones, muscles, and internal organs beneath its surface. The skin works with other body systems to sense touch and maintain body temperature. It also plays a role in producing and storing some nutrients and getting rid of body waste. Compare the siding on a house to the skin covering your body. What do you think they have in common?

The skin has three layers—the epidermis, dermis, and hypodermis (Figure 9.4). The **epidermis** (eh-puh-DER-muhs) [*epi* = upon, *derm* = skin, *is* = pertaining to] is the thin, outer layer that is mostly made up of dead

epidermis
the thin, outer layer of the skin

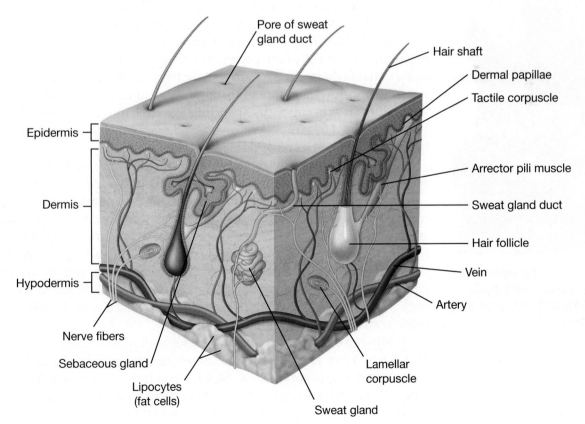

Figure 9.4   The epidermis is the outermost layer of skin, followed by the dermis and hypodermis. Which layer contains most of the skin's structures?

Label Art

dermis
the middle layer of the skin, which contains most of the skin's structures

hypodermis
the innermost layer of the skin, which stores fat

skin cells. The **dermis** lies below the epidermis and contains the skin's sensory organs, blood vessels, hair follicles, oil glands, and sweat glands. The **hypodermis** (hI-puh-DER-muhs) [*hypo* = below] lies beneath the dermis and contains a layer of fat and connective tissue that attaches the skin to the muscle tissue and provides padding for the structures underneath. Each layer of the skin has a different role in covering and protecting the body.

The Epidermis

The epidermis is the thin, outer layer of the skin. New skin cells are constantly being pushed up to the surface of the skin. This layer contains no blood vessels, so as the cells move away from their blood supply, they become dehydrated [*de* = lack of, *hydr* = water, *ate* = having]. As the cells dry out, their cytoplasm changes to keratin (KAIR-uh-tihn), a tough, orange-colored protein. This dried outer layer of keratin-filled skin cells makes it difficult for bacteria to get through the skin and holds in moisture to prevent dehydration of the body.

Skin, hair, and eye colors normally vary from very light to very dark (Figure 9.5). Albinism is a genetic condition that prevents the skin from making its dark **pigment**, or *color*. As a result, the skin of a person with albinism is fair, the hair is whitish-blonde, and the eyes appear pale blue to pink. Skin, hair, and eye color depend on how much pigment is in the underlying tissue.

Melanin (MEH-luh-nihn) [*melan* = black, *in* = within] is the brownish-black pigment produced by melanocytes (MUH-la-nuh-sItz), which are special cells in the epidermis. When your skin is exposed to ultraviolet radiation, these cells make more melanin. Think of a tan as a big melanin umbrella that comes out to protect the DNA in your skin cells from the sun's radiation. A mole is a clump of melanocyte pigment cells that can become cancerous and spread through the skin layers. You can protect yourself from skin cancer by spending less time in the sun between 10:00 a.m. and 4:00 p.m., covering up, and reapplying sunscreen often. A tan or sunburn are signs of damage to your skin.

Skin cancer can be detected with regular skin checks. You can remember the signs of skin cancer with the acronym *ABCDE* (Figure 9.6).

The most deadly skin cancer is malignant melanoma (muh-LIHG-nuhnt meh-luh-NOH-muh). It usually appears dark and asymmetrical and grows rapidly. The fact that it spreads easily makes it very dangerous. Basal cell carcinoma (BAY-suhl sehl kahr-sih-NOH-muh) is the most common type of skin cancer. It typically appears as a raised bump with an indentation in the center and it is most often found on the face or neck. If you have a suspicious skin growth that fits any of the ABCDE symptoms, see a dermatologist.

Warts can also form lumps on the skin, but most are not cancerous. They result from an infection that causes an overgrowth of cells in the epidermis. Cryosurgery (krI-oh-SER-jeh-ree) [*cryo* = cold] uses freezing temperatures to destroy warts, moles, and other diseased tissues.

Dead cells are constantly being scraped off the skin's surface, and they make up the majority of our household dust. When dead skin cells fall from the scalp in clumps, we call them *dandruff*. An abrasion (uh-BRAY-zhuhn) is

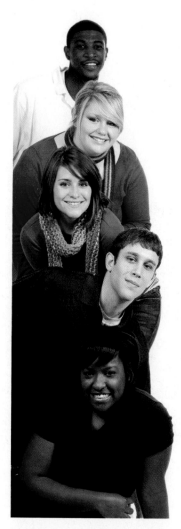

Figure 9.5 The amount of melanin produced by your skin cells determines your skin color.

a scrape on the skin's surface, and dermabrasion (der-muh-BRAY-zhuhn) is the process of scraping off the top layers of the skin. Dermabrasion is used to remove superficial scars, wrinkles, hair, or unwanted tattoos from the epidermis. An abrasion of the epidermal layer will heal well with no scar, but a laceration (la-suh-RAY-shuhn), or *cut*, into the layers below is more serious and will usually cause scarring.

Notice that skin characteristics vary on different areas of the body. Skin cells can specialize in absorption, protection, or secretion. The ability to absorb chemicals through thin areas of the skin makes certain medications deliverable through a patch instead of a pill. The medication in the patch, such as nicotine to help you stop smoking, can be absorbed transdermally, or *through the skin*. Skin on the soles of the feet lacks hair and forms thick calluses to cushion the bones as you walk. Skin on the

Figure 9.6 Normal and Cancerous Skin Growths

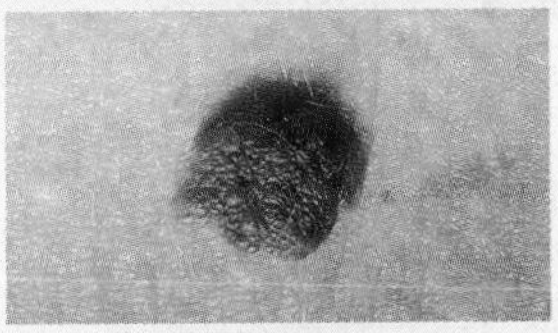	Normal mole

Cancerous Skin Growth	Sign	Characteristic
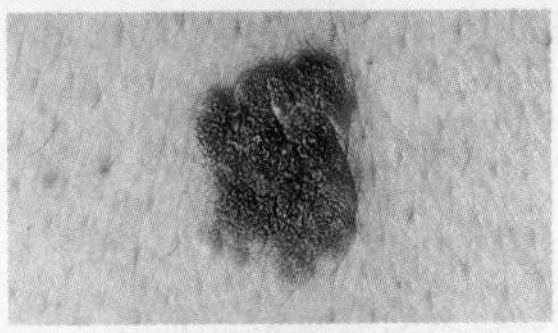	**A**symmetry	If you draw a line down the center of the marking, the two sides are different shapes.
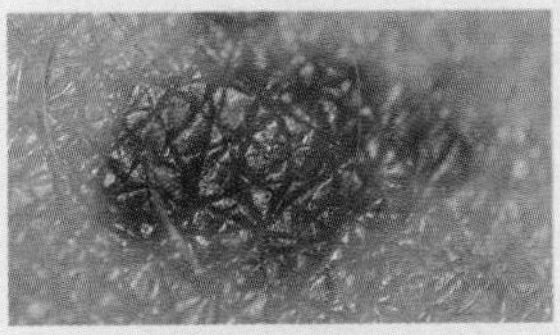	**B**order irregularity	The borders (edges) of the marking are blurry or uneven in shape rather than smooth.
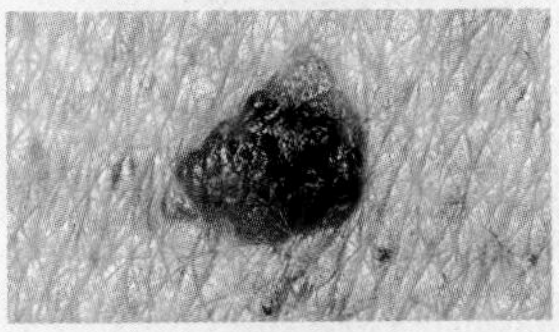	**C**olor changes	The marking changes color from one area to another (tan, brown, black, pink, blue, or white).
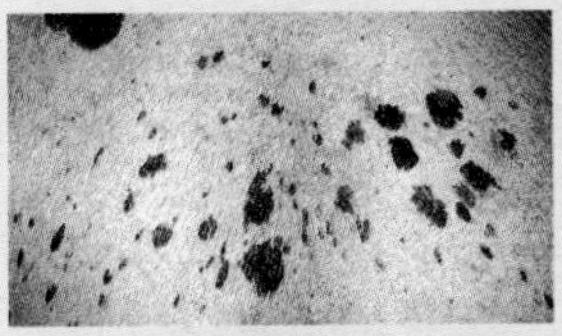	**D**iameter	The marking is larger across than a pencil's eraser (¼ inch).
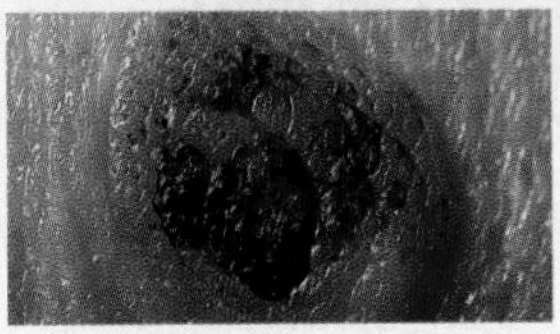	**E**volving	The marking changes over time in size, shape, color, bleeding, or other symptoms.

palms of the hands produces sweat more quickly than other areas of the body. What differences do you see between the skin on your face and the skin on your arms?

The Dermis

The dermis is the second layer of the skin, just beneath the epidermis. It is made of connective tissue and contains most of the skin's structures, including sensory organs, blood vessels, hair follicles, oil glands, and sweat glands. Dermal papillae (puh-PIH-lee) are small bumps that connect the epidermis to the dermis. These papillae group together on the fingertips and feet to form ridges that make the patterns of our fingerprints and footprints. Three basic shapes—arch, whorl, and loop—in different combinations make each person's prints unique (Figure 9.7). This uniqueness is important in many ways. For example, babies' footprints are recorded at birth for identification, and forensic investigators use fingerprints to help solve crimes. Take a minute to examine your own fingerprints. What shapes and patterns do you see? Is the print on each finger different?

There are many nerve endings in the dermis. These sensors are more concentrated in some areas than in others. Different types of nerve endings sense different things, including light touch, heavy pressure, vibration, temperature, and pain. Many nerve endings are found at the base of each hair, fingernail, and toenail.

Hair and nails both grow from living roots in the dermis, but the hair and nails seen on the outside of the body are formed from dead keratinized cells, like the skin's surface (Figure 9.8). Hair growth begins in the **root** at the bottom of a tube called the **hair follicle**. The shaft of dead cells pushes up through the epidermis where we see it as hair. Similarly, the nail root produces a hard, dead "shell" called the *nail plate*

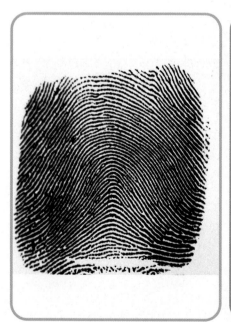
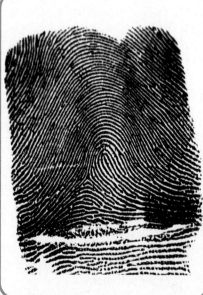
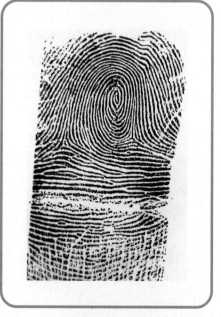

Figure 9.7   Though everyone's fingerprints are unique, they all contain the basic shapes of the arch, whorl, and loop. Which shapes do you see in your own fingerprints?

as protection for the sensitive **nail bed** at the tips of our fingers and toes. The phrase "you cut me to the quick" means that someone has hurt you deeply—like when you cut your nail too close and the sensitive nail bed is exposed. But we know there are no nerve endings in hair shafts or nail plates themselves because there is no pain when we cut them.

A muscle and oil gland are also connected to each hair follicle. Tiny *arrector pili* muscles raise the body hair and cause goose bumps when we are cold or scared. The **sebaceous** (sih-BAY-shuhs) **gland** provides sebum, an oily secretion that coats the hair and skin with a softening, waterproof film. As we grow from babies to teens and adults, our sebaceous glands become more active, providing more moisture and protection to the skin so it is less sensitive. When sebum traps dead skin cells in a pore, it can form a plug that becomes infected. This pus-filled pore is called *acne*. When the hair follicle or sebaceous gland is infected, it's called a *boil*. In old age, the sebaceous glands become less active, and dry skin may become a problem.

The skin gets rid of waste through its pores. Perspiration comes from **sudoriferous** (soo-duh-RIH-fuh-ruhs), or *sweat*, **glands** in the dermis that empty through sweat pores on the skin's surface. You can remember the

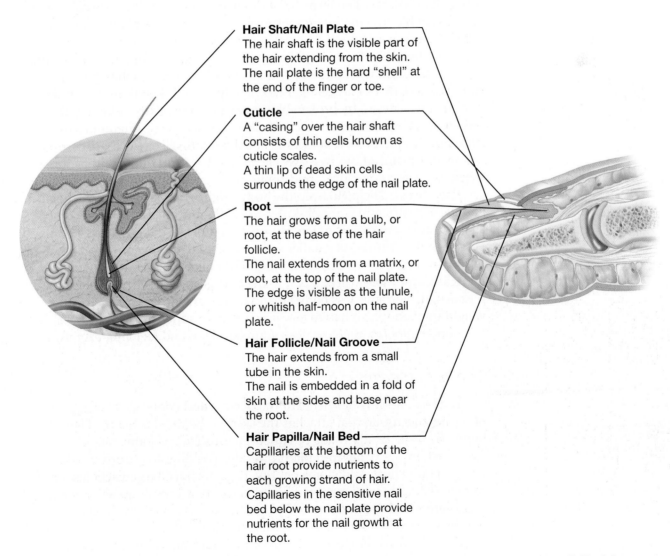

Hair Shaft/Nail Plate
The hair shaft is the visible part of the hair extending from the skin.
The nail plate is the hard "shell" at the end of the finger or toe.

Cuticle
A "casing" over the hair shaft consists of thin cells known as cuticle scales.
A thin lip of dead skin cells surrounds the edge of the nail plate.

Root
The hair grows from a bulb, or root, at the base of the hair follicle.
The nail extends from a matrix, or root, at the top of the nail plate. The edge is visible as the lunule, or whitish half-moon on the nail plate.

Hair Follicle/Nail Groove
The hair extends from a small tube in the skin.
The nail is embedded in a fold of skin at the sides and base near the root.

Hair Papilla/Nail Bed
Capillaries at the bottom of the hair root provide nutrients to each growing strand of hair.
Capillaries in the sensitive nail bed below the nail plate provide nutrients for the nail growth at the root.

Figure 9.8   Hair and nails have a similar structural makeup. Are your nails and hair alive or dead? Explain your answer.

difference between *sebaceous* and *sudoriferous* glands by remembering that sudoriferous can be "*odor*-iferous!" During puberty, the sudoriferous glands begin to produce perspiration and body odor increases. Perspiration helps cool the body through evaporation, drawing warmth out of the skin. An active person can produce as much as one quart of perspiration per hour. Perspiration also helps get rid of body waste such as excess salt and other minerals. This waste provides food for bacteria and fungi that live on the skin's surface. In turn, these microorganisms produce lactic acid that discourages the growth of harmful bacteria such as *Salmonella*.

Many kinds of skin irritation can occur from acne and chicken pox to insect bites and blisters. Figure 9.9 describes some common skin eruptions, or *lesions*. Aging brings an increase in skin tabs, moles, and other skin irregularities. These conditions may cause pain, itching, and embarrassment. Some skin conditions, like crusts, may clear up on their own. Others, like scales and polyps, may require treatment.

Blood vessels running through the dermis affect skin color. Although their purpose is to deliver nutrients and carry away waste, these vessels show through the skin in areas with less pigment and cause a variety of skin color changes. The term *pallor* describes skin that is a pale color due to a lack of blood, which is sometimes seen on the face before a person faints. Cyanosis (sI-uh-NOH-sihs) is the blue color seen in the lips, skin, or nails when the blood is low in oxygen. Erythema (ehr-uh-THEE-muh), or *redness*, occurs with increased blood flow to the skin when you are embarrassed, ill, or exercising. Petechiae (puh-TEE-kee-I) are tiny red or purple spots caused by broken blood vessels in the skin. A hematoma (hee-muh-TOH-muh), or *bruise*, gets its color from bleeding under the skin, not from the blood vessels themselves. Jaundice (JAWN-dihs) is the yellow color caused by liver disease. Skin color is an important factor when assessing a person's condition.

The skin also helps to keep the body's temperature at 98.6°F. Body fat and vasoconstriction (vay-soh-kuhn-STRIHK-shuhn) [*vaso* = vessel, *con* = against, *strict* = narrow, tighten, *ion* = action of] hold in body heat. The blood vessels in the dermis get smaller when we are cold, preventing heat loss. Vasodilation [*vaso* = vessel, *dilate* = expand] makes blood vessels wider so they can carry more warm blood to the body's surface where heat can be released. Babies have less body fat and more surface area for their body weight than adults, so babies are more likely to suffer from *hypothermia*, or low body temperature. How does your skin look and feel after exercising?

The Hypodermis

The hypodermis lies beneath the dermis and contains a layer of connective tissue that attaches the skin to the muscle below. The hypodermis is mostly made of **subcutaneous** [*sub* = below, *cutane* = skin, *ous* = pertaining to, having] **fat**. It provides padding to absorb shock, holds in body heat, and stores energy. Fat cells have large vacuoles for fat storage. They shrink when you diet and exercise but fill up again when you overeat and are not active. One pound of excess fat on the body requires an extra mile of blood vessels to supply that area with nutrients. This layer of fat builds up as we grow into adulthood but decreases again in old age, when the loss of fat and elasticity causes the skin to sag and wrinkle. Body fat distribution, which describes where fat is stored

Figure 9.9 Common Skin Conditions

Condition	Drawing	Appearance	Description
Crusts	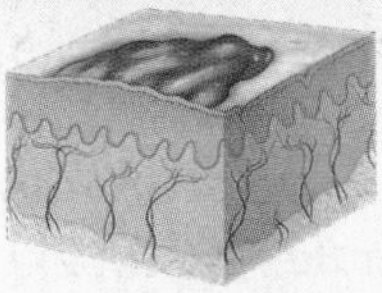	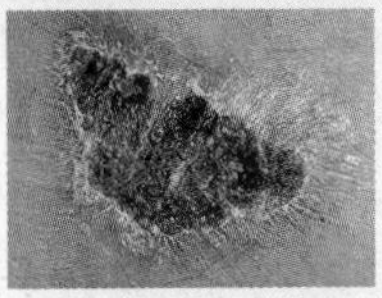	**Crusts** are dried blood and body fluid that scab over on the skin surface.
Scales	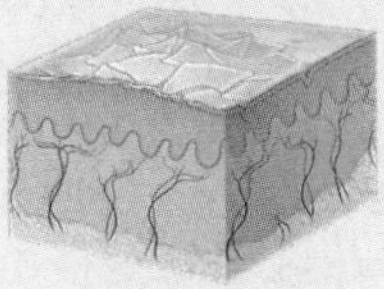	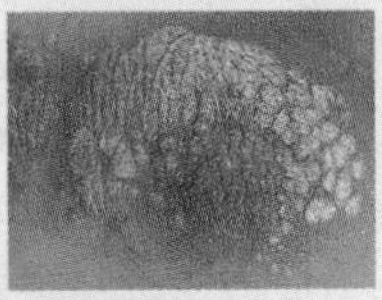	**Scales** are dry skin flakes that remain attached to the skin surface, as with eczema and psoriasis.
Seborrhea	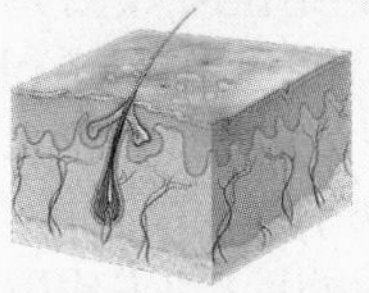	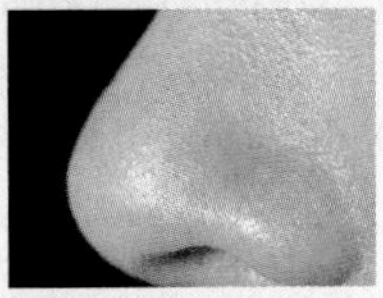	**Seborrhea** is the problem of oily skin, often seen during puberty when the sebaceous glands produce too much sebum.
Polyps	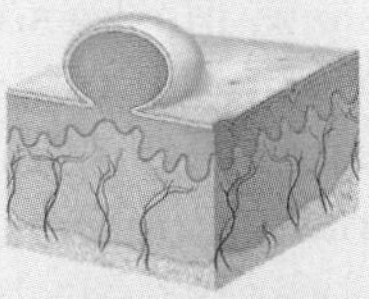	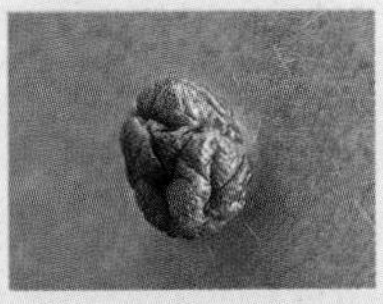	**Polyps**, or *skin tabs*, are small flaps of skin attached to the epidermis by a thin stalk. They are common on the neck, chest, armpits, and eyelids.
Macules	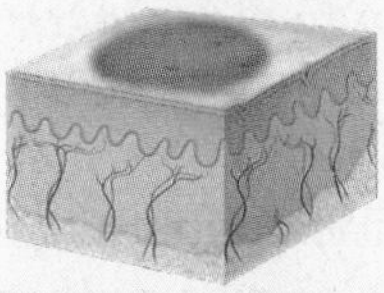	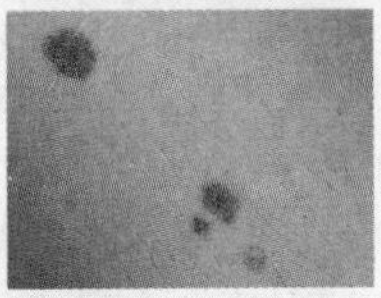	**Macules** are flat, colored spots on the skin surface, such as freckles.
Wheals	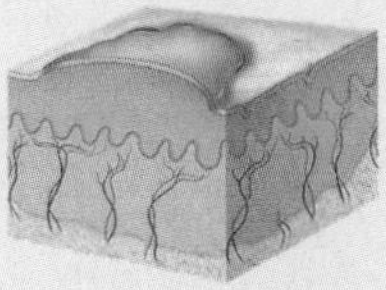		**Wheals**, or *welts*, are large, red, raised, itchy bumps, often seen in an allergic reaction called *hives*.
Papules	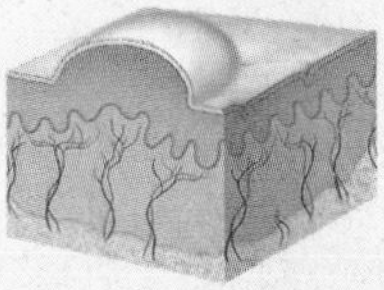	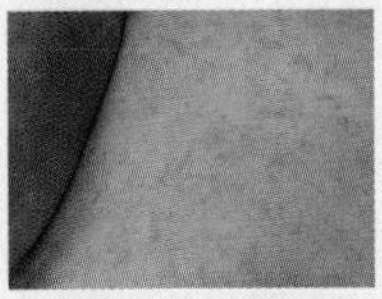	**Papules** are small, solid, raised bumps on the surface of the skin, like those seen with heat rash.
Pustules	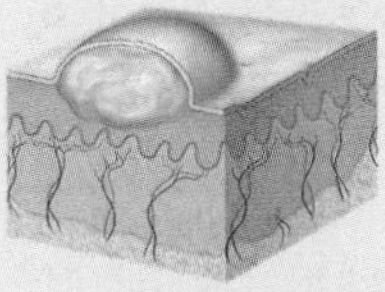	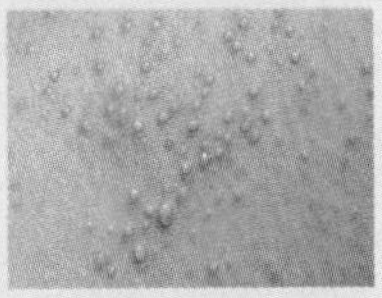	**Pustules**, or *pus-filled pimples*, like acne, are most common on the face, neck, and back.
Vesicles	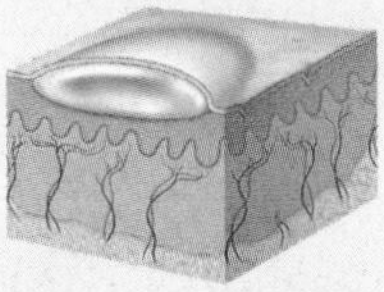	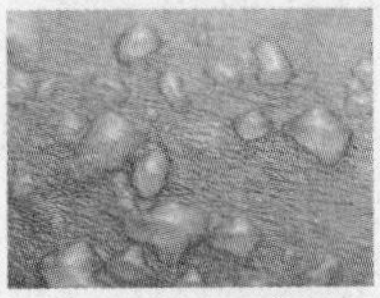	**Vesicles** are blisters filled with clear fluid that can burst and ooze.
Nodules	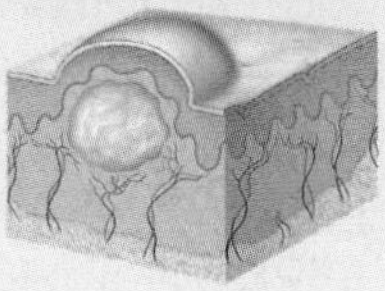	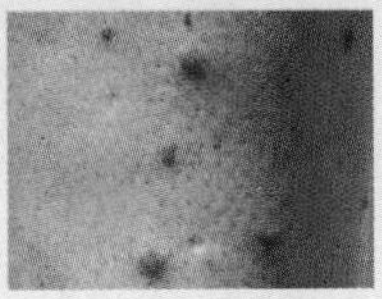	**Nodules** are filled sacs, or *cysts*, that form a firm bump going down into the dermis.

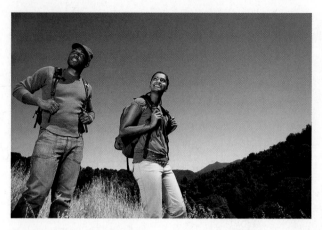

Figure 9.10   Some daily sun exposure can be healthy, but too much sun can damage the skin. What are the benefits of sun exposure? How can you protect your skin from overexposure?

on the body, is important. Excess fat around the abdomen, for example, is related to a higher risk for diabetes, heart disease, and cancer.

Some fat is required for normal body functions. Fat-soluble vitamins such as vitamins A, D, E, and K are stored in body fat. Vitamin D is formed when cholesterol in the skin is exposed to ultraviolet (UV) light. Just five minutes of sun exposure on the face and arms each day will provide the recommended daily allowance of vitamin D (Figure 9.10). The body needs some fat to store these nutrients, as well as provide insulation from cold and pad other body structures.

Plastic surgery repairs, reshapes, or rebuilds skin and the structures below it. Cosmetic surgery is the best-known form of plastic surgery. However, not all forms of plastic surgery are about beauty-related enhancements. Reconstructive surgery helps to repair damage and improve function after accidents and disease. For example, an accident victim may need a surgeon to rebuild his jaw. Plastic surgery is a growing field for employment, research, and new technology.

Both pressure ulcers (UHL-serz) and burns cause damage to all layers of the skin. Pressure ulcers occur when something presses against the skin long and hard enough to prevent blood from reaching the skin cells, causing them to die. Patients who are in wheelchairs or confined to bed should be repositioned or reminded to shift their weight regularly to increase circulation and prevent these sores.

Burns can be caused by heat, electricity, or chemicals (Figure 9.11). Both first-degree burns and pressure sores cause redness and affect only

Figure 9.11   Pressure, heat, electricity, and chemicals can all damage the skin layers. What degree of damage does each of these images represent—first, second, third, or fourth?

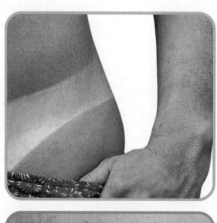

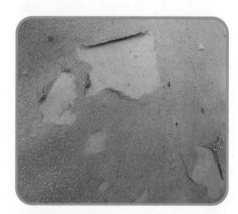

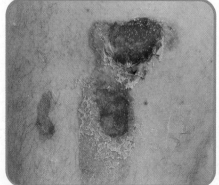

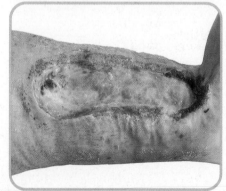

the epidermis. Second-degree injuries result in blisters and damage to the dermis that may take several weeks or longer to heal. Third-degree injuries damage the full thickness of the skin, including the subcutaneous layer (hypodermis). Fourth-degree injuries extend into the muscle, tendons, and bone. Third- and fourth-degree injuries are serious enough to require surgery to remove dead skin, place skin grafts, and manage the scars and skin tightening that occur.

The size of a burn is estimated using the "rule of nines" (Figure 9.12). The total body surface is divided into sections representing multiples of nine. The larger the area affected, the more likely a patient is to suffer complications such as infection or dehydration. Always seek medical attention for a burn if your skin is broken, the injury covers an area larger than the palm of your hand, or it doesn't heal within a week.

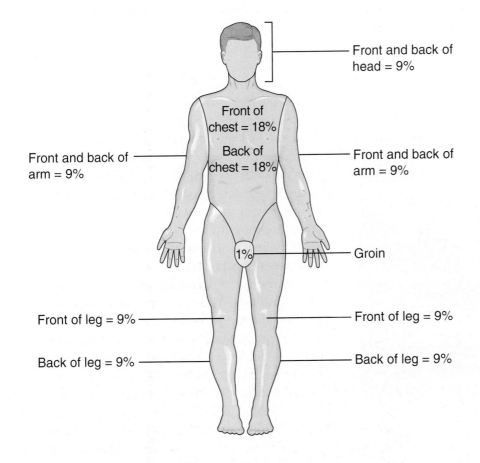

Front and back of head = 9%

Front of chest = 18%

Back of chest = 18%

Front and back of arm = 9%

Front and back of arm = 9%

1%

Groin

Front of leg = 9%

Front of leg = 9%

Back of leg = 9%

Back of leg = 9%

Figure 9.12   The rule of nines divides the body as shown here to determine what percentage of the body was damaged by a burn.

Animation

RECALL YOUR READING

1. Collagen in the _____ of the integumentary, skeletal, and muscular systems provides structure and _____ for the body.

2. Functions of the integumentary system include providing a _____ to protect the body, maintaining body _____, producing and storing _____, and eliminating body _____.

3. The three layers of skin include the _____, dermis, and _____.

4. Skin _____ are important to observe when assessing a patient's condition.

Complete the *Map Your Reading* graphic organizer for the section you just read.

The Skeletal System

The skeletal system includes bones, joints, and cartilage named for their shape and function. Bones work with the muscular, circulatory, nervous, and digestive systems. Together, they provide support, protection, movement, blood cell production, and nutrient storage. Collagen provides structure, support, and strength for the skeletal system.

Orthopedic [*ortho* = to straighten, *ped* = foot] **surgeons** work closely with bones. The name for this field comes from early procedures that focused on straightening the feet. These surgeons now correct a wide variety of misshaped bones and complicated breaks. The field of orthopedics is constantly developing new techniques to relieve pain and improve function. For example, in arthroscopy (ahr-THRAHS-kuh-pee) [*arthr* = joint, *scopy* = process of viewing, examination], surgical tools are inserted through several small openings in the skin instead of one large cut. This allows faster healing and less exposure to infection. Joint replacement, or *arthroplasty* (AHR-thruh-plas-tee) [*plasty* = surgical repair], is a major surgery used to improve movement and relieve joint pain. A five-year residency is required to train an orthopedic surgeon, and surgeons will work an average of 50 to 55 hours per week for their $400,000 annual salary. These doctors may also specialize in sports medicine or hand, spine, or microsurgery.

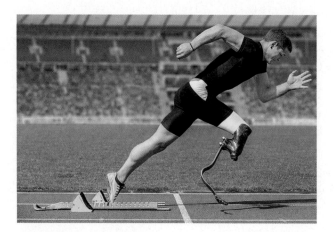

Figure 9.13   Artificial limbs made by prosthetists can help people walk, lift objects, or even compete in sports. What injuries or diseases might cause someone to lose a limb?

If you don't see yourself as a future surgeon but are interested in working with bone structure, you may want to think about a more creative type of therapeutic career. A prosthetist (PRAHS-theht-ihst) makes custom-built artificial limbs, or **prostheses** (prahs-THEE-seez), for patients who are missing body parts (Figure 9.13). Orthotists (OR-thah-tihsts) make a variety of braces, or *orthotics*, to support weak bones or correct physical problems. Pedorthists (PEHD-orth-ihsts) specialize in devices that relieve foot problems caused by disease, birth defects, overuse, or injury. People in these careers are caring, social, and detail-oriented. They like to work with their hands and have a strong background in science and computers. They may work in a clinic, hospital, or rehabilitation center. A master's degree and one year of residency are required for certification in orthotics, prosthetics, and pedorthics.

Although you cannot actually see your bones, you can see their outline and feel them through their covering of skin, muscle, and fat. You will understand the skeletal system better if you use your own body as a model. As you read this section, try to find the different types of bones on your own body and feel how they move together.

Parts of a Bone

A bone has many parts, each with a different function (Figure 9.14). Bones provide mineral and fat storage, and they enable red and white

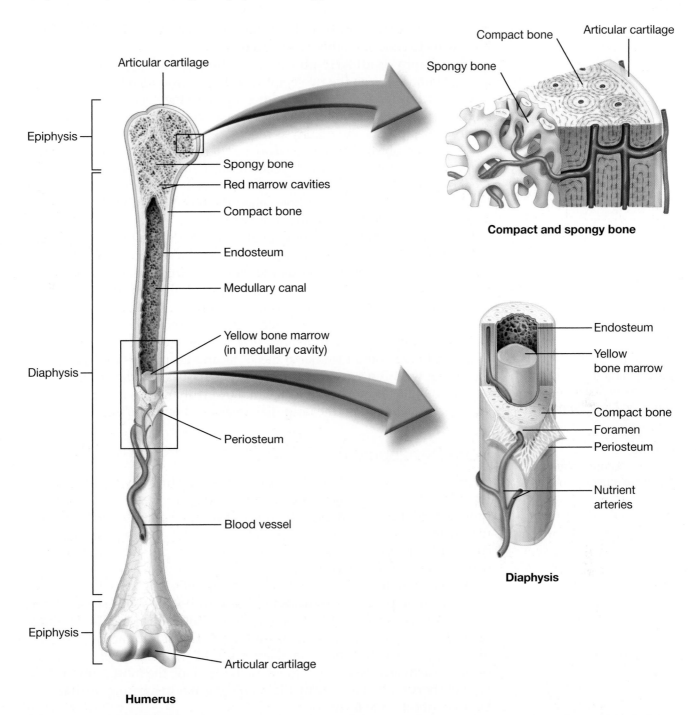

Compact and spongy bone

Diaphysis

Humerus

Figure 9.14   Bones, which appear very simple on the outside, contain important structures and materials such as bone marrow and blood vessels. Can you identify the functions of spongy bone and compact bone?

blood cell production. Each of these jobs takes place in a different part of the bone.

Each end of a long bone forms a knob called the **epiphysis** (eh-PIHF-uh-sihs) [*epi* = upon, *physis* = to grow]. The epiphysis is mostly **spongy bone**, a lighter and less dense structure than compact bone. Blood cells are made in the red bone marrow of the epiphysis. Bone marrow is sometimes transplanted to cure diseases like leukemia (loo-KEE-mee-uh), a blood disorder. The epiphysis is covered with articular **cartilage**, which is found where two bones meet to form a joint. This cartilage allows the bone ends to slide smoothly across each other.

The **diaphysis** (dI-AHF-uh-sihs) [*dia* = through, across] is the long shaft of bone between the two epiphyses. It is surrounded by **compact bone**, which is made of bone cells lined up close together to withstand stress. Bone growth occurs in the epiphyseal (ehp-ih-FIHZ-ee-ahl) plate where the epiphysis and diaphysis meet.

A hollow tube called the *medullary cavity* runs down the center of the diaphysis and stores the fat-rich yellow bone marrow. This soft center is what dogs like to lick out of a bone. Blood vessels and nerves run through this cavity and an opening or hole called the **foramen** (fuh-RAY-mehn) allows them to pass through the compact bone.

Try to find one of your supraorbital foramen. Press a fingertip against the inner third of one of your eyebrows (the end near your nose). When you press on the foramen, you should feel a tingling sensation because you are compressing the nerve that runs through the foramen.

The diaphysis is wrapped in a thin membrane called the *periosteum* (pair-ee-AHS-tee-uhm). This is where ligaments and tendons attach to a bone. **Ligaments** (LIHG-uh-mehnts) [*liga* = to tie] are straps of connective tissue that hold bones together at the joints and keep joints from moving the wrong way. **Tendons** are also connective tissues, but they connect muscle to bone for movement at a joint. Powerful muscles get their strongest attachment on the large, flat areas of a bone's surface.

ligament
a tough, fibrous tissue that connects bones to other bones and holds organs in place

tendon
a tough, fibrous tissue that connects muscles to bones

Bone Development

Bones begin as tough, rubbery cartilage in the first few weeks of a fetus' development. Collagen fibers in the cartilage give it strength and provide the structure for making bones. Osteogenesis (ahs-tee-oh-JEHN-uh-sihs) [*osteo* = bone, *genesis* = origin, formation, producing] imperfecta, commonly known as *brittle bone disease*, is a genetic mutation caused by defective or insufficient collagen.

Osteoblasts are specialized bone-forming cells that begin the mineralization process. **Ossification** (ahs-uh-fuh-KAY-shuhn) [*osse* = bone, *fic* = making, causing, *ation* = action of, process of] is the process of taking calcium from what we eat or drink and depositing it into cartilage to form bone. In achondroplasia (ay-kahn-droh-PLAY-zhee-uh) [*a* = without, *chondr* = cartilage, *plasia* = development, formation], the most common type of short-limbed dwarfism, the problem is not in forming cartilage, but in ossification to form bone.

Our bones need vitamin D for calcium to deposit into the bones as they grow. Children with a poor diet or lack of exposure to the sun may develop *rickets* because they don't get enough vitamin D. Rickets causes bowed legs, more fragile bones, delayed growth, and muscle weakness. This condition is commonly prevented in the United States by fortifying milk with vitamin D so it provides the vitamins and minerals needed for healthy bones.

Bones continue to change as we grow older. **Osteoclast** cells break down bone during exercise, so it can be remodeled into new bone cells. Stress on the bones, such as jogging, helps bones deposit more calcium where it is needed to become stronger. We reach our maximum bone density by 25 years of age. After about 40 years of age, we begin to lose more bone mass than we usually gain through diet and exercise. Hormone changes during pregnancy and menopause also pull calcium out of the bones.

Osteoporosis [*osteo* = bone, *por* = pores, *osis* = condition, process] is a loss of bone mass, which weakens the bones so they break easily. Osteoporosis affects spongy bone more severely than compact bone because spongy bone is less dense. Absorptiometry (ab-sorp-shee-AHM-eh-tree) uses X-ray beams to measure bone mineral density. Elderly white women, especially those with a petite build, are at the greatest risk for osteoporosis (Figure 9.15).

At birth, we have about 300 soft bones that ossify and fuse together to become about 206 hard and permanent bones as we grow (Figure 9.16 on the next page). Some bones, such as the cranium [*crani* = skull, *ium* = structure], become **sutured** (SOO-churd), growing together like interlaced fingers to form a strong and immovable joint. The frontal bone at the forehead, parietal bones on the top of the head, temporal bones above the ears, and occipital bone at the back of the head begin as separate bones in a fetus. This allows a baby's head to flex as it goes through the birth canal. The soft spot, or **fontanel**, on an infant's head is where the bones have not yet grown together. Twenty-one bones become sutured and ossified to create the adult skull. This skull forms a protective shield around the brain, eyes, nose, and mouth, including the maxilla of the upper jaw. The lower jaw, or *mandible*, is the only bone in the skull that moves freely.

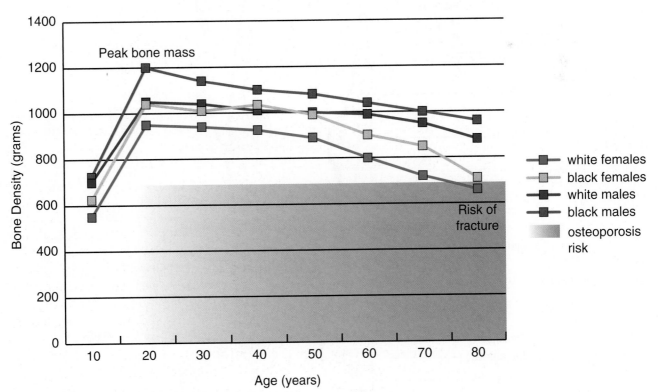

Figure 9.15   Risk for osteoporosis depends on age and ethnicity. According to this chart, which group of people is most at risk for developing osteoporosis?

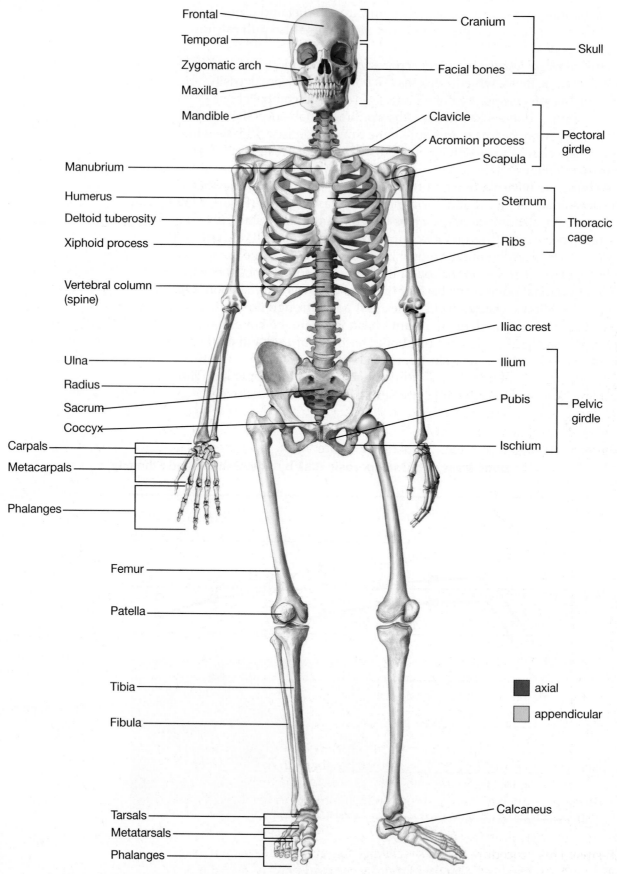

Frontal — Cranium
Temporal — Skull
Zygomatic arch —
Maxilla — Facial bones
Mandible —

Clavicle
Acromion process — Pectoral girdle
Scapula

Manubrium —
Humerus — Sternum
Deltoid tuberosity — Thoracic cage
Xiphoid process — Ribs
Vertebral column (spine) —

Iliac crest
Ilium
Pubis — Pelvic girdle
Ischium

Ulna —
Radius —
Sacrum —
Coccyx —
Carpals —
Metacarpals —
Phalanges —

Femur —
Patella —

Tibia —
Fibula —

■ axial
□ appendicular

Tarsals —
Metatarsals —
Phalanges —
Calcaneus

Figure 9.16   A fully-grown adult has approximately 206 bones in his or her body, while a baby who was just born has 300 bones. Why do babies have more bones in their bodies than adults?

Label Art

Types of Bones

Bones provide support for the body, with different types of bones performing different roles. The **flat bones** of the cranium, sternum, scapula, and ribs sandwich a layer of spongy bone between two layers of compact bone (Figure 9.17). These bones are thin, flat, and effective as protective shells.

Long bones, like the femur in the thigh and humerus in the upper arm, are longer than they are wide (Figure 9.18). The hollow design of their diaphysis provides strength without excess weight. If the skeleton was built out of steel to an equivalent strength, it would weigh five times as much! Long bones act as levers for muscles to raise and lower different parts of the body.

Larger, stronger bones are also used to bear weight. Compare the size of the femur, tibia, and fibula in the leg to the size of the humerus, ulna, and radius in the arm. These bones have the same basic structure, but the stronger leg bones have more mass than the arm bones to carry the body's weight. In Figure 9.16, compare the tibia and fibula in the lower leg of the skeleton. Which one bears the body's weight and which one is only used for muscle attachments?

Not all long bones are large. The metacarpals in the palm of the hand, the metatarsals in the arch of the foot, and the phalanges (fuh-LAN-jeez) of the fingers and toes are all long bones. Notice that the fingers and toes have a similar structure and the same name. Directional terms are used to name the different segments: proximal phalanges are closer to the palm or sole, medial phalanges are in the middle, and distal phalanges are at the ends of the fingers and toes. Although they are small, phalanges are still longer than they are wide, and they act as levers for muscles that move the body.

Short bones, such as the carpals and tarsals of the wrists and ankles, are useful as bridges (Figure 9.19). They are as long as they are wide, and they are made of spongy bone covered by a thin layer of compact bone. Notice again that the tarsals are larger than the carpals because they are weight bearing.

People can develop different numbers of sesamoid (SEHS-uh-moyd) bones. These are small, flat, sesame seed-shaped bones embedded within tendons or joint capsules. Most people have two patella (puh-TEHL-uh) bones, which form the two kneecaps. Sometimes additional sesamoid bones form during fetal development or fail to fuse together, so we say an adult has "about" 206 bones.

Irregular bones, like the vertebrae (VERT-uh-bray) of the spine and the ilium (IHL-ee-uhm) of the hip, are complex shapes (Figure 9.20). They provide many surfaces to which tendons and ligaments can attach. Irregular bones contain mostly spongy bone with a thin covering of compact bone. This higher proportion of spongy bone makes irregular bones more prone to osteoporosis. Elderly people with osteoporosis may develop a hunched back and lose an inch or more in height as their vertebrae lose mass and compact together. As a large irregular bone, the ilium is an ideal site for performing osteocentesis (ahs-tee-oh-sehn-TEE-sihs). This procedure uses a special needle to remove bone marrow for biopsy or transplants. The thin layer of compact bone on the ilium is more easily penetrated than in long bones, and there is more red marrow available in the hip than in long bones.

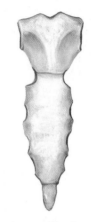

Figure 9.17   Flat bone

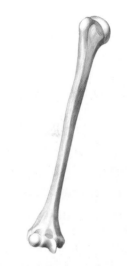

Figure 9.18   Long bone

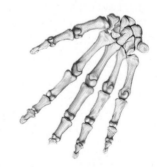

Figure 9.19   Short bones

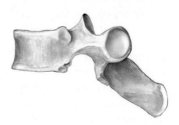

Figure 9.20   Irregular bone

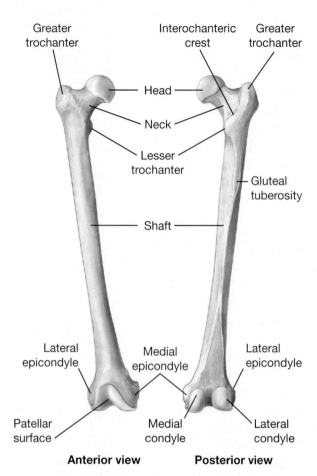

Figure 9.21 Bone markings such as condyles and tuberosities are used to describe locations on bones, as shown on the femur above. How does Wolff's Law explain the development of these markings?

Bone Markings

A variety of markings—usually bumps and grooves—are used to describe locations on bones. The condyles (KAHN-dIlz), or rounded knobs at the ends of bones, can be seen where two bones meet to form a joint, such as where the tibia and femur meet at the knee (Figure 9.21). These condyles are named for their anatomical positions—the *medial condyle* is located toward the midline of the body and the *lateral condyle* is located on the outer side of the knee. The elbow has similar but smaller bumps, called *epicondyles* (ehp-ih-KAHN-dIlz), where the ulna and humerus meet. The medial and lateral *malleoli* (mah-LEE-oh-lI) are bumps that form the ankle where the tibia and fibula connect to the tarsals. These bumps provide attachment sites for ligaments and muscles.

A *process* is a part of the bone that projects out like a bridge. For example, the acromion (ay-KROH-mee-ahn) process connects the scapula and clavicle in the shoulder. The process forming the cheekbone at the zygomatic (zI-goh-MAT-ihk) arch can be seen and felt through the skin. A *tuberosity* (too-buh-RAHS-uht-ee) is a long bump, but it doesn't project out as far as a process, so it is more difficult to see or feel. A *crest* is a raised ridge at the edge of a bone. The iliac crest is the ridge you feel when you rest your hand on your hip. It is thicker and more prominent than a tuberosity, but it doesn't stand out as far as a process.

These bumps and ridges form as attachment sites for skeletal muscles. Wolff's law says that a bone is shaped by the forces that put stress on it. This means that the greater the impact or stress, the more calcium the bone stores through the actions of osteoclasts and osteoblasts. This is why exercise is important for forming and maintaining strong bones. The areas where muscles pull on bones to create movement will cause bumps to form on the bones over time. The stronger the muscles, the larger the bumps formed. Anthropologists (an-thruh-PAHL-uh-jihsts) use these bumps found on skeletons—and other signs such as bone breaks and the weight or length of bones—to gather information about how people lived.

Divisions of the Skeleton

The skeleton is divided into two parts called the *axial* (AK-see-uhl) *skeleton* and the *appendicular* (ap-ehn-DIHK-yuh-luhr) *skeleton*. The **axial skeleton**, or center "axis" of the body, is formed by the skull, spine, and rib cage. The "appendages," or arms and legs, are part of the **appendicular skeleton**. The shading in Figure 9.16 shows these two divisions.

The axial skeleton forms a line down the center of the body. The vertebral column, or *spine*, supports the skull and ribs. The spine is made of 33 bones divided into five groups (Figure 9.22). There are seven small cervical bones in the neck that connect the skull to the chest. The chest

axial skeleton
term that applies to the skull, spine, and rib cage, which rotate around an imaginary center line of the body

appendicular skeleton
term that describes the bones of the arms and legs, including the shoulder and hip bones where they are attached

is attached in the back to 12 slightly larger thoracic vertebrae. Five large lumbar vertebrae make up the lower back. Just above the buttocks, five bones are fused together into the *sacrum*, a flat triangular bone. The tailbone, or *coccyx* (KAHK-sihks), is made up of four more tiny bones fused together below the sacrum. Many small muscles stabilize the bones of the vertebral column to keep you upright.

The vertebral column has natural curves that help it support the weight of the body. More extreme curves can be caused by birth defects, poor posture, weak abdominal muscles, or a breakdown of the vertebrae (Figure 9.23 on the next page). Lordosis is an inward swayback, which causes the buttocks to stick out and the hips to tilt too far forward. Kyphosis (kI-FOH-sihs) is an outward hunchback, which causes the shoulders to slump forward and makes it difficult to raise the head. Scoliosis (skoh-lee-OH-sihs) is a sideways (lateral) curve that may require a brace to stabilize the spine. These conditions can require surgery when they limit movement, compress internal organs, or cause pain.

The axial skeleton protects the body. Three different types of ribs form a protective cage around the internal organs. The first seven on each side are *true ribs* because they are attached directly to the sternum in front and to the thoracic vertebrae in back. The next three are called *false ribs* because they are attached to thoracic vertebrae in the back but only by cartilage in the front. There are also two *floating ribs* on each side that attach only to the last two thoracic vertebrae in back. The ribs are strong enough to protect the heart and lungs, but they flex and spring back when someone presses on the chest, such as during cardiopulmonary resuscitation (CPR).

The sternum, or *breastbone*, where the ribs connect helps to complete the cage around the chest. The breastbone also has three interconnected parts. The upper section near the neck looks like the knot of a man's tie and is called the *manubrium* (muh-NOO-bree-uhm). This is fused to the long, tie-shaped middle section called the *body*. The *xiphoid* (ZI-foyd) *process* is a small point at the bottom of the breastbone that can sometimes break off under pressure, such as during CPR.

While the axial skeleton provides protection, the appendicular skeleton allows us to move our appendages. In addition to the bones of the arms and legs, it includes the shoulder and hip bones. These are the bones that attach the arms and legs to the axial skeleton.

The shoulder, or *pectoral* [*pector* = chest] *girdle*, is made up of three bones that connect the arm to the axial skeleton. The clavicle, or *collarbone*, supports the arm from the front. The scapula, or *shoulder blade*, provides extra surface area for attaching powerful shoulder muscles in the back. The acromion process forms a bridge between the clavicle and the scapula

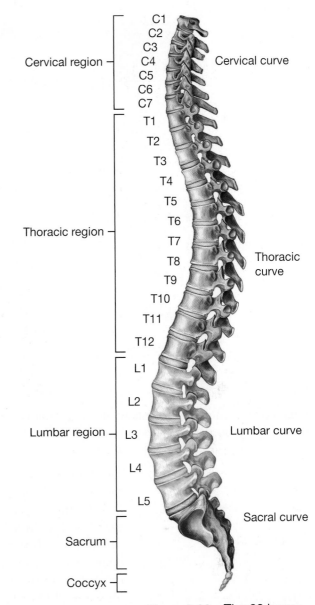

Figure 9.22   The 33 bones of the spine are divided into five regions. Within these regions, each bone is assigned a number. Which section of the spine would you expect to be the most flexible? Why?

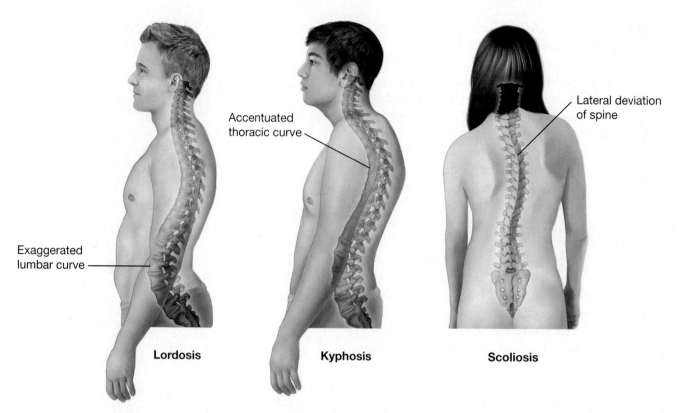

Accentuated
thoracic curve

Lateral deviation
of spine

Exaggerated
lumbar curve

Lordosis   **Kyphosis**   **Scoliosis**

Figure 9.23   The three conditions illustrated here change the shape of the spine. What can cause these conditions to occur?

for extra stability. The clavicle, acromion process, and scapula are fused together to make a "cup" for the shoulder joint.

The hip, or *pelvic girdle*, is also a combination of three bones fused together. Put your hands on your hips. The large, rounded top of each side of the pelvis is the ilium. The *ischia* (IHS-kee-uh) are the boney rings below each buttock. The pubis connects the left and right hip structures in the pubic region. This bowl-shaped shell of the pelvic girdle protects the intestines, bladder, rectum, and—in the female—reproductive organs.

Types of Joints

The connection of two bones creates a joint. Different types of joints allow different types of movement. Diarthroses (dI-ahr-THROH-seez) [*dia* = through, across, *arthr* = joint, *osis* = condition, process], or *synovial joints*, are the most freely movable joints. The ends of these joints are covered with cartilage, and they are enclosed in a bursa, or *capsule*, containing synovial fluid to help the bones slide against each other smoothly without pain.

A variety of problems can occur in the joints. When the cartilage wears out, as in arthritis [*arthr* = joint, *itis* = inflammation], the joints become swollen and movement can be painful. Bursitis is an inflammation of the joint capsule that causes pain. Joint replacements made from a combination of metals and plastics are often used to replace worn-out cartilage and bone in hips, knees, and other joints.

There are several different types of diarthroses (Figure 9.24). **Ball-and-socket joints**, like the hip and shoulder, have a rounded head

Gliding joint (intercarpal)

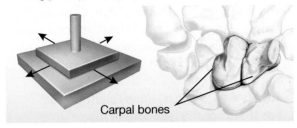

Carpal bones

Hinge joint (humeroulnar)

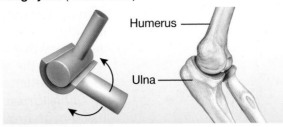

Humerus

Ulna

Pivot joint (radioulnar)

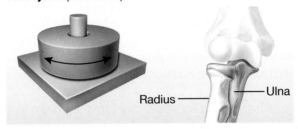

Radius — Ulna

Condylar joint (metacarpophalangeal)

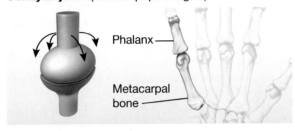

Phalanx —

Metacarpal bone —

Saddle joint (trapeziometacarpal)

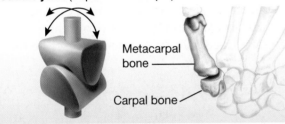

Metacarpal bone —

Carpal bone —

Ball-and-socket joint (humeroscapular)

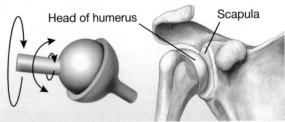

Head of humerus   Scapula

Figure 9.24   Diarthroses are joints that can move freely. Test out the range of motion for each of these joints yourself.

Animation

of bone that fits into a cup-shaped cavity of bone. This allows for the widest range of motion in many directions. **Condylar** (KAHN-dih-lahr), or *ellipsoidal* (ih-lihp-SOY-duhl), joints like the wrist and fingers can bend, straighten, and move side to side, but they move in the shape of an ellipse rather than a full circle. The first metacarpal bone of the thumb forms a saddle joint, which allows our opposable thumb to touch the other fingers and grasp things.

Hinge joints, like the elbow or jaw, only bend and straighten or open and close with no side-to-side motion. The flat wrist and anklebone surfaces slide over each other in a gliding joint, but their movement is limited by strong ligaments. The pivot joint formed by the top two cervical vertebrae allows you to turn your head from side to side to say no. At the elbow, the radius pivots in the notch at the base of the humerus. Bend your fingers—what type of joint allows you to do this?

Amphiarthroses (am-fee-ahr-THROH-seez) [*amphi* = around] are slightly movable joints. The 7 cervical, 12 thoracic, and 5 lumbar vertebrae are all able to move a little bit backward, forward, and to each side. They are separated by disks made of cartilage that pad the joints. Although each individual joint moves only slightly, these many small movements allow us to bend comfortably. A herniated (HER-nee-ayt-ed) disk, which occurs when the soft center of the disk bulges out between the vertebrae, puts pressure on the nerves running through the spine. This causes pain up and down the back and along the shoulder or thigh. Treatments include injections to reduce inflammation, removal of the damaged tissue, or surgery that fuses the vertebrae together. A chiropractor (KI-roh-prak-ter) adjusts the alignment of the vertebrae to help the muscles and joints function better and relieve pain.

Synarthroses (sihn-ahr-THROH-seez) [*syn* = same, together] are fused in an immovable joint. For instance, the sacrum is made up of five bones located below the lumbar vertebrae that are fused into a flat triangle at the small of the back. The tailbone is four fused bones located at the end of the vertebral column. The skull is another example of a synarthrosis. A cleft palate occurs when the hard palate bones in the roof of the mouth fail to fuse into their synarthrosis during embryonic development. On the other hand, orthodontists sometimes use an expander to spread the synarthrosis of the hard palate to provide more space for growing teeth.

When a bone "jumps out" of its normal location in a joint, damage to bones, ligaments, nerves, and blood vessels may occur. A dislocated joint is a separation of two bones that are normally held together by ligaments and muscles. A **fracture**, or *break*, in the bone may occur with or without dislocation (Figure 9.25). Simple fractures leave the bone in its original position, while compound fractures break through the surrounding tissues and skin. The geometry of a fracture is often used to describe the

Figure 9.25 Some fractures are more serious than others. Which of these types of fractures is common in children?

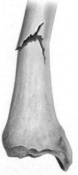

A *greenstick fracture* is incomplete. The break occurs on the convex surface of the bend in the bone.

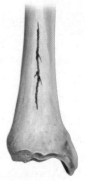

A *stress fracture* involves an incomplete break.

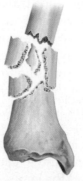

A *comminuted fracture* is complete and splinters the bone.

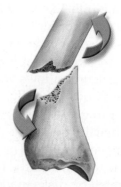

A *spiral fracture* is caused by twisting a bone.

direction of the break. Transverse fractures break straight across the bone, oblique fractures break at an angle, and spiral fractures twist around the bone. Comminuted fractures break into many small pieces, while stress fractures are a crack in a bone that stays in one piece. Greenstick fractures, in which only one side of the bone breaks, are common in young children because they have more cartilage in their bones.

Both dislocations and fractures must be repositioned and immobilized until healed. Surgery may be required to realign, stabilize, or reattach tissues that have been damaged. The body heals fractures by bringing in osteoclasts to fill the gap and create a "callus" on the bone. After the injury has healed, strengthening exercises may help to reduce the chance of another injury by ensuring that the surrounding muscles support the bones.

RECALL YOUR READING

1. At birth, our bones are mostly soft _____, but they have fused and _____ by adulthood.
2. The _____ bones provide protection while the _____ bones provide support and movement.
3. Bones store fat and _____, produce _____, connect with muscles for _____, and protect us from _____.
4. The different types of bones include _____, short, flat, and _____.
5. _____ connect bone to bone and _____ connect muscle to bone.

Complete the *Map Your Reading* graphic organizer for the section you just read.

The Muscular System

Muscles interact with the skeletal, nervous, digestive, and circulatory systems to produce stability, movement, breathing, body heat, and digestive functions. Collagen surrounds each muscle fiber and gives it strength. Collagen is also the main component of tendons that connect muscles to bones to allow movement. The work of many different healthcare professionals is focused on building and maintaining the health and function of the muscular system.

The Therapeutic Worker: Pat

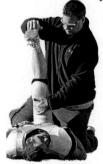

Pat is a certified athletic trainer. He works nights and weekends, educating high school athletes on injury prevention, assessing sports injuries, and providing appropriate treatment and rehabilitation of bone and muscle injuries. He also works as a physical education and health teacher during the day. He completed his bachelor's degree in education and obtained his certification in athletic training through an internship program. The certification test was challenging but is required for this job in most states. Today, many states also require a degree in athletic training to qualify.

Pat works under the direction of a licensed physician and coordinates the care of his athletes with other healthcare providers. He likes the variety of work settings and personal interactions that are involved with his job, but he finds the variable schedule and long hours on his feet a challenge. He knows that athletic trainers for professional athletes may earn a little more than his $40 per hour, but those jobs are difficult to get. Many of the new jobs in this growing profession will be in healthcare facilities as a cost-effective way to increase healthcare and injury prevention services, but Pat prefers to work with high school students on the playing field and in the locker room.

As mentioned in chapter 6, a physical therapy assistant is able to obtain employment after just two years of education, but many physical therapist (PT) training programs now require a doctoral degree. Most physical therapists work in a hospital or healthcare office, but some also work in home health, nursing homes, schools, and industrial settings. They provide therapy treatments to patients with physical disabilities, teaching these patients proper exercise techniques and using a variety of exercise equipment and activities to help strengthen muscles, improve mobility, restore function, and relieve pain.

The Therapeutic Worker: Kim

As a recreational therapist in a nursing home, Kim uses a variety of activities—such as crafts, sports, dance, and interaction with animals—to reduce residents' stress, stimulate their minds, help them recover basic motor functions, and build their socialization skills. She previously worked in a hospital and rehabilitation center, but she really enjoys working with the elderly. Jobs in nursing care facilities and outpatient settings have been increasing as the aging population requires more services. Kim completed a bachelor's degree in therapeutic recreation, and she would like to specialize in art therapy. Her state requires certification, but not all states do.

cardiac muscle
an involuntary, striated muscle tissue located in the walls of the heart

smooth muscle
an involuntary muscle located in the body's visceral organs and blood vessels; also known as *visceral muscle*

skeletal muscle
a voluntary, striated muscle that connects to bones and is responsible for movement

Types of Muscle

There are three types of muscle in the body—cardiac, smooth, and skeletal. Each muscle type has a different function. The walls of the heart that pump blood throughout the body are made of **cardiac muscle**. You will learn more about cardiac muscle and the circulatory system in chapter 13. **Smooth muscle**, or *visceral muscle*, is used to move food and drink along the alimentary canal and blood through the blood vessels. This will be discussed again in chapter 17 when we focus on the digestive system. The main focus in this section is **skeletal muscle**, which attaches to bones to produce movement and provide stability to the body (Figure 9.26 and Figure 9.27 on page 318).

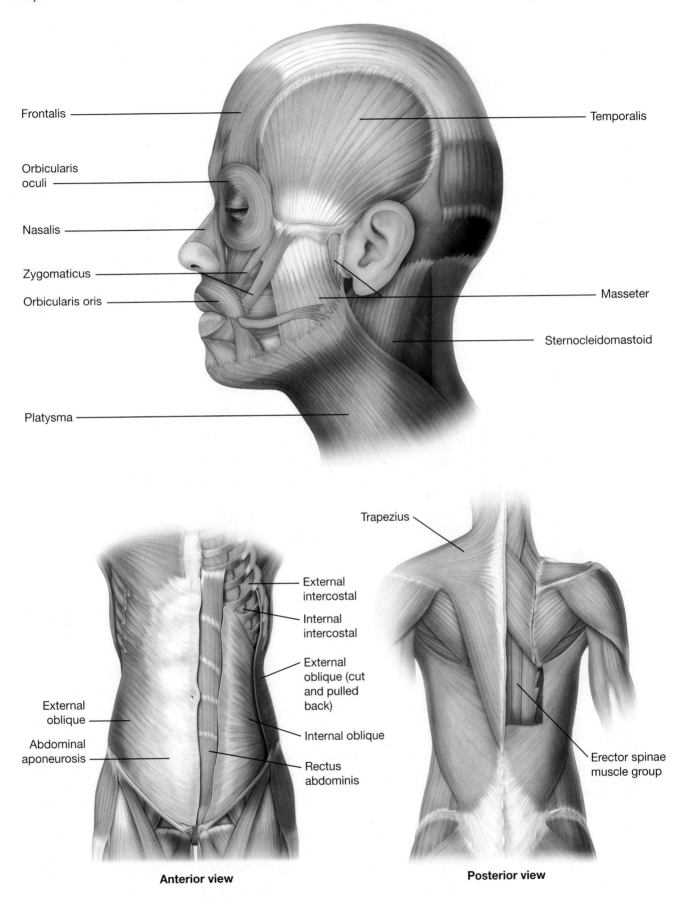

Frontalis

Orbicularis oculi

Nasalis

Zygomaticus

Orbicularis oris

Platysma

Temporalis

Masseter

Sternocleidomastoid

Trapezius

External intercostal

Internal intercostal

External oblique (cut and pulled back)

Internal oblique

Rectus abdominis

External oblique

Abdominal aponeurosis

Erector spinae muscle group

Anterior view

Posterior view

Figure 9.26   Skeletal muscles of the head and torso.

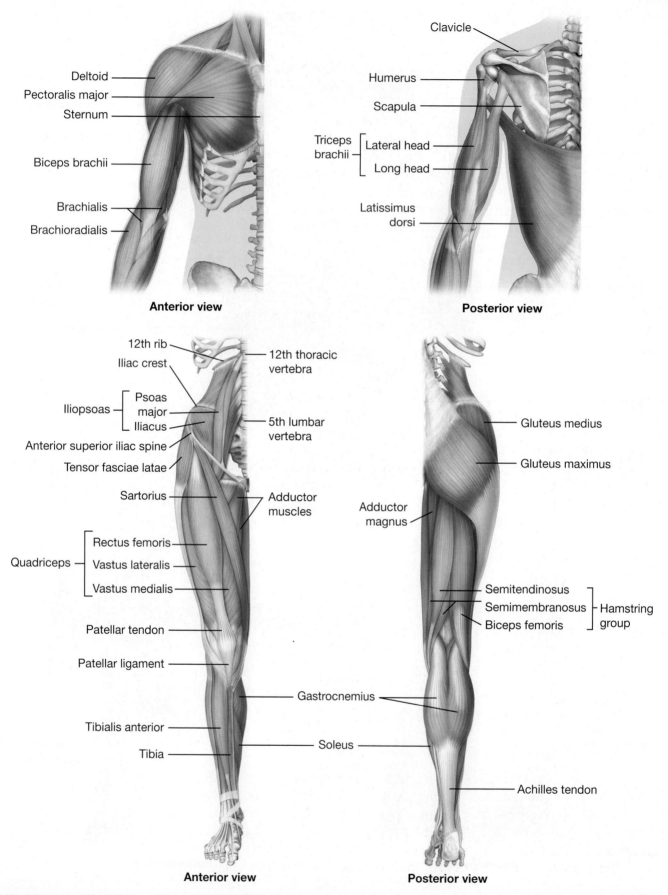

Deltoid
Pectoralis major
Sternum

Biceps brachii

Brachialis
Brachioradialis

Anterior view

Clavicle

Humerus

Scapula

Triceps
brachii — Lateral head

Long head

Latissimus
dorsi

Posterior view

12th rib
Iliac crest

12th thoracic
vertebra

Iliopsoas — Psoas
major
Iliacus

5th lumbar
vertebra

Anterior superior iliac spine
Tensor fasciae latae

Sartorius

Adductor
muscles

Quadriceps — Rectus femoris

Vastus lateralis

Vastus medialis

Patellar tendon

Patellar ligament

Gastrocnemius

Tibialis anterior

Soleus

Tibia

Anterior view

Gluteus medius

Gluteus maximus

Adductor
magnus

Semitendinosus
Semimembranosus — Hamstring
group
Biceps femoris

Gastrocnemius

Soleus

Achilles tendon

Posterior view

Figure 9.27   Skeletal muscles of the arms and legs.

Movement. All muscles contract when they are stimulated, then return to their original size and shape when they relax. Muscles depend on this stimulation. Just as bones are shaped by the forces placed on them, muscles also remodel to fit their tasks. The more a muscle is used, or *stimulated*, the stronger and larger it grows, like the muscles of a bodybuilder. In contrast, a muscle that is not used will shrink, or *atrophy* [*a* = without, *trophy* = development].

A nerve and blood vessel accompany each muscle. The nerve carries electrical impulses from the brain to stimulate the muscle and cause it to move. The blood vessel brings the muscle protein and other nutrients needed for growth and energy and carries away waste products. If a muscle loses the nerve connection that provides its stimulus or the blood supply that carries its nutrients, the muscle will atrophy within a few months.

Muscles are also described as *striated* or *smooth*. Both cardiac and skeletal muscle are called **striated** muscle because their protein fibers are arranged in a striped pattern. Visceral muscle is sometimes called *smooth muscle* because it does not have a striped appearance when viewed under a microscope. Striated muscle produces a single, short, "twitch" contraction, like the beating of the heart. Smooth muscle gives a long, sustained contraction when it is stimulated. Skeletal muscle is capable of both sustained and twitch contractions.

Control. The source of control for muscle contractions varies. Both cardiac and smooth muscle are *involuntary*. This means they respond to signals from the nervous and endocrine systems, but we cannot consciously control them. These muscles are always working, even when we are asleep. In contrast, skeletal muscles are *voluntary* and under our conscious control, unless excited by a "reflex." Some voluntary muscle movements have been practiced for such a long time that they become automatic and seem to occur without thought. We are able to decide and choose to move the muscles attached to our bones, but not the muscle that makes up our heart or the insides of our organs and blood vessels.

Control of skeletal muscles develops in an organized pattern. The body contains more than 600 skeletal muscles, which account for about half of our body weight. As children develop, they first learn to control their large motor muscles, and then they gain fine motor skills. This control develops from the head down and from the center of the body outward. Babies will hold up their head and control the muscles used to eat before they learn to coordinate the muscles used for speech. Babies will reach with their arms before learning to grasp with their hands, and they will later learn the finger coordination necessary to write. They will also sit before standing and walk before skipping or riding a bike. After about 30 years of age, the amount, size, and tone of muscle tissues begin to decrease again, resulting in a gradual loss of strength.

Disease and Injury. *Muscular dystrophy* [*dys* = bad, *trophy* = development] is the name for a group of diseases that cause atrophy and weakness in skeletal muscles (Figure 9.28 on the next page). Some forms of muscular dystrophy are caused by a defect in the structural protein—collagen—that gives muscles their strength. These diseases are more common in young males than females. Many forms also affect cardiac muscles, which may result in an early death. Muscular dystrophy is treated with physical therapy, but there is no cure.

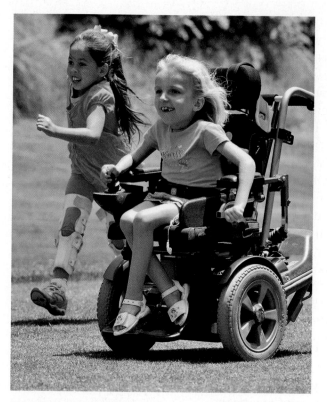

Figure 9.28 Muscular dystrophy can occur in childhood or adulthood. The disease often requires that a person use a wheelchair.

Muscle injury, which is often due to overexertion, repetitive movement, or sudden movement, is more common than muscle disease. Tendinitis is an inflammation of the tendon due to stretching, stress, or repeated friction that irritates either the lining of the sheath enclosing the tendon or the tendon itself. This condition may cause pain, swelling, and reduced range of motion. Treatment usually includes eliminating the cause to prevent recurrence.

Muscle strain can cause a moderate amount of damage to a muscle or tendon. The symptoms of tenderness and swelling are treated with *RICE*—an acronym that means *Rest, Ice, Compression,* and *Elevation*. Muscle tears are more severe than strains and can include detachment from the bone. Surgery may be required to repair these injuries. Collagen is generated first after an injury, and then myofibers are regenerated to rebuild the muscle. Understanding how muscles are structured and how they work is important to understanding muscular disorders.

Muscle Shape and Attachment

Muscles have a "belly" in the middle and tendons at the ends. The belly is the meaty bulk of muscle tissue that can be felt when muscle contractions occur. It is made from muscle fibers gathered together in **fascicles**, or *bundles* (Figure 9.29). Fascicles are wrapped with perimysium (pair-uh-MIHZ-ee-uhm) [*peri* = around, *my* = muscle, *ium* = structure], a thin layer of collagen-based connective tissue. Epimysium [*epi* = upon] surrounds groups of fascicles. These connective tissues extend beyond the muscle belly into cordlike tendons at the ends to attach the muscle to bone.

Tendons have less bulk than muscle fibers, but their collagen base makes them very strong. They attach skeletal muscles to the periosteum that covers bones. Some of the best-known tendons are those of the ankle and wrist. The large Achilles tendon on the back of the lower leg attaches the *soleus* and *gastrocnemius* (gas-trahk-NEE-mee-uhs) muscles to the heel (see Figure 9.27). Many separate tendons in the lower arm attach to muscles for the fingers. These tendons pass through a tunnel in the wrist bones. Carpal tunnel syndrome is a painful inflammation that squeezes the tendons, blood vessels, and nerves in the wrist. This interrupts the movement of tendons and muscles, as well as their nerve connection and blood supply.

Differently shaped muscles have different attachments. Muscle fibers form striation lines that point to the muscle attachments and show the direction in which the muscle will move. Strap muscles are long and narrow with parallel muscle fibers, like the *sartorius* in the thigh. They have small tendon attachment sites at both ends. Round muscles, or

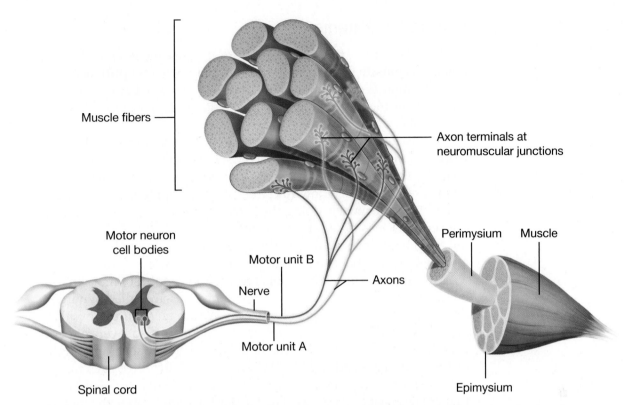

Figure 9.29   A fascicle is a bundle of muscle fibers wrapped with perimysium. The epimysium encloses a group of fascicles.

sphincters, such as the *orbicularis oculi* (or-bihk-yuh-LAIR-uhs AHK-yuh-lI) of the eye, have many short attachments around their outer edge, forming a circle that pull together to close an opening.

Convergent muscles are fan-shaped, with the muscle bundles spread over a broad attachment area on one end and coming to a point on the other end. This allows muscles like the *pectoralis major* to produce motion in different directions by contracting different portions of the muscle set. Muscle fibers in pennate muscles, such as the *biceps brachii* are parallel, but they attach to their tendons at an angle and have larger attachment sites. This allows more muscle fibers to attach for more power than strap muscles. Compare the shape and attachments of the long, thin *sartorius* with the large, fan-shaped *gluteus maximus.* Which muscle do you think is more powerful? Why?

Each muscle must have at least two points of attachment and must cross at least one joint to create movement. These muscle attachments are identified as the *point of origin* and the *point of insertion.* The point of origin is on the stationary bone. The point of insertion is on the bone that moves. For example, when you contract the *biceps brachii,* the humerus in the upper arm remains still and the radius in the lower arm moves toward it. The point of origin for the *biceps brachii* is the attachment at the humerus, the point of insertion is the attachment on the radius, and the muscle crosses over the elbow joint to flex the arm. You can predict this direction of movement by following the direction of the muscle striations.

Muscle Movements

Muscles always pull and get shorter to cause movement; they never push. The muscle fibers contain protein filaments that pull together during a muscle contraction. This makes the muscle belly shorter and wider. After the contraction is complete, the muscle relaxes back to its normal shape.

If muscles always pull, then how do our joints unbend? Our muscles work together in opposing pairs to create movement and maintain posture. The biceps and triceps are an opposing muscle pair: the biceps bends the arm at the elbow, and the triceps straightens it. In concentric contraction, the muscle doing the work is called the *agonist*, while the relaxed muscle is called the *antagonist*. Notice that the skeletal muscles of the trunk and limbs always maintain a partly contracted state known as **muscle tone** that helps maintain the body's balance.

Most of our body movements require the support of more than one muscle. These functional groups of muscles are called **synergists**. The body has several layers of muscles. We are most familiar with the superficial muscles near the surface, but there are also layers of deep muscles below this, closer to the bone. Each layer attaches at a slightly different angle to add stability. When they pull together, each muscle gets some help from the other muscles in the group. This work uses energy that creates heat in the body. The harder the body works, the more energy is used and the more heat is created. For example, the body burns about 200 calories per hour walking but about 500 calories per hour running. You need to burn about 3,500 calories of energy to work off a pound of body weight.

Joint movements are most easily understood as pairs of opposing actions (Figure 9.30). **Flexion** [*flex* = bend] moves a ventral surface toward a ventral surface, decreasing the angle of the joint. **Extension** [*ex* = out, beyond, *tens* = stretch] moves a dorsal surface toward a dorsal surface and increases the angle of the ventral surfaces of a joint. Hyperflexion and hyperextension [*hyper* = more than normal, excessive] continue these movements beyond normal anatomical position, sometimes through the use of force, and can add stress to the joint. **Abduction** [*ab* = away, *duct* = to lead] moves a limb laterally away from the side of the body, while **adduction** [*ad* = to, toward] returns a limb to the side of the body. These movements can be seen with the arms, legs, fingers, and toes.

Ball-and-socket joints are capable of the greatest range of motion. In addition to flexion, extension, abduction, and adduction, they can also rotate and circumduct. **Rotation** means turning on an axis. The limb does not bend during this movement, but performs more of a twisting motion. **Circumduction** is a motion that makes circles rather than twisting. This increased range of motion in a joint means less stability is provided by the bone structure, so these joints use more muscle to return stability to the joint.

Muscles and tendons must be flexible to work well together. Heavy exercise or lack of use can cause a muscle to become tight and stiff. At that point, sudden movement can tear the muscle or tendon. Warm-up and cool-down stretches help to avoid this problem, and the elasticity of muscles allows them to return to their original shape after stretching. Contractures are a permanent shortening of muscles and tendons that

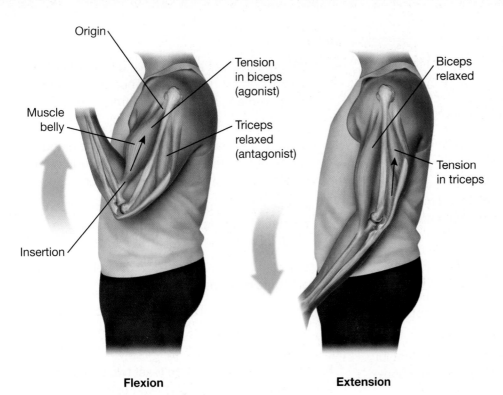

Figure 9.30   Flexion and extension, shown here, make up one pair of opposing actions that result in joint movement.

Flexion   **Extension**

can develop from lack of movement. Range-of-motion (ROM) exercises that move the joint to its fullest extent are important for those who are immobile.

The Logic of Muscle Names

Not all muscle names are easy to remember or pronounce, but they make sense when you apply a few simple rules. Many muscle names indicate their action, structure, location, shape, or size. The adductor *longus* is a *long* muscle in the thigh that brings the leg toward the body. The *extensor* digitorum *straightens* and *extends* the fingers. The *inter*costals run *between* the ribs. The *tibialis* anterior is located on the front of the *tibia*. The *triceps* brachii has *three* attachments on the upper arm. The *deltoid* is a *triangular* shape. The gluteus *maximus* is a *large* muscle. When faced with a muscle name you don't know, look for descriptive words, directional terms, bone names, and words referring to muscle actions. These clues will help you find, understand, and remember muscle names.

RECALL YOUR READING

1. The three types of muscle are _____, _____, and _____.
2. The body contains over 600 _____ muscles, which account for about half our body weight.
3. To create movement, muscles _____ at two or more points and cross at least one _____.
4. _____ and _____ muscles pull in opposite directions.

Complete the *Map Your Reading* graphic organizer for the section you just read.

Chapter 9 Review

SUMMARY

Assess your understanding with chapter tests

- As you read an assignment, highlight the main ideas and take notes to gather the most important information. Review the information often to get the most from your reading.

- There are many styles you can use for taking notes and organizing your thoughts.

- The collagen in connective tissue is important for the integumentary, skeletal, and muscular systems. It helps provide structure and support for the body.

- The integumentary system, or *skin*, has three layers that cover the body. The structures of the skin provide protection, maintain body temperature, produce and store nutrients, and get rid of body waste.

- Observing changes in the skin is important for detecting many different disorders of the body.

- Our bones ossify and fuse together from about 300 soft and separated bones that are mostly cartilage at birth to about 206 hard calcified bones in adulthood.

- The two sections of the skeleton show the different roles of bones. Axial bones are for protection while appendicular bones are for support and movement.

- Different parts of a bone have different functions such as providing storage of nutrients, support for movement, and protection from injury.

- The shape and structure of long bones, short bones, flat bones, irregular bones, and sesamoid bones are all used in different ways to create movement and provide support.

- At the joints, ligaments connect bone to bone for stability and tendons connect muscle to bone for movement.

- Different types of joints allow different types and amounts of movement.

- The three types of muscle—cardiac, smooth, and skeletal—each have a different structure and purpose.

- Muscles always have at least two points of attachment and cross at least one joint to create movement.

- Agonist and antagonist muscles pull in opposite directions to create muscle tone, movement, and maintain posture. Synergistic muscle groups work together.

- Muscle names describe the action, structure, location, shape, or size of each muscle.

MAXIMIZE YOUR PROFESSIONAL VOCABULARY

Build vocabulary with e-flash cards, games, and audio glossary

Listed below are the essential, yellow-highlighted terms and the additional professional vocabulary that you encountered in this chapter. Complete the activities that follow the list to make all of these terms part of your everyday professional vocabulary.

abduction	compact bone	flexion
adduction	condylar	fontanel
appendicular skeleton	dermis	foramen
axial skeleton	diaphysis	fracture
ball-and-socket joint	epidermis	hair follicle
cardiac muscle	epiphysis	hinge joint
cartilage	extension	hypodermis
circumduction	fascicle	integumentary
collagen	flat bone	irregular bone

ligament

long bone

melanin

muscle tone

nail bed

orthopedic surgeon

ossification

osteoblast

osteoclast

osteoporosis

pigment

prostheses

root

rotation

sebaceous gland

short bone

skeletal muscle

smooth muscle

spongy bone

striated

subcutaneous fat

sudoriferous gland

sutured

synergist

tendon

VOCABULARY DEVELOPMENT

Matching. Match each essential term from this chapter with the correct definition below by writing the letter of the description next to the number of the essential term on a separate sheet of paper.

1. appendicular skeleton
2. axial skeleton
3. cardiac muscle
4. collagen
5. dermis
6. epidermis
7. hypodermis
8. integumentary
9. ligament
10. skeletal muscle
11. smooth muscle
12. tendon

a. a protein fiber that connects, supports, and gives strength to body tissues such as the skin, muscle tendons, and bone ligaments

b. an involuntary muscle located in the body's visceral organs and blood vessels; also known as *visceral muscle*

c. related to the skin

d. the innermost layer of the skin, which stores fat

e. term that applies to the skull, spine, and rib cage, which rotate around an imaginary center line of the body

f. a tough, fibrous tissue that connects muscles to bones

g. the middle layer of the skin, which contains most of the skin's structures

h. a voluntary, striated muscle that connects to bones and is responsible for movement

i. an involuntary, striated muscle tissue located in the walls of the heart

j. the thin, outer layer of the skin

k. a tough, fibrous tissue that connects bones to other bones and holds organs in place

l. term that describes the bones of the arms and legs, including the shoulder and hip bones where they are attached

13. Term Snap. Make flash cards for each word part listed in the table on the next page. Sit in circles of 3 to 5 students and shuffle your cards, keeping them all facing in the same direction. The first player turns over a term card to reveal the definition and places it in the center, "term side" facing up. Other players go around the circle, taking turns to discard one card at a time with the definition side facing up.

When the definition matching the term card in the center of the circle is discarded, the first to notice must slap the matching card. That player takes all the cards in the middle and draws the next term card. Play continues until the time is up or players run out of cards. The player with the most term cards at the end of play is the winner.

Medical Word Parts

Prefixes		Root Words			Suffixes	
a-	ex-	arthr/o	integument/o	ped/o	-ary	-ium
ab-	hyper-	coll/a	lig/a	por/o	-ate	-osis
ad-	sub-	cry/o	melan/o	strict/o	-ation	-ous
amphi-	syn-	cutane/o	my/o	tens/i	-fic	-plasia
con-		derm/o, dermat/o	orth/o	vas/o	-gen, -genesis	-plasty
de-		duct/o	osse/o, oste/o		-in	-scopy
dia-		flex/o	path/o		-is	-trophy
dys-		hydr/o	pector/o		-it is	

REFLECT ON YOUR READING

14. Revisit the answers you gave for the *Connect with Your Reading* activity. Share one of the *text to self*, *text to text*, or *text to world* connections you made to your reading. Discuss how your reading of the chapter deepened, strengthened, or made you rethink your understanding of one of the connections you made.

BUILD CORE SKILLS

15. **Listening.** Watch the narrated bones review on *The Virtual Body* at the MEDtropolis website. According to this video, how is calcium from bones used in the body? How are vitamins used by the skeletal system?

16. **Writing.** Find the human skeleton on the *E-Skeletons* website. View the skull from the posterior angle. Draw the suture lines as shown and describe them.

17. **Math.** Suppose you are a doctor. You have a male patient who is 19 years of age and weighs 170 pounds (77 kg). He slipped and fell onto a hot grill with his arms outstretched, resulting in second-degree burns down the back of both his arms and on his face. Use the rule of nines in Figure 9.12 and the Parkland Formula below to calculate how much fluid to give him to prevent dehydration from his wounds.

V (fluid volume) = % TBSA (% total body surface area) × body weight (kg) × 4 mL

18. **Math.** Examine Figure 9.15, which shows bone mass density and osteoporosis risk by age, gender, and ethnicity. Use the graph to answer the following questions:
    a. Who is at the lowest risk for osteoporosis?
    b. At what age does risk of fracture begin?
    c. Approximately how many years sooner would you expect a white woman to develop osteoporosis than a black woman?

19. **Critical Thinking.** Combine what you learned about the skin layers with what you learned about burns to explain why a third- or fourth-degree burn is more likely to cause dehydration and infection than a first- or second-degree burn.

20. **Writing.** Imagine that you are a bone. Write a love note to a muscle, telling it why you love it and how empty your life would be without it. Alternatively, imagine that you are a muscle. Write a thank-you note to a bone, explaining why you appreciate it and how your life has been improved by its existence.

ACTIVATE YOUR LEARNING

21. Make a model of a pair of opposing muscles using four wooden craft sticks, two pieces of duct tape, and four clumps of clay. Tape two of the wooden sticks together, end to end, to represent bones at a joint that is able to bend. Then follow the steps listed here:

    Step 1—making a muscle

    - Roll a gumball-sized piece of clay into a ball. Then roll the clay ball between your palms to form a short tube of clay that looks like a AA battery.

    - Press on one end of the tube and roll to form a carrot-shaped "tendon" on the end. Repeat this process on the other side so it becomes a "strap-shaped muscle." The thick middle represents the "belly" of the muscle. Attach one end of this muscle to one of the wooden sticks and the other end to another, crossing over the joint.

    - Examine your own arm and consider where the belly of each muscle is in order to avoid excess bulk at the joint.

    Step 2—making an opposing muscle

    - Roll another ball of clay. Apply pressure to just one side to make a teardrop shape. Roll a carrot-shape to make a "tendon" on one end. Flatten the teardrop to make a "fleshy attachment." Press the fleshy attachment to the backside of one wooden stick from step 1. Press the tendon end to the other wooden stick, crossing over the joint.

    - From what you know of different types of muscle attachments, which of these two muscle types would you expect to do more work—the tendinous attachment or the fleshy attachment?

    Step 3—showing muscles in resting and working positions

    - Repeat this process to make a second set of muscles.

    - Now, modify the muscle shapes to show the muscle shapes when the joint is flexed instead of at rest.

    - Examine your own arm as you flex and relax your muscles. Compare the difference between the two muscle sets in each position, flexed and relaxed.

22. Collect your fingerprints by rubbing pencil lead onto a scrap of paper, then rubbing each finger over the penciled area, pressing each pencil-soiled finger onto a piece of cellophane tape, and taping it down to a piece of paper. Label each print as the type of fingerprint it is—arch, whorl, or loop. Compare your own prints to each other, then compare them to other students' prints and answer the questions listed here.

    - Are the prints the same on both hands?

    - Which pattern is most common?

    - Which pattern is least common?

    - How might this information be important to an investigator?

THINK AND ACT LIKE A HEALTHCARE WORKER

23. Imagine you are a dermatologist. Your 15-year-old patient has neglected his skin care and has severe acne. You are concerned that he will not follow the recommended treatment plan and is just looking for an easy solution. Your treatment will include washing the face with a medicated soap twice a day, applying a medicated cream, and avoiding contact with the pimples. How will you tactfully explain the treatment program and the importance of washing your face twice a day?

GO TO THE SOURCE

24. Search the Internet for "Gray's Anatomy classification of joints." Print the section on synarthroses and the four varieties. Begin by surveying the section you printed. The purpose for your reading is to compare features of synarthroses as immovable joints. Create a question to guide your reading. Underline main ideas and circle key terms as you read. Take notes in Cornell style. On the left side of your notes, compare this passage to chapter 9's information on joint classifications. In the summary section of your notes, state what you learned in your own words.

Unit 3

Diagnostic

While studying, look for the online icon to:
- **Listen** to the audio Glossary and review e-flash cards
- **Assess** learning with quizzes and online exercises
- **Expand** knowledge with animations and activities
- **Simulate** healthcare tasks and employability skills

Companion
G-W Learning

www.g-wlearning.com/healthsciences

Mobile
G-W Learning

Study on the Go
Use your mobile device to practice vocabulary and assess learning
www.m.g-wlearning.com

Career Pathway

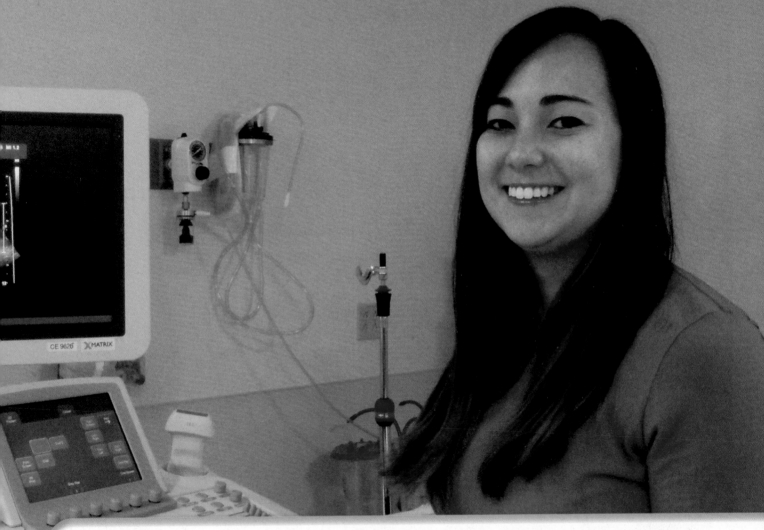

Healthcare Insider:

Mindy, BS, ARDMS (ABD, OB/GYN, RVT)
Ultrasonographer

"I chose sonography as a career because I like anatomy, physiology, pathology, and imaging. As an ultrasonographer, I take images for the radiologist using an ultrasound scanner. I also find the pathology that goes along with each patient's signs and symptoms. I enjoy sonography because I have direct patient contact every day, but every interaction is different. I have to be creative when taking images for the radiologist, making sure they include all the information the radiologist needs to make a diagnosis. I am able to work independently as well as with a team of other sonographers and radiologists."

Chapter 10
Career Skills in Diagnostic Services

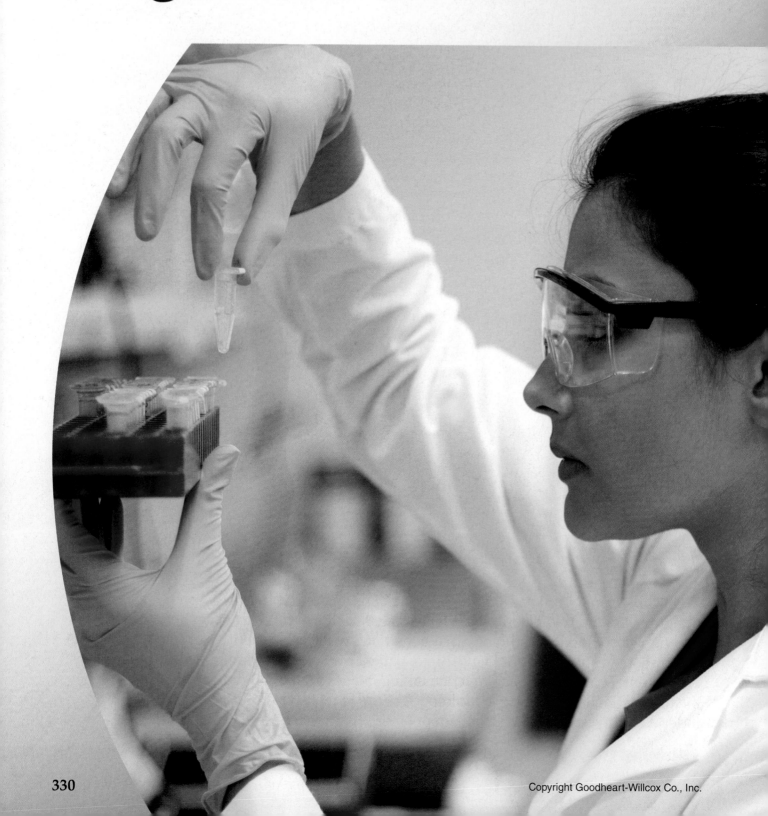

PROFESSIONAL VOCABULARY

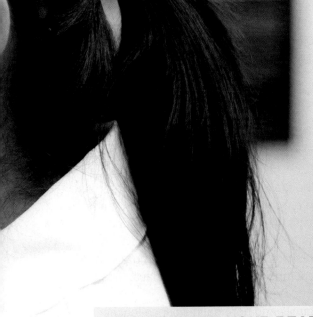

E-flash
Cards

You will need to learn the essential terms listed below before you begin your reading. These terms will help you understand the main concepts of the chapter. These terms, which will be highlighted in yellow within the text, will become part of your professional vocabulary.

In addition to these essential terms, you will see bold terms throughout the chapter. The meanings of these terms are explained where the terms first appear. The bold terms, like the essential terms listed here, will become part of your professional vocabulary and deepen your understanding of the topics presented.

body alignment   term used to describe a position of the body in which the spine is not crooked or twisted

diagnostic   pertaining to the identification of a disease or syndrome

discretion   the ability to know when to keep sensitive information private

first aid   emergency treatment given before regular medical services can be obtained

gross pay   the total amount of money earned in a pay period

incompetence   a lack of qualifications or ability to perform job tasks

integrity   adherence to ethical principles and professional standards

invasive procedure   a test or treatment that requires incisions to the skin or the insertion of instruments or other materials into the body

net pay   the amount of money received in a pay period after all deductions have been taken out; also known as *take-home pay*

noninvasive procedure   a test or treatment that does not require incisions to the skin or the insertion of instruments or other materials into the body

radiographers   healthcare professionals who create medical images or treat diseases by passing radiation, such as X-rays or gamma rays, through an object

sonographers   healthcare professionals who create medical images or treat diseases through the use of high-frequency sound waves

vital signs   the key measurements that provide information about a person's health, including temperature, pulse, respiration, and blood pressure

CONNECT WITH YOUR READING

Think of a time when you or someone you know was injured, such as a car accident or an athletic injury. Which healthcare professionals helped to figure out or diagnose the damage? Patients meet some diagnostic healthcare workers but never even see others who play a part in their diagnosis. Can you identify diagnostic workers who are unseen as well as those who are seen by patients?

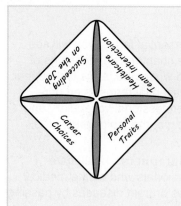

MAP YOUR READING

Create a visual summary of this chapter, just as you did in chapter 2. Begin with a square sheet of paper—an 8½-inch square works well. Fold each of the four points of the square to the center. Label each of the four resulting flaps with one of these topics: *Personal Traits*, *Career Choices*, *Healthcare Team Interaction*, and *Succeeding on the Job*. When you finish reading each of these sections in the chapter, open the corresponding flap and draw a picture or symbol to illustrate what you have read. Ask yourself what each topic looks like, how you could draw it, and what graphic or symbol best represents it. Finally, for each of the four topics, write two words that explain how the topic relates to you personally in the center square of your visual summary.

Unlike doctors, nurses, or other therapeutic workers, those who work in the diagnostic services career pathway are often unseen. These behind-the-scenes workers help determine diagnoses through clinical tests and medical imaging. Diagnostic workers often interact with machines more than they interact with patients. If you're interested in the technology and equipment involved in the healthcare field, the diagnostic services pathway may be the right choice for you.

This chapter illustrates the important role that diagnostic healthcare workers perform in clinical laboratory and imaging careers. You will learn about healthcare opportunities in vision- and hearing-related careers, and see how some healthcare workers complete both diagnostic and therapeutic tasks. You will also learn how healthcare team members interact to share patient care tasks and information while protecting patient privacy. This chapter also discusses the value of building positive team relationships. In this chapter, you will find multiple opportunities for expanding your technical skills through measuring vital signs, providing emergency care, and performing vision and hearing screening tests.

The Diagnostic Worker: Briana

Briana always knew that she wanted to work in healthcare, specifically as a nurse. She signed up for challenging science and math classes, and she took all of the health science courses available to her until it was time to register for a nursing assistant class. Briana wanted to help people, and her aunt always talked positively about her own nursing career. However, the more Briana thought about the nursing assistant class, the more uncertain she became.

She shared her concerns with her family and her health science teacher. They had observed her preference for working in an organized environment with a predictable schedule. Since she enjoyed her science lab classes, Briana's health science teacher suggested medical laboratory careers. Briana did some research and met with her guidance counselor to learn more about college programs in her state. She decided not to take the nursing assistant course and went on to major in clinical laboratory science in college.

The more courses Briana completed in college, the more convinced she became that medical technology was the career for her. She even noticed that other students in her courses seemed to be a lot like her in terms of their interests and aptitudes. When asked how she found such a good career match for herself, she would say that she just sort of fell into it. However, the reality is that Briana took some important steps to find a good career fit. Instead of sticking to her first health career choice, she paid attention to her own uncertain feelings about nursing. She talked to people who knew her well to get their advice. She took the time to research careers with an open mind, and it paid off.

Today Briana is a medical technologist at a major research hospital. She has met her goal of helping people, but she does this by analyzing laboratory findings that lead to the detection and diagnosis of disease rather than by interacting directly with patients. Briana is a diagnostic healthcare worker.

Personal Traits

Do you enjoy working with equipment? Are you interested in operating machines? **Diagnostic** workers are experts in using machines to create the best possible images so that a correct diagnosis can be made (Figure 10.1). Mechanical aptitude is an asset for this career pathway.

Diagnostic workers follow detailed instructions to complete laboratory tests and record and organize data in precise ways. They must be accurate and reliable, and must remain calm and focused in stressful situations.

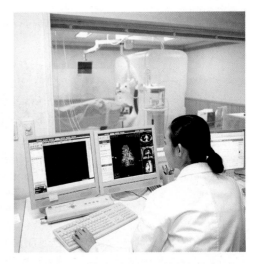

Figure 10.1   Diagnostic workers use equipment such as this MRI machine to provide images that will lead to a diagnosis.

diagnostic
pertaining to the identification of a disease or syndrome

The Diagnostic Worker: Jack

It was a busy day in the lab. Jack was labeling blood specimens in preparation for testing when he was interrupted by a question from a fellow worker. When he turned back to the labels, Jack couldn't remember which specimen belonged to which patient. Now he had to contact both patients and have them return to the clinic to leave a second specimen. As you can imagine, they weren't pleased. However, a correct diagnosis relies on the accuracy of the diagnostic test.

Being willing to admit your mistakes and correct your errors demonstrates honesty and **integrity**. Workers with integrity do what is right even when they think no one will notice. Honest healthcare workers earn the trust and respect of their patients and fellow workers.

Workers with a realistic, "doer" personality can perform repeat procedures with a high degree of accuracy, which can be an asset in the diagnostic field. However, as diagnostic tests become more computerized, the role of the diagnostic worker is becoming more analytical, which means it involves more thinking and reasoning. Workers with an

integrity
adherence to ethical principles and professional standards

investigative, "thinker" personality will enjoy the problem-solving parts of diagnostic work. This might involve asking questions, such as: *How can I position this car accident victim to get the clearest image without causing further injury? If I arrange the images in a specific order, will the physician be able to examine the characteristics of the entire tumor? How can I organize the data to make the results easier to read and interpret?*

When diagnostic workers interact with patients, they should demonstrate a pleasant and relaxed manner. Patients may be in pain or worried about what the results of their test might reveal. Workers need to be articulate (ar-TIHK-yuh-leht), or able to communicate clearly and effectively, so they can explain the test and answer the patient's questions about it. These workers must also show **discretion** by not revealing information that is outside their scope of practice.

discretion
the ability to know when to keep sensitive information private

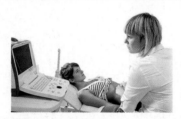

The Diagnostic Worker: Mital

Mital performed an ultrasound for a patient with a suspected miscarriage. She was careful to turn the screen away from her patient. She spoke calmly to the patient but did not reveal what was shown on the screen. The ultrasound technician does not diagnose; that is the job of the physician. Mital provided information about how soon the results would be sent to the patient's physician and encouraged the woman to contact her doctor.

Many diagnostic careers require physical **stamina**, or *endurance*. Diagnostic workers may be on their feet operating equipment for the entire workday. They may also need to lift and position patients for imaging tests or be required to transport heavy equipment to a patient to complete a test.

The diagnostic worker must be committed to lifelong learning because technology is always advancing. Diagnostic workers learn to use automated equipment and computerized instruments capable of performing a number of tests simultaneously. They may specialize in the fast-growing fields of microbiology, immunology, and molecular biology. In addition to traditional X-ray radiography, diagnostic workers who specialize in medical imaging may learn ultrasonography (uhl-trah-sah-NAHG-rah-fee), magnetic resonance imaging (MRI), computed tomography (toh-MAHG-ruh-fee), or other specialized imaging techniques (Figure 10.2).

Figure 10.2 Computed tomography (CT) is just one type of imaging technology with which diagnostic workers may be familiar. What are some other types of imaging technology?

Diagnostic Career Choices

Diagnostic workers create a picture of a patient's health status at a single point in time by using a variety of tests and imaging techniques.

They may evaluate diseases for genetic links or analyze laboratory findings. Some diagnostic workers administer radiation intravenously, while others examine microscopic tissue samples for abnormalities.

Clinical laboratory workers perform diagnostic laboratory testing. These tests play an important role in medical care. They are often the least expensive healthcare procedures, but they influence more than 70 percent of healthcare decisions. They provide objective information that is used for many purposes. Test results can assess a patient's risk of developing a disease, monitor the course of a disease, or measure a patient's response to medical treatment.

Medical imaging professionals are important to the healthcare industry because the images they obtain help doctors to diagnose health issues. Medical imaging professionals work with a variety of diagnostic imaging procedures and technologies. In addition to requiring knowledge of medical equipment and technology, these jobs may include direct contact with patients. Therefore, medical imaging professionals must be caring and empathetic to patients' needs. Figure 10.3 shows how clinical

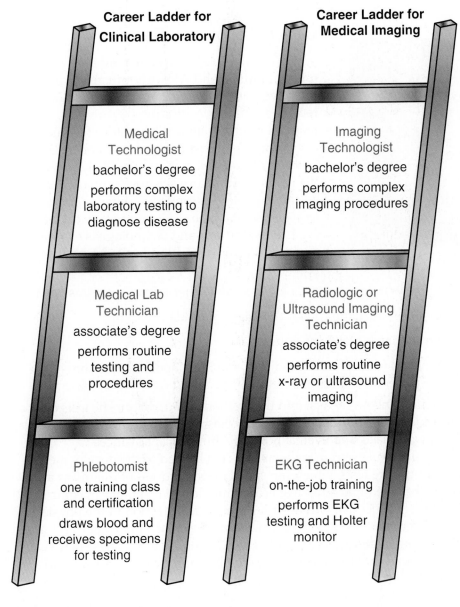

Career Ladder for Clinical Laboratory

Medical Technologist

bachelor's degree

performs complex laboratory testing to diagnose disease

Medical Lab Technician

associate's degree

performs routine testing and procedures

Phlebotomist

one training class and certification

draws blood and receives specimens for testing

Career Ladder for Medical Imaging

Imaging Technologist

bachelor's degree

performs complex imaging procedures

Radiologic or Ultrasound Imaging Technician

associate's degree

performs routine x-ray or ultrasound imaging

EKG Technician

on-the-job training

performs EKG testing and Holter monitor

Figure 10.3   Tests performed by diagnostic healthcare workers influence more than 70 percent of healthcare decisions. This means it's important for diagnostic workers to have the appropriate training and education for their position. Which diagnostic career interests you the most? What education and training is required for that job?

laboratory and medical imaging professionals can advance in their careers and the level of education needed for each stage.

The fields of audiology and ophthalmology use many diagnostic tests to assess changes in hearing and vision. You may have observed that several medical careers have overlapping diagnostic and therapeutic roles. For example, physicians both diagnose and treat diseases. Some technicians in the ophthalmologist's (ahf-thal-MAHL-uh-jihst) office perform tests to diagnose vision changes, while others fit eyeglasses or contact lenses to treat vision changes.

The job outlook for diagnostic workers is above average overall and excellent for some specific careers. There is currently a shortage of clinical laboratory workers. Many people don't know about these "behind-the-scenes" workers, who often don't interact directly with patients. Medical imaging professionals who are trained in more than one kind of imaging will have better job opportunities. While many diagnostic workers are employed in hospitals, employment is expected to grow rapidly in physicians' offices and other ambulatory healthcare facilities such as blood banks, dialysis centers, and medical laboratories.

Clinical Laboratory Careers

In a healthcare lab, you may meet a **phlebotomist** (fleh-BAHT-uh-mihst) or a medical assistant, both of whom can draw your blood and receive specimens for testing (Figure 10.4). You may not meet the clinical laboratory technician— also known as the *medical technician* or *medical laboratory technician*. Nor are you likely to meet the medical laboratory scientist, who may also be called a *clinical laboratory scientist*, a *medical technologist*, or a *medical laboratory technologist*.

Lab technicians and technologists examine and analyze body fluids and cells for a variety of reasons:

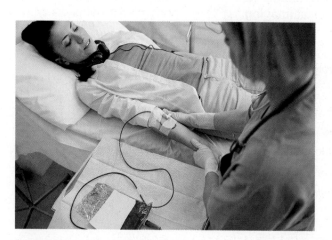

Figure 10.4   A phlebotomist is one kind of diagnostic worker who may work in a clinical laboratory. Phlebotomists draw blood for testing.

- to look for bacteria, parasites, and other microorganisms

- to analyze the chemical content of fluids

- to match blood for transfusions

- to test for levels of medication in the bloodstream to measure a patient's response to treatment

Depending on the test and the methods used, diagnostic tests can be performed at a centralized laboratory, hospital bedside, physician's office, clinic, workplace, and even at home. Technological advances have made tests easier to use and more accurate. This has led to the development of point-of-care tests, which can speed up the process of diagnosis and treatment. The rapid strep test is an example of a test that can confirm a positive streptococcal (strehp-tuh-KAHK-uhl) infection in the physician's office. Pregnancy tests, which can be purchased at a pharmacy and used at home, are another example of easier diagnostic tests. These new types of tests mean that those who choose a clinical lab career can work in a variety of settings.

Not only is progress in technology changing the way diagnostic tests are performed, it is actually causing changes in the practice of medicine. Advances based on the mapping of the human genome have led to gene-based and other molecular diagnostic tests. These tests can predict the likelihood that a patient will develop a specific disease even before symptoms appear. For example, genetic testing for specific gene mutations can indicate an individual's risk for developing breast or ovarian cancer. This allows physicians to focus on prevention or early treatment to reduce the negative effects of a disease.

Diagnostic tests that involve the molecular analysis of genes, proteins, and metabolites will lead to more personalized medical care. Doctors will be able to use test results to select the best medication in the right amount for a particular patient, thereby avoiding adverse reactions to treatment.

Public health laboratory professionals are highly educated specialists with knowledge of one or more scientific disciplines. They have advanced skills in laboratory practice, and they use their skills to solve complex problems that affect human health. When health risks emerge, public health laboratories analyze the threat, provide prevention and treatment information, and act to protect the public. These labs are found in every state and can focus on environmental health concerns as well as disease detection. Figure 10.5 shows the variety of services provided by a public health laboratory scientist.

Lab technologists use microscopes, cell counters, and other specialized laboratory equipment. Manual dexterity and normal color vision are assets for these workers. Computer skills are essential because the use of automated equipment and computerized instruments capable of performing several tests simultaneously is becoming more common. Technologists working in large laboratories often become specialists in specific testing procedures (Figure 10.6 on the next page).

Lab technicians perform less complex tests and laboratory procedures than technologists. Technicians may prepare specimens, operate automated analyzers, or perform manual tests under the supervision of

Figure 10.5 Services Provided by Public Health Laboratories	
Service	**Description**
Environmental Health	• testing drinking and some recreational water for bacteria, parasites, pesticides, and other harmful substances • testing air quality
Food Safety	• detecting foodborne illness • developing policies to limit the spread of foodborne illness
Infectious Diseases	• identifying outbreaks of infectious disease • detecting new diseases such as SARS and West Nile virus
Newborn Screening	• screening 97% of the babies born in the United States for potentially life-threatening metabolic and genetic disorders
Public Health Preparedness and Response	• rapidly identifying suspect agents, such as testing more than 1,200 specimens a day during the anthrax attacks

Figure 10.6 Areas of Specialization for Laboratory Technologists

Area of Specialization	Duties
Clinical Chemistry	prepare specimens and analyze the chemical and hormonal contents of body fluids
Microbiology	examine and identify bacteria and other microorganisms
Immunohematology (Blood Bank)	collect, type, and prepare blood and its components for transfusions
Immunology	examine elements of the human immune system and its response to foreign bodies
Cytotechnology	prepare slides of body cells and examine these cells microscopically for abnormalities that may signal the beginning of a cancerous growth
Molecular Biology	perform complex protein and nucleic acid testing on cell samples

the technologist. Because clinical laboratory workers handle infectious specimens, they must be skilled in infection control and sterilization techniques. Personal protective equipment is required for laboratory work.

Job opportunities for laboratory technicians and technologists are expected to be excellent. Technologists need a bachelor's degree in medical technology or a life science for entry-level positions. A graduate degree promotes advancement to the positions of lab supervisor, manager, or director. Technicians generally need an associate's degree from a technical or community college or a certificate from a hospital training program. Phlebotomists and medical assistants must complete technical training to receive a program certificate or diploma. Some states may require licensure for these positions and employers prefer to hire certified workers.

Medical Imaging Careers

Medical imaging has come a long way since 1895, when Wilhelm Roentgen accidentally discovered an image cast from his cathode ray generator (Figure 10.7). Today, **radiographers** perform a wide variety of imaging exams. Radiologic technicians, previously called *X-ray technicians*, perform X-ray imaging examinations (Figure 10.8 on page 340). Radiologic technologists use other methods of examination such as mammography, computed tomography (CT), and magnetic resonance imaging (MRI). Radiographers produce X-ray images, or *radiographs*, of the human body for use in diagnosing medical problems. Their duties include the following:

radiographers
healthcare professionals who create medical images or treat diseases by passing radiation, such as X-rays or gamma rays, through an object

- positioning a patient to obtain the proper projection for the body part being imaged

- aligning the X-ray beam to limit radiation exposure and using shielding techniques to prevent exposure

- selecting the correct control settings to get clear, detailed images

- working with physicians to decide if additional images need to be taken

- storing and retrieving images

Figure 10.7 Imaging Techniques

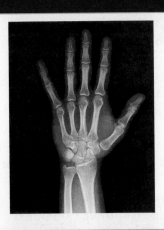

X-Ray: produces images of the structures inside your body, particularly your bones

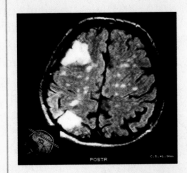

Magnetic Resonance Imaging (MRI): produces clear images of soft tissues in the body

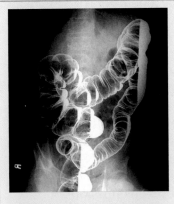

Fluoroscopy: shows a continuous X-ray image of moving body structures on a monitor, much like an X-ray movie

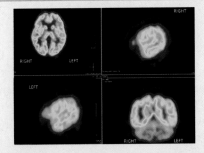

Positron Emission Tomography (PET): shows functional processes in the body and can show the development of a condition

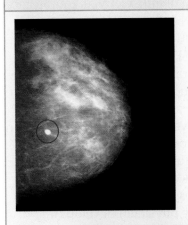

Mammography: uses a low-dose X-ray system to examine the breasts

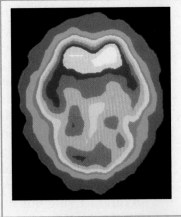

Single Photon Emission Computed Tomography (SPECT): shows how blood flows to tissues and organs

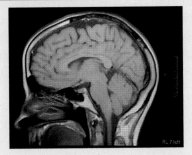

Computed Tomography (CT): uses a narrow beam of X-rays and high-powered computers to generate images of bones and soft tissues in the body

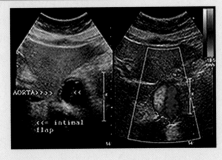

Sonography: uses sound waves to create a computerized picture

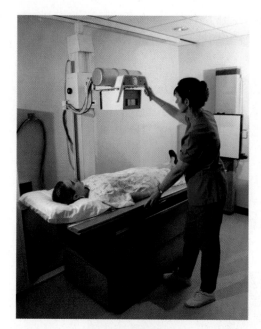

Figure 10.8 Radiographers work with medical imaging equipment. These are the diagnostic workers who take X-rays of broken bones and other internal injuries or health issues.

sonographers
healthcare professionals who create medical images or treat diseases through the use of high-frequency sound waves

Today X-ray images are captured digitally, which results in sharper images. These images can be enhanced on a computer and sent or stored electronically. This means patients can allow their images to be readily available to several caregivers.

Radiologic technologists perform more complex imaging procedures than radiologic technicians. A fluoroscopy, for example, requires the patient to drink a special solution that will result in an image that clearly shows soft tissues in the body. Technologists who specialize in mammography use low-dose X-rays to produce images of the breast to screen for abnormalities.

Specialization in computed tomography or magnetic resonance imaging is becoming more common. Computed tomography takes multiple cross-sectional X-rays. The computer processes these to produce virtual images that show what a surgeon would see during an operation. Computed tomography allows doctors to examine the inside of a patient's body without having to operate. Magnetic resonance imaging uses radio frequency to produce an image contrast.

Nuclear medicine technologists administer radioactive substances as part of the imaging process. Nuclear medicine scans can detect disease based on metabolic changes and focus on physiology, or how the body is functioning. These scans can detect tumors, aneurysms (AN-yuh-rihz-uhms), poor blood flow to tissues, and other diseases.

Two types of nuclear medicine scans are positron emission tomography (PET) and single photon emission computed tomography (SPECT). PET scans create a 3-D image of the body and can show the process of glucose metabolism in the brain. PET scans are used to detect cancer, heart problems, and brain disorders. SPECT scans create a similar image but do so through the use of different radioactive chemicals. These scans are useful for showing blood flow through the brain and help doctors diagnose brain injury.

The job of the **radiation therapist** has evolved with the advancements in radiography. Radiation therapy is a treatment procedure that projects high-energy X-rays at targeted cells to shrink and eliminate cancerous tumors.

Working as part of a medical radiation oncology team, a radiation therapist uses CT or other imaging techniques to pinpoint a tumor's location. Using this information, the oncology physician develops a treatment plan for the patient. Then the radiation therapist uses the treatment plan to position the patient and deliver the radiation treatment. The radiation therapist monitors both the physical and emotional reactions of the patient. Because cancer patients experience high levels of stress, radiation therapists must be able to maintain a positive attitude and provide emotional support.

Diagnostic medical **sonographers** use sound waves to generate an image (Figure 10.9). Sonography or ultrasonography is often associated with imaging during pregnancy, but there are many other uses for this method of medical imaging. Areas of specialty for sonographers include the following:

- abdomen—evaluation of all the soft tissues, blood vessels, and organs of the abdominal cavities such as the liver, spleen, urinary tract, and pancreas

- breast—frequently used to evaluate breast abnormalities that are found with mammography

- obstetrics/gynecology—evaluation of the female reproductive system

- echocardiography (ehk-oh-kard-ee-AHG-ruh-fee)—evaluation of the anatomy and blood flow of the heart

- vascular technology—evaluation of the blood flow in peripheral and abdominal blood vessels

- neurosonography—evaluation of the brain and spinal cord

- ophthalmology—evaluation of the eye

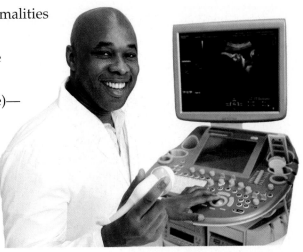

Figure 10.9 Sonographers can specialize in certain areas of the body. Why is sonography safer than radiography?

Because sonography does not involve the risk of radiation exposure, it is considered safer than imaging methods that use X-rays. However, its use is limited because it can't image through air. As a result, sonography is not used for lung or bowel imaging.

Cardiovascular technologists and technicians assist physicians in diagnosing heart and blood vessel disorders. Cardiac diagnostics may require **invasive** or **noninvasive procedures**. For example, cardiovascular technologists assist physicians with cardiac catheterization procedures, which are invasive (Figure 10.10A on the next page). During this procedure, a small tube or *catheter* is threaded through an artery from the groin to the heart. The catheter can locate blocked blood vessels and may open them using a balloon angioplasty process. Catheterization procedures can also help to locate areas of heart tissue that are causing abnormal rhythms. Cardiovascular technologists may also assist physicians during open-heart surgery or during the insertion of pacemakers or stents.

Cardiographic technicians perform electrocardiogram (EKG) tests and Holter monitor procedures. These tests measure the electrical impulses of the heart and help to detect abnormal rhythms of the heartbeat. They are noninvasive procedures (Figure 10.10B on the next page). These technicians may also perform stress tests to measure the effect of physical exertion on the function of the heart.

Electroencephalographic (ee-lehk-troh-ehn-sehf-uh-luh-GRAF-ihk) (EEG) technologists, electroneurodiagnostic (ee-lehk-troh-noo-roh-dI-ag-NAHS-tihk) (END) technologists, and polysomnographic (pahl-ee-sahm-nuh-GRAF-ihk) technologists all perform tests that measure brain activity and responses. Results of these tests can help doctors diagnose brain-related disorders such as tumors, strokes, epilepsy, and sleep disorders. All of these tests are noninvasive procedures.

Most diagnostic workers are employed in hospitals, but a growing number work in medical clinics and in medical and diagnostic laboratories. While a 40-hour workweek is typical, hospital employees commonly work overtime, evening, and weekend hours, and maintain on-call schedules.

Medical imaging technicians typically complete a technical training program through a community college or a hospital-sponsored program. Unlike other healthcare technicians, most EKG technicians are trained

invasive procedure
a test or treatment that requires incisions to the skin or the insertion of instruments or other materials into the body

noninvasive procedure
a test or treatment that does not require incisions to the skin or the insertion of instruments or other materials into the body

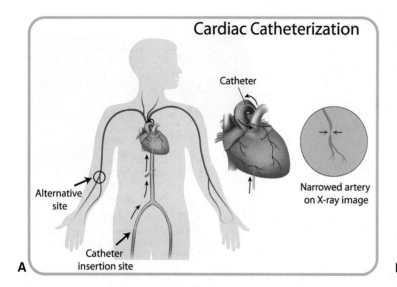

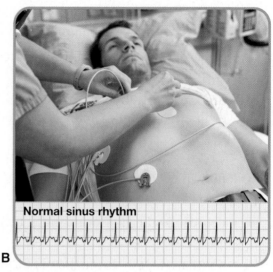

Figure 10.10   Cardiac catheterization (A) and electrocardiograms provide valuable information about the functioning of the heart. Catheterization is an invasive procedure. EKG (B) is a noninvasive procedure. What makes a procedure invasive?

on the job. Employers prefer to train workers who are already in the healthcare field, such as nursing assistants. The majority of imaging technologists complete an associate's degree, but four-year bachelor's degree programs are becoming more common.

Vision- and Hearing-Related Careers

An **ophthalmologist** is an eye specialist and an **otolaryngologist** (oh-toh-lair-uhn-GAHL-uh-jihst) is an ear specialist, but many patients never see these doctors when they have their hearing or vision checked. Routine vision testing and correction are performed in the office of an **optometrist**.

An optometrist holds a doctor of optometry (O.D.s) degree that requires a minimum of seven years of postsecondary study. Optometrists pass state and national examinations to maintain licensure. In addition to vision care, they can test for glaucoma and diagnose eye problems caused by diabetes and high blood pressure. They refer patients with eye diseases and those who need surgery to an ophthalmologist.

Optometrists, who often operate independent businesses, need business management skills and the ability to deal tactfully with patients. Job opportunities for optometrists are expected to grow rapidly, but there is tough competition for admission to the limited number of required training programs. Optometrists often employ optometric technicians so they can serve a larger number of patients. These technical jobs have a variety of titles and may have separate duties, depending on the organization of the office (Figure 10.11).

An **audiologist** works with people who have hearing and balance problems. Audiologists can identify the symptoms of hearing loss as well as related sensory and neural problems. They use audiometers (awd-ee-AHM-eh-ters) and other equipment to assess patients' hearing disorders and develop treatment plans. Treatments may include cleaning the ear canal, fitting hearing aids, and programming cochlear implants.

Audiologists also work to develop and present programs about hearing loss prevention for factory workers and students.

Audiologists complete eight years of postsecondary training and receive the doctor of audiology degree (Au.D.). Like optometrists, they are licensed and complete continuing education to learn new diagnostic and treatment technologies. While employment is expected to grow in this field, there are relatively few job openings due to the small size of this field. For instance, there are more than twice as many optometrists as compared to audiologists in the United States.

Audiologists may employ assistants who work with patients to fit hearing aids. These technicians may be called *hearing aid specialists* or *audioprosthologists* (aw-dee-oh-prahs-THAHL-oh-jihst). They generally have six months to two years of supervised training or a two-year college degree. These technicians must pass licensing tests in most states and can seek national certification.

Diagnostic services careers are worth a closer look if you enjoy working with equipment and are interested in learning about advances in technology. Whether you want to work directly with patients or prefer a laboratory setting, there are many interesting job opportunities in the diagnostic career pathway.

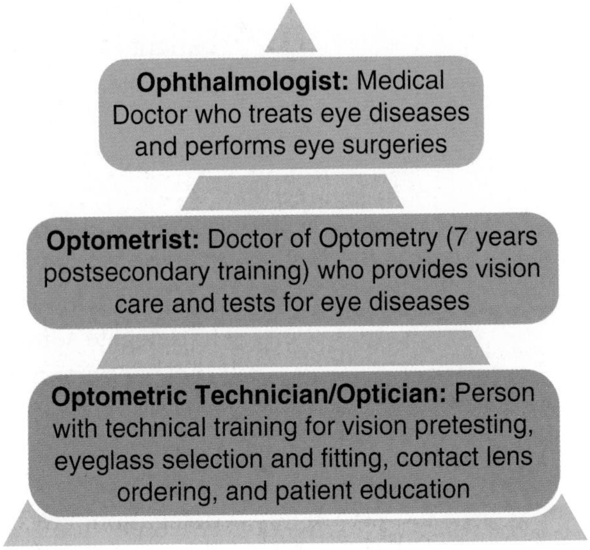

Ophthalmologist: Medical Doctor who treats eye diseases and performs eye surgeries

Optometrist: Doctor of Optometry (7 years postsecondary training) who provides vision care and tests for eye diseases

Optometric Technician/Optician: Person with technical training for vision pretesting, eyeglass selection and fitting, contact lens ordering, and patient education

Figure 10.11   The diagnostic pathway includes vision-related careers such as the ones shown here. What is the difference between an ophthalmologist and an optometrist?

RECALL YOUR READING

1. Diagnostic services workers perform laboratory tests and use _____ techniques to create a picture of the patient's _____ at a specific time.
2. Mechanical aptitude and physical _____ can lead to success in imaging careers.
3. Diagnostic workers must be _____ learners to keep pace with advancing technologies.
4. Some medical careers have overlapping _____ and _____ roles.
5. _____ storage of diagnostic images allows for quicker sharing of test results with patients and other care providers.
6. Because some healthcare workers, such as _____, operate their own businesses, they need business management skills as well as diagnostic skills.

Complete the *Map Your Reading* graphic organizer for the section you just read.

Healthcare Team Interaction

As healthcare team members work with each other, they follow a set of important guidelines for assigning tasks to each team member. This process is called **delegation**. Even the sharing of patient information follows a set of established guidelines or protocols. Following these guidelines ensures that patient care is safe and effective and protects each patient's right to confidential treatment of personal health information.

Productive relationships among team members promote high-quality patient care, and having a positive attitude at work makes your workday more pleasant and calm. Since people spend about one-third of their lives at work, learning how to build and maintain positive team relationships is worth the time and effort.

Delegating Tasks

Healthcare workers who supervise other workers may have the right to delegate some work tasks. To *delegate* means to give permission for another person to complete a specific task for you. For example, licensed nurses (RNs or LPNs) may delegate tasks to nursing assistants or medical assistants. Physicians may delegate tasks to physician assistants or nurse practitioners. State laws and facility policies guide the practice of delegation. Physicians and nurses have the authority to delegate tasks, but they are still responsible for the quality of patient care.

A worker's scope of practice always determines which tasks are delegated (Figure 10.12). If a nurse delegates a task that the nursing assistant is not qualified to perform and fails to supervise the assistant, the nurse is liable if the patient is harmed. However, if a nurse delegates a task that is within the assistant's scope of practice, but the assistant does not complete the task correctly, then the assistant is liable for patient injury.

Figure 10.12: Tasks that Can and Cannot Be Delegated	
Tasks that Physicians CAN Delegate to Physician Assistants and Nurse Practitioners	• examining patients • interpreting diagnostic test results • obtaining and recording patient medical data • performing therapeutic procedures, such as injections and wound sutures • instructing and counseling patients
Tasks that Physicians CANNOT delegate to Physician Assistants or Nurse Practitioners	• assuming responsibility for total care of the patient • supervising other physician assistants and nurse practitioners • prescribing medication • performing tasks outside the physician's scope of practice
Tasks that Registered Nurses or Practical Nurses CAN Delegate to Nursing Assistants	• assisting with activities of daily living • measuring vital signs • ambulating patients • changing bed linens • repositioning patients
Tasks that Registered Nurses or Practical Nurses CANNOT Delegate to Nursing Assistants	• administering medications • receiving verbal orders from doctors • supervising other nursing assistants • inserting or removing catheters

Workers protect patients and themselves when they carefully consider work assignments. Healthcare workers never refuse a task because they don't want to do it, but they may refuse a task for valid reasons, including the following:

- The task is illegal or unethical.

- The task is outside their scope of practice.

- They can't perform the task safely because they lack clear directions, proper equipment, or adequate supervision.

- They have not been trained for the task.

- The task is not part of their job description at the facility where they are working.

While healthcare team members follow the organizational chain of command when reporting problems, they also adhere to a chain of command for accepting work assignments. They know when they can take directions from another worker and when they can't. For example, a nursing assistant may not supervise or delegate tasks to another nursing assistant.

Sharing Information

The healthcare worker's scope of practice also guides the process of sharing information. For instance, a dental assistant does not diagnose patient conditions. When a patient asks if her tooth can be repaired, the dental assistant refers the question to the dentist (Figure 10.13). If a physician calls to give orders regarding the care of a particular patient, an RN or an LPN must take the phone call.

Healthcare workers are cautious about what patient information they share and with whom they share it. They must work to protect the privacy of each patient's medical information according to the guidelines of the HIPAA Privacy Rule. As a general guideline, physicians will disclose an individual's information for three purposes: treatment, payment, and healthcare operations such as quality assessment or medical reviews.

Healthcare workers only share medical information that is important to a patient's care with other members of the healthcare team. For example, a physician will give orders for patient care following surgery but will not discuss any previous medical procedures unless they affect current care. A nurse caring for a patient who has had an appendectomy (removal of the appendix) does not need to know about the patient's history of depression unless the patient exhibits signs of depression that require nursing observation and care.

Healthcare workers must also follow guidelines for sharing medical information with a patient's friends and family members. If the patient does not object, a healthcare provider may share information with family, friends, or others involved in providing or paying for that person's care. However, they may only discuss the information the third party needs to

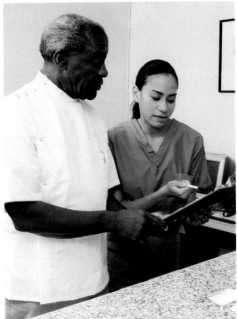

Figure 10.13 Because of her scope of practice, this dental assistant must ask the dentist to answer diagnostic questions from patients.

know about the care. Healthcare providers have policies regarding this type of information sharing. These policies may require a patient's verbal or written permission to share information. If a patient objects to the sharing of his or her information, providers are not allowed to share it.

Building Positive Team Relationships

Team members rely on each other as they work together to provide quality care. When team members don't work well together, workers' stress levels increase, which causes the quality of care to decrease. Successful healthcare teams make a constant effort to maintain positive working relationships.

Team members understand that each member is unique. Members will have different ages, sexes, socioeconomic statuses, lifestyle preferences, beliefs, education, and cultural backgrounds. These differences affect each person's attitudes and work preferences. Team members must be sensitive to and respectful of these differences to build positive relationships.

Productive and positive relationships result when team members are friendly and willing to assist each other (Figure 10.14). They keep their communication positive and encourage rather than criticize fellow team members. Finally, they work hard and perform job tasks to the best of their ability. Their actions show that they are reliable and can be trusted.

Figure 10.14 Dos and Don'ts for Building Positive Relationships

Do	Don't
be sensitive to the feelings of all team members	assume that everyone thinks the way you do
be honest	demand that others compromise before you will
be patient	assume that all of your expectations will be met
listen to all members	expect everyone to participate equally
be willing to compromise	give up at the first sign of disagreement

Complete the *Map Your Reading* graphic organizer for the section you just read.

RECALL YOUR READING

1. _____ refers to the assignment of tasks to each team member.
2. Healthcare workers' _____ of practice directs their ability to share information with patients.
3. Aides and assistants should _____ questions about a diagnosis to the healthcare professional in charge of the patient's care.
4. All workers follow the policies established by the _____ when sharing patient information.
5. Positive team relationships reduce worker stress and promote _____.

Technical Skills for Diagnostic Workers

Clinical technologists can perform literally thousands of different laboratory tests. Imaging specialists operate extremely advanced technological equipment as they assist medical specialists in diagnosing or monitoring a patient's illness or injury. Yet the basics of health assessment begin with measuring vital signs, height, and weight, and routine screening of vision and hearing. As you practice these skills and learn basic first aid techniques, consider whether you would enjoy a career in diagnostic services.

Measuring Vital Signs

The term *vital* means "needed for life." **Vital signs** measure temperature, pulse (heartbeat), respiration (breathing), and blood pressure. Healthcare workers must know the normal ranges for each vital sign as well as the techniques for accurately measuring them. When caring for patients, workers must know how to record vital sign measurements in the medical record and when to report changes that may indicate a need for prompt medical care.

Temperature. The human body works to balance the heat it loses and the heat it produces to maintain a temperature that varies only slightly. As a result, when we're hot, we sweat to cool the body, and when we're cold, we shiver to warm the body. Activities like sleeping, exercising, and anything that creates excitement cause temperatures to fluctuate slightly. These are normal variations. However, an abnormally increased temperature signals a fever. Fever is a sign that the body is fighting infection. Figure 10.15 shows the normal ranges for temperatures taken in different body locations for children and adults. Healthcare workers report temperatures outside these normal ranges. They also report changes outside the typical range of temperatures for a particular patient. Even though a temperature may be within average normal ranges, it can still signal illness because it is not normal for a specific patient.

Temperature can be measured at various sites in the body. Measurement in the mouth, which is called *oral temperature*, is common. For accuracy, an oral temperature can't be measured if the person has recently smoked, chewed gum, or had something to eat or drink. In these cases, wait at least 15 minutes before taking the oral temperature.

vital signs
the key measurements that provide information about a person's health, including temperature, pulse, respiration, and blood pressure

Figure 10.15 Normal Temperature Ranges for Adults and Children (°Fahrenheit)				
Method	**0–2 years of age**	**3–10 years of age**	**11–65 years of age**	**65 years of age and older**
oral	—	95.9°–99.5°	97.6°–99.6°	96.4°–98.5°
rectal	97.9°–100.4°	97.9°–100.4°	98.6°–100.6°	97.1°–99.2°
axillary	94.5°–99.1°	96.6°–98.0°	95.3°–98.4°	96.0°–97.4°
tympanic/temporal	97.5°–100.4°	97.0°–100.0°	96.6°–99.7°	96.4°–99.5°

Glass thermometers (not containing mercury) and digital thermometers are used to measure oral temperature in all types of settings, including the home. In a healthcare facility, an electronic thermometer may be used to measure temperature in just a few seconds. Electronic thermometers are also easier to read because the temperature appears in large numbers on the viewing screen. Figure 10.16 shows different types of oral thermometers.

Follow these steps when taking an oral temperature:

1. Complete your beginning procedure steps, including washing your hands. Wear gloves for this procedure.

2. Check to make sure the person has not had anything to eat or drink, smoked, or chewed gum within the last 15 minutes.

3. Prepare the thermometer.

   Glass. Remove the clean thermometer from its case, holding it at the stem end only. Never hold a thermometer at the bulb end. Rinse it in cool water and dry with a paper towel. Shake the thermometer down using a "snap of the wrist" action until it reads below 94°F. Put a disposable sheath (a clear vinyl cover used to prevent infection) over the thermometer.

   Digital/Electronic. Cover the probe with a sheath. Turn the thermometer on and wait until it beeps or the "ready" sign appears on the viewing screen.

4. Ask the patient to open his or her mouth and carefully place the thermometer under the tongue and to one side. Have the patient gently close his or her mouth to hold the thermometer in place and breathe through his or her nose.

5. Leave the glass thermometer in place for three to five minutes. Leave the digital or electronic thermometer in place until it blinks or beeps.

6. Ask the patient to open his or her mouth and carefully remove the thermometer while holding it at the stem end.

7. Remove the sheath or eject the probe cover and discard it in an approved waste container.

8. Read the temperature.

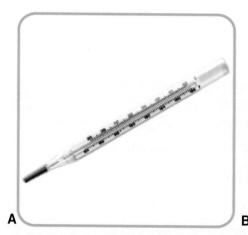
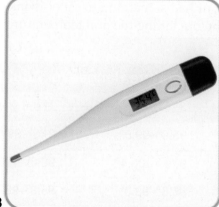
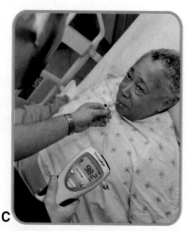

A   B   C

Figure 10.16   Glass thermometers (A) and digital thermometers (B) are often used at home. In the hospital, you are likely to have your temperature taken with an electronic thermometer (C).

Glass. Hold the thermometer at eye level and rotate it until you see the indicator line. Read the temperature, adding 0.2°F for each mark on the thermometer (Figure 10.17).

Digital or Electronic. Read the temperature on the display screen.

9. Store the thermometer.

Glass. Shake the thermometer down and clean it according to your facility's policy. Return it to its storage case.

Digital or Electronic. Turn off thermometer. Clean as required by facility policy, and push the probe back into the thermometer case. Remove gloves and wash hands.

10. Record the patient's name, the time you took the temperature, the temperature, and the method used (in this case, *O* for *oral*). Report an abnormal temperature immediately.

11. Complete your end-of-procedure steps.

Some situations require a different method of temperature measurement, such as axillary (armpit), tympanic (eardrum), or temporal (forehead). For example, young children are likely to bite an oral thermometer and an unconscious person can't hold an oral thermometer in the mouth.

A **rectal temperature** is taken by placing the thermometer in the rectum. Because the data comparing different methods is mixed, a rectal temperature is still considered the most accurate temperature reading. For this reason, a physician may indicate that a patient's temperature should be measured rectally in critical situations.

Pulse. Pulse measures heartbeats. With each beat, blood moves through the arteries in a wave or pulse. When you touch or *palpate* an artery near the surface of the skin, you will feel these waves. All of our arteries have a pulse, but we can feel the pulse in only a few of the arteries (Figure 10.18 on the next page).

You measure the pulse rate by counting the number of beats or pulses in one minute. This tells you the heart rate, which is how fast the heart is beating. In addition to measuring the pulse rate, you will assess the pulse rhythm and the pulse volume, or *amplitude*. Pay attention to the pattern of pulsations and the pauses between them. Normally, the pulse rhythm is smooth and regular, with the same amount of time between each pulsation. Pulse amplitude measures the force or quality of the pulse; it describes how the pulse feels. A normal pulse is easy to feel and each pulsation is strong. Report and record any pulse rate that is higher or lower than normal, is irregular, or feels weak or faint.

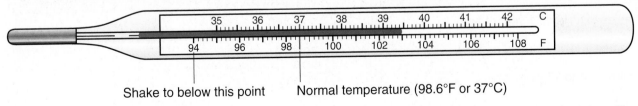

Shake to below this point   Normal temperature (98.6°F or 37°C)

Figure 10.17   To read temperature on a glass thermometer, hold the thermometer at eye level and rotate until you see the indicator line. Add 0.2 degrees for each mark on the thermometer. What temperature is shown on this thermometer?

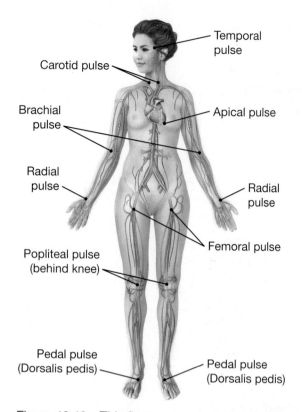

Temporal pulse

Carotid pulse

Brachial pulse

Apical pulse

Radial pulse

Radial pulse

Femoral pulse

Popliteal pulse (behind knee)

Pedal pulse (Dorsalis pedis)

Pedal pulse (Dorsalis pedis)

Figure 10.18   This figure shows pulse points on the body. Which pulse requires a stethoscope for its measurement?

Pulse rate varies with age (Figure 10.19). An infant's heart beats much faster than an adult's does. Pulse rates are normally affected by exercise, when the heart speeds up to supply more oxygen to body tissues. Heart rates also increase due to anger, excitement, illness, pain, or fever. Medications may increase or decrease the heart rate. Hypothermia, lowered oxygen levels, physical conditioning, and sleep will decrease the heart rate.

Two common sites for pulse measurement are the radial artery and the apex of the heart. These are known as *radial pulse* and *apical pulse*. **Radial pulse** is measured by placing two or three fingers over the radial artery on the inside of the wrist. Follow these steps to measure radial pulse:

1. Complete your beginning procedures steps, including washing your hands.

2. Rest the patient's arm on a table or on the bed. Locate the radial pulse on the thumb side of the wrist using two or three fingers. Do *not* use your thumb because this may cause you to feel your own pulse.

3. Count the number of pulses for one full minute to assess rhythm and amplitude. For pulse rate only, you may count pulses for 30 seconds and multiply by two.

4. Record the patient's name; the time you took the pulse; and the pulse rate, rhythm, and amplitude. Report an abnormal pulse rate, rhythm, or amplitude immediately.

5. Complete your end-of-procedure steps.

Apical pulse is measured by listening over the apex (lower tip) of the heart using a stethoscope. A **stethoscope** makes sound louder (Figure 10.20). You will hear, rather than feel, each beat of the patient's heart. The apex is located in the left fifth intercostal space on the midclavicular line, or approximately two inches below the left nipple. An apical pulse is taken when the patient has a weak or irregular pulse that may be difficult to feel. An apical pulse is also used to measure heart rate in infants.

Figure 10.19 The Range of Normal Pulse Rates	
Age or Fitness Level	**Beats per Minute (bpm) in Resting Heart Rate**
babies to children 1 year of age	100–160
children 1 to 10 years of age	70–120
children 11 to 17 years of age	60–100
adults	60–100
well-conditioned athletes	40–60

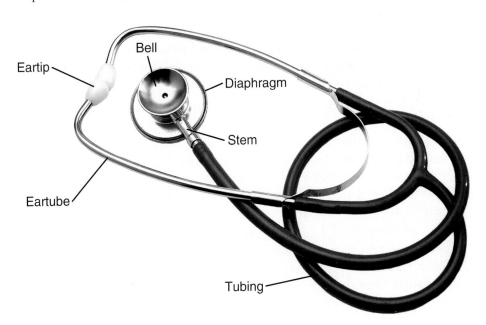

Eartip

Bell

Diaphragm

Stem

Eartube

Tubing

Figure 10.20   Before using a stethoscope, clean the earpieces, bell, and diaphragm with alcohol wipes. Rotate the diaphragm until you can hear sound through the earpieces.

Respiration. Counting breaths for one minute is the simplest way to assess a person's respiratory function. As you watch the patient's chest move, count one breath in (inhalation) and one breath out (exhalation) as a single **respiration** or breath. If it is difficult to see chest or abdominal movement, you can place your hand near the collarbone to feel the patient's breathing. Try to measure respiration right after measuring pulse. Keep your fingers on the patient's wrist as though you were still counting the pulse (Figure 10.21). In this case, you don't want the patient to know you are measuring respirations because a person can consciously change breathing rates, which will result in an inaccurate measurement. Your measurement will be more accurate when the patient doesn't know that his or her breaths are being counted.

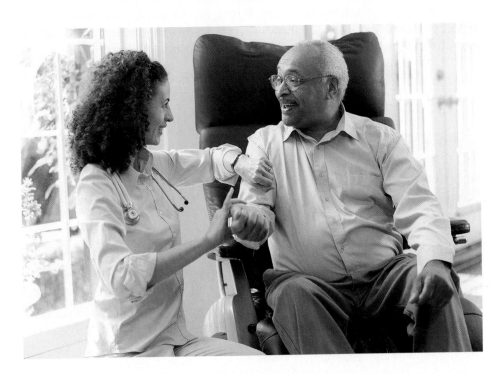

Figure 10.21   To check a patient's respiration, pretend to continue taking a pulse reading as you observe and count his or her breaths.

A healthy resting adult will breathe about 16 to 20 times per minute. During normal breathing, the chest rises and falls evenly in a regular rhythm and breathing is quiet and easy. Measure respirations using the following steps:

1. Complete your beginning procedure steps, including washing your hands.

2. Measure respiration right after measuring the pulse. Without telling the patient, begin counting each rise and fall of the chest as one breath. For regular respirations, you may count for 30 seconds and multiply by two. If breathing is irregular, you should count respirations for a full minute.

3. Record the patient's name, the time you measured the respiration, and the respiratory rate. Report a respiratory rate that is greater than 24 or less than 10 breaths per minute. Report any breathing that is irregular, very deep or very shallow, difficult, or painful.

4. Complete your end-of-procedure steps.

Expand

Blood Pressure. Blood pressure is the force of blood pushing against the inside of the blood vessel (artery) walls. When you take someone's blood pressure, you record two measurements—systolic and diastolic. The systolic (sihs-TAHL-ihk) pressure is the force caused by the contracting heart muscle pushing blood through the arteries. The diastolic (dI-uh-STAHL-ihk) pressure is the lesser force of the blood when the heart muscle relaxes. Blood pressure is measured in millimeters of mercury (mmHg) and is recorded as a fraction. Write the higher (systolic) number first and the lower (diastolic) number second. A systolic pressure of 115 mmHg and a diastolic pressure of 70 mmHg are written as 115/70.

Blood pressure readings provide vital information about a person's current health and future risk for disease. Normal blood pressure varies throughout the day, with readings being lower in the morning and when lying down. Readings are typically higher when sitting or standing, after eating a meal, and when exercising. Stress, anxiety, and pain all increase blood pressure. Figure 10.22 shows several factors that influence blood pressure, including some that are related to lifestyle choices.

Figure 10.22   The factors shown here influence blood pressure readings. Which of these factors can be changed by lifestyle choices?

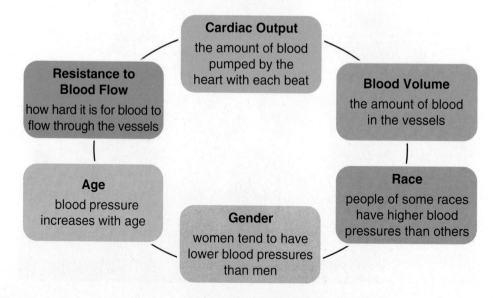

When blood pressure is too low (**hypotension**), the body tissues don't get enough nutrients and oxygen. When blood pressure is too high (**hypertension**), the heart works harder to push blood through the arteries. Eventually, this causes damage to the heart muscle. High blood pressure also stresses the kidneys and blood vessels, which can lead to kidney failure and stroke. Figure 10.23 lists the readings that indicate normal blood pressure, hypertension, and hypotension.

A **sphygmomanometer** (sfihg-moh-muh-NAHM-eht-er) measures blood pressure and comes in three types—mercury, aneroid, and digital (Figure 10.24). The mercury sphygmomanometer is the most accurate, but a column of mercury is difficult to carry around, and mercury is not an environmentally friendly substance. Aneroid sphygmomanometers are very common. They use a small mechanical device with a convenient dial to measure pressure. Aneroid sphygmomanometers do require recalibration, which means the equipment must be checked regularly to ensure that its measurements remain accurate. The manometer, or *gauge*, should point to zero when the cuff is deflated. When using either of these pieces of equipment, you are trying to "hear" the blood pressure.

Digital sphygmomanometers are even more convenient than the aneroid version, especially in noisy places. Instead of sound, digital instruments use vibration to determine diastolic and systolic pressures. When blood pressure is high, arterial walls vibrate as blood flows through

Figure 10.23 Blood Pressure Classifications for Adults				
	Hypotension	**Normal**	**Prehypertension**	**Hypertension**
SYSTOLIC	<90 mmHg	<120 mmHg	120–139 mmHg	140+ mmHg
DIASTOLIC	<60 mmHg	<80 mmHg	80–89 mmHg	90+ mmHg

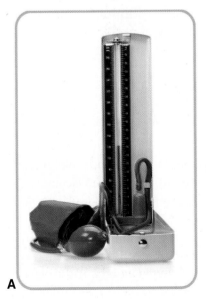

A

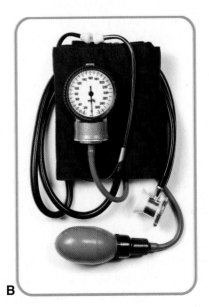

B

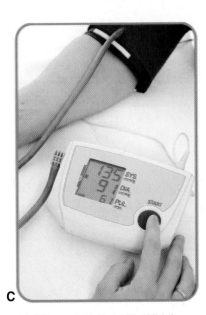

C

Figure 10.24   The different types of sphygmanometers include mercury (A), aneroid (B), and digital (C). Which type is most accurate? most convenient?

them. Digital sphygmomanometers detect the changes in these vibrations as the pressure in the cuff is released.

The sounds that you hear through the stethoscope as you auscultate (AW-skuhl-tayt), or listen to, a blood pressure on a mercury or aneroid

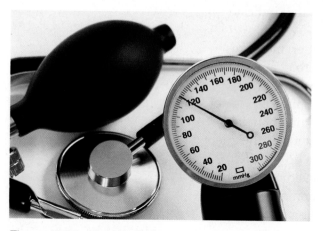

sphygmomanometer are named for Nikolai Korotkoff (koh-RAHT-kohf), the Russian surgeon who first identified them. As you slowly release the valve, you will hear tapping sounds that gradually become louder. The first tapping sound is the systolic pressure. Next, you will hear a sequence of swishing and tapping sounds. Finally, the sound will become muffled and very soft. The last sound is the diastolic pressure.

Sphygmomanometers consist of a bulb that is squeezed to fill the cuff with air, a manometer that measures the pressure in the cuff, the cuff itself, and flexible tubing to connect all the parts. Cuffs come in different sizes, designed to fit children, adults, large adults, and the thigh. The cuff must fit correctly or the blood pressure reading will not be accurate. The manometer measures the pressure of the air in the cuff (Figure 10.25). The longer dark lines mark increments of 10 mmHg, and the short lines in between mark increments of 2 mmHg.

Figure 10.25 Each long line on the manometer gauge represents 10 mmHg. What pressure measurement is shown on this gauge?

Measuring Height and Weight

Height and weight are not considered vital signs, but they are measured periodically because the relationship between a person's weight and height provides information about that person's overall health. A baseline height and weight can be compared to future changes.

Height is typically measured on admission to a healthcare facility or at a yearly exam. Individuals with osteoporosis, a degeneration of the spinal column, will have more frequent height measurements. However, weight is measured at most physician visits and on admission, transfer, and discharge at a healthcare facility for a variety of reasons:

- Weight indicates nutritional status.

- When the patient retains fluid, weight will increase. This is an indication of heart and kidney function.

- Unexplained weight loss can signal a disease such as cancer or diabetes.

- Since many medications are prescribed based on body weight, a change in weight may require a change in medication dosage.

Several types of scales are used in healthcare facilities (Figure 10.26). Both the mechanical scale and the digital scale are commonly used for patients who can stand independently. To use the mechanical scale, you slide metal weights along a bar until the bar is balanced. Once turned on, the digital scale automatically measures the patient's weight and displays it on a screen. Height measurements are recorded in feet (') and inches ("), or meters (m) and centimeters (cm). Weight is recorded in pounds (lb) or kilograms (kg).

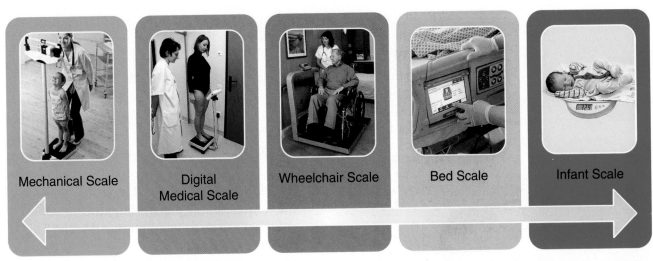

Figure 10.26   Different patients require different types of scales. When might it be necessary to use the bed scale?

Follow these steps to measure height and weight using a mechanical, upright scale:

1. Complete your beginning procedure steps, including washing your hands.

2. Place paper toweling on the stand area of the scale. Move both weights to the zero position.

3. Ask the patient to remove his or her shoes and coat and to put aside anything he or she is carrying. Help the patient onto the scale platform, facing the balance bar. Check to see that the patient is not holding on to you or the scale.

4. Move the large weight to the right until the balance bar drops down on the lower guide. Slide the weight back one notch. Move the small weight on the upper scale bar to the right until the balance pointer is centered between the two scale bars (Figure 10.27).

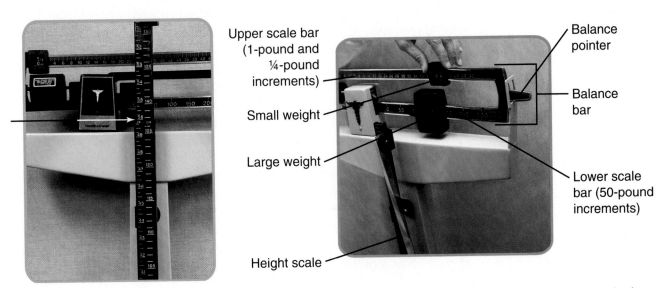

Figure 10.27   To measure height, observe the point at which the movable ruler bar meets the stationary ruler bar. To measure weight, slide the small and large weights along the balance bar until the balance pointer is centered between the two scale bars. Then read the weight displayed by adding both numbers.

5. Read the numbers on the upper and lower scale bars where each weight is positioned and add these two numbers together. This is the patient's weight.

6. Help the patient turn and face away from the scale bar. Keep safety in mind by observing the patient and assisting as necessary to prevent falls. Slide the height rod up until you can open the measuring bar without hitting the patient. Seek assistance if you can't safely operate the height bar when a patient is taller than you.

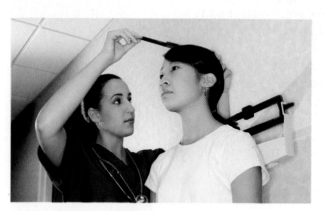

Figure 10.28   It is safer to raise the height bar with the patient facing away from the scale, as shown here.

7. Slide the height rod down until it touches the top of the patient's head (Figure 10.28). Read the number at the place where the movable ruler bar meets the stationary ruler bar. This is the patient's height.

8. Help the patient step off the scale.

9. Record the patient's name, the time you took measurements, and the height and weight measurements.

10. Discard the paper toweling, lower the height rod, and slide the weights to zero.

11. Complete your end-of-procedure steps.

When patients are unable to stand independently, a wheelchair scale is used to measure weight. Wheelchair scales allow you to roll the chair onto a platform, which weighs the patient and the chair. Next, you weigh the empty chair. Subtracting the weight of the chair from the first measurement gives you the patient's weight. Patients who are confined to bed can be measured and weighed using a bed scale. Infants are weighed using a special scale that features a tray to support the baby.

Positioning a Patient

Medical examinations and imaging procedures require specific patient positions. In simple terms, a person needing examination on the front part of the body will lie on his back. However, each position has a specific name and the position descriptions become more detailed as the imaging requirements become more specific.

For example, suppose a physician orders an upright chest X-ray with two views of an ambulatory patient. *Upright* means that the patient will stand during the X-ray. The standard positions are *posterior/anterior* (P/A), which means back to front, and *lateral*, which means from the side. The radiographer positions the patient standing and facing the X-ray image receptor for a posterior/anterior projection (the X-rays pass through the patient's body from back to the front) and a left lateral projection (the patient stands with the left side closest to the image receptor, and the X-rays pass through the body from right to left). Body positioning may also require steps such as moving the patient's arms out of the imaging area.

Positions also describe patients resting in bed. Those who cannot move independently need to be repositioned frequently to prevent skin breakdown. As you position patients, pay close attention to **body alignment**. Position your patient so that the spine is not twisted or crooked. Imagine a line going down the middle of the patient's body. The line should be straight in any position (Figure 10.29). Proper body alignment makes the patient more comfortable by relieving strain on muscles and joints.

Patients are positioned on a wide variety of tables for surgery, examinations, or imaging procedures. You must learn how to operate each kind of table to provide for the safety of your patient. Tables are cleaned or disinfected and often covered with table paper before the patient enters the examination room.

As you position your patient, protect his or her privacy by closing the door or pulling the curtain. Drape or cover the patient to avoid unnecessary exposure. Watch the patient closely and observe safety precautions to prevent falls and injuries. Always provide for your own safety by using proper body mechanics.

Figure 10.30 on the next page provides the descriptions and uses for a few basic patient positions. Remember to use your beginning and end-of-procedure steps as you practice positioning a patient.

body alignment
term used to describe a position of the body in which the spine is not crooked or twisted

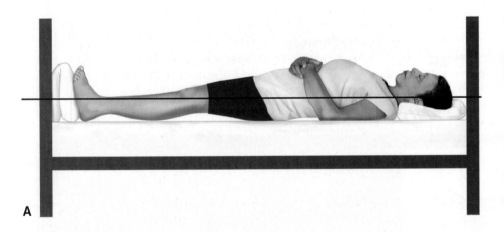

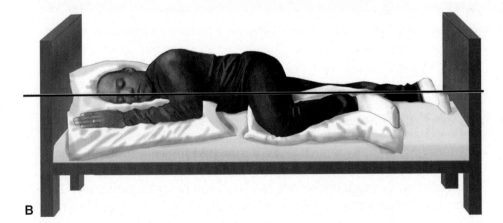

Figure 10.29   When a patient is in proper body alignment, the spine is not twisted or crooked, regardless of the position. In the supine position (A), the patient's hip, shoulder, and ear will form a straight line. In Sim's position (B), you can draw an imaginary line connecting the patient's nose, sternum, and pubic bone. Note that pillows provide comfort and help the patient to maintain correct alignment.

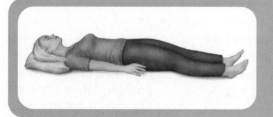

Supine/Dorsal Recumbent Position
- Lying on the back with the bed flat
- Used for physical examinations and surgeries of the chest, heart, and abdomen

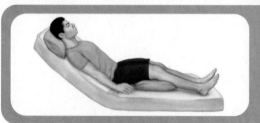

Fowler's Position
- A sitting position with the head of the bed elevated
- High Fowler's is 60–90 degrees, Fowler's is 45–60 degrees, low or semi-Fowler's is 30–45 degrees
- Used for eating in bed, reading or watching TV, and to make breathing easier

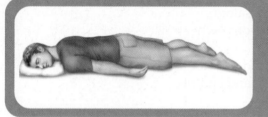

Prone Position
- Lying face down
- Used when examining the spine or back

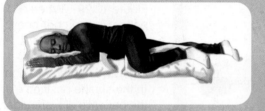

Sim's Position
- Halfway between lateral position and prone position, with upper knee bent
- Used for rectal examinations and enemas

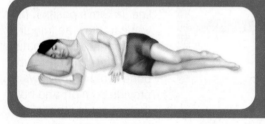

Lateral/ Lateral Recumbent Position
- Lying on the side
- Used to relieve pressure on the spine, tailbone, and hips and to reduce back pain

Figure 10.30 These patient positions are each used in specific situations, such as surgery, exams, or imaging procedures.

Screening Vision and Hearing

Vision and hearing screening helps identify children who need further evaluation, diagnosis, and treatment for vision and hearing problems. Many state departments of public health set guidelines for the routine screening of school-age children. Because learning is mostly accomplished through the senses of vision and hearing, screenings help determine barriers that would interfere with a child's ability to learn. Identifying children with impaired hearing or vision when they are just entering school can prevent or reduce many of the learning problems that result from these impairments. Screening all children is the most practical approach to identifying those in need of professional services.

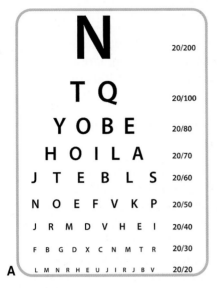
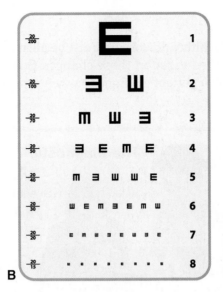
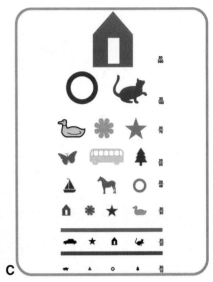

Figure 10.31   Vision can be tested using several different charts. These include a simple letter chart (A), the Snellen chart (B), and a simple shapes chart for children (C).

Expand

Visual acuity tests in the school setting screen for distance vision, or *nearsightedness* (myopia). The child reads from a chart with letters or pictures that is mounted on a wall 20 feet away. There are several different types of charts that may be used for this screening (Figure 10.31). Other vision tests include the test for close vision, or *farsightedness* (hyperopia), and for color blindness.

Hearing screenings conducted in schools use an instrument called an **audiometer** (awd-ee-AHM-eht-er). This machine has a set of headphones for the child to wear and it makes sounds at different frequencies to test hearing. A quiet area is necessary for accurate results. Again, this test is a screening, which means that students who fail the test will be referred to a medical professional for follow-up testing. Generally, a child is tested twice with at least a week between each test before a referral is made. Temporary hearing loss can be the result of an upper respiratory infection. An exam by a medical professional is necessary to determine the cause of hearing loss (Figure 10.32).

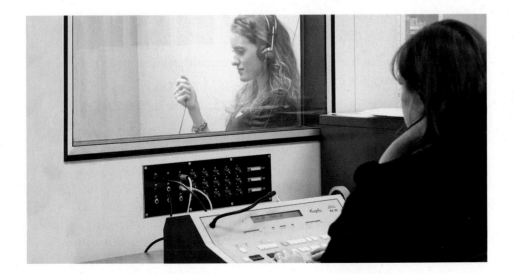

Figure 10.32   Hearing screenings can detect hearing problems, but a professional hearing exam is needed to identify the cause of hearing loss and to determine appropriate treatment.

Providing First Aid

Healthcare workers must be alert to changes in patient status and prepared to report those changes. Sometimes a healthcare worker will detect a patient emergency when others don't notice a serious problem.

The Diagnostic Worker: Erin

Erin works in a long-term care facility. She knows the normal signs of health for the residents in her care and realizes that a change in status can signal an emergency. For example, Mr. Lyon usually has above-normal blood pressure readings, Mrs. Siemens is always hungry at mealtime, and Mr. Frederick complains about his arthritis most often in the evening. Erin observes her residents closely to notice when something is different.

Could Mrs. Siemens' tiredness and indigestion be signs of a heart attack? Does Mr. Frederick's slurred speech indicate a stroke? Does Mr. Lyon's drop in blood pressure mean something is wrong? Erin reports signs and symptoms that are unusual or alarming so her residents receive needed emergency care at the earliest opportunity.

Healthcare workers must also be prepared to act in the case of a sudden illness or injury. All workers can seek **first aid** training. The goal of first aid is to minimize the effects of an injury or illness until more advanced medical help arrives. Appropriate first aid responses can mean the difference between life and death. The following are emergency health situations that healthcare workers must be prepared to treat:

first aid
emergency treatment given before regular medical services can be obtained

- cardiac emergencies (heart attack and cardiac arrest)
- breathing emergencies (respiratory distress, respiratory arrest, choking, asthma, or anaphylaxis (an-uh-fuh-LAK-sihs), which is a life-threatening allergic reaction)
- sudden illness (poisoning, fainting, seizures, stroke, allergic reactions, or diabetic emergencies)
- environmental emergencies (heat- or cold-related emergencies, bites, stings, or lightning strikes)
- soft tissue injuries (wounds, burns, or external bleeding)
- muscle, bone, and joint injuries (fractures; dislocations; sprains; strains; or head, neck, and spinal injuries)

The American Heart Association and the American Red Cross offer several levels of first aid training courses (Figure 10.33). At a minimum, health science students will want to learn basic first aid procedures for responding to a medical emergency. Course skills include, but are not limited to, checking an injured or ill person; performing **cardiopulmonary resuscitation**, also known as *CPR*, which keeps the brain and other vital organs supplied with oxygen until advanced medical care arrives; and using an **automated external defibrillator** (dee-FIHB-ruh-layt-er), also known as an *AED,* to deliver an electric shock to the heart and restore its normal rhythm. Trainees will also learn how to clear a foreign body airway obstruction (FBAO), apply dressings and bandages to wounds, and detect signs of a stroke.

When people encounter emergencies, they are often afraid to help because they feel unprepared or are afraid of being sued. Good Samaritan laws encourage people to help others in emergencies. These laws protect people who provide emergency care to ill or injured individuals. The responder cannot be sued or found financially responsible for the victim's injury as long as the responder acted reasonably and within his or her level of training. The following are some reasonable actions responders can take:

- moving a victim only if his or her life is in danger

- asking a conscious person for permission before giving care

- calling for professional help

- providing care until more highly trained help arrives

In many schools and workplaces, employers sponsor first aid training for employees. They may establish an emergency response team of volunteers who can provide assistance when an emergency occurs. The Good Samaritan law continues to protect these workplace volunteers.

Many healthcare workers complete a more extensive training program designed for professional rescuers, and certain healthcare workers have a duty to respond to an emergency. Individuals who perform rescues as a part of their jobs have a legal duty to respond and rescue in an emergency. In addition, when emergency medical technicians (EMTs) are on duty, they are legally responsible for the care they provide to victims of an accident or sudden illness. The training for EMTs includes each of the following:

- making primary assessments

- giving ventilations

- performing advanced CPR and AED

- using epinephrine autoinjectors and asthma inhalers

- using emergency oxygen and breathing devices

Whether you are learning basic first aid or professional rescue techniques, you will want to earn certification to show that you have passed a test demonstrating your new skills. The American Red Cross and the American Heart Association are the two agencies that certify first aid skills. To become certified, your first aid course must be taught

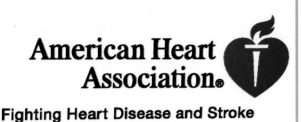

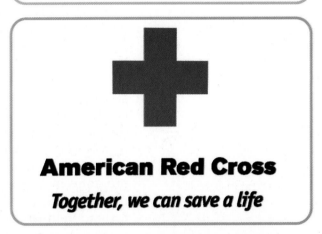

Figure 10.33 You can take many first aid courses through the American Heart Association and American Red Cross. What skills might these courses cover?

by an approved trainer. You are required to complete the entire course curriculum and to pass a written test as well as a skills demonstration.

In all situations, healthcare workers should provide emergency care within their scope of practice based on their training and certification (Figure 10.34). They also follow their facilities' policies for responding to emergencies. For example, Cindy works as a CNA in a hospital. When she identifies a patient emergency, a special code alerts hospital personnel to respond with medical assistance. Janice, on the other hand, works at an assisted living facility. She is required to maintain first aid certification. In an emergency, she calls 911 and provides appropriate first aid until emergency medical personnel arrive. Both workers must know a patient's wishes for resuscitation before providing life support. For example, patients who have a no code, or *do not resuscitate (DNR)*, order have chosen not to receive resuscitation in the event of respiratory or cardiac arrest.

The following sections will introduce you to a few of the basic first aid techniques. These sections provide essential information about the goals of each procedure according to the guidelines of the American Red Cross. However, these sections will not teach you the skills for performing first aid procedures. You will want to seek out the appropriate training and certification required for your current or future career.

For example, emergency medical responder programs require professional level coursework and training. Some college nursing programs include a professional level course in their entrance requirements. Nursing assistants may or may not be required to complete first aid training based on individual state certification requirements, but employers appreciate CNAs who take the initiative to seek this training on their own. Employers often require home care and assisted living aides to maintain first aid certification since they may be the only ones available to act when a medical emergency occurs. Students who work as lifeguards are required to take a specialized water safety training course.

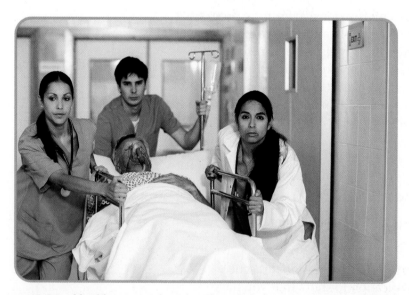
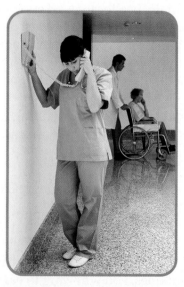

Figure 10.34   Healthcare workers in a hospital must alert personnel in the hospital when an emergency occurs. In contrast, healthcare workers at an assisted living facility should call 911 if an emergency occurs. What concept does this illustrate?

Checking an Injured or Ill Adult. When responding to an emergency, you must be alert to dangers in the environment (Figure 10.35). For example, when you see smoke billowing from your client's home, are there downed wires or a fire in the kitchen stove? Is the home even safe for you to enter? Do you see broken glass or an open medication container? You can check the victim once you know the scene is safe, but you must continue to keep safety in mind as you provide care during an emergency. Remember to practice standard precautions and use appropriate personal protective equipment (PPE) to prevent disease transmission before checking a victim.

Once you have done everything you can to maintain safety, you are ready to assess the victim and try to diagnose the problem before providing care. When more than one person is injured in an emergency, you will need to determine which person to help first. This process is called *triage*, which means that you treat life-threatening emergencies before any others. For instance, a breathing problem takes priority over a broken bone. Remember the first rule of rescue and do no further harm to the victim. Never move a seriously injured person unless there is an immediate danger such as fire or flooding. Check the victim for life-threatening conditions such as the following:

- unconsciousness
- trouble breathing
- no breathing or movement
- severe bleeding

Call 911 immediately if you observe any of these conditions.

When checking an unconscious victim, you should follow an ABC sequence. First, check the *airway* to make sure it is open. Next, check the victim's *breathing*. Finally, check *circulation* by looking for any signs of severe bleeding

---

Figure 10.35 Being Alert to Environmental Dangers

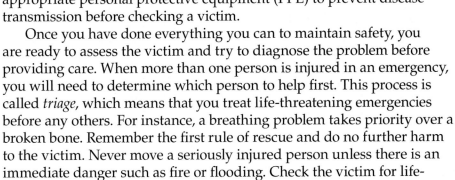

Unusual sights, appearances, and behaviors
- spilled medicine container
- sparks, smoke, or fire
- unexplained confusion or drowsiness

Unusual noises
- breaking glass, crashing metal, screeching tires
- screaming, yelling, calling for help
- unusual silence

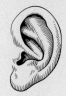

Unusual odors
- strong odors
- unrecognizable odors
- inappropriate odors

Treating a Choking Victim. Choking or airway obstruction is the most common respiratory emergency. Common situations that result in choking include children who take large bites of food and don't chew them completely. When adults drink alcohol, they dull the nerves that help with swallowing and are more likely to choke. People who wear dentures can't always sense when food is completely chewed and swallow before they should. Eating rapidly, eating while talking or laughing, and playing or running while eating can also lead to choking.

When a person begins to choke, the airway may be partially blocked. If the person can cough or speak, stay with him while he tries to cough up the object. Call 911 if he can't cough it up.

If the airway is completely blocked, the person cannot cough, speak, or breathe. You must act immediately to provide care. Let the person know you can help. Get a parent's consent if a child is choking or a nonverbal sign of permission from a choking adult. Deliver a combination of five back blows followed by five abdominal thrusts (Figure 10.36). Your goal is to clear the airway obstruction. The back blows will help to loosen the object, while the abdominal thrusts force air out of the lungs. This helps to expel the object from the airway.

To give back blows, lean the person forward while supporting the chest. Strike the person between the shoulder blades with the heel of your hand. Follow these steps to give abdominal thrusts:

1. Stand behind the person and wrap your arms around the waist.

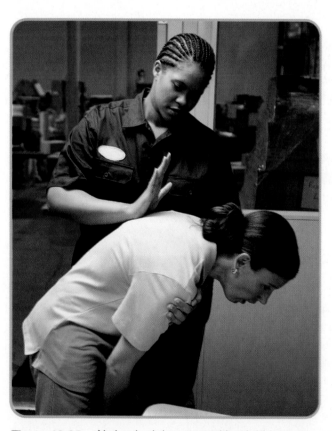
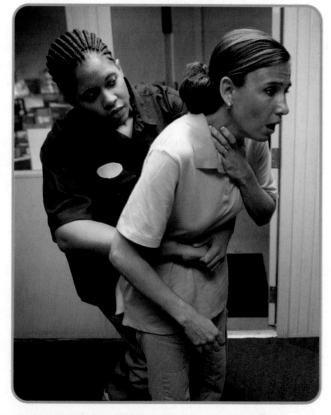

Figure 10.36 Abdominal thrusts and back blows are used when a person is choking. Because there is a risk of injury, you should *never* practice back blows or abdominal thrusts on another person. Always use a choking mannequin to practice these procedures.

2. Make a fist with one hand and place the thumb side against the middle of the person's abdomen—above the navel and below the breastbone.

3. Place your other hand over your fist and give quick, upward thrusts.

Continue with back blows and abdominal thrusts until the object is dislodged or the person becomes unconscious. As with many first aid procedures, this one is different when a child or infant is choking. You must know the correct first aid procedure for the age of the victim.

The American Heart Association teaches only the abdominal thrust procedures, not the back blow technique. If you haven't learned the technique for back blows, you don't have to use them. Either method is acceptable.

Performing Cardiopulmonary Resuscitation. Cardiopulmonary resuscitation is used to respond to **cardiac arrest**. In cardiac arrest, a person's heart stops beating or does not beat well enough to circulate blood to the brain and other vital organs. When this occurs, a person also stops breathing. For a short time after breathing stops, the cells of the brain and other vital organs will continue to live until all the oxygen in the blood is used up. Performing CPR supplies oxygen to the victim through rescue breathing and circulates oxygenated blood through chest compressions. CPR increases the victim's chances of survival by keeping the brain and other vital organs supplied with oxygen until advanced medical care arrives.

Drowning, choking, drugs, brain injury, or electric shock can all cause cardiac arrest. However, the most common cause is cardiovascular disease. When the coronary arteries, which supply blood to the heart, become stiff or clogged, blood can't get to the heart muscle. As a result, the person suffers a heart attack. Learn to recognize the signs and symptoms of a heart attack so you can call 911 immediately when necessary (Figure 10.37 on the next page).

Early treatment reduces damage to the heart muscle and improves the person's chance of survival, but many people delay seeking care. While the key symptom of a heart attack is chest discomfort that does not go away in a few minutes, or goes away and comes back, about one-third of women don't have any chest pain when experiencing a heart attack. Women are more likely to deny that their symptoms are serious than men are. Women may believe they are merely suffering from heartburn or indigestion.

Using an Automated External Defibrillator. An automated external defibrillator (AED) is a machine that delivers an electric shock to the heart. In many cardiac arrest situations, the person's heart is in *fibrillation*. This means that the heart has an abnormal rhythm (arrhythmia) and can't pump blood effectively. An AED defibrillates the heart and restores its normal rhythm. The sooner the shock is given, the greater the chance of survival. Healthcare facilities and many public buildings such as schools, fitness clubs, and athletic facilities now have on-site AEDs.

You can make a difference before EMS personnel arrive by learning how to use an AED as part of your first aid training.

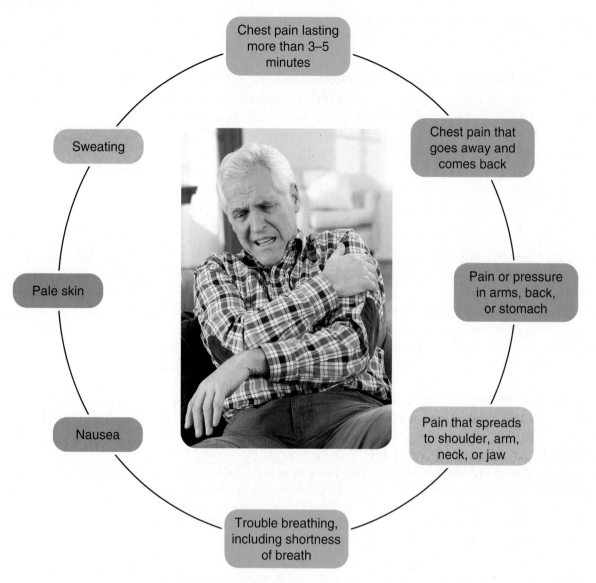

Figure 10.37   These are the common signs and symptoms of a heart attack. Knowing how to recognize these can help you respond quickly to a person in need of medical attention.

Stroke. Stroke occurs when blood flow to a part of the brain is cut off. Recognizing the signals of a stroke and getting emergency care quickly can reduce the damage caused by a stroke (Figure 10.38). Most strokes occur when a vessel supplying blood to the brain is blocked. Blood clots traveling from other parts of the body or arteries damaged by diabetes and heart disease can cause the blockage. A smaller number of strokes are caused by bleeding in the brain from a broken blood vessel or a bulging aneurysm that breaks open.

In a *mini-stroke*, a person experiences the signals of a stroke, but they go away. When someone has a mini-stroke, or *transient ischemic* (ihs-KEE-mihk) *attack* (TIA), emergency care is needed because that person has a high risk of experiencing a major stroke.

Sudden weakness or numbness of the face, arm, or leg—usually on one side of the body—signals a stroke. Additional signs may include trouble speaking clearly, blurred vision, or a severe headache. Using the **FAST** mnemonic (*Face, Arm, Speech,* and *Time*) can help you identify a stroke:

- **F**ace: Ask the person to smile to see if one side of his or her face droops.

- **A**rm: Ask the person to raise both arms to see if one arm drifts downward.

- **S**peech: Ask the person to repeat a simple sentence to see if his or her speech is slurred, and if he or she can repeat the sentence correctly.

- **T**ime: Determine when the signals began and call 911 immediately. Tell the dispatcher when the signals started.

Follow these steps to provide care to a stroke victim:

1. Call 911 and note the time when the signals started.

2. If the person is unconscious, make sure the airway is open and check for life-threatening conditions. Position the person on his or her side if vomiting occurs.

3. Stay with the person, monitor breathing, and don't give food or drink.

4. Offer comfort and reassurance.

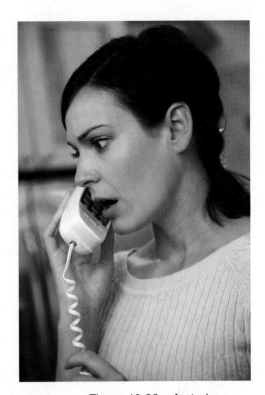

Figure 10.38   A stroke is a medical emergency that requires immediate attention. You can identify a stroke by using the *FAST* method—Face, Arm, Speech, and Time.

The most important step you can take to prepare for an emergency is completing a CPR and first aid training course. Continue to take refresher courses to maintain your certification. Care procedures change as newer and more effective treatments for illness and injury are developed. The AED is an example of a fairly recent improvement in emergency care. **Continuous compression resuscitation (CCR)** is a technique recently developed to encourage more people to take action immediately when they witness cardiac arrest in an adult.

The American Heart Association has developed a first aid and CPR mobile app that provides text and video care instructions. Since it can be downloaded and stored on a mobile device, the app can be accessed even without a Wi-Fi signal. Recently, an earthquake victim with basic first aid knowledge used the information in his phone to care for his wounds and signals of shock while he waited for rescue personnel to arrive.

The American Red Cross also has a free first aid mobile app with advice for everyday emergencies. It offers videos and interactive quizzes for reviewing first aid information. In addition, the complete American Red Cross first aid training manual can be accessed through the agency's website for further reading and study.

Complete the
Map Your Reading
graphic organizer for the
section you just read.

Employability Skills for Healthcare Workers

Congratulations, you got the job! You filled out several applications and had a few interviews. Finally, your work paid off and you have a job. Breathe a sigh of relief and pat yourself on the back. Then take a deep breath and get ready to succeed on the job (Figure 10.39).

You are probably thinking about all of the benefits that a job will bring you such as your first paycheck, work experience for your résumé, and the chance to learn new skills. Yet to succeed on the job, you will need to focus on meeting your employer's expectations. Your employer will evaluate your work and decide on your future job responsibilities, which can impact your future career opportunities.

Succeeding on the Job

Feeling nervous about your first day at work is normal. Get plenty of rest and allow extra time for getting to work. On your first day, you may attend an orientation and complete employment forms, or your supervisor or a coworker may train you. During your first week, try to focus on these guidelines:

- Be on time. Show up to work on time and take only the time allowed for breaks and lunches.

- Dress appropriately and be well groomed every day. Learn the facility's dress code policies and follow them exactly.

- Make an effort to learn as many names as possible. Focus on the names of your supervisor and coworkers in your immediate area.

- Listen closely and follow instructions. Show enthusiasm for and interest in learning your job duties. Ask questions if you don't completely understand a task.

- Work hard and be productive. Make a positive first impression by focusing on being accurate. Do your best work.

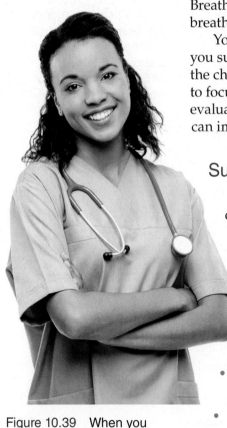

Figure 10.39 When you secure a job, you must focus on meeting your employer's expectations and succeeding on the job.

As you gain experience, learn any facility policies that affect your work. Demonstrate an increase in the work you complete and a decrease in the supervision you need. Show initiative and become self-directed in your work. Employers will expect you to complete your own job and then seek out other tasks you are able to complete while waiting for your next instruction. Workers who stand around waiting become a burden to their supervisors. Finally, be positive and enthusiastic. No one enjoys working with a complainer.

Learning your duties leads to job success, but working well with other people is just as important. You can expect to be assigned tasks that you don't want to do. Since the work needs to be done, you must accept this and do a good job without complaining. Supervisors have different personalities and leadership styles. It's up to you to make the effort to cooperate with your supervisor. Listen respectfully and follow through on your supervisor's suggestions (Figure 10.40).

Keep your eyes and ears open to observe how your facility operates as well as the social interactions of your coworkers. Always be friendly and cooperative, but resist the temptation to gossip, repeat rumors, or take rumors seriously. In other words, avoid workplace drama.

These job success skills are just as important as knowing how to perform the tasks you're assigned. Ninety percent of job firings are due to personal reasons such as poor conduct and problems working with others. The following are the most common reasons employers give for firing employees:

- not showing up for work on a regular basis (especially problematic in the healthcare setting where patients require around-the-clock care)

- laziness on the job (taking long breaks, leaving the work area without reason, texting friends while working, or avoiding less pleasant job tasks)

- personality conflicts (not getting along or collaborating effectively with the supervisor or coworkers)

- violating facility rules (smoking, using alcohol, and ignoring safety regulations)

- **incompetence**

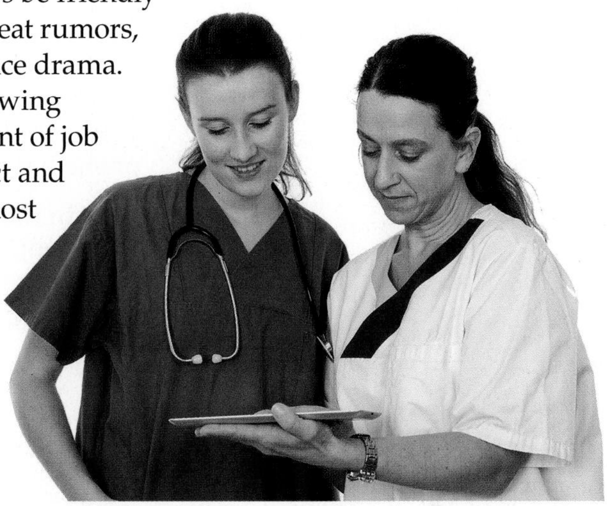

Figure 10.40   Listen respectfully and follow through on your supervisor's suggestions.

incompetence
a lack of qualifications or ability to perform job tasks

Following Professional Standards for Healthcare Workers

When you follow the employability skills described in the last section, you are practicing the professional behaviors that apply to all workers. However, healthcare workers have an additional set of behaviors that support patient rights and advance directives. Following these professional standards protects you, your employer, and your patients.

As you study these standards, you will recognize some of the beginning and end-of-procedure steps you generally perform. Notice how these standards fulfill the ethical guidelines and legal obligations required in the delivery of healthcare.

- **Work within your scope of practice.** This means that you will perform only the procedures for which you have been trained and that you are legally permitted to perform. You must refuse to perform any procedure for which you are not qualified. This is a legal obligation.

- **Use correct, approved methods for all procedures.** Follow the approved procedure manual for your place of employment. Complete procedures according to the methods learned in your training program.

- **Seek proper authorization for all procedures.** Your supervisor may authorize a procedure by assigning a patient care task to you. Some healthcare professionals, such as nurses, will receive verbal authorization from a physician or therapist. For other workers, such as those in a pharmacy, a written order provides the authorization for a procedure.

- **Address patients by name.** If you work in a hospital, you may check the name or scan the bar code on a patient's wristband. If you work in a clinic, you may verify a patient's birthday after he or she has provided a photo ID at reception.

- **Obtain the patient's consent.** Patients have the right to refuse treatment. You must explain each procedure and get the patient's permission before proceeding. For some procedures, like surgery, written consent is required (Figure 10.41).

Figure 10.41   Some healthcare procedures require written consent from the patient.

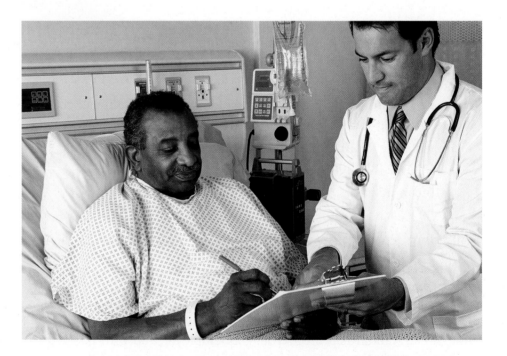

- **Maintain confidentiality.** Choose a private area when reporting patient information to your supervisor. Keep written records where unauthorized individuals can't view them. Do not discuss patient information with other patients, your own friends and family, or even other healthcare workers who are not part of the care team.

- **Provide high-quality care at all times and to all people.** Healthcare workers do not accept tips because the quality of healthcare is not based on payment. Patients receive high-quality care regardless of their social or economic status, race, age, religion, gender, nationality, or other protected category.

- **Report errors to your supervisor immediately.** Take responsibility for your actions by reporting errors and correcting your errors whenever possible. This is important because mistakes made by healthcare workers can affect a patient's health status.

- **Stay calm.** Even during an emergency, healthcare workers must remain calm to reassure patients and allow themselves to think more clearly. When you are frustrated by the actions of a coworker, calm yourself before trying to resolve the problem. Follow the chain of command by reporting a problem to your supervisor rather than complaining to your coworkers.

- **Act with integrity.** Healthcare workers with integrity fulfill their legal and ethical obligations. They are loyal and dedicated employees. They provide empathetic care and maintain a positive attitude.

Understanding Your Paycheck

When you enter the world of work, you begin to earn an income. Knowing how your income is calculated is important, and you will want to understand why money is taken out of your paycheck in the form of deductions.

The Diagnostic Worker: Stacy

Stacy couldn't wait to pick up her check on the first payday at her new job. After two weeks of work, she had carefully calculated her wages. She was excited to celebrate her hard work by splurging on a few special purchases. However, she received a shock when she looked at her check. It was less than half of the wages she had earned! She needed some information to help her understand her paycheck.

Every business has an established pay-period schedule. You may be paid each week, every other week, twice each month, or once each month. Pay will lag behind actual hours worked. This allows the business time to calculate the hours you've worked and the appropriate deductions and to prepare paychecks or transfer automatic deposits to employee accounts. In the scenario presented here, Stacy was paid for the first week she worked. On her next check, she will receive the pay for her second and third weeks of work. She would then have been working a total of four weeks.

Gross pay is the amount that you will find if you calculate the number of hours you've worked multiplied by your hourly wage. Your **net pay** (take-home pay) is that amount with deductions subtracted (Figure 10.42). At least two deductions will appear on your check stub—Federal Insurance Contributions Act (FICA) and federal withholding tax.

Federal Insurance Contributions Act (FICA) is a tax to fund **Social Security**. Social Security provides retirement income, disability, and survivors' benefits. It also supports Medicare, which is a health insurance plan for elderly and disabled citizens.

Federal withholding tax is a tax on your personal income. Taxes are payments that citizens are required to pay so governments can provide a wide range of public services, including police and fire protection, libraries, parks and recreation, hospitals, schools, road maintenance, garbage collection, unemployment insurance, Medicare, and Medicaid. Additional deductions may be made for state income tax, retirement savings plans, union dues, or insurance premiums.

Plan for spending based on your net income rather than your gross income. When you file your tax return, you may receive a refund if

gross pay
the total amount of money earned in a pay period

net pay
the amount of money received in a pay period after all deductions have been taken out; also known as *take-home pay*

Figure 10.42 Deductions are listed on your pay statement so you can understand how your net pay amount was determined.

My Paycheck

Employee Irma M. Payne	Employee Identification 123-45-6789	Check # 164	Net Pay $1,102.98
Employee Address 012 Canal Street Star Prairie, TX 74260			

	Pay Type– Gross Pay	Deductions	Current	Year-to-date
	$1,353.33	Federal Withholding	$106.00	$2,120.00
		State Withholding	$40.82	$816.40
		Fed OASDI/EE or Social Security	$83.91	$1,678.20
		Fed MED/EE or Medicare	$19.62	$392.40
		Medical	$0.00	$0.00
		401k	$0.00	$0.00
		Totals	$250.35	$5,007.00

Pay Period 10/12/2015 – 10/26/2015

more money was withheld than required for the tax you owe. When you change jobs, you will usually receive one final paycheck from the facility at which you no longer work. That is the pay that lagged behind the hours you actually worked, which appeared to be missing from your first paycheck.

HOSA Connections

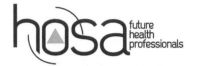

HOSA conferences provide a great opportunity for networking. At these conferences, you will meet healthcare professionals and fellow HOSA members from around your state or the entire nation. Get to know these people because they may be your future employers or coworkers. As your career advances, you will use this network of healthcare workers to seek out information and advice about career opportunities. Figure 10.43 provides a list of competitive events that will strengthen your diagnostic skills. You can read about these events in the competitive events section of the HOSA website.

Figure 10.43 HOSA Events	
Event Name	**Event Description**
CPR/First Aid	Written test and skills demonstration
Creative Problem Solving	Written test and group presentation
Pathophysiology	Written test
EMT/Life Support Skills	Written test, patient assessment and treatment
CERT Skills	Written test and disaster response skills
Healthcare Issues Exam	Written test

RECALL YOUR READING

1. As a new employee, your job success is determined by how well you meet your _____ expectations.
2. Healthcare workers protect patient rights when they follow _____ for the delivery of healthcare.
3. Your take-home or _____ pay is less than your _____ pay because _____ for items such as taxes have been subtracted.
4. Attending HOSA conferences provides valuable opportunities for building your _____ of potential future _____ or coworkers.

Complete the
Map Your Reading
graphic organizer for the
section you just read.

SUMMARY

Assess your understanding
with chapter tests

- Diagnostic workers use a variety of laboratory tests and imaging techniques to create a picture a patient's health status.

- Mechanical aptitude, physical stamina, and the ability to follow detailed instructions with precision and accuracy lead to success in diagnostic careers.

- Improvements in diagnostic testing are speeding up patient diagnosis and leading to more personalized medical care.

- The diagnostic images used in healthcare today can be sent or stored electronically.

- Healthcare supervisors may delegate tasks that are within a worker's scope of practice.

- Successful healthcare teams make a constant effort to maintain positive working relationships in order to promote quality care.

- Healthcare workers must know how to measure temperature, pulse, respiration, and blood

pressure accurately, and when to report changes that may indicate a need for prompt medical care.

- Healthcare workers must check for correct body alignment when positioning patients.

- Vision and hearing screenings reduce learning problems by identifying children who need further evaluation, diagnosis, and treatment.

- The most important step you can take to prepare for an emergency is to complete CPR and first aid certification training.

- Healthcare workers follow a set of professional standards that fulfill the ethical and legal guidelines required in the delivery of healthcare.

- Gross pay is the total amount earned in a pay period, and net pay, or *take-home pay*, is the amount a worker receives after deductions are subtracted.

MAXIMIZE YOUR PROFESSIONAL VOCABULARY

Build vocabulary with
e-flash cards, games,
and audio glossary

Listed below are the essential, yellow-highlighted terms and the additional professional vocabulary that you encountered in this chapter. Complete the activities that follow the list to make all of these terms part of your everyday professional vocabulary.

apical pulse

audiologist

audiometer

automated external
   defibrillator (AED)

blood pressure

body alignment

cardiac arrest

cardiopulmonary resuscitation
   (CPR)

cardiovascular technologists

continuous compression
   resuscitation (CCR)

delegation

diagnostic

discretion

FAST (Face, Arm, Speech,
   Time)

Federal Insurance
   Contributions Act (FICA)

federal withholding tax

first aid

gross pay

hypertension

hypotension

incompetence

integrity

invasive procedure

net pay

noninvasive procedure

nuclear medicine technologists

ophthalmologist

optometrist

otolaryngologist

phlebotomist

public health laboratory
   professionals

radial pulse

radiation therapist

radiographers

rectal temperature	sonographers	stethoscope
respiration	sphygmomanometer	stroke
Social Security	stamina	vital signs

VOCABULARY DEVELOPMENT

Matching. Match each essential term from this chapter with the correct definition below by writing the letter of the description next to the number of the essential term on a separate sheet of paper.

1. body alignment
2. diagnostic
3. discretion
4. first aid
5. gross pay
6. incompetence
7. integrity
8. invasive procedure
9. net pay
10. noninvasive procedure
11. radiographers
12. sonographers
13. vital signs

a. healthcare professionals who create medical images or treat diseases through the use of high-frequency sound waves
b. a lack of qualifications or ability to perform job tasks
c. term used to describe a position of the body in which the spine is not crooked or twisted
d. the key measurements that provide information about a person's health, including temperature, pulse, respiration, and blood pressure
e. the ability to know when to keep sensitive information private
f. adherence to ethical principles and professional standards
g. a test or treatment that does not require incisions to the skin or the insertion of instruments or other materials into the body
h. the total amount of money earned in a pay period
i. the amount of money received in a pay period after all deductions have been taken out; also known as *take-home pay*
j. healthcare professionals who create medical images or treat diseases by passing radiation, such as X-rays or gamma rays, through an object
k. emergency treatment given before regular medical services can be obtained
l. pertaining to the identification of a disease or syndrome
m. a test or treatment that requires incisions to the skin or the insertion of instruments or other materials into the body

14. **Diagnostic Dialogue.** Work in pairs to create a vocabulary chart that lists each vocabulary term under one of these categories: *Careers, Personal Traits, Knowledge (Things to Know),* and *Skills (Things to Do).* As your instructor reads a term definition, you and your partner will compete against each other to cross off the correct term first. Whoever crosses off the most terms is the winner.

15. **Walk the Plank.** Write each of the vocabulary terms for this chapter on a note card. Line up the cards in a row on the floor. "Walk the plank" by stepping on each card as you define its term. How many terms caused you to "fall off

the plank" because you couldn't define them? Take these terms and review their meanings. Then create a new plank and try "walking the plank" again until you can define all the terms.

REFLECT ON YOUR READING

16. Review the diagnostic careers that were discussed in this chapter. Which diagnostic career area has the best opportunities for employment? Would you consider a career in this area? Be prepared to explain the reasons for your choice.

BUILD CORE SKILLS

17. **Critical Thinking.** Some healthcare jobs involve both diagnostic and therapeutic tasks. Identify the following workers as *D* for diagnostic, *T* for therapeutic, or *D/T* for both diagnostic and therapeutic. List a job task to illustrate your choice for each worker.

    audiologist

    dentist

    physician

    nursing assistant

    dental hygienist

    optometrist

    radiation therapist

    emergency medical technician

18. **Writing.** Write a paragraph explaining the concept of personalized medical care. How is it different from the current medical care model? Include technological advances in your explanation.

19. **Speaking and Listening.** Review the chart of services provided by public health laboratories in Figure 10.5. Describe three instances in which you have personally benefitted from the work of a public health laboratory employee.

20. **Critical Thinking.** Identify an imaging technique that could be used in each of the following patient situations:

    a. Jane, age 40, is being seen for a regular physical examination.

    b. John is complaining of heart palpitations.

    c. Lea is a patient with a history of heart disease. She is complaining of pain in her calf muscle but has no apparent injury.

    d. Dylan is receiving treatment to shrink a brain tumor.

    e. Lily has passed out a few times in the past couple of months and the doctor wants to rule out a seizure disorder.

21. **Writing.** Write a paragraph explaining how to succeed on the job. Distinguish between "doing a good job" and "getting along on the job." Use examples to illustrate your explanations.

22. **Reading.** List the healthcare workers you meet when receiving a routine eye exam. Reread the section on vision-related careers.

If necessary, search the Internet for additional information. Identify the required level of training for each worker.

23. **Problem Solving.** Review the following situations. Make changes as needed so that they reflect an appropriate delegation of tasks.

    a. A nursing assistant tells a coworker to complete vital signs for his patients.

    b. A pharmacy technician answers a patient's question about the side effects of her medication.

    c. The supervising RN asks the nursing assistant to finish delivering medications to patients.

    d. A nursing assistant answers the phone and writes down the patient orders for a physician who is in a hurry to get to a surgical appointment.

    e. A physician assistant writes a prescription.

    f. An RN asks a fellow RN to administer medication to her patients while she responds to a patient emergency.

24. **Problem Solving.** Suppose you come upon a car accident. Create a list of five possible injuries you may encounter. Now triage those injuries. Which victims will receive care first, second, and so on? Why?

25. **Math.** Sue works as a pharmacy technician earning $9.50 per hour. She worked 40 hours during her two-week pay period. What is her gross pay? Calculate these deductions: federal withholding tax = 10%; FICA = 6.2%; Medicare = 1.45%. Subtract those deductions from her gross pay. What is her net pay?

26. **Critical Thinking.** List the professional standard that applies to each of these situations.

    a. A friend of your grandmother is a resident at the nursing home where you work. Your grandmother asks you what's wrong with her friend.

    b. As your patient is discharged from the hospital, he offers you a tip for the good care you provided.

    c. At lunch in the hospital cafeteria, your friend begins to tell you about the diagnosis and treatment for a specific patient who is not in your care.

ACTIVATE YOUR LEARNING

27. Review the guidelines for observing standard precautions and measuring vital signs. Then assemble supplies and follow the procedure steps in this chapter to practice measuring temperature, radial pulse, and respiration. Practice locating and measuring your own apical pulse.

28. Review the guidelines for responding to an emergency. Read the section about choking. Use a choking mannequin to practice responding to a choking emergency.

29. Review the guidelines for positioning patients. Then assemble supplies and follow the procedure steps in this chapter to practice patient positioning.

THINK AND ACT LIKE A HEALTHCARE WORKER

30. Shannon has been working at an assisted living center for a month. She likes working with the residents and really enjoys the time she spends assisting them, but getting along with the rest of the staff has been difficult. As a senior in high school, Shannon is the youngest worker at the assisted living center. Every time she asks a question, Shannon feels like the other employees are annoyed, and she has begun to think they are talking about her when she can't hear. Sometimes she just feels like giving up and quitting. Create a dos and don'ts chart with specific steps Shannon can take to improve relationships with her coworkers.

GO TO THE SOURCE

31. Jarod was attending a college hockey game. Suddenly he noticed a student slumped over the back of his seat. The student's sister asked Jarod to get a doctor. Jarod texted the security office to ask for medical assistance. The student was having a seizure. When the seizure stopped, Jarod could not find a pulse and the student had stopped breathing. Jarod got help from another bystander to carry the student to the area near the concessions booth, where Jarod could perform CPR.

The paramedics arrived and took over chest compressions while they attached the AED electrode pads. Triggering the AED produced a heartbeat and the student opened his eyes. The paramedics transported him to the hospital by ambulance and he was released a few days later. Use the Internet to research the steps included in the chain of survival. Identify each step in this case study.

32. Use the Internet to learn more about diagnostic services careers. Select two careers of interest to you and complete a career profile for each one. Use at least one site that ends in ".gov" and one site that ends in ".org." Record the following information for each career:

    • name of career
    • tasks involved in this career
    • personal traits and abilities needed
    • educational requirements
    • type of credential needed and how it is obtained
    • work conditions
    • wages and benefits
    • job outlook for the future
    • the websites you accessed

    How do the two careers compare? Why might you prefer one to the other?

DEVELOP YOUR HEALTH SCIENCE CAREER PORTFOLIO

33. Use the HOSA website to research the HOSA competitive events listed in this chapter. Select and note which event would be your first choice. Explain why you chose this event.

34. Begin to build your career network. List all the people you know who could help you with educational information, volunteer opportunities, job shadowing, or employment in the field of healthcare. Place this list in your career portfolio.

35. Diagnostic careers involve working with laboratory equipment and imaging machines. Do you like to repair cars or machinery, build items from wood or other materials, or operate a cash register or video equipment? What is the connection between these activities and diagnostic careers? How can you use the answers to these questions to guide your health career selection process?

Chapter 11
Fundamental Skills in Diagnostic Services

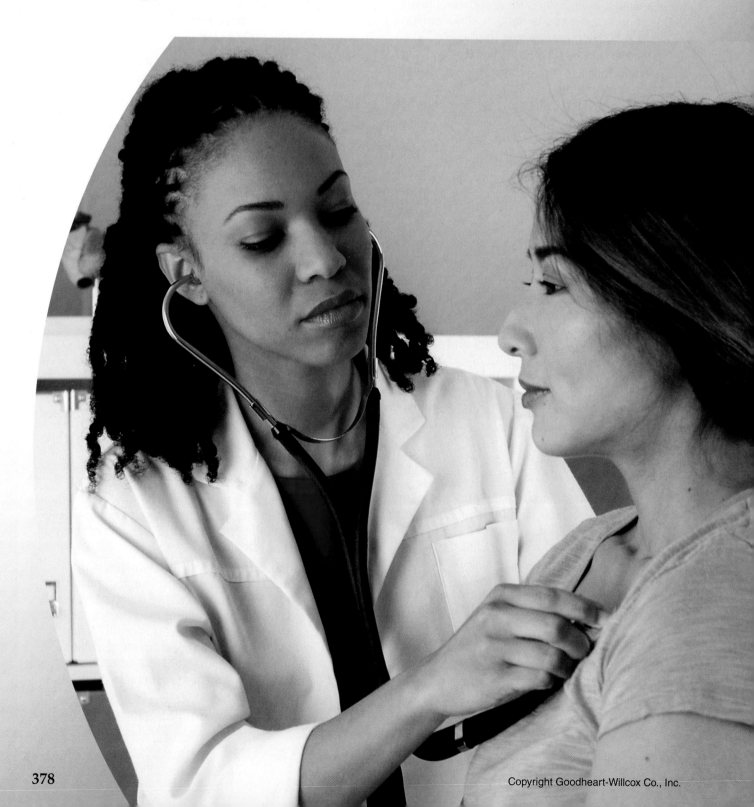

PROFESSIONAL VOCABULARY

 E-flash
Cards

You will need to learn the essential terms listed below before you begin your reading. These terms will help you understand the main concepts of the chapter. These terms, which will be highlighted in yellow within the text, will become part of your professional vocabulary.

In addition to these essential terms, you will see bold terms throughout the chapter. The meanings of these terms are explained where the terms first appear. The bold terms, like the essential terms listed here, will become part of your professional vocabulary and deepen your understanding of the topics presented.

auscultation   the use of a stethoscope to listen to sounds made by a patient's internal organs (heart, lungs, abdominal organs) to make a diagnosis

body mass index (BMI)   a method of relating weight to height used to define normal weight, overweight, and obesity

breach   access, use, or disclosure of protected health information that compromises the security or privacy of that information

cultural competence   the ability to interact effectively with people of different cultures

de-identified information   health documents from which specified personal data has been removed

differential diagnosis   a determination made by a doctor that distinguishes a disease or condition from others that present with similar symptoms

inspection   visual examination used to assess parts of the body by looking for abnormal color, shape, size, or texture

medical diagnosis   a determination made by a doctor that identifies the cause of a patient's illness

nursing diagnosis   the description of a client's health problem that a nurse is licensed and competent to treat

palpation   a medical examination that uses touch to detect growths, changes in the size of organs, or tissue reactions to pressure

percussion   the process of tapping various body parts during examination and using resulting sounds to assess the condition of internal organs

personal bias   an unfair preference for, or dislike of, something or someone

prejudice   a strong feeling or belief about a person or subject that is not based on reason or actual experience

sign   evidence of a health condition that can be seen or measured

stereotype   the assumption that everyone in a particular group is the same

symptom   an indication of a disease or disorder experienced by the patient, such as pain

telehealth   the use of electronic information and telecommunications technologies to support long-distance clinical healthcare, health-related education, public health, and health administration

CONNECT WITH YOUR READING

Think about the last time you saw a physician. During your appointment, what steps did the medical assistant and physician take to assess your health? Some assessments, such as measuring vital signs, are obvious. But you should also consider what the doctor asked you and watched you do. Make a list describing each assessment you can recall.

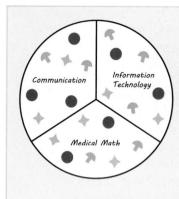

MAP YOUR READING

Create a visual summary by drawing a large circle on a blank sheet of paper. Divide the circle into three pizza slices. Label one slice *Communication*, another *Information Technology*, and the third *Medical Math*. As you finish reading each section of the chapter, place the following "toppings" on your pizza:

- Draw "pepperoni" circles containing the main ideas or the "meat" of the information.
- Draw "mushroom" shapes containing bits of information that are new or interesting for you and kept you from "vegging out" as you read.
- Draw "mystery" toppings (you create the shapes) that contain questions you still have about your reading.

All medical treatments begin with a diagnosis. Healthcare workers in the diagnostic services pathway contribute to the process of diagnosing a patient's illness or injury. Many fundamental skills are important to the diagnostic worker's job, including communication, confidentiality, information technology, and math.

This chapter introduces the communication skills healthcare workers use to examine patients and diagnose their illnesses. You will learn how a person's culture influences this process. You will also learn about the requirements for protecting patient health information that is stored or exchanged electronically and the ways in which healthcare technology is changing diagnostic techniques. Finally, you will enhance your math skills as you convert temperatures between the Fahrenheit and Celsius scales; learn to graph vital signs; and chart height, weight, and body mass index.

Communication Skills for Patient Diagnosis

Diagnostic communication skills focus on patient observation and the process of physical examination and assessment. Healthcare workers must know how to record their observations and when it is important to report those observations to a supervisor. Effective healthcare workers are alert to cultural differences and competent in adapting care to meet the unique needs of the individuals they serve.

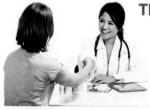

The Diagnostic Worker: Trinity

Trinity was surprised that she was feeling nervous. After 12 years of preparation, she was starting her first full-time job as a medical doctor. Of course, she had already worked with many patients during her internship and residency, but this felt different. Today she would see patients as a newly licensed, board-certified physician working independently instead of under the supervision of another doctor.

Starting today, patients would rely on her examination, diagnosis, and treatment to restore their good health. It was a sobering realization, but it was exciting at the same time. Helping people and curing disease had been Trinity's dream job for as long as she could remember.

Checking her schedule, she reviewed the first patient's record and headed to the exam room. She knocked, entered, smiled, and said, "Hello, I'm Dr. O'Dell. What seems to be the problem?"

Communicating Observations

In the process of diagnosis, physicians use reading skills as they review entries in the patient record. They use speaking and listening skills as they interview patients using open-ended questions. Perhaps most importantly, they use the powerful skill of observation as they examine patients.

Healthcare workers use nearly all of their senses when they observe a patient:

- **Sight.** Healthcare workers look for the **signs** of injury or illness using **inspection**. Also called **objective observations**, signs can be seen (as with bruises, swelling, rashes, or cuts) or measured (as with vital signs, such as temperature and blood pressure).

- **Hearing.** Listening to a patient's statements or complaints reveals **symptoms**. Also called **subjective observations**, symptoms cannot be seen or measured by a healthcare worker. For example, only the patient can detect stomachache, back pain, and fatigue. Healthcare workers won't learn about symptoms unless the patient tells them.

  In the process of examination, healthcare providers also use hearing as they listen to respirations and abnormal body sounds. Through **auscultation** (aw-skuhl-TAY-shuhn), healthcare workers can hear the sounds of the heart and lungs, listen to bowel sounds, and hear the flow of blood through arteries.

- **Touch.** Healthcare providers use **palpation**, or touching and applying pressure, to measure pulse rates and assess blood flow to many areas of the body. They also use palpation to identify abnormal conditions such as swelling, unusual hardness, body parts that are out of place, and the location of pain. They can feel dryness, perspiration, heat, and unusual skin texture through touch.

  Percussion is a method of tapping body parts with fingers, hands, or small instruments while listening for sounds coming from body organs. Through percussion, healthcare workers learn the size, density, and position of internal organs. They can also detect the presence or absence of fluid in specific body areas.

  Using percussion on a body part is similar to playing a drum. A healthcare provider can interpret differences in sound to determine the kind of tissue within the body. For example, healthy lungs sound hollow because they are filled with air. Bones and joints sound solid, but the abdomen sounds like a hollow organ filled with air, fluid, or solids.

sign
evidence of a health condition that can be seen or measured

inspection
visual examination used to assess parts of the body by looking for abnormal color, shape, size, or texture

symptom
an indication of a disease or disorder experienced by the patient, such as pain

auscultation
the use of a stethoscope to listen to sounds made by a patient's internal organs (heart, lungs, abdominal organs) to make a diagnosis

palpation
a medical examination that uses touch to detect growths, changes in the size of organs, or tissue reactions to pressure

percussion
the process of tapping various body parts during examination and using resulting sounds to assess the condition of internal organs

- **Smell.** Healthcare workers pay attention to body odors, as well as unusual breath, wound, urine, or **stool** (waste material released during a bowel movement) odors. While the concept of using odors in patient assessment may not be appealing, odors do provide important signals about a patient's health. For example, breath that smells fruity may mean the patient is experiencing **ketoacidosis**, a serious condition that can lead to diabetic coma and needs further medical care.

Performing a Physical Examination and Assessment

During a physical examination, the medical provider follows four basic steps: inspection, palpation, percussion, and auscultation (Figure 11.1). Moving from head to foot, the provider checks each area of the body and documents findings in the patient's medical record.

Examinations may be preventive, as in the case of a yearly physical, or they may be done to determine the cause of problematic symptoms a patient is experiencing. When a patient *presents* (comes to the provider) with signs of illness, the provider begins the process of forming a **differential diagnosis**. The physician completes a physical examination and takes a medical history. The results of the examination along with the patient's medical history are used to formulate a list of all the possible causes of the patient's symptoms.

differential diagnosis
a determination made by a doctor that distinguishes a disease or condition from others that have similar symptoms

Figure 11.1   The four basic steps in a physical examination are shown here. Which of these steps uses a stethoscope?

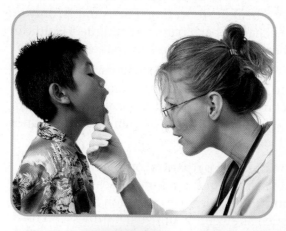
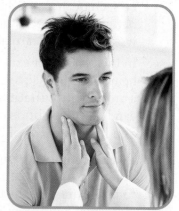
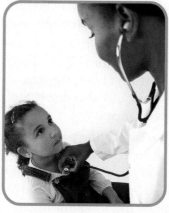
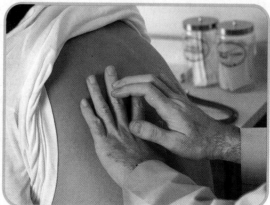

Next, the physician works to develop a **medical diagnosis**. He or she orders specific diagnostic tests to confirm the cause or identify other previously overlooked causes before beginning treatment. The physician interprets the results of these tests to determine the medical diagnosis.

Physical examinations vary according to the needs of each patient. Specialists focus on a particular body system or organ. For example, a cardiologist will focus an examination on the patient's heart-related symptoms. The patient's chief complaint, or most important health concern, also guides the examination. For example, a patient who complains of hearing problems may be given Weber and Rinne tests to screen for conductive hearing loss.

Nursing staff members also **assess**, or evaluate patients to determine a **nursing diagnosis** and develop a patient care plan. This diagnosis may be made using patient and family interviews, medical records, and a physical examination to identify a patient's problems. The nursing diagnosis states the patient's problem and the cause of the problem. For example, a nursing diagnosis could be "impaired mobility caused by stroke." The nursing staff members use the diagnosis to develop a care plan that identifies solutions for this problem and techniques that team members will use to help the patient overcome the problem.

As the care plan is implemented, staff members use observation skills to evaluate the patient's progress. A nursing assistant, for example, looks for changes in the patient's skin to prevent the development of skin ulcers and reports any observations of skin redness and warmth at pressure points. The nursing process—which consists of assessment, problem identification, planning, implementation, and evaluation— relies on careful observation to promote patient recovery.

When a resident enters a long-term care facility, a special **minimum data set (MDS)** assessment is completed. This minimum data set is part of a government requirement for the clinical assessment of all residents in a long-term care facility (Figure 11.2). The MDS provides a comprehensive evaluation of each resident's functional capabilities. This helps nursing home staff identify health problems. MDS assessments are required for residents on admission to the facility and are repeated periodically.

Licensed healthcare professionals, usually registered nurses employed by the long-term care facility, complete the MDS. These professionals transmit MDS information electronically to the state MDS database and, from there, it becomes part of the national MDS database at the Centers for Medicare and Medicaid Services (CMS). CMS uses the data to generate reports concerning resident status and indicators of quality care.

medical diagnosis
a determination made by a doctor that identifies the cause of a patient's illness

nursing diagnosis
the description of a client's health problem that a nurse is licensed and competent to treat

	Figure 11.2 Categories of the Minimum Data Set (MDS)
1	cognitive patterns
2	communication and hearing patterns
3	vision patterns
4	physical functioning and structural problems
5	continence
6	psychosocial well-being
7	mood and behavior patterns
8	activity pursuit patterns
9	disease diagnosis
10	other health conditions
11	oral/nutritional status
12	oral/dental status
13	skin condition
14	medication use
15	treatments and procedures

Reporting and Recording Observations

All healthcare workers are responsible for reporting unusual events or changes in a patient's behavior or physical condition. For example, an observant receptionist may notice a person in the waiting room who is having trouble breathing and needs immediate help. Take your reporting obligation seriously and do not wait for someone else to report an unusual situation. You may prevent a more serious problem by quickly calling attention to unusual behavior.

In a care facility, health team members report changes in a patient's or resident's status throughout the shift by giving a verbal report to a supervising team member. In general, the following patient or resident observations are reported:

- changes in the person's condition (vital signs, skin color, breathing, or behavior—confusion, agitation, restlessness, or lethargy)

- reactions to a new treatment or therapy

- complaints of pain or discomfort such as weakness, dizziness, or nausea

- refusal of treatment

- request for a clergy visit

Specific signs and symptoms of illness should be reported, as should specific signs and symptoms of infection (Figure 11.3). Always ask the patient about pain; do not assume that patients will tell you on their own. Use a **pain scale** to help you assess a patient's level of pain (Figure 11.4).

Figure 11.3 Observations to Be Reported	
Signs and Symptoms of Infection	**Indications and Symptoms of Pain**
• elevated temperature • sweating/chills • skin is hot, cold, red, or swollen • drainage from wounds or body cavities • discharge of mucus or pus	• chest pain • radiating pain • pain when moving • pain during urination or bowel movement • any pain is not normal; report all complaints of pain

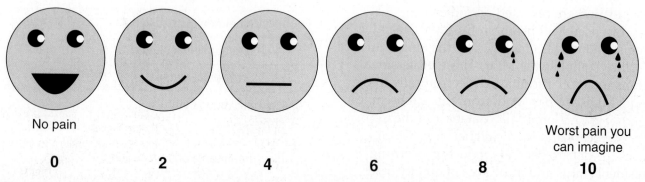

Figure 11.4   Pain scales can be helpful in assessing your patient's pain level.

When you make a report, state the patient's name and room number. Make your report orderly and concise by giving actual vital sign measurements and reporting only what you observe. Because symptoms can't be observed or measured by others, you should always report exactly what a resident tells you when he or she complains of symptoms.

Correct: Jane Smith in Room 602 has a right arm that is red, swollen, and warm to the touch.

Correct: Jane Smith in Room 602 says her left ear aches.

Incorrect: Mrs. Smith has an ear infection.

Incorrect: Mrs. Smith's vital signs don't look good.

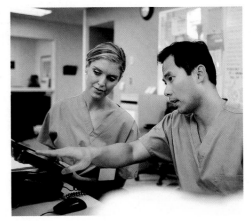

Figure 11.5 Communication is essential for providing the best possible care. When the workers on one shift at a healthcare facility leave, they must report to the new shift to explain the current status and care needs for each patient.

At the end of each shift, workers present a **shift report** that tells the oncoming staff the information necessary for a smooth continuation of patient care (Figure 11.5). During the shift report, the oncoming staff members learn about new patients or residents and their care plans. Outgoing staff highlight changes in the care plans for current patients, such as new medication orders or treatments, and share changes in the status of patients, such as a change in appetite or level of alertness.

Record all observations in the patient record and, just as importantly, record the fact that you reported an observation. For example: *Right arm is red, swollen, and warm to touch. Reported to charge nurse.*

Abbreviations are less common when charting in an electronic health record, but remember to use only the abbreviations approved by your facility whether you are documenting by hand or electronically. If you do not know the meaning of an abbreviation that appears in a resident's care plan, look it up or ask your supervisor for clarification. Never guess or assume that you know the meaning. You can find more detailed information about using abbreviations in chapter 5.

cultural competence
the ability to interact effectively with people of different cultures

Developing Cultural Competence

Cultural competence is an important component of communication (Figure 11.6). You can begin to develop your knowledge and skills for working with diverse populations by following basic guidelines for showing sensitivity to cultural differences. Continue to expand your knowledge by studying the cultural backgrounds and customs of your coworkers and patients. Finally, as you get to know the individual personalities and beliefs of patients and coworkers, adjust your own communication style to accommodate their individual preferences.

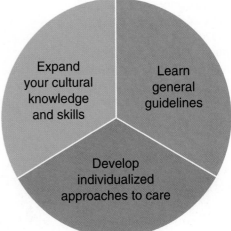

Figure 11.6 Learning these three aspects of cultural competence will help you give the best possible care to patients of diverse cultures.

Learning General Guidelines. Chapter 7 mentioned an employer who only hired applicants who looked her in the eye. She turned away two excellent nursing assistants because she didn't know they looked down as a sign of respect. While you certainly will not know the culture and customs of all your future patients and coworkers, following these general guidelines will help you avoid unintentionally insulting patients and colleagues.

Figure 11.7 Eye Contact in Different Cultures	
Anglo-American	• direct eye contact shows interest, honesty, and attention to the speaker
Asian, Hispanic, Navajo, Nigerian	• avoiding eye contact shows respect
Middle Eastern	• direct eye contact between a man and woman may be seen as a sexual invitation

Eye Contact

Sit next to—instead of facing—a patient or coworker who appears uncomfortable with direct eye contact. Figure 11.7 shows several different cultures' feelings about eye contact.

Body Language

Regarding physical distance and touching, you should always follow the lead of the person with whom you are speaking (Figure 11.8). Be sensitive to those who are uncomfortable with close contact, and ask permission before touching a patient during an examination.

Use gestures cautiously because they can have very different meanings in different cultures. Ask patients about their reactions to a gesture if you are uncertain.

Do not interpret pain or fear based solely on facial expressions. Appropriate expressions of physical or emotional feelings are closely guided by a person's cultural and personal background (Figure 11.9). Remember that pain is an individual experience. Do not assume that a patient is exaggerating pain. Always check for all possible causes for pain.

Figure 11.8   In closer cultures, friends of the same sex may hold hands, and kissing is a common greeting. In more distant cultures, the handshake is a common greeting, with hugs reserved for close friends and family members.

Closer Contact Areas of the World
- Africa
- Indonesia
- Latin America
- Mediterranean
- Southern Europe

Distant Contact Areas of the World
- North America
- Northern Europe
- Great Britain
- Middle East
- Asia

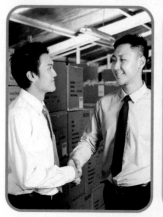
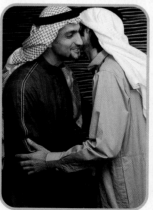
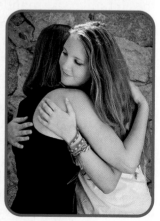

Figure 11.9 Pain Responses	
Stoic Cultural Background	**Expressive Cultural Background**
• Northern European • Asian • American Indian	• Hispanic • Middle Eastern • Mediterranean

Sense of Time

Understand that healthcare facilities operate on "clock" time, but many people operate on "activity" time. For example, arriving at 3:30 p.m. for a 2:45 p.m. appointment is late to a clinic, but it's still midafternoon to a person with "activity" time orientation. This person will not see himself or herself as late. Someone with "activity" time orientation might simply come to the appointment when the morning work is finished rather than when the clock says it's time.

In this type of situation, avoid showing frustration. Respectfully explain why clock time is important. For example, you could say, "Our clinic policy is to reschedule appointments when patients are more than 15 minutes late. This prevents long waits for patients."

Speech and Communication

Address patients and coworkers using their last name. Then follow their lead if they ask you to use their first name. Ask patients how they would like to be addressed if you feel uncertain.

Match the volume and speed of your speech to those of the patient. This will make the patient feel more comfortable. Avoid interrupting and showing impatience, which is disrespectful in nearly every culture.

Use an interpreter when language differences interfere with the patient's ability to understand healthcare information or your ability to understand the patient's description of signs and symptoms. Provide written information and directions in the patient's own language whenever possible.

While most Americans prefer independent decision making, many cultures defer to the head of the household to make decisions for family members. For example, a woman may look to her husband for permission to speak.

Modesty

Provide complete privacy for all patients when they are changing clothing. Knock before entering the exam room to avoid interrupting a patient who is changing. Keep the patient covered as much as possible during the examination, diagnosis, and treatment process. Use a provider of the same sex when culture forbids a person of the opposite sex from touching a patient. For example, in some Middle Eastern countries, men may not touch females who are not immediate family members.

Expanding Your Knowledge and Skills. Your challenge, as you improve your cultural competence, is to develop a balance between knowing about specific cultural groups and using skills and attitudes that are not specific to any cultural group.

Learning your patients' religious customs, their views on death and dying, and how they explain illness and its causes is valuable to the delivery of healthcare. For example, in the United States, we value telling patients the truth, whether the news is good or bad. However, this is not the case for all cultures. Did you know that some cultures believe that talking about death actually leads to death? Figure 11.10 gives an overview of elements of belief systems that may differ among cultures. The chart also presents healthcare-related examples from specific cultures to help you develop your cultural competence. You will need to complete more research as you work with specific patients.

Developing Individualized Approaches to Care. Even though we are products of our culture, we are all unique individuals with our own set of preferences. Never presume to know a patient's preferences based on your personal understanding of the patient's culture. Spend time learning about the specific cultural beliefs of groups in your community but also strive to develop individual **rapport** (ra-POR), or understanding with

Figure 11.10 Interacting with Patients When Belief Systems Influence Healthcare

Element	Actions to Take	Selected Examples That May Influence Healthcare
Religion and spirituality	• Acknowledge and respect all religious and spiritual beliefs. • Remember that religion may also influence dietary choices.	• Jehovah's Witnesses cannot receive blood products or blood transfusions. • Orthodox Judaism forbids healthcare procedures on the Sabbath. • Christian Scientists accept no medication or surgery.
Explaining health and disease	• Ask about the cultural meaning of illness for your patient. • Present problems in ways that reflect the patient's model of illness.	• Native Americans believe that an imbalance between man and nature causes illness. • Hispanic cultures believe that fear, evil, or envy may lead to illness. • Several cultural groups view illness as a punishment from God.
Death and communicating "bad news"	• Understand that beliefs will vary. • Ask for patient preferences.	• In Asian cultures, it is proper to reveal a terminal diagnosis to the patient's family. They will decide whether to tell the patient. • Many cultural groups oppose removing life support for reasons related to God's will. • Muslims and Hmong may refuse organ donation or autopsy.
Role of the family	• Understand that interdependence may be valued more than independence. • Ask patients with whom they will consult regarding medical decisions.	• In Asian and Hispanic cultures, families want to help care for the patient. The patient should not be alone. • Several cultural groups view the eldest male as the spokesperson and decision maker for all family members.

the patients you serve (Figure 11.11). A positive relationship enhances the delivery of healthcare. When you make patients feel comfortable and show respect and caring, they will begin to trust you. When patients trust you, they will share their healthcare concerns, and your diagnosis, treatment, and care will be far more effective.

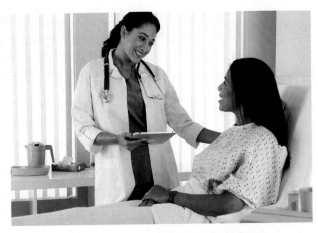

Figure 11.11 Maintaining a positive relationship with patients can improve the quality of care being administered. What can you do to create a friendly rapport with patients?

Developing rapport begins with making patients feel comfortable. Do you focus your attention on patients when talking to them, or are you looking at the computer screen to enter their information? Could you learn a couple of simple phrases to greet patients in their own language? Do you assume that patients know whom they will see and what these individuals will do as part of patient care, or do you take the time to explain? Do all patients know how to learn the results of their lab tests and when those results will be available? Do you make sure that patients clearly understand follow-up procedures before they leave the facility? Taking the time to show these courtesies to all patients illustrates cultural competence. Notice that culturally competent medical receptionists are just as important as culturally competent care providers.

As you develop rapport with the patients you serve, seek to know them as individuals. Take the time to ask about their views and preferences. Record these for future reference and use them in your interactions with your patients. This shows respect, care, and concern. This kind of individualized approach to care leads to a higher quality of care. Healthcare professionals sometimes use mnemonic tools to remember detailed guidelines. As you record health history, you can use the UNIQUE mnemonic shown in Figure 11.12 on the next page to learn your patients' individual preferences.

Exhibiting Cultural Competence with Coworkers. As our workforce becomes more diverse, we must expand our viewpoints regarding the delivery of care. Expecting others to think exactly as you do invites misunderstanding and damages working relationships. You need to extend the same respect, care, and concern to coworkers that you show to patients. Take the time to know your colleagues' beliefs and preferences so you can work as a team that takes advantage of each member's unique skills. Of course, this leads to a higher quality of care for your patients. Remember, providing the best care for your patients is the primary goal of all coworker communication.

Overcoming Barriers to Cultural Competence. Healthcare workers have their own cultural beliefs, attitudes, and viewpoints that can influence their feelings about and their diagnosis and treatment of patients. These personal preferences can be **conscious**, meaning you are aware of them, or they can be **unconscious** preferences that you don't know you possess. Though most healthcare workers do not purposely ignore the beliefs and preferences of their patients, all workers can benefit from examining their own personal biases and prejudices to learn how these affect their interactions with patients.

	Figure 11.12 UNIQUE Mnemonic for Charting Patient Preferences	
	Assessment Categories	**Sample Questions**
U	**U**ncover cultural background	1. Where were you born? 2. How long have you lived in the United States? 3. What is your age? (also note gender)
N	**N**ote religious and spiritual traditions	1. How might religious observances affect your treatment? 2. Do you avoid any particular foods or change your diet during religious observances?
I	**I**dentify healthcare beliefs and treatment preferences	1. What do you believe causes illness/preserves good health? 2. What traditional/home health remedies do you use? 3. Are there any healthcare procedures that are unacceptable to you? 4. What alternative healing methods do you use?
Q	**Q**uestions and concerns for care	1. Do you find it easier to talk with a man or a woman? Someone older or younger? 2. What do you want to accomplish from today's visit/treatment?
U	**U**nmet language needs	1. What language do you prefer to speak/read? 2. Do you need an interpreter? 3. Do you prefer printed or spoken instructions?
E	**E**nvironment	1. With whom do you live? 2. Who helps you when you are ill? 3. When do you usually eat? 4. Can you shop and cook for yourself?

Personal Bias

personal bias
an unfair preference for, or dislike of, something or someone

Your **personal biases** may interfere with patient care if you are unaware of them. For example, consider pain treatment. If you expect patients to be stoic and put up with pain, do you ignore those who express pain because they are just being "difficult"? On the other hand, if you expect patients to express pain, do you ignore stoic patients because you assume their silence means they have no pain?

Prejudice

prejudice
a strong feeling or belief about a person or subject that is not based on reason or actual experience

Prejudice is a pre-established opinion based on a lack of individual knowledge or irrational feelings. Prejudice can lead to an unfounded dislike, fear, or mistrust of a person or cultural group.

Suppose a female Hispanic patient came to the surgical recovery room and, as her sedation wore off, began to scream loudly and complain of terrible pain. The nurse, Dale, administered the prescribed pain medication, but the woman's screaming continued. He checked her vital signs and examined the surgical site but did not find any unusual signs. He was frustrated with the patient's loud cries. He thought to himself,

"Looks like another loud female complainer. I wish she would quit exaggerating her pain."

After another hour of her cries, Dale finally decided to call the surgeon. An examination showed pressure on nerves near the patient's surgical site, which was causing excruciating pain. Further surgery was completed to fix this problem. This time, the patient was calm and cooperative in the recovery room. Dale's prejudice caused him to mistrust the patient's expression of pain. Fortunately, he eventually reported her pain and the patient received the necessary treatment.

Stereotypes

When you buy into **stereotypes**, you view everyone in a cultural group as identical to each other. We use the phrase "as American as apple pie," but does that mean that all Americans love to eat apple pie? Though this stereotype is untrue, it is also fairly harmless. You might encounter more serious or offensive stereotypes in the healthcare setting.

Mrs. Carter is an African-American mother with young children. Like many families, her family has health insurance through her husband's employer. Yet when she approaches the clinic reception desk, she is automatically asked for her Medicaid card. She is irritated that the reception staff automatically assumes that because she is African-American, she is poor. You should avoid making assumptions and using harmful stereotypes such as this one.

Assimilation and Acculturation. Assimilation is the process by which members of a new cultural group adopt all the beliefs and customs of the majority group. The United States does not require assimilation from its immigrants. We are all free to choose our own religion and celebrate holidays according to our own customs. Citizens, however, are expected to appreciate and respect cultural differences.

Over time, **acculturation** (uh-kuhl-chuh-RAY-shun) will occur. This is the process by which immigrants learn the beliefs and customs of the dominant culture and adopt some of them, while maintaining beliefs and customs of their own culture (Figure 11.13). As healthcare workers, we must not assume that all people of the same culture will have the same beliefs and follow the same customs.

stereotype
the assumption that everyone in a particular group is the same

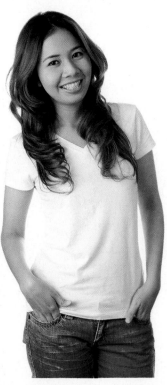

Figure 11.13   Over time, many immigrants adopt some of the customs of the dominant culture. What is the term for this process?

The Diagnostic Worker: Celia

Celia works as a nutritionist in a senior apartment complex. Two of the Asian residents have terminal illnesses. Celia is familiar with the customs of Asian families in her community and assumes the families of these two residents won't share the diagnosis with their loved ones. One family followed the traditional custom of not telling the resident about the terminal diagnosis. They were happy that she lived out her last days without the burden of knowing she was dying. However, the other family shared the terminal diagnosis. Celia was surprised when the resident said goodbye and thanked her for her careful work and helpful manner. The resident's family was happy that he was able to make final arrangements and say goodbye to everyone.

Dealing with Difficult People

Considering the stress, worry, and pain that illness brings to patients and the harried and stressful environments that healthcare workers can experience, you are sure to encounter some difficult interactions. While you can't directly change the behavior of another person, the way you interpret and react to a situation can lead to solving the problem.

The first step in dealing with difficult people is to not label them as difficult! Using that label creates a barrier in your thinking that keeps you from looking more closely at the reason for the behavior that you want to change. People usually have a reason for acting the way they do. However, they might not be able to explain their reason logically or even know the reason.

People who are being "difficult" typically need something. Look at the situation from the patient's point of view and ask yourself what has changed in the patient's environment. Try to diagnose the individual's unmet need. Is it physical, social, emotional, or intellectual? Once you figure out what that need is and satisfy it to the best of your ability, the behavior may change.

For example, Mrs. Stevens usually enjoys a relaxing bath, but she has recently refused her bath, saying she's too tired or in too much pain. Yet she's not too tired or in too much pain to participate in other activities at the care center. This has gone on too long, and now she really needs that bath.

Taking a careful look at the bath schedule, you see that Jake, a new employee, was assigned to give Mrs. Stevens her baths around the same time that she began to refuse them. You review her chart and notice that all of her physicians are female. You speak with Mrs. Stevens privately to ask if she would like to have a female bath aide. She looks relieved and immediately says yes. She didn't want to make Jake feel bad, but she was embarrassed to have a man help her bathe.

Suppose you have just worked 11 hours of a 12-hour nursing shift and are feeling exhausted. Mr. Matthews, who is recovering from a partial **prostatectomy** (surgical removal of the prostate gland), presses his call light every couple of minutes. He complains about everything: your care, the food, and even the other patients in his room. What is wrong with him? You'd like to tell him to grow up and act his age! Instead, you take a deep breath and put yourself in his place. He's the head of a large company and is used to giving orders to other people. How do you think he feels having to lie in bed and wait for someone else to take care of him? Consider his surgery. What other feelings might he be experiencing?

Feelings of helplessness, frustration, and fear may be expressed with loud and angry complaints. Try not to take it personally. These complaints certainly aren't about you. They are caused by the emotional stress the patient is experiencing. Remain calm and listen to your patient's requests. Offer as many choices as possible to help your patient regain a sense of control. Instead of avoiding a demanding patient, use your observation and listening skills to learn more about him or her (Figure 11.14). You may be surprised by the power of careful listening. It allows your patient to express worries, which may begin to calm his or her fears.

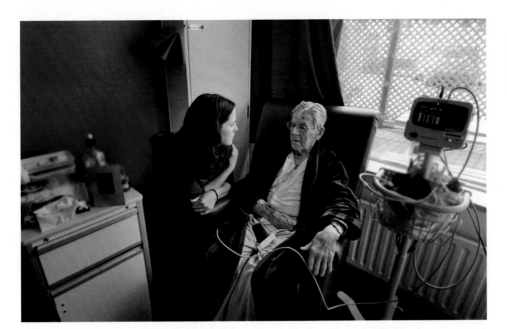

Figure 11.14   Listening to your patients' needs and concerns will help you understand why they may be acting uncooperatively.

RECALL YOUR READING

1. _____ skills are important when healthcare workers are examining patients.
2. Inspection, _____, percussion, and _____ are used when a medical provider does a(n) _____.
3. In a long-term care facility, nurses use a(n) _____ clinical assessment to evaluate each resident's capabilities.
4. One step in developing _____ is using skills and attitudes that build _____ with patients.
5. Healthcare workers must avoid prejudice, _____, and stereotypes.

Complete the *Map Your Reading* graphic organizer for the section you just read.

Information Technology

The increased use of electronic records and electronic forms of communication raises concerns about the privacy and security of patient information. The provisions of the Health Information Technology for Economic and Clinical Health (HITECH) Act address those concerns. Meanwhile, the expansion of new technologies is changing diagnostic techniques and shortening the time frame for making a medical diagnosis.

Electronic Health Records: Addressing Privacy Concerns

As discussed in chapter 7, the HITECH Act made significant changes to privacy and security regulations. These changes address the concerns many patients have regarding the privacy and confidentiality of personal information when it is stored in electronic health records. The law strengthens the rules for securing the data set called *protected health information (PHI)*. The PHI data set includes any information that could be used to identify a person (Figure 11.15 on the next page).

Figure 11.15 Types of Protected Health Information

1	name
2	address (identifiers more specific than a state)
3	dates (other than year)
4	phone numbers
5	fax numbers
6	e-mail addresses
7	Social Security number
8	medical record number
9	health insurance beneficiary number
10	account number
11	certificate and license numbers
12	vehicle identifiers and serial numbers, including license plate numbers
13	device identifiers and serial numbers
14	URLs
15	IP addresses
16	biometric identifiers, including finger, retinal, and voice prints
17	full-face photographic images
18	any other unique identifying number or code

The basic guideline for protecting the rights of clients is to keep all health information confidential. Confidential information and PHI are kept private when access to information is restricted to need-to-know situations as defined by the HITECH Act. All healthcare workers who access patient data must adhere to the privacy rule as they work with healthcare records (Figure 11.16). Think carefully before you leave papers lying on your desk, when you use your phone in a hospital hallway, or when you have a discussion with another healthcare worker in the elevator. Are you protecting the patient's PHI?

Releasing PHI in other situations, such as for marketing purposes or medical research, requires patient authorization. However, **de-identified information** can be released because it is no longer considered PHI. The process of de-identifying health information removes all patient-specific information so there is no reasonable basis on which a person can be identified. Once information is certified as de-identified, it may be shared and used for marketing or research purposes.

de-identified information
health documents from which specified personal data has been removed

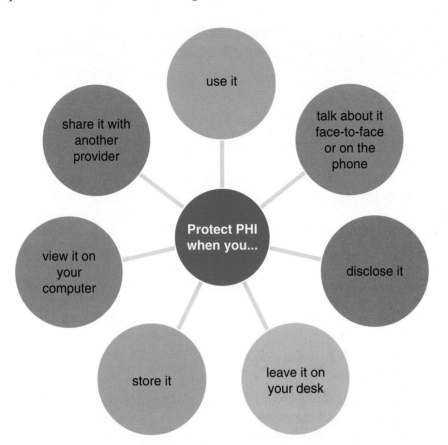

Figure 11.16   All healthcare workers must protect PHI at all times.

breach
access, use, or disclosure of protected health information that compromises the security or privacy of that information

Under the HITECH Act, healthcare providers must notify the Department of Health and Human Services (HHS) of any **breach** of privacy or security regarding patient information. Breaches can occur in many different ways. For example, sending an e-mail to the wrong person, a fax to the wrong number, or a letter to the wrong address is a breach (Figure 11.17). Losing a file that contains PHI is a breach. Sharing or posting passwords that allow account access or letting a fellow worker use your login to gain access to more patient information is a breach. Losing a laptop that is not encrypted is a breach. Accessing information that you do not need to know for your job but are simply curious about is a breach.

The HHS Office of Civil Rights oversees the investigation of breaches and enforces privacy rules. HHS is authorized to levy fines against healthcare businesses when a breach occurs (Figure 11.18 on the next page). As you can imagine, the resulting publicity from a breach has a negative impact on a business. As a result, healthcare facilities carefully focus on protocols that protect PHI and prevent breaches of confidential information.

Protecting your password also protects you. Since you are responsible for all actions taken using your user ID and password, never publicly post

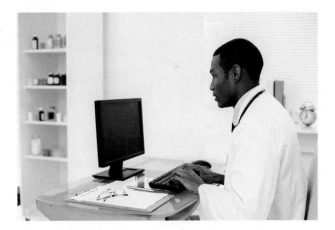

Figure 11.17   A simple mistake when sending an e-mail can cause a breach of privacy or security. What happens to a healthcare facility when it experiences a breach of privacy?

Figure 11.18 HHS Fines for Breaches of Privacy or Security

Description of Violation	Minimum Penalty
The healthcare business was unaware of the breach.	$100 per violation $25,000 per year
There was a reasonable cause for the breach and no willful neglect.	$1,000 per violation $100,000 per year
There was neglect, but it was corrected.	$10,000 per violation $250,000 per year
There was neglect that was not corrected.	$50,000 per violation $1.5 million per year

or share this information. Take these steps to avoid breaches of privacy and security:

- Diligently double-check addresses before sending confidential information.

- Always include a confidentiality statement in the signature block of your e-mail messages and send all messages using encrypted e-mail services (Figure 11.19).

- Store confidential information on network drives rather than your local hard drive.

- Make sure that papers containing confidential information are shredded. Always follow appropriate techniques for the destruction of sensitive information stored on mobile devices and verify the status of the information to ensure it has been destroyed.

- Store backup files that are on CDs, USB flash drives, or portable hard drives in a locked storage area.

Finally, take a yearly refresher course to learn about updates in HIPAA privacy rules so you maintain the best practices for safeguarding PHI and confidential information.

Figure 11.19 Sample Confidentiality Statement

Confidentiality Notice: *This e-mail transmission, and any documents, files, or previous e-mail messages attached to it, may contain confidential information. If you are not the intended recipient, or a person responsible for delivering it to the intended recipient, you are hereby notified that any disclosure, copying, distribution or use of any of the information contained in or attached to this message is STRICTLY PROHIBITED. **If you have received this transmission in error, please immediately notify us by reply e-mail or by telephone at (111) 900-9000, and destroy the original transmission and its attachments without reading them or saving them to disk.***

Diagnostic Applications

New technologies continue to change diagnostic techniques. Bailey, a medical technologist, says that IT is now a part of everything done in a medical lab. The entire lab is automated, from specimen receiving and processing to running samples through analyzers that are linked to patient medical records. Efforts to reduce costs, increased lab testing volumes, and a shortage of medical technologists have encouraged the automation of medical laboratory functions. Single specimens that were traditionally handled three or four times during processing may now be handled only once as they are placed on an automated line that processes samples using an **automated analyzer** (Figure 11.20).

Software systems produce bar-coded specimen labels that are scanned by the analyzer to read identification numbers and perform the necessary lab tests. Test results can be uploaded into the **lab information system (LIS)**, which manages data about patients, lab test requests, and lab test results. This system allows the automated lab equipment, computers, and staff members to see what tests are pending. An LIS tracks every detail about patients, from the time they arrive until they leave, and keeps the information stored in its database for future reference. The system also directs test results to the appropriate hospital department or directly to the physician. Some labs use robotic sample handlers. This improves workflow and reduces the risk of pathogen exposure for lab workers.

Just as new and improved imaging technologies are continuously being developed, the requirements for digitizing images have improved access for patients and medical providers. **Digital Imaging Communications in Medicine (DICOM)** is a standard for handling, storing, printing, and transmitting information that enhances the distribution and viewing of medical images such as MRIs, CT scans, ultrasound images, and X-rays. The DICOM standard format and communications protocol allows medical images to be accessed and transferred between devices designed by different manufacturers and among medical staff at different locations. When healthcare facilities follow the DICOM standard, patients don't have to carry images from one

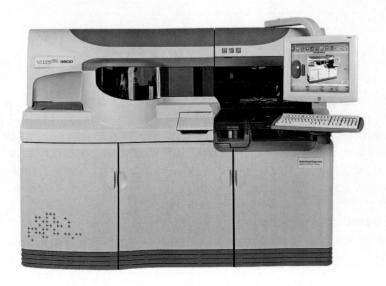

Figure 11.20   Automated analyzing equipment like the machine shown here can quickly sort and prepare samples for analysis.

doctor to another. Instead, the images can be sent electronically as part of the EHR.

Telehealth is an area of medicine that seeks to bring healthcare to patients who might otherwise have difficulty accessing healthcare by using electronic information and telecommunications technologies to support long-distance diagnosis, care, and consultation. For patients who live in rural areas without specialty clinics, telehealth can provide specialty diagnostics through local clinics.

As a telehealth technician, Tanya operates the mobile video cart (Figure 11.21). The cart includes **peripheral** (puh-RIH-fuh-ruhl) **devices** such as an exam camera, a video otoscope with an optic cable and light source, tongue depressor attachments, stethoscope, pulmonary function test equipment, and capture software for storing and forwarding data and images in the medical record. A separate cart contains audiology equipment with attachments for remote hearing aid programming.

Traditionally, a patient who needed hearing aids had to travel to a distant specialty clinic four different times. With the implementation of telehealth, the patient only has to travel to the specialty clinic for the initial hearing assessment. For the following three appointments, the patient sees Tanya, the telehealth technician, at the local clinic. She connects the patient to the verification equipment and enters the patient's audiogram into the computer link. From there, the audiologist at the specialty clinic many miles away takes over and remotely adjusts hearing aid settings for the patient.

In addition to audiology, telehealth can be used for rheumatology, pulmonary function testing, retinal imaging, and infectious disease assessment. More applications are being developed for future use. Patients who use telehealth report improved satisfaction with healthcare services and enjoy reduced personal costs for specialty care.

telehealth
the use of electronic information and telecommunications technologies to support long-distance clinical healthcare, health-related education, public health, and health administration

Figure 11.21   Using a media cart with an exam camera allows a patient in a local clinic to be examined by a specialist in a distant location.

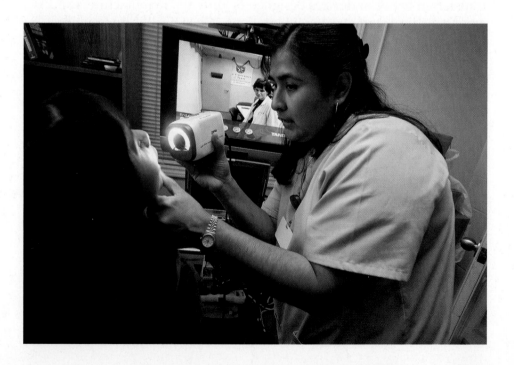

RECALL YOUR READING

1. Healthcare workers should only share protected health information in _____ situations.
2. When a privacy or security breach occurs, the Department of _____ levies fines against the _____ where the breach occurred.
3. _____ are used in medical labs to reduce the handling of specimens.
4. The _____ standard has improved access to digital medical images.
5. Telecommunications technologies help support long-distance _____, care, and _____.

Complete the *Map Your Reading* graphic organizer for the section you just read.

Medical Math

Accurately reading, recording, and interpreting vital sign measurements is a basic diagnostic skill. This means that healthcare workers must frequently apply data from tables, charts, and graphs to provide solutions to health-related problems. For example, US temperature readings typically use the **Fahrenheit scale**. But some US facilities and most facilities in other countries use the **Celsius scale**, or *Centigrade scale*. Healthcare workers must understand temperature readings in both scales and be able to convert between the two scales.

Temperature Conversions

Knowledge of both the Fahrenheit and Celsius temperature scales is especially important when providing service to patients who are familiar with the Celsius scale. Using only the Fahrenheit temperature scale that you are comfortable with, rather than the scale the patient is more likely to know, can cause confusion.

Here are two basic comparisons: water boils at 212 degrees Fahrenheit (°F) and 100 degrees Celsius (°C), and water freezes at 32°F and 0°C. If you tell a patient from another country that his temperature is 100 degrees, don't be surprised if he thinks his blood is boiling. While 98.6 degrees is an average adult temperature in the Fahrenheit scale, 37 degrees is the average temperature in the Celsius scale (Figure 11.22). Temperatures are typically written as 98.6°F or 37°C and read as "ninety-eight point six degrees Fahrenheit" or "thirty-seven degrees Celsius."

Figure 11.22 Average Temperature Ranges		
Method Used to Obtain Temperature	**Fahrenheit (°F)**	**Celsius (°C)**
oral	97.6 to 99.6	36.5 to 37.5
rectal	98.6 to 100.6	37 to 38.1
axillary	96.6 to 98.6	36 to 37
tympanic	98.6	37
temporal	98.6	37

To express degrees Fahrenheit in the Celsius scale, use this formula:
$$°C = \frac{5}{9}(°F - 32).$$

Example: To express 98°F in the Celsius scale:

1. Write the formula. $°C = \frac{5}{9}(°F - 32)$

2. Substitute the specific value. $°C = \frac{5}{9}(98 - 32)$

3. Calculate: $°C = \frac{5}{9}(66)$

$$5 \div 9 \times 66 = 36.7°C$$

To express degrees Celsius in the Fahrenheit scale, use this formula:
$$°F = \frac{9}{5}°C + 32.$$

Example: To express 36°C in the Fahrenheit scale:

1. Write the formula. $°F = \frac{9}{5}°C + 32$

2. Substitute the specific value. $°F = \frac{9}{5}36 + 32$

3. Calculate: $9 \div 5 \times 36 + 32 = 96.8°F$

It may be easier for you to remember a conversion guide expressed in words. For °F to °C, subtract 32, then multiply by 5, then divide by 9.

Example: To express 98.6°F in the Celsius scale:

1. $98.6 - 32 = 66.6$
2. $66.6 \times 5 = 333$
3. $333 \div 9 = 37°C$

For °C to °F, multiply by 9, then divide by 5, then add 32.

Example: To express 37°C in the Fahrenheit scale:

1. $37 \times 9 = 333$
2. $333 \div 5 = 66.6$
3. $66.6 + 32 = 98.6°F$

There are a few tips that can help you "think" in Celsius and recognize abnormal body temperatures. First, to compare Celsius to Fahrenheit, remember that 16°C is about 61°F, and 28°C is about 82°F. Second, use this rhyme to remember key temperatures on the Celsius scale:

39 is too hot
37 is nice
35 is too cold
Because 0 is ice

Graphing Vital Signs

Vital signs are routinely recorded in a patient's medical record. When paper records are used, the measurements may be written in a table or recorded on a graph. Graphic charts provide a visual diagram of a patient's progress and can be easier to read than a list of numbers containing the same information. Figure 11.23 shows two formats of the vital signs taken for a patient who has just returned from surgery.

Before the development of electronic records, all vital signs were graphed on paper charts and written by hand. This process took time and great attention to detail when locating the correct spot on a grid. When recording temperatures, healthcare workers would also flag any temperature not taken orally. For example, an oral temperature is recorded as 98.6°F, but a rectal temperature is recorded as 99.6°F followed by the letter *R* in a circle. A temporal artery temperature may read like an oral temperature or a rectal temperature depending upon the individual thermometer. Record the temperature reading followed by the letters *TA* in a circle.

Figure 11.23 Postoperative Vital Signs

Time	Temperature (°F)	Pulse Rate per Minute	Respiration Rate per Minute	Blood Pressure (mmHg)
1200	98.6	95	16	110/70
1215	98.6	90	16	110/75
1230	98.0	92	14	115/75
1245	98.2	90	13	120/82
1300	98.6	92	13	120/80
1315	100 (TA)	94	12	124/82
1345	98.6	88	12	124/82
1400	97.6	86	13	124/82
1415	98.0	82	12	125/80
1430	98.2	80	13	125/80
1445	98.6	82	14	120/80
1500	99 (R)	82	15	120/82

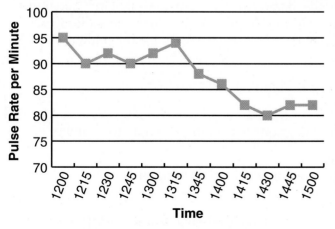

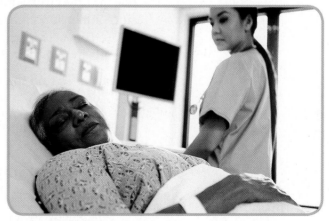

Figure 11.23   This table shows vital signs measurements taken for Jane Simmons following surgery. When individual vital signs are charted on a graph, as shown here for the pulse rate, it is easier to track the patient's progress. The line graph shows that Jane's pulse rate became more normal as she recovered from surgery.

Remember that temperature readings vary based on the site. A rectal temperature will be higher than an oral temperature because it measures temperature closer to the core of the body. Facilities that still use handwritten charts often require workers to note medications that affect vital signs or hospital events such as admission, delivery, surgery, and discharge on the graphic chart (Figure 11.24). Specific graphic forms vary by facility, but the basic steps for graphing vital signs remain the same:

1. Fill in patient identification information and dates.

2. Note the admitting date (ADM) and number the days after admission. Day 1 is the first day after admission.

3. Note the date of surgery (OR) and number the days after surgery (PO for *postoperative*). For a new mother, note the date of delivery (DEL) and number the days after delivery (PP for *postpartum*).

4. Find the correct date and time column for your vital sign reading (x-axis). Move down the column until you reach the correct number on the left side (y-axis) and mark the reading with a dot. When you have made dots for each vital sign reading, connect the dots for each vital sign to make a line graph.

5. Flag temperatures not taken orally by writing the correct abbreviation on the graph. Circle the abbreviation for emphasis.

Today, most facilities use electronic health records, which automatically chart vital signs. Once you have entered the vital sign values, they can be viewed as line or bar graphs to show comparisons with previous entries. New technologies are connecting vital signs equipment with the EHR. When the equipment measures the patient's vital signs, the readings are sent electronically to the patient's electronic health record. This avoids possible recording errors.

Charting Height, Weight, and BMI

For adult patients, height and weight are recorded to provide an indication of overall health. Height should be recorded in feet and inches. For example, 5'3" indicates a height of five feet and three inches. Weight should be recorded in pounds. For example, 130 lbs indicates a weight of one hundred thirty pounds. Be prepared to convert weight into kilograms, since a metric weight may be needed to calculate medication dosages.

To convert weight in pounds to kilograms, divide the number of pounds by 2.2.

Example: To find the metric weight of 130 pounds:

130 ÷ 2.2 = 59.09 kg

To convert weight in kilograms to pounds, multiply the number of kilograms by 2.2.

Example: To find the pound equivalent of 60 kilograms:

60 × 2.2 = 132 lbs

body mass index (BMI)
a method of relating weight to height used to define normal weight, overweight, and obesity

Healthcare providers now use the **body mass index (BMI)** to screen for weight measurements that may lead to health problems. Body mass index is a number calculated from a person's weight and height (Figure 11.25 on page 404). It provides a reliable indicator of weight

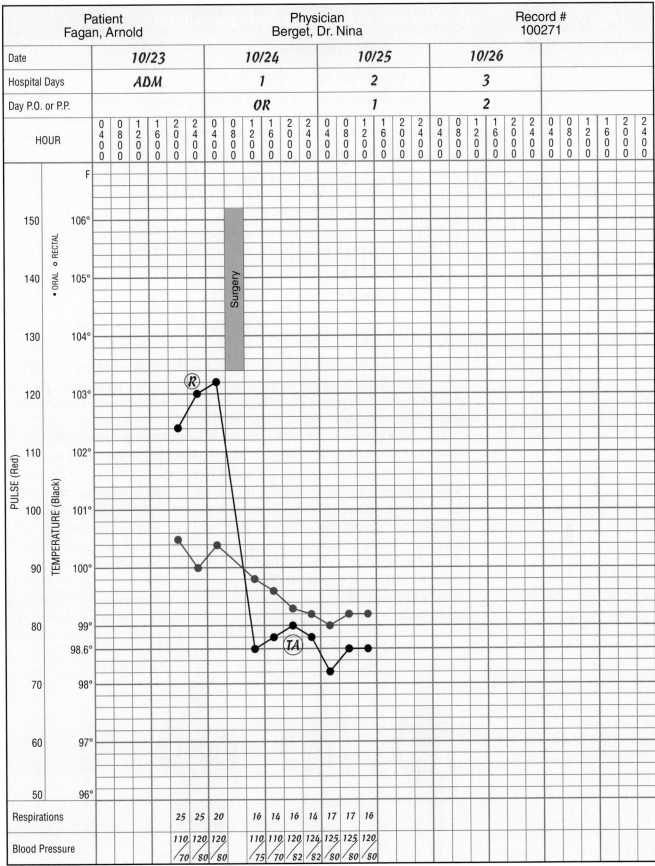

Figure 11.24   The red line traces pulse; the black line traces temperature. Respirations and blood pressure have been listed below. Hand charting of vital signs requires close attention to detail to produce an accurate record.

Simulate
EHR

Figure 11.25 How to Calculate Body Mass Index	
Measurement Units	**Formula and Calculation**
kilograms and meters (or centimeters)	**Formula:** weight (kg)/[height (m)]^2 In the metric system, the formula for BMI is weight in kilograms divided by height in meters squared. Since height is commonly measured in centimeters, divide height in centimeters by 100 to obtain height in meters. **Example:** Weight = 68 kg, Height = 165 cm (1.65 m) **Calculation:** 68 ÷ (1.65)^2 = 24.98
pounds and inches	**Formula:** weight (lb)/[height (in)]^2 × 703 Calculate BMI by dividing weight in pounds (lb) by height in inches (in) squared and multiplying by a conversion factor of 703. **Example:** Weight = 150 lbs, Height = 5'5" (65") **Calculation:** [150 ÷ (65)^2] × 703 = 24.96

Courtesy of the Centers for Disease Control and Prevention

category for most people. Since BMI is not a diagnostic tool, providers will use additional assessments such as skin-fold thickness measurements and evaluations of diet, physical activity, and family history to determine the health risks associated with a high BMI.

Standard categories showing underweight, normal, overweight, and obese BMI measurements are used for all adults beginning at 20 years of age (Figure 11.26). However, for teens and children (2 years of age to 19 years of age), the categories are interpreted using both age and gender. The BMI and age of the child are recorded on the CDC's "body mass index for age percentiles" chart for the child's gender to determine a percentile number. The percentile number is compared to a graph that assesses weight status for children. Figure 11.27 shows the ranges for assessing BMI in both age groups.

In addition to BMI, providers use waist circumference and risk factors for diseases and conditions associated with obesity to assess weight and health risks. While the BMI is accurate for most people, it can overestimate

Figure 11.26   These images show visual estimations of the standard BMI categories of underweight, normal, overweight, and obese.

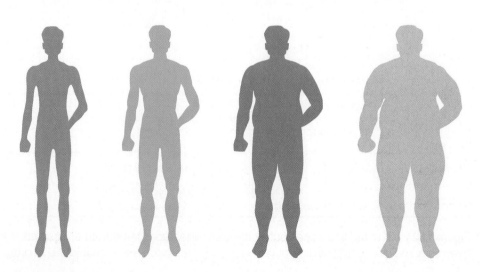

Figure 11.27 Assessing Weight Status in Adults	
BMI	**Weight Status**
below 18.5	underweight
18.5–24.9	normal
25.0–29.9	overweight
30.0 and above	obese

Courtesy of the Centers for Disease Control and Prevention

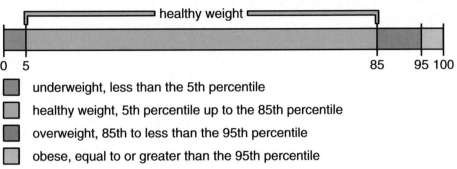

underweight, less than the 5th percentile

healthy weight, 5th percentile up to the 85th percentile

overweight, 85th to less than the 95th percentile

obese, equal to or greater than the 95th percentile

Figure 11.27   For adults, these standard categories of BMI indicate weight status. For children and teens, both age and gender are used along with the BMI to assess weight status. Comparisons to other children of the same age and gender provide a percentile ranking. BMIs between the 5th and 85th percentiles are considered healthy.

body fat in athletes and others who have a muscular build. It may also underestimate body fat in older persons and others who have lost muscle.

Waist circumference measurements provide another method of screening for health risks due to obesity. Patients have a higher risk for type 2 diabetes and heart disease when most of their body fat is located around the waist rather than at the hips. Risk increases when the waist size is greater than 35 inches for women or greater than 40 inches for men (Figure 11.28 on the next page). Measure your waist size while standing by placing a tape measure around your middle, just above your hipbones. Breathe out and take the measurement.

When you are overweight or obese, the following conditions put you at greater risk for heart disease:

- hypertension
- high LDL or low HDL cholesterol
- high triglycerides
- high blood glucose
- family history of early heart disease
- lack of exercise
- cigarette smoking

Patients who are overweight or obese and experience two of these risk factors can improve their future health by losing weight. Even a loss of 5 or 10 percent of your current weight will lower your risk of developing diseases associated with obesity.

Healthcare providers record and track patient BMIs over time in the same way they track vital signs. BMI readings, just like blood pressure readings, can provide signals for changing lifestyle choices to improve the

Figure 11.28 Classification of Overweight and Obesity by BMI, Waist Circumference, and Associated Disease Risks

Weight Classification	BMI (kg/m²)	Obesity Class	Risk for Type 2 Diabetes, Hypertension, and Cardiovascular Disease Relative to Normal Weight and Waist Circumference	
			Men 102 cm (40 in) or less Women 88 cm (35 in) or less	Men greater than 102 cm (40 in) Women greater than 88 cm (35 in)
Underweight	<18.5		-	-
Normal	18.5–24.9		-	-
Overweight	25.0–29.9		increased	high
Obesity	30.0–34.9	I	high	very high
	35.0–39.9	II	very high	very high
Extreme Obesity	40.0	III	extremely high	extremely high

Courtesy of the National Heart, Lung, and Blood Institute

patient's future health. Electronic health record systems can automatically calculate a patient's BMI and will graph changes over time to illustrate an increased risk for disease development.

For infants and children, height and weight measurements are charted on graphs from the Centers for Disease Control and Prevention (CDC) that show the average height and weight of children based on age and gender (Figure 11.29). Healthcare providers use these charts to compare growth in infants, children, and adolescents with a reference tool that is based on measurements of children of all ages and racial or ethnic groups. Follow these steps to chart height and weight for infants and children:

1. Select the correct growth chart based on the age and gender of the child. Enter the child's name and medical record number.

2. Record all historical data. This may include the height of the parents, the child's birth date, and the child's weight and length at birth.

3. Record current data, including today's date, the child's current age (to calculate current age, subtract birth date from the date of the measurement), and the height and weight measurements.

4. Convert the weight and height measurements to decimal values using the charts shown in Figure 11.30 on page 408. For example, 25 lbs 4 oz = 25.25 lbs and 30½ in = 30.5 in.

5. Calculate the child's BMI using the appropriate formula.

BMI = weight (kg) ÷ stature (cm) ÷ stature (cm) × 10,000

or

BMI = weight (lb) ÷ stature (in) ÷ stature (in) × 703

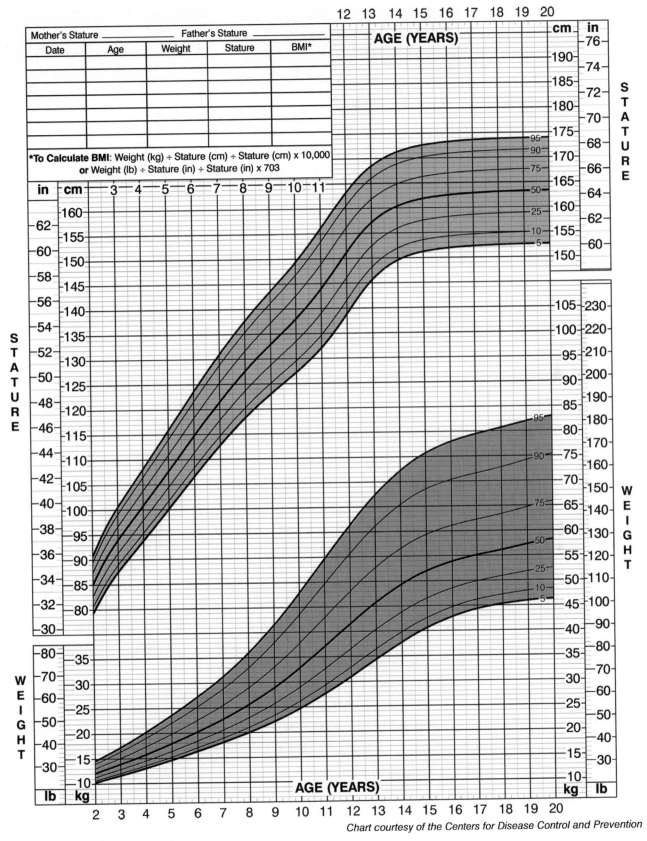

To Calculate BMI: Weight (kg) ÷ Stature (cm) ÷ Stature (cm) x 10,000
or Weight (lb) ÷ Stature (in) ÷ Stature (in) x 703

Chart courtesy of the Centers for Disease Control and Prevention

Figure 11.29   The CDC's National Center for Health Statistics provides charts for monitoring the growth of infants and children. The sample chart shown here tracks height and weight for girls from 2 to 20 years of age. In addition to height and weight, charts are available for monitoring head circumference and BMI. Separate charts are developed for boys and girls, and they cover 0 to 2 years of age and 2 to 20 years of age.

Simulate EHR

Figure 11.30A Ounces with Decimal Equivalents		
Ounces	Fraction	Decimal
1	1/16	.0625
2	1/8	.125
3	3/16	.1875
4	1/4	.25
5	5/16	.3125
6	3/8	.375
7	7/16	.4375
8	1/2	.5
9	9/16	.5625
10	5/8	.625
11	11/16	.6875
12	3/4	.75
13	13/16	.8125
14	7/8	.875
15	15/16	.9375

Figure 11.30B Inches with Decimal Equivalents		
Inches	Fraction	Decimal
1	1/12	.0833
2	1/6	.1667
3	1/4	.25
4	1/3	.3333
5	5/12	.4167
6	1/2	.5
7	7/12	.5833
8	2/3	.6667
9	3/4	.75
10	5/6	.8333
11	11/12	.9167

6. Record the BMI to one place after the decimal point (for example, $25.325 = 25.3$). While this formula varies slightly from the method described in Figure 11.25, the results will be the same using either method.

7. Plot the measurements you have recorded in the data table.

- Find the child's age on the horizontal axis. Use a straight edge to draw a vertical line up from that point.

- Find the appropriate measurement on the vertical axis (weight, height, or BMI) and use a straight edge to draw a line from that point until it intersects the vertical line.

- Make a small dot where the two lines intersect.

These measurements are recorded at each subsequent visit. Once again, electronic records can automatically graph measurements once you have entered the data.

The curved lines on the growth chart show selected **percentiles** that define the rank of the child's measurement. A dot that is plotted on the 50th percentile line for height by age means that 50 out of 100 (50 percent) of children of the same age and gender are taller.

Healthcare providers compare a child's measurements with percentile indicators to determine whether a health concern exists. They also compare the child's current percentile rank with the rank from previous visits to identify any major changes in the child's growth pattern that point to the need for further assessment (Figure 11.31).

Figure 11.31 Percentile Ranking for Child Growth Rate

Anthropometric Index *	Percentile Cut-off Value**	Nutritional Status Indicator
BMI-for-Age	≥95th percentile	overweight
Weight-for-Length	>95th percentile	
BMI-for-Age	≥85th and <95th percentile	at risk of overweight
BMI-for-Age Weight-for-Length	<5th percentile	underweight
Stature/Length-for-Age	<5th percentile	short stature
Head Circumference-for-Age	<5th and >95th percentile	developmental problems

*This is an *Anthropometric Index,* which means that it pertains to human body measurements used for comparison.
**Cut-off value* means "a measurement that indicates a dividing line between average development and a health concern."

Courtesy of the Centers for Disease Control and Prevention

RECALL YOUR READING

1. Knowledge of the _____ and _____ temperature scales is important for those working in healthcare.
2. Vital signs measurements are sometimes presented in _____ to show a visual representation of a patient's progress.
3. To calculate medication _____, healthcare workers may need to convert patients' weight from _____ to _____.
4. Children's _____, weight, and _____ are plotted on gender- and age-specific charts.

Complete the *Map Your Reading* graphic organizer for the section you just read.

SUMMARY

Assess your understanding with chapter tests

- A physical examination includes inspection, palpation, percussion, and auscultation.

- Nurses complete a minimum data set clinical assessment for long-term care residents as required by the Centers for Medicare and Medicaid Services (CMS).

- All healthcare workers are responsible for reporting unusual events or changes in the behavior or physical condition of a patient.

- Developing cultural competence is a three-step process that includes following general guidelines to avoid unintentionally insulting patients, learning about specific cultural groups, and using skills and attitudes that build rapport with individual patients.

- Healthcare workers can examine their personal biases to avoid creating barriers when communicating with their patients.

- Identifying the unmet needs of a patient is a powerful tool for changing "difficult" behaviors.

- Protected health information (PHI) can only be shared within a healthcare provider network on a "need to know" basis.

- When a breach of privacy or security of PHI occurs, HHS must be notified and they may levy fines against the healthcare business where the breach occurred.

- Medical labs use automated analyzers to reduce the handling of specimens and to increase the number of specimens labs can process.

- The DICOM standard formats allow digital medical images to be easily transferred between healthcare facilities and accessed by different providers.

- Telehealth brings healthcare to patients through the use of information and telecommunications technologies.

- Vital signs graphs provide a visual diagram of a patient's progress and can be easier to interpret than a list of numbers containing the same information.

- Height, weight, and BMI measurements for children are plotted on gender- and age-specific charts. These charts provide a percentile rank used to evaluate a child's growth pattern.

MAXIMIZE YOUR PROFESSIONAL VOCABULARY

Build vocabulary with e-flash cards, games, and audio glossary

Listed below are the essential, yellow-highlighted terms and the additional professional vocabulary that you encountered in this chapter. Complete the activities that follow the list to make all of these terms part of your everyday professional vocabulary.

acculturation	de-identified information	nursing diagnosis
assess	differential diagnosis	objective observation
assimilation	Digital Imaging Communications in Medicine (DICOM)	pain scale
auscultation		palpation
automated analyzer	Fahrenheit scale	percentiles
body mass index (BMI)	inspection	percussion
breach	ketoacidosis	peripheral devices
Celsius scale	lab information system (LIS)	personal bias
conscious	medical diagnosis	prejudice
cultural competence	minimum data set (MDS)	prostatectomy

rapport	stereotype	symptom
shift report	stool	telehealth
sign	subjective observation	unconscious

VOCABULARY DEVELOPMENT

Matching. Match the professional terms from this chapter with the best descriptions below by writing the letter of the description next to the number of the professional term on your answer sheet.

1. auscultation
2. body mass index (BMI)
3. breach
4. de-identified information
5. differential diagnosis
6. inspection
7. medical diagnosis
8. nursing diagnosis
9. palpation
10. percussion
11. personal bias
12. prejudice
13. sign
14. stereotype
15. symptom
16. telehealth

a. a determination made by a doctor that distinguishes a disease or condition from others that present with similar symptoms

b. the process of tapping various body parts during examination and using resulting sounds to assess the condition of internal organs

c. an unfair preference for, or dislike of, something or someone

d. the description of a client's health problem that a nurse is licensed and competent to treat

e. the use of electronic information and telecommunications technologies to support long-distance clinical healthcare, health-related education, public health, and health administration

f. a strong feeling or belief about a person or subject that is not based on reason or actual experience

g. the use of a stethoscope to listen to sounds made by a patient's internal organs (heart, lungs, abdominal organs) to make a diagnosis

h. access, use, or disclosure of protected health information that compromises the security or privacy of that information

i. a medical examination that uses touch to detect growths, changes in the size of organs, or tissue reactions to pressure

j. health documents from which specified personal data has been removed

k. an indication of a disease or disorder experienced by the patient, such as pain

l. a method of relating weight to height used to define normal weight, overweight, and obesity

m. the assumption that everyone in a particular group is the same

n. a determination made by a doctor that identifies the cause of a patient's illness

o. evidence of a health condition that can be seen or measured

p. visual examination used to assess parts of the body by looking for abnormal color, shape, size, or texture

17. **Taking on Terms.** Review the professional vocabulary list and select the five most difficult terms and the five most familiar terms. Use each of these terms correctly in a sentence. Then share your sentences with your classmates.

18. **Picture It.** Select five professional vocabulary terms and draw a picture to represent each one. Trade pictures with a classmate and see if you can identify the terms used.

REFLECT ON YOUR READING

19. Review the list of assessments you recorded from your last physician visit in the *Connect with Your Reading* activity. Create a table like the sample shown below. For each assessment, mark the technique or techniques and the senses used during your examination. Key to numbers: 1 = objective observation/sign, 2 = subjective observation/symptom, 3 = auscultation, 4 = palpation, 5 = percussion, 6 = sense of sight, 7 = sense of hearing, 8 = sense of touch, and 9 = sense of smell.

BUILD CORE SKILLS

20. Critical Thinking. Review each patient description. Mark those which are signs with an "x" and those which are symptoms with a "v." For each sign, determine which diagnostic technique (inspection, auscultation, palpation, percussion) would be used to identify the medical issue.

    * patient complains of wrist pain
    * patient has a wet cough
    * patient has a sore on his tongue
    * patient has a lump under the skin near the wrist
    * patient complains of severe pain on the right side of the abdomen
    * patient has a temperature of 102°F with a rapid pulse, complains of chills, and has trouble breathing
    * baby cries loudly and pulls legs up to chest

21. Reading. Use the Internet to research a cultural group represented in your community. What are the cultural beliefs of this group? Be sure to research specific healthcare-related beliefs in this group

22. Speaking and Listening. Interview a member of the cultural group you researched to learn the individual customs of this person. Use the UNIQUE chart in Figure 11.12 to guide the interview. Once you have finished your interview, study the information you have gathered and provide examples of the person's acculturation. Report your findings to the class.

23. Problem Solving. Sarah, an R.N., and Jake, a P.A., are in the hallway of Glen Grove Medical Clinic. Sarah is typing information related to a patient, Gorge, into the EHR. She calls down the hallway to ask Jake about information regarding Gorge's diagnosis. When Jake doesn't respond, Sarah leaves the computer screen on and goes down to Jake's office to get the details. When she returns with her notes, Sarah leaves them by the computer and quickly goes to the restroom. List the breaches of privacy and security that have taken place in this scenario. Explain the correct actions for Sarah to take to protect the privacy and security of patient information.

24. Writing. Clarence is an elderly man who is uncooperative when the nurse wants to take his blood pressure and draw a blood sample. Since his wife died several months ago, Clarence has gained a considerable amount of weight. He has had to rely on restaurant food because his late wife did all the cooking.

Description of Assessment Used	1	2	3	4	5	6	7	8	9
Example: measured pulse rate	X			X				X	

Write a response for this scenario that identifies Clarence's potential unmet needs and propose ways to meet those needs.

25. Reading. Use the Internet to find an article about telehealth, such as a description of what a telehealth technician's job entails or the latest advances in telehealth applications. Then write a paragraph about the pros and cons of working in telehealth or with a specific telehealth application.

26. Math. Convert each of the following Fahrenheit temperatures to Celsius and the Celsius temperatures to Fahrenheit.
   - 98°F
   - 102°F
   - 83.8°F
   - 44°C
   - 33.9°C
   - 15.5°C

27. Math. Record these temperature readings on a graphic chart as shown in Figure 11.24. Flag the readings where necessary.

   6:45 p.m.—99°

   12:35 a.m.—102°

   9:30 a.m.—103° (rectal)

   2:20 p.m.—100.6°

   5:45 p.m.—99.3°

28. Math. Convert each of the following weights from pounds (lb) to kilograms (kg).
   - 185 lbs
   - 248 lbs
   - 34 lbs
   - 194 lbs
   - 215 lbs
   - 62 lbs
   - 150 lbs
   - 26 lbs

ACTIVATE YOUR LEARNING

29. Chester is a 25-year-old male who weighs 175 lbs and is 6' tall. Calculate his BMI. Find a website that will calculate BMI to check your answer. Once you know Chester's BMI, classify him as normal weight, overweight, underweight, or obese.

30. Choose a classmate to be your partner. Take your partner's vital signs measurements over a five-day period, once each day. Graph your partner's vital signs and then check each other's graphs to make sure the vital signs were recorded correctly, as described in this chapter.

31. Imagine you have a 4-year-old patient who weighs 38 pounds and is 40 inches tall. Plot the height and weight for this young girl using a chart like the one in Figure 11.29 and determine percentiles for height and weight.

THINK AND ACT LIKE A HEALTHCARE WORKER

32. Add details as needed to make these oral reports complete, orderly, and concise.

   I think Mr. Crawford has a fever.

   Mrs. Krueger's blood pressure is pretty high.

   Mrs. Patel's leg hurts.

33. Suppose a Hispanic mother visiting from Mexico brings her sick child to the emergency room while you are working there. She only knows enough English to tell you that her child has a fever. The child appears fatigued and has a cough. You need to examine the child further to diagnose his illness, but the mother is very protective and won't let you come too close to the child. Review the general guidelines for developing cultural competence given in the text and describe the steps you would take to complete this examination in a culturally competent manner.

GO TO THE SOURCE

34. As a pediatrician, you will have patients of varying ages, genders, weights, heights, and BMIs. Imagine that a young girl named Corina is one of your female patients. She is 6 years of age, her height is 4'10", and she weighs 57 lbs. Calculate Corina's BMI. Then go to the CDC website and print out the correct children's BMI for age percentiles chart for Corina's gender. Graph the data and determine whether the data indicates cause for concern about Corina's growth.

Chapter 12
Professional Knowledge in Diagnostic Services

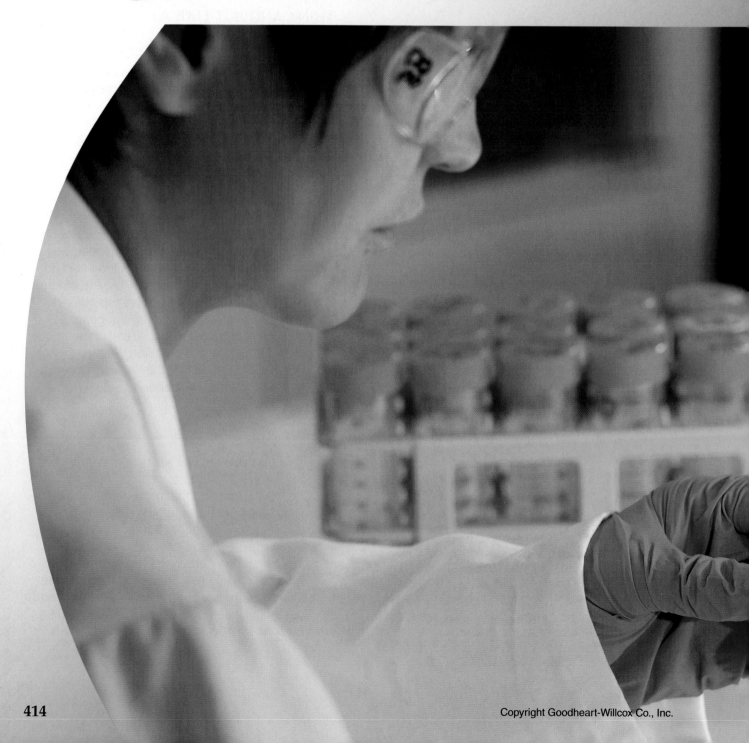

PROFESSIONAL VOCABULARY

 E-flash Cards

You will need to learn the essential terms listed below before you begin your reading. These terms will help you understand the main concepts of the chapter. These terms, which will be highlighted in yellow within the text, will become part of your professional vocabulary.

In addition to these essential terms, you will see bold terms throughout the chapter. The meanings of these terms are explained where the terms first appear. The bold terms, like the essential terms listed here, will become part of your professional vocabulary and deepen your understanding of the topics presented.

aseptic techniques practices used by healthcare professionals to maintain a pathogen-free environment and prevent the transmission of disease

Bloodborne Pathogens Standard an OSHA regulation that protects employees from exposure to blood and other potentially infectious materials

chain of infection the elements required for an infection to spread from one source to another

drug-resistant bacteria strains of a bacterium that have adapted and are no longer controlled or killed by normal antibiotic treatment

Hazard Communication Standard (HCS) an OSHA regulation aimed at promoting awareness of hazardous substances and understanding of safe handling practices

healthcare-associated infection (HAI) an infection that is not present when a patient is admitted to a hospital or healthcare facility but develops 48 hours or more after admission

occupational exposure term for the reasonable expectation for contact with blood or other potentially infectious materials during the performance of job duties

pathogen a disease-causing microorganism

resistant not susceptible; able to survive in negative conditions

Safety Data Sheet (SDS) an OSHA-required document that explains the hazards of a chemical product

transmission-based precautions heightened care techniques that are performed in addition to standard precautions based on how the patient's infection is spread

CONNECT WITH YOUR READING

How do healthcare workers' actions affect a patient's experience? Consider the following scenario:

Ellen Tate went to the women's clinic for a mammogram one morning. The admissions worker noted that she seemed nervous and asked her about it. Ellen said it was the first time she had ever had a mammogram and she was worried about what it would entail. She asked how much it would cost, whether it would hurt, and how soon she would know if it revealed any tumors. Ellen had cause to be concerned; women in her family had a history of breast cancer, putting her at a higher risk for developing the disease. The admissions worker tried to calm her down and gave her a brochure about mammograms to read while she waited.

When it was Ellen's turn, a radiologic technician named Dennis called her into the exam room. Ellen was taken aback that a man would do the test. She did not feel comfortable exposing herself to him. She said nothing, but Dennis sensed her unease. Following the policy of the women's clinic, he asked if she would be more comfortable with a female technologist, pointing out that she might have to wait a bit longer in that case. Relieved, Ellen readily agreed to wait. Dennis asked her to take her seat and said she would be the next one called when a female technologist was available.

Ten minutes later, a radiologic technician named Sharon came to get Ellen. Dennis had mentioned the patient's unease, so Sharon tried to use humor and reassurance to make her more comfortable. Sharon washed her hands and began explaining the procedure. She provided privacy for Ellen to change and kept her covered as much as possible during the procedure. Although Sharon was not able to give Ellen any results, she explained how the test worked and how soon Ellen would be notified of the results. By the time the test was done, Ellen felt much better. Although she was still concerned about the possible results of the test, she felt much less alarmed about the exam process.

What difference did the actions of these healthcare workers make to Ellen's experience? As you read this chapter, look for additional information to support or reject your assumptions about the specific role of diagnostic workers.

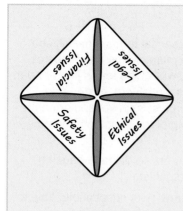

MAP YOUR READING

Can you identify the important role of diagnostic workers in healthcare? Make a visual summary to record your ideas. Begin with a square sheet of paper—an 8½-inch square works well. Fold each of the four points of the square to the center. Label each of the four resulting flaps with one of these topics: *Financial Issues*, *Legal Issues*, *Ethical Issues*, and *Safety Issues*. When you finish reading each of these sections in the chapter, open the corresponding flap and draw a picture or symbol to illustrate Dennis and Sharon's roles in this situation. Ask yourself how diagnostic workers affect financial, legal, ethical, and safety issues. Include three or four key words below each drawing that help to highlight these important topics. Finally, for each of the four topics, write two words that explain how the topic relates to you personally in the center square of your visual summary.

As you learned in previous chapters, diagnostic workers include clinical laboratory workers and medical imaging professionals. These healthcare workers often come into contact with patients as they perform diagnostic procedures. They fulfill an important part of the diagnostic process and are valued members of any healthcare facility. They are also involved in some important issues within the healthcare system.

In this chapter, you will consider the impact that diagnostic workers have on safety issues in healthcare and how these workers can help to control healthcare costs. You will focus on legal and ethical issues related to diagnostic services, such as access to care. Finally, you will examine the safety issues that diagnostic workers face, such as how to control the spread of infection.

Diagnostic Workers in the Healthcare System

Workers in the diagnostic career pathway are an integral part of the healthcare system. They help to detect medical conditions, diagnose diseases, assess health, and document a patient's condition at a specific point in time. They use specialized equipment to create images and conduct tests. The way they perform their jobs has a direct effect on patient outcomes. These workers are affected by concerns about costs and by recommendations regarding certain tests and screenings they perform.

Cost Control

For many Americans, the cost of healthcare is covered by a combination of healthcare insurance and out-of-pocket payments. Healthcare insurance may be provided by employers, purchased by individual consumers, or obtained through government health insurance programs such as Medicare and Medicaid.

In 2009, about 50 million Americans—one-sixth of the population—had no health insurance. That number dropped to about 40 million in 2013 and 31 million in 2014. Much of this change is due to the Affordable Care Act (ACA). The ACA requires all citizens and legal immigrants to obtain healthcare insurance. This may be done through an employer, by purchasing private insurance, or by taking part in health insurance exchanges.

Cost is an increasingly important issue in healthcare. Healthcare costs have risen significantly over the last few decades, from $75 billion in 1970 to $2.6 trillion in 2010 (Figure 12.1). According to the Aetna Foundation, an organization dedicated to improving access to high-quality healthcare, costs are expected to reach $4.8 trillion in 2021. Patients may ask questions about healthcare costs and insurance coverage for their diagnostic tests. They may also ask why a particular test is necessary. If you cannot answer these questions, you can refer patients to your supervisor or the billing office.

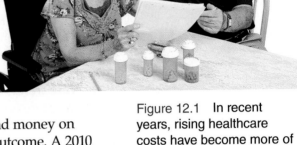

One reason costs are increasing is the practice of *defensive medicine*. This occurs when healthcare professionals recommend diagnostic tests that are not medically necessary in order to protect themselves from possible malpractice lawsuits. It is wasteful to spend money on healthcare services that do not produce a better health outcome. A 2010 study led by Stanford University estimated that more than $50 billion was spent on medical liability and defensive medicine in 2008.

Figure 12.1   In recent years, rising healthcare costs have become more of a concern for many people.

There are two reasons why insurers have focused cost controls on diagnostic services. First, several studies have found that early diagnosis of many conditions can lead to improved—and less costly—care. Advocates of testing argue that prescreening for conditions such as breast or colon cancer can detect tumors in early stages, when they can be treated at a lower cost and with a better chance for positive outcomes.

On the other hand, sophisticated testing can be expensive. Increased screening has also led to an increase in the number of *false positives*, meaning tests that suggest a cancer or other condition is present when it is not. Medicare costs for diagnostic imaging tests, such as MRIs, PET scans, and computed tomography (CT) scans, rose nearly 20 percent every year from 2000 to 2006. As a result, Medicare cut the amount it pays for imaging studies and proposed new rules to further limit medical imaging reimbursement. Many healthcare professional associations fiercely opposed the original cuts and have tried to convince Congress to pass a law reinstating them, believing that patients are being deprived of medically necessary tests.

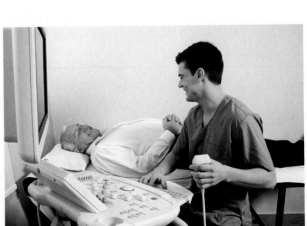

These policy changes may impact the future development of diagnostic tests and the number of imaging studies that doctors order in the coming years. However, the US Bureau of Labor Statistics (BLS) estimates that the number of jobs held by nuclear medicine technologists will still continue to grow by 19 percent over the next 10 years—somewhat faster than the average for all occupations. They also estimate that the number of radiologic technicians will grow by nearly 28 percent over the next 10 years—about double the average for all occupations (Figure 12.2). These predictions suggest that the BLS does not think diagnostic workers will be adversely affected by the push for cost control.

Figure 12.2   Radiologic technician is one diagnostic occupation for which the job outlook is improving.

Another reason for rising healthcare costs is the inefficiency of the healthcare system as a whole. Many hours are spent on extra paperwork and repeating tests because information is not communicated from one doctor to another. However, this inefficiency should begin to improve with new innovations and advances in technology. Although the Health Information Portability and Accountability Act (HIPAA) has increased the amount of paperwork and regulation for healthcare workers, the current investment in information technology and electronic health records (EHRs) is improving the coordination of care. Diagnostic test results and clinical information can be shared between providers and accessed from a variety of locations through the EHR. Electronic prescriptions reduce medication errors caused by messy handwriting and improve cross-checks for drug interactions and allergies. The database of patient information can even be used to send patient reminders and track the healthcare trends of a large population.

Healthcare errors, such as medical injuries and preventable infections, also increase the cost of healthcare. A 2012 study published in the *Journal of the American Medical Association (JAMA)* estimated that these types of avoidable errors cost between $100 and $150 billion in 2011. Adopting best practices for preventive care and patient safety can reduce the time patients spend in the hospital and the care needed to correct errors, thereby decreasing costs. Furthermore, an estimated $25 to $45 billion is spent annually on hospital readmissions and avoidable complications caused by fragmented care and poor management of patient transitions from one care setting to another. Diagnostic workers can help keep costs down by following accepted practices during procedures, avoiding injuries and the spread of infection, and charting patient information accurately.

Consumer Responsibilities

Chapter 8 identified healthcare consumer rights that a presidential panel recommended in 1998. In addition to those rights, the panel identified certain consumer responsibilities. Among these responsibilities is the need to "maximize healthy habits, such as exercising, not smoking, and eating a healthy diet."

As part of meeting these responsibilities, consumers should follow through on diagnostic tests ordered by their physicians. Doctors recommend that people in their 30s and 40s have a physical every other year and that those 50 years of age and older have an annual checkup. Many physicians order blood tests as part of these checkups. Blood tests can reveal health issues such as high cholesterol or diabetes, which require treatment (Figure 12.3).

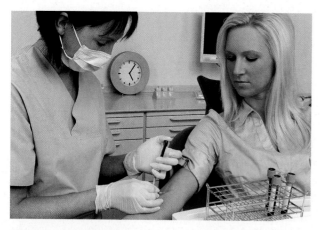

Figure 12.3 Blood tests, which are performed by diagnostic workers such as phlebotomists and medical assistants, can provide important health information.

In addition to blood tests, other tests are recommended for certain groups of people. The US Preventive Services Task Force (USPSTF) recommends that women have Pap smears, which can detect cervical cancer, every one to three years after they reach 21 years of age. The task force also suggests that women 50 years of age and older have a mammogram every other year. Some physicians hold to an older standard that called for mammograms to be performed annually beginning at 40 years of age. The USPSTF recommends that women 65 years of age and older be screened for osteoporosis, a disease that causes bones to break easily. Once they reach their 50s, both men and women should have routine colonoscopies. This test can detect and remove small growths, called *polyps* (PAHL-uhps), which can be checked for signs of colon cancer.

Taking an active role in your own healthcare can have other positive effects. Patients who are involved in their care are more likely to ask questions that keep them healthy. They are also more likely to follow their doctor's recommendations. A combination of lifestyle changes, preventive care, and compliance can all help keep healthcare costs down.

RECALL YOUR READING

1. There are many factors increasing the cost of healthcare, such as _____, _____, and _____.
2. It is difficult to predict the impact of _____ control on diagnostic workers.
3. In 1998, a presidential panel recommended a national set of rights and _____ for consumers that apply to healthcare.
4. Consumers who follow their doctor's recommendations for _____ care are more likely to request specific kinds of tests performed by _____ workers.

Complete the *Map Your Reading* graphic organizer for the section you just read.

Legal and Ethical Issues for Diagnostic Workers

The chief legal requirements for diagnostic pathway careers are the laws regulating the right to practice. These include licensing, certification, and registration laws. In addition, careers in this pathway are affected by their scope of practice and safety regulations.

Licensure, Certification, and Registration

As with other healthcare pathways, many workers in the diagnostic services pathway must gain some level of official recognition to be able to work. The most stringent requirement is licensure, which is usually issued by states. State licensure laws vary greatly from career to career and from state to state. Thirty-nine states have licensure requirements for radiographers or radiologic technicians, who take X-rays. On the other hand, only 13 states currently require medical technologists or medical laboratory technicians to obtain licenses.

One type of diagnostic technologist, the neurodiagnostic technologist, is still allowed to perform a variety of procedures for monitoring neural function without a license, and certification and registration are voluntary. That may change as the American Society of Electroencephalographic Technicians (ASET) works to convince state legislatures to adopt licensing requirements.

Even within closely related careers and specialties, licensure requirements can vary widely. Radiologic technicians who specialize in nuclear medicine images—such as PET, MRI, CT, or nuclear cardiology technology (NCT)—have to be licensed in 31 states. Mammographers, who use medical imaging to screen for breast cancer, are required to be licensed in only a handful of states. In some states, technicians are not required to be licensed because they work under the supervision of a radiologist (Figure 12.4).

Licensing for diagnostic careers typically involves passing an examination. These exams are often given by professional organizations, not by the states themselves. For instance, the American Registry of Radiologic Technologists (ARRT) gives exams in radiology, nuclear medicine technology, radiation therapy, and sonography that are recognized by those states that require a license.

As with other careers, diagnostic workers must renew their licenses regularly. To renew a license, you will need to show that you have completed the continuing education requirements. A background check may also be required to verify that you have not violated the standards of practice established for your profession. Biennial renewal (every other year) is the most common, but requirements will vary. Renewal for radiologic technicians is required annually by ARRT, while the period for respiratory therapists and pulmonary function technologists is every five years through the National Board for Respiratory Care.

In addition to a license, many careers in the diagnostic field require certification. Certification is typically granted by professional organizations. For many diagnostic careers, such as radiologic technologists, certification is required in most states. Even in states where it is not required, employers prefer to hire workers who are certified. One reason that employers might insist on certification is that insurers— including Medicare—refuse to pay for services provided by noncertified workers. As with licensure, continuing education is usually required to

Figure 12.4   Some states require that radiologic technicians work under the supervision of a radiologist. Why might supervision be required for unlicensed workers?

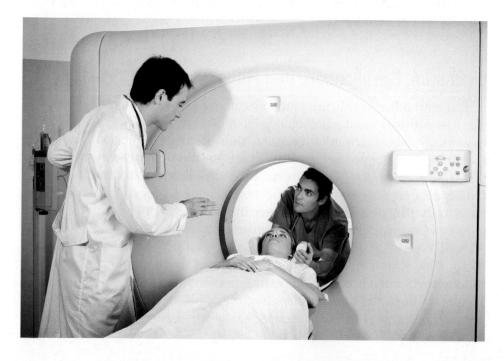

renew your certification. This ensures that professionals remain aware of current practices and are proficient in current technology.

Licensure grants a healthcare worker permission to operate within a specific scope of practice. Just like workers in other career pathways, diagnostic workers must adhere carefully to the legal boundaries of their scope of practice. For example, their scope of practice does not allow technicians to diagnose, so they are not able to interpret results for patients. A physician or radiologist uses information provided by the technician to make a diagnosis. Diagnostic workers do not have the authority to decide which tests to perform. They must be sure to perform all of the tests ordered by a physician. They cannot leave an image study out because the patient is tired or cranky that day. Workers also need to meet the quality standards of their profession. Lab technicians and technologists have to perform the correct tests, use equipment properly, and read and report results carefully and accurately to ensure that physicians and patients are fully and accurately informed about patients' conditions and can make the best decisions.

Laws Regulating Health and Safety

Some professionals in the diagnostic services pathway work with blood and blood products, biomedical waste products, and other materials that increase the risk of infection (Figure 12.5). As a result, the federal government has passed several laws that strictly regulate the handling of these potentially dangerous materials.

Two federal agencies oversee adherence to these laws. The Centers for Disease Control and Prevention (CDC) is a public health agency that conducts research to track and promote public health, respond to health problems, and promote the creation and maintenance of safe and healthy workplaces. The CDC is also an excellent source of information on disease prevention and health promotion. The **Occupational Safety and Health Administration (OSHA)** creates regulations to prevent work-related injuries, illnesses, and deaths. OSHA is also the primary federal agency responsible for workplace safety. It closely follows CDC recommendations in regulating these areas.

Bloodborne Pathogens. One important OSHA standard is related to **occupational exposure** to bloodborne pathogens and other potentially infectious materials. **Pathogens** are disease-causing organisms, such as bacteria and viruses. OSHA's **Bloodborne Pathogens Standard** is designed to protect employees who are at risk of being exposed to blood and other potentially infectious materials. The regulation is aimed chiefly at the human immunodeficiency virus (HIV), which causes acquired immune deficiency syndrome (AIDS), the hepatitis B virus (HBV), and the hepatitis C virus (HCV).

According to this regulation, employers must have a written Exposure Control Plan, train employees at risk for occupational exposure to bloodborne pathogens, offer HBV vaccination to employees with potential

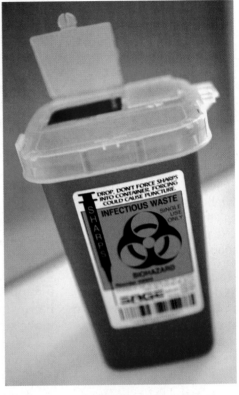

Figure 12.5   Biomedical waste must be kept in a container like the one shown here to prevent risk of infection for healthcare workers.

occupational exposure
term for the reasonable expectation for contact with blood or other potentially infectious materials during the performance of job duties

pathogen
a disease-causing microorganism

Bloodborne Pathogens Standard
an OSHA regulation that protects employees from exposure to blood and other potentially infectious materials

occupational exposure, provide personal protective equipment (PPE) such as gloves and gowns as a barrier to prevent contact with pathogens, and use devices to decrease exposure to needlesticks and other sharps. In relation to this requirement, the **Federal Needlestick Safety and Prevention Act** of 2000 also requires healthcare facilities to use needles specially engineered for safer injections and blood draws.

Medical Waste. In 1988, Congress passed the **Medical Waste Tracking Act,** which empowers OSHA to investigate workplaces' storage and disposal methods for medical waste. Regulations require workers to discard sharp objects, such as needles, in solid containers that cannot be punctured and to dispose of chemicals and blood products in secure containers. Biohazard signs must be posted in areas where medical waste may be found to alert all healthcare workers to use necessary precautions (Figure 12.6). In addition, facilities that have biohazards must contract with disposal companies specially equipped to handle these materials.

Hazardous Chemicals. In 2012, OSHA revised its **Hazard Communication Standard (HCS)**, which was aimed at promoting awareness about and safe handling of hazardous substances. The regulation is relevant to many healthcare settings because it includes blood and other body fluids, disinfectant sprays, and **reagents**. Reagents are chemicals often used in diagnostic tests to trigger desired chemical reactions. If employers have hazardous substances on their premises, this regulation requires them to make sure their workers are aware of these substances and their risks.

In addition, the regulation also requires employers to obtain a document called a **Safety Data Sheet (SDS)**, formerly known as a *material safety data sheet (MSDS)*, from the manufacturer for each hazardous substance. A substance's SDS must be readily accessible to employees in the work area where it is needed (Figure 12.7). In addition, a label containing condensed SDS information has to be placed on packages containing the hazardous substance. Beginning in 2015, uniform SDS formatting regulations required 16 sections of information, including the following:

- identification of the product, its manufacturer, and recommended uses and restrictions

- a statement of the physical and health hazards the substance poses

- legally allowed exposure limits and PPE for the substance

- emergency and first aid procedures to use if someone is exposed to the hazardous substance

- handling and storage precautions

- a statement of whether any chemical in the product is **carcinogenic** (cancer-causing) or **toxic** (poisonous), including routes of exposure and related symptoms

- safety precautions for handling the substance

Clinical Laboratory Testing. Diagnostic workers frequently use laboratory-developed tests. These tests are considered medical "devices" and must be approved by the Food and Drug Administration (FDA)

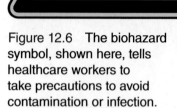

Figure 12.6   The biohazard symbol, shown here, tells healthcare workers to take precautions to avoid contamination or infection.

Hazard Communication Standard (HCS)
an OSHA regulation aimed at promoting awareness of hazardous substances and understanding of safe handling practices

Safety Data Sheet (SDS)
an OSHA-required document that explains the hazards of a chemical product

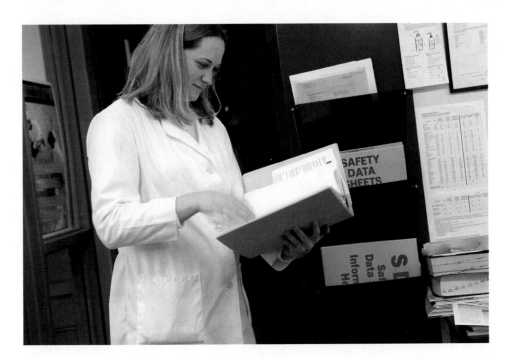

Figure 12.7   Safety Data Sheets (SDS) must always be accessible to healthcare workers. What information does an SDS contain?

before being used to diagnose patients. This is to ensure each test's safety, effectiveness, reliability, and accuracy. The FDA evaluates the clinical validity of medical testing procedures to determine if they are able to find the diseases or injuries for which they claim to test.

Clinical laboratories and their workers must engage in practices that conform to the **Clinical Laboratory Improvement Act (CLIA)**. First passed in 1988 and subsequently amended several times, CLIA applies to all laboratory facilities across the country. The federal government defines *laboratory* as any facility that does testing on specimens derived from humans to give information for the diagnosis, prevention, treatment of disease or impairment, or assessment of health. CLIA regulates how a laboratory test is performed and how the test results are interpreted and reported. Under CLIA, labs are required to do the following:

- use materials and equipment for testing that meet basic performance standards

- maintain equipment to meet the manufacturer's performance specifications

- create procedure manuals and quality control procedures

- ensure that employees are properly educated and trained to do their assigned work

Laboratories have to be certified and maintain compliance with CLIA regulations. Employers are required to provide training in the law and potential hazards to all employees. Facilities have to maintain detailed records of the training provided and document any accidents or other incidents in which CLIA regulations are violated.

The CDC is studying best practices for laboratory quality improvement. The agency found that blood culture samples are less likely to be contaminated if they are collected through a needle inserted in the vein by dedicated phlebotomy teams than if they are collected through a catheter or by a non-phlebotomist. The use of smaller needles, syringes, and full-suction vacuum tubes causes unnecessary damage to red blood cells during blood draws. Electronic bar coding has been proven to reduce patient specimen and laboratory testing identification errors. Translating test results into common reporting formats allows faster automated reporting and follow-up of critical results. These best practices may eventually become part of new regulations for diagnostic procedures.

Ethical Issues in Diagnostic Careers

Professional associations for careers in the diagnostic pathway, like those in other pathways, have codes of ethics to guide their members' professional behavior. For example, the first item in the National Society for Histotechnology's code requires members to work with dignity and integrity. The second item echoes the patient-centered concern of many healthcare professions, as members pledge to "place the welfare of the patient above all else, with the full realization of personal responsibility for the patient's best interest." The code of ethics of the American Academy of Audiology requires audiologists—who diagnose and treat hearing disorders—to provide services to any person without discrimination and forbids them from limiting the services provided without a justifiable reason.

These ethical codes are enforced by requiring professionals to report any violations. Healthcare workers also pledge to cooperate in any investigations of ethical violations by themselves or others.

Maintaining Privacy. One ethical concern for diagnostic workers who interact with patients is ensuring respect for patients' sense of privacy. When radiologists or technicians need to obtain images that require the patient to exchange clothes for a hospital gown, they need to respect the patient's privacy and leave the room while he or she changes (Figure 12.8). During the procedure, they should keep the patient covered as much as possible. Some facilities have policies that require a female chaperone to be present when a male radiologist takes a mammogram of a female patient. This policy is aimed at ensuring the patient's comfort.

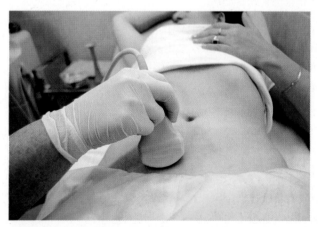

Figure 12.8 Radiologists should always respect patients' privacy and modesty. What can a radiologist do to protect a pregnant woman's privacy?

After diagnostic tests are completed, you should only share results with members of the care team who need to know. Privacy and discrimination resulting from others' knowledge of their condition are very real concerns for patients undergoing medical testing. They may be concerned about how family, friends, or employers will react if they test positive for a disease. Patients may also worry about being overlooked for a promotion or turned down for a new job based on information in their test results. There are even cases of healthcare workers treating patients differently or refusing to provide care for patients who test positive for contagious diseases. This misuse of health information is both unethical and illegal.

Accessibility of Diagnostic Tests. One of the factors that differentiates care in one region of the United States from another is the availability of health services. People who live in large cities with teaching hospitals that are fully up-to-date with current best practices have more diagnostic and therapeutic options readily available than those who live in rural areas. These differences raise ethical questions. How can we assure equal access to healthcare for everyone?

Some governmental agencies, healthcare institutions, and nonprofit organizations have taken steps to try to improve healthcare access for individuals who don't have it. The state of Arizona, for example, provides mobile mammography testing services for low-income women who don't have health insurance. The Seton Healthcare Family system provides similar services for women in central Texas. Many pharmacies have blood pressure monitors that people can use for free to check their blood pressure regularly (Figure 12.9). Some pharmacies also occasionally offer free blood testing for diabetes. These kinds of programs improve access for people who cannot afford healthcare or those living in rural areas.

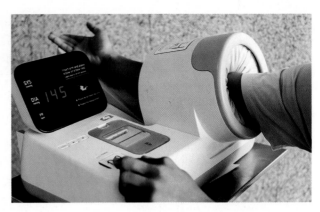

Figure 12.9   Blood pressure monitors are often available in pharmacies for self-testing. What other healthcare services do pharmacies offer?

RECALL YOUR READING

1. Some jobs in the diagnostic pathway may require _____ or _____. Laws will vary from state to state as well as within and between careers.

2. To protect the safety of workers, patients, and others, federal laws govern _____ and _____ to minimize the spread of _____.

3. Certain laws also relate to disposal of _____ waste and _____ objects.

4. The _____ standards of diagnostic workers include respect for _____ and freedom from discrimination.

5. An important ethical concern in diagnostic medicine is equal _____ to testing and treatment facilities.

Complete the *Map Your Reading* graphic organizer for the section you just read.

Safety and Infection Control

A key area of concern for several occupations in the diagnostic pathway is infection control. Phlebotomists, who take blood samples for evaluation, must be careful about exposure to bloodborne infections. The same is true of lab workers who handle those samples. Infectious waste—any item or product with the potential to transmit disease—must be handled carefully as well. Before learning the precautions that diagnostic workers should follow, you will learn about the basics of infection.

The Chain of Infection

Infections are caused by microorganisms. As you read earlier, some microorganisms are pathogens, or *disease-causing agents*. Figure 12.10 on the next page lists the major pathogens, some of the diseases they cause, and common treatments for these types of infection.

Figure 12.10 Major Pathogens, Diseases They Cause, and Treatment Options

Pathogen	Description	Sample Diseases	Common Treatments
Bacteria	one-celled organisms that come in three types determined by shape: cocci, bacilli, and spirilla	MRSA, tuberculosis, tetanus, syphilis, gonorrhea	antibiotics
Virus	a nonliving pathogen that invades living cells and uses their metabolic processes to reproduce	colds, influenza, chickenpox, measles, mumps, hepatitis B, HIV	treatment of symptoms; some viruses can be effectively prevented through vaccination
Fungi	plantlike organisms	ringworm, athlete's foot, yeast infections	antifungal medications
Protozoa	animals that live in infected water supplies or decaying organic matter	malaria, giardiasis, trichomoniasis, sleeping sickness	antiprotozoal medications

chain of infection
the elements required for an infection to spread from one source to another

The **chain of infection** describes all of the elements that must be present for infectious diseases to spread (Figure 12.11). Because all the elements must be present, each link in the chain presents an opportunity to prevent the spread of infection.

The first element is the **infectious agent**, or pathogen causing the infection. Rapid diagnosis and identification through diagnostic testing helps a pathologist know how best to control the pathogen. Remember that different pathogens are controlled with different medications. More detailed information about pathogens can be found in chapter 13.

The next link in the chain is the **reservoir**, which is a place where the pathogen can live, such as the human body, animals, food, or **fomites** (contaminated objects). Microorganisms like to live in places that are moist, warm, dark, and have a food source. This means it is important to keep skin, equipment, and the environment clean and dry so pathogens don't have a place to live. Using good personal hygiene such as hand washing helps to remove pathogens from the skin, while **pasteurization** uses heat to kill pathogens that cause foodborne illnesses.

A pathogen leaves its reservoir through a **portal of exit**, the next link in the chain of infection. Both natural body openings and breaks in the skin provide a way for pathogens to leave the body. It is important to cover wounds with a bandage, cover the mouth when coughing or sneezing, and control body fluids. Covering portals of exit protects both patients and the people around them.

The **mode of transmission** describes how a pathogen moves from its reservoir to a new host. There are several different modes of transmission. **Direct contact** with infected body fluid, which is achieved by touching it, is a common way to spread pathogens such as the cold virus and HBV. **Indirect contact** through a fomite, or contaminated object, can also transfer pathogens. Droplet transmissions from a cough, sneeze, or spray of body fluids can travel several feet. Small airborne pathogens can hang in the air for some time before they are inhaled by others. Some pathogens are also transferred by the bite of a *vector*, or animal host. Malaria, which is transmitted by mosquito bites, is one example. Lyme

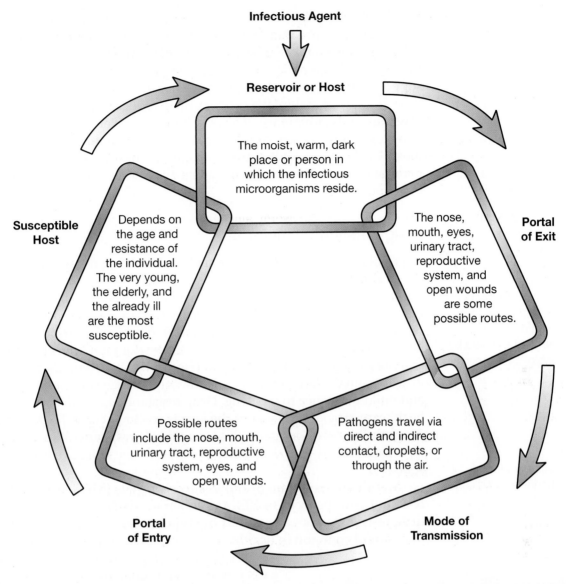

Infectious Agent

Reservoir or Host

The moist, warm, dark place or person in which the infectious microorganisms reside.

Susceptible Host

Depends on the age and resistance of the individual. The very young, the elderly, and the already ill are the most susceptible.

Portal of Exit

The nose, mouth, eyes, urinary tract, reproductive system, and open wounds are some possible routes.

Portal of Entry

Possible routes include the nose, mouth, urinary tract, reproductive system, eyes, and open wounds.

Mode of Transmission

Pathogens travel via direct and indirect contact, droplets, or through the air.

Figure 12.11   All of the elements in this chain must be present for an infection to occur. How can healthcare workers break this chain to prevent infection?

disease, which is transmitted by the bite of a deer tick, is another. Fluids from a vector carry the pathogen from one infected host's bloodstream to another, spreading the infection. Using hand washing and the appropriate PPE can prevent most disease transmission. You can't tell if someone is infected by just looking at them, so it is important to use the appropriate standard precautions for every person in your care.

The next link in the chain of infection is the **portal of entry**, which is a way for the pathogen to enter a new reservoir or host. Breaks in the skin can be covered and the use of PPE will reduce the number of portals available for pathogens to enter the body. If you are working with patients who have contagious conditions, you will need to follow specific precautions, including using the appropriate PPE and procedures to prevent the spread of infection.

Finally, a **susceptible host** is needed to complete the chain of infection. A susceptible host is anyone who can contract a disease.

People who are very old, very young, or already ill are most susceptible to infection because they have a weaker immune system for fighting infection. Hormonal changes, poor nutrition, and stress can also lower the immune system's ability to fight disease. Healthcare workers must support patients' natural defenses by ensuring good hygiene, proper fluid and nutritional intake, and efforts to reduce stress. **Opportunistic infections** take advantage of a weak immune system. A person with a weak immune system can die from a pathogen that would not make most people seriously ill. Immunizations, natural body defenses, and maintaining good health all reduce the likelihood of contracting an infection.

Drug-Resistant Bacteria

drug-resistant bacteria
strains of a bacterium that have adapted and are no longer controlled or killed by normal antibiotic treatment

While antibiotics have been effective in treating many infections, the rise of **drug-resistant bacteria** has become a growing concern. These are strains of a treatable bacterium that have developed the ability to resist normal antibiotic treatment. Drug-resistant bacteria are created when antibiotics are used inappropriately. A patient contributes to the development of these strains when he or she does not take all of the pills in a prescribed antibiotic treatment (Figure 12.12). By not taking the full dosage of medication, the patient allows the strongest bacteria to survive and build resistance to the drug. Drug resistance can also develop if a healthcare provider prescribes the wrong treatment or if the patient takes drugs that are of poor quality. If a strain that is **resistant** to treatment is identified, lab tests can determine which antibiotic will have the best results against it.

resistant
not susceptible; able to survive in negative conditions

Methicillin-resistant *Staphylococcus aureus* (MRSA), vancomycin-resistant *Enterococcus* (VRE), and **tuberculosis (TB)** are examples of drug-resistant pathogens. MRSA is a type of staph, or *bacterial*, infection that is most common in healthcare settings but is increasingly found in the community at large. Washing your hands with a disinfectant that is effective against the *S. aureus* bacterium can help prevent the disease. MRSA can be treated with increasingly stronger courses of antibiotics. VRE is another bacterial infection that is most often contracted in healthcare settings. While the VRE bacterium has developed immunity to vancomycin (van-kuh-MI-suhn)—the usual treatment for *Enterococcus* (en-ter-oh-KAHK-uhs)—other antibiotics can be effective against it.

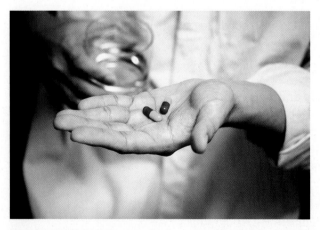

Figure 12.12   Patients must take all pills prescribed in an antibiotic treatment to help prevent drug-resistant bacteria from developing. What are some types of drug-resistant bacteria?

Tuberculosis (too-ber-kyuh-LOH-suhs) is a very serious infection that most commonly affects the lungs and, before the development of antibiotics, was generally fatal. There are two forms of drug-resistant TB. The first is called *multidrug-resistant TB (MDR TB)* because this strain cannot be killed by the two principle medications used to treat tuberculosis, which are known as the *first-line medications*. Patients with MDR TB can still be successfully treated with a course of second-line medications, the next best treatment for this infection. The second and more serious form is called *extensively drug-resistant TB (XDR TB)*, which is resistant to both the first-line and at least one of the three second-line medications. Patients with XDR TB have few treatment options, and those that exist are less likely to be successful.

Aseptic Practices

Aseptic techniques maintain a clean environment to prevent **healthcare-associated infections (HAIs)**, formerly known as *nosocomial infections*, that occur during the process of caring for patients. Preventing infection is a matter of breaking the chain of infection, which can occur at any step in the process. Proper hand washing and wearing the appropriate PPE are standard precautions that can prevent most transmissions of infection (Figure 12.13). These precautions break the chain of infection by interrupting the mode of transmission and blocking

aseptic techniques
practices used by healthcare professionals to maintain a pathogen-free environment and prevent the transmission of disease

healthcare-associated infection (HAI)
an infection that is not present when a patient is admitted to a hospital or healthcare facility but develops 48 hours or more after admission

Figure 12.13 Standard Precautions Recommended by the CDC	
Precaution	**Recommendation**
hand washing	Perform after touching blood, body fluids, secretions, excretions, contaminated items; immediately after removing gloves; and between patient contacts.
PPE gloves	Use when touching blood, body fluids, secretions, excretions, contaminated items; also when touching mucous membranes and non-intact skin.
gown	Use during procedures and patient-care activities when contact of clothing/exposed skin with blood/body fluids, secretions, and excretions is anticipated.
mask, eye protection (goggles), face shield	Use during procedures and patient-care activities likely to generate splashes or sprays of blood, body fluids, and secretions, especially suctioning and endotracheal intubation.
removal of soiled patient-care equipment	Handle in a manner that prevents the transfer of microorganisms to others and to the environment; wear gloves if visibly contaminated; perform hand hygiene.
environmental control	Develop procedures for routine care, cleaning, and disinfection of environmental surfaces, especially frequently touched surfaces in patient-care areas.
textiles and laundry	Handle in a manner that prevents the transfer of microorganisms to others and to the environment.
needles and other sharps	Do not recap, bend, break, or hand-manipulate used needles; if recapping is required, use a one-handed scoop technique only; use safety features when available; place used sharps in a puncture-resistant container.
patient resuscitation	Use a mouthpiece, a resuscitation bag, or other ventilation devices to prevent contact with the patient's mouth and oral secretions.
patient placement	Prioritize patient for a single-patient room if he or she is at increased risk of transmission, is likely to contaminate the environment, does not maintain appropriate hygiene, or is at increased risk of acquiring infection or developing an adverse outcome following infection.
respiratory hygiene/cough etiquette	Instruct symptomatic persons to cover their mouth/nose when sneezing/coughing; use tissues and dispose of them in a no-touch receptacle; use hand hygiene after hands are soiled with respiratory secretions; wear a surgical mask if tolerated or stay at least three feet away from the symptomatic person, if possible.

portals of exit and entry. Other precautions include covering wounds with bandages, covering your mouth when you cough or sneeze, and carefully handling body fluids.

You cannot tell if people are infected just by looking at them, so you should use the standard precautions for every person in your care. Most healthcare settings require some level of *asepsis*, or elimination of pathogens, through **clean technique** to limit the spread of infection. If an object or a surface has come in contact with pathogens, it has been contaminated. In that case, disinfectants are required. Disinfection uses powerful chemicals, such as bleach, to kill pathogens. Medical asepsis uses handwashing, disinfection of contaminated surfaces, standard precautions, and PPE whenever exposure to blood and body fluids is expected to prevent the spread of infection.

Surgical asepsis is achieved through **sterile technique**, which uses sterilization to prevent the introduction of pathogens during invasive procedures. This process is required for surgery, the care of open wounds, the use of urinary catheters, the insertion of intravenous tubes, and any procedure that breaks the patient's skin. The implementation of sterile technique creates what is called a *sterile field*. Sterilization with heat or chemicals destroys all microorganisms on objects and surfaces. Surgical tools are sterilized in an autoclave, and operating rooms are kept dry, cool, and well lit to deter pathogens from living there. Can you think of other ways that you can prevent a healthcare facility from providing a reservoir for pathogens?

Preventing Exposure to Bloodborne Pathogens. OSHA requires specific protections when there is a potential for exposure to bloodborne pathogens. The first step in preventing the spread of these pathogens is to use standard precautions for all patients at all times. These precautions include the following:

- Wear PPE such as gloves, a gown, and a mask, and avoid contact with contaminated objects.

- Prevent contact with body fluids, secretions, and excretions by carefully handling open wounds, patients' bodies, and soiled equipment.

- Clean and disinfect the environment when necessary.

- Deposit soiled sheets, towels, hospital gowns, scrubs, and other cloth items in laundry containers in ways that prevent the spread of infection.

- Use sharps properly, including making use of safety features, and dispose of them in appropriate sharps containers.

- Use a mouth shield when resuscitating a patient.

- Advise patients to cover their mouths when coughing or sneezing and practice the same behavior yourself.

- Above all, wash your hands when required—which is often (see Figure 12.13).

The CDC has launched the "Stop Sticks" campaign, which is aimed at preventing another cause of bloodborne infections—injuries from **sharps**. Sharps are needles, scalpels, or other sharp-edged objects found in healthcare settings that can puncture the skin. Injuries from sharps introduce the possibility of infection by bloodborne pathogens.

According to the CDC, healthcare workers suffer more than 380,000 sharps injuries each year. Many infections due to sharps injuries occur in laboratory or autopsy settings. Nearly half of these injuries occur while the sharp is being used. Just under a third of these injuries take place after use but before the sharp is disposed of properly. The risk of serious infection from hollow-bore needles used in phlebotomy is high because these needles can carry blood from the patient, which increases the risk of transmitting infections such as HIV and hepatitis.

The CDC makes several recommendations for preventing sharps injuries. One is for healthcare facilities to develop a culture that encourages safety. The CDC recommends that administrators adopt the following practices to promote this safety culture:

- Ensure that there is a commitment to safety at all levels of the organization, beginning with management.

- Involve employees in planning and implementing activities that promote a safe healthcare environment.

- Identify and remove sharps injury hazards in the work environment.

- Develop communication and feedback links to increase safety awareness.

- Hold individuals accountable for their roles in maintaining a safe environment.

In recent years, healthcare facilities have taken several steps to reduce sharps injuries. One approach has been to reduce the use of sharps. For instance, needleless intravenous connection systems have greatly reduced the use of needles. Similarly, the use of safer hinged needles and winged-steel needles has been shown to reduce sharps injuries for phlebotomists (Figure 12.14). Use of these needles has been mandated by the federal government as a result of the Needlestick Safety and Prevention Act. Workers are also cautioned not to recap needles because this increases the chances of sticking themselves.

Careful disposal of sharps is another key to preventing injuries. To comply with federal regulations, sharps must be disposed of in durable, puncture-proof containers that can be closed. These containers must be easily available, positioned away from doors, and fixed to prevent them from tipping over. The containers must be easy to dispose of and visible. They must also allow healthcare workers to put sharps inside with just one hand (Figure 12.15 on the next page). Workers must take care not to fill a container past the level specified on the outside.

Transmission-Based Precautions. In addition to the standard precautions listed in Figure 12.13, the CDC recommends taking heightened care with patients who are or may be infected with certain serious pathogens. These

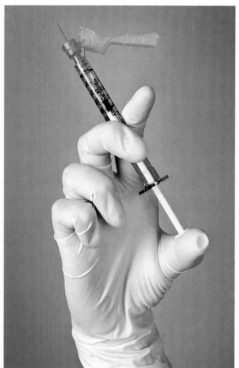

Figure 12.14   Hinged needles have a cap that can be removed and replaced easily, preventing accidental needlesticks.

transmission-based precautions focus on how the identified infection is spread. The goal is to anticipate and prevent the transmission of infection before it even begins.

Transmission-based precautions are used when standard precautions are not enough to prevent the possible spread of a pathogen. Based on how a pathogen is spread, transmission-based precautions are divided into three categories:

- **Contact precautions.** These are used when the infection can be spread by direct or indirect contact with the patient or his environment. These precautions are employed in the case of infections such as *Staphylococcus aureus* or diarrhea, when contact with waste matter can result in infection. When contact precautions are necessary, the patient should be in a single-person room or have his bed at least three feet from the bed of another patient. Healthcare workers should put on PPE before entering the room of a patient for whom contact precautions are necessary. They should also take off and dispose of that PPE before leaving the room.

- **Droplet precautions.** When a pathogen can be transmitted by close contact with the respiratory system or mucous membranes, droplet precautions are required. Certain respiratory infections in children warrant these precautions. These patients should also be in a single-person room or in a bed at least three feet away from that of another patient. In addition, curtains should be drawn around the bed of a patient under droplet precautions. Healthcare workers should wear masks when in the patient's presence. If the patient must be taken out of the room and moved through the facility, he should also wear a mask as a form of reverse-isolation if he can tolerate it. If the patient cannot tolerate a mask due to their age or respiratory status, he should be instructed on cough etiquette and hand hygiene.

- **Airborne precautions.** These precautions are needed for infections that can spread over a great distance, such as the viruses causing measles; chickenpox; and possibly severe acute respiratory syndrome (SARS), a viral respiratory disease. These patients should be placed in a special single-patient room called an *airborne infection isolation room (AIIR)*, which has special filtration and ventilation equipment. Healthcare workers caring for these patients need to wear a mask or respirator, depending on the particular pathogen that is present. TB pathogens are so small that they require a special N95 respirator mask to filter them.

Transmission-based precautions can be implemented before a pathogen is identified, based on the symptoms of a disease. These symptoms may call for specific precautions. When a symptom can indicate more than one possible pathogen, multiple transmission-based precautions may be needed. For instance, a patient with a rash of an unknown origin who, in the past 10 days, has traveled to a country with outbreaks of very high fever should receive both airborne and contact precautions. This is because the possible viruses causing the symptoms are spread in different ways.

transmission-based precautions
heightened care techniques that are performed in addition to standard precautions based on how the patient's infection is spread

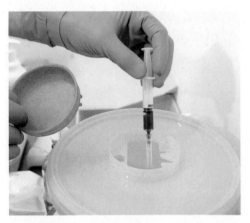

Figure 12.15   Containers for sharps disposal must be easily available so healthcare workers can dispose of needles and other sharps quickly and safely.

Transmission-based precautions are used in addition to standard precautions when the risk of transmitting a disease is high. A patient with symptoms of coughing or diarrhea, for example, will require transmission-based precautions as long as those symptoms persist. Patients with drug-resistant infections may require transmission-based precautions for a specific period of time, even after they have been treated or no longer display symptoms. This allows time to ensure that the drug-resistant infection has not returned. If **isolation** in a private room is required, healthcare workers must maintain regular contact so that the patient's needs are not ignored and he or she doesn't become depressed. Care can return to standard precautions after the heightened risk of infection has passed.

Safety Procedures for Radiation

Radiologic technicians are at some risk for radiation exposure while performing their jobs. Radiation can cause cell mutations that may be passed on to future generations and can lead to cancer and other health conditions. To guard against overexposure to harmful radiation, the federal government requires technicians to wear protective gear, including lead aprons and gloves (Figure 12.16). Technicians are also required to wear badges that indicate the amount of radiation they are receiving and to track lifetime exposure to radiation.

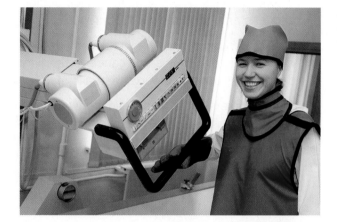

Figure 12.16 Radiologic technicians must wear protective gear to prevent over-exposure to radiation. What protection is provided for patients receiving X-rays?

To minimize the risk to patients undergoing imaging exams, technicians must be careful to set radiation to the prescribed levels and limit exposure to the predetermined amount of time. Lead aprons provide localized shielding of the reproductive organs during X-ray procedures. If proper precautions are used when directing the beam and the number of exposures is minimized, the risk for patients is low.

As new techniques for diagnostic care are developed, safety procedures will continue to adapt. It is important to stay up-to-date with the latest safety and health risks in all healthcare careers. That is why safety and infection control are studied when you complete your continuing education units to remain certified.

RECALL YOUR READING

1. Four broad types of pathogens include _____, _____, fungi, and _____.

2. Hand washing and wearing protective equipment are part of standard _____ recommended by the _____.

3. Any objects that can cut or puncture the skin are called _____, such as _____ and _____.

4. Stronger measures of infection prevention are used when there is potential that a patient is carrying certain serious _____.

5. Patients and diagnostic workers must be monitored for the amount of _____ they receive.

Complete the *Map Your Reading* graphic organizer for the section you just read.

Chapter 12 Review

SUMMARY

 Assess your understanding with chapter tests

- Insurance, defensive medicine, inefficiency, and medical errors are all driving up the cost of healthcare.

- Efforts to control the cost of healthcare services have focused on diagnostic testing, which may affect workers in the diagnostic pathway in the future, but the exact impact is difficult to predict.

- Healthcare consumers have a responsibility to demonstrate healthy habits, complete the diagnostic tests recommended by their doctor, and take an active role in their care.

- Recommended annual diagnostic tests, which may include blood tests and cancer screenings, depend on your age group and health status.

- Some workers in the diagnostic pathway need to obtain licensure or certification to practice.

- Several federal laws govern procedures and practices in diagnostic careers to protect the safety of workers, patients, and others by minimizing the likelihood of the spread of infection.

- Certain laws pertain to the handling of blood and other body fluids, the disposal of medical waste, the use of harmful chemicals, and the quality and cleanliness of laboratory practices.

- Respect for privacy and the goal of high quality and accurate performance of duty are among

the ethical standards important to workers in the diagnostic pathway.

- The chain of infection outlines the steps by which any of the four broad types of pathogens—bacteria, viruses, fungi, and protozoa—cause an infection.

- Some pathogens have developed resistance to standard treatments and require alternative treatments.

- The government recommends practices called *standard precautions* to try to prevent or interrupt the chain of infection. These standard practices include hand washing and wearing proper protective equipment.

- The safe use and disposal of sharps—needles, scalpels, and other objects that can cut or puncture—are important elements of preventing infection.

- Having symptoms or evidence that a patient is carrying certain serious pathogens calls for stronger measures of infection prevention.

- The type of transmission-based precaution used depends on how each type of infection is transmitted.

- Radiologic technicians must monitor the amount of radiation they and their patients receive to prevent harm.

MAXIMIZE YOUR PROFESSIONAL VOCABULARY

 Build vocabulary with e-flash cards, games, and audio glossary

Listed below are the essential, yellow-highlighted terms and the additional professional vocabulary that you encountered in this chapter. Complete the activities that follow the list to make all of these terms part of your everyday professional vocabulary.

airborne precautions

aseptic techniques

Bloodborne Pathogens
    Standard

carcinogenic

chain of infection

clean technique

Clinical Laboratory
    Improvement Act (CLIA)

contact precautions

direct contact

droplet precautions

drug-resistant bacteria

Federal Needlestick Safety and
    Prevention Act

fomites

Hazard Communication
    Standard (HCS)

healthcare-associated infection (HAI)

indirect contact

infectious agent

isolation

Medical Waste Tracking Act

methicillin-resistant *Staphylococcus aureus* (MRSA)

mode of transmission

occupational exposure

Occupational Safety and Health Administration (OSHA)

opportunistic infections

pasteurization

pathogen

portal of entry

portal of exit

reagents

reservoir

resistant

Safety Data Sheet (SDS)

sharps

sterile technique

susceptible host

toxic

transmission-based precautions

tuberculosis (TB)

vancomycin-resistant *Enterococcus* (VRE)

VOCABULARY DEVELOPMENT

Matching. Match the essential terms from this chapter with the best descriptions below by writing the letter of the description next to the number of the essential term on your answer sheet.

1. aseptic techniques
2. Bloodborne Pathogens Standard
3. chain of infection
4. drug-resistant bacteria
5. Hazard Communications Standard (HCS)
6. healthcare-associated infection (HAI)
7. occupational exposure
8. pathogen
9. resistant
10. Safety Data Sheet (SDS)
11. transmission-based precautions

a. an OSHA-required document that explains the hazards of a chemical product

b. the elements required for an infection to spread from one source to another

c. practices used by healthcare professionals to maintain a pathogen-free environment and prevent the transmission of disease

d. term for the reasonable expectation for contact with blood or other potentially infectious materials during the performance of job duties

e. an infection that is not present when a patient is admitted to a hospital or healthcare facility but develops 48 hours or more after admission

f. not susceptible; able to survive in negative conditions

g. strains of a bacterium that have adapted and are no longer controlled or killed by normal antibiotic treatment

h. heightened care techniques that are performed in addition to standard precautions based on how the patient's infection is spread

i. an OSHA regulation that protects employees from exposure to blood and other potentially infectious materials

j. an OSHA regulation aimed at promoting awareness of hazardous substances and understanding of safe handling practices

k. a disease-causing microorganism

12. **Connecting Terms.** Fold a sheet of paper in half. List half of this chapter's professional vocabulary terms on one side of the paper and the other half on the other side. Draw lines between terms that you think are connected or closely related to each other. Explain to a partner or the class why or how you think the terms are related to each other.

13. **Least Familiar Vocabulary.** Select eight to ten of the professional vocabulary terms in this chapter that are least familiar to you. In your own words, write a statement of

explanation for each term that does not use the term itself. Have a partner guess the professional vocabulary terms you are describing.

REFLECT ON YOUR READING

14. Review the story about Ellen Tate at the beginning of the chapter. Use the notes you took in the *Map Your Reading* activity to identify what issues were involved in Ellen Tate's situation, how they were handled, and whether they were handled correctly. Try to use your new professional vocabulary as you support your points.

BUILD CORE SKILLS

15. **Critical Thinking.** Choose three different types of diagnostic workers. Describe the different environments in which these three professionals carry out their responsibilities. Compare and contrast these workers according to how much they interact with consumers.

16. **Critical Thinking.** Using the systems theory model discussed in chapter 4, consider how changes in federal regulation of safety procedures would affect the behavior of diagnostic workers, the cost of healthcare, and the safety of healthcare professionals and the public. How would changes to safety procedures affect the input, throughput, output, and feedback loops in a healthcare facility?

17. **Speaking and Listening.** Explain why defensive medicine can cause healthcare costs to increase. Debate the pros and cons of practicing defensive medicine. Why do insurance companies focus on this issue?

18. **Problem Solving.** Describe how you personally take an active role in your own healthcare or your family's healthcare. Overall, what are your healthcare goals and activities? What suggestions do you have for improving your own healthcare or your family's healthcare? What areas are more challenging to improve than others? Why? How can you improve these challenging areas for you or your family? How might small improvements benefit your personal health and healthcare costs?

19. **Reading.** Reread the section of this chapter that covers licensure, certification, and registration. Recall that diagnostic workers must carefully follow strict guidelines in their scope of practice. Choose a diagnostic occupation that interests you. Research that occupation's scope of practice. On a note card, list five guidelines in the scope of practice that you found. Compare your list with the list of a classmate who chose a different occupation.

20. **Reading.** Refer to Figure 12.10. Select one of the pathogen categories and research a disease caused by this type of pathogen. Read about the disease and fill in a chart similar to Figure 12.10. Add a *Signs and Symptoms* category to replace the *Sample Diseases* category.

21. **Writing.** Use the information from your pathogen research in the previous question. Create a poster or brochure for patients, describing the pathogen, signs and symptoms of infection, and how the infection may be treated.

22. **Problem Solving.** In your own words, describe the chain of infection and the steps that can be taken at each point in the chain to prevent the occurrence of infection. How can diagnostic workers help to interrupt the chain of infection?

23. **Writing.** Find an actual SDS binder in your school, a local business, a healthcare facility, or on the Internet. Select a sheet that covers a hazardous substance. Record information for the required sections listed on page 422 in the chapter. Report your findings to the class.

24. **Math.** Visit the CDC website. Find statistics on healthcare-associated infections (HAIs) occurring in acute care hospitals in the United States. Record the number of people infected in each of the categories listed here. Which type of HAI is the most common? least common?

    - pneumonia
    - gastrointestinal illness
    - urinary tract infections
    - primary bloodstream infections
    - surgical site infections from any inpatient surgery
    - other types of infections
    - estimated total number of infections in hospitals

25. **Math.** The CDC's HAI prevalence survey in 2011 found that approximately 1 in 25 hospital patients in any given day had an HAI. If a hospital was the size of your school, how many patients would have an HAI today?

26. **Writing.** Using what you have learned in this chapter, develop a procedure for properly disposing of sharps. Write up the steps of the procedure. Check that your procedure fits with current recommendations for sharps disposal.

27. **Speaking and Listening.** Share the procedure that you developed in the previous activity with a classmate. Listen to your classmate's feedback about what they don't understand in your procedure. Then use that feedback to create a short training video that could be used to teach healthcare workers your procedure. Present your video to the class.

28. **Critical Thinking.** Compare and contrast standard precautions and transmission-based precautions. When are transmission-based precautions necessary? What can they achieve that standard precautions cannot?

ACTIVATE YOUR LEARNING

29. Patient responsibilities to "maximize healthy habits" include exercising, eating a healthy diet, following your doctor's recommended diagnostic testing, and not smoking. Conduct a survey of at least 20 people. Which of these responsibilities are they willing to comply with? Which are they not willing to do? Summarize your findings. What does this mean to you as a future healthcare worker?

30. Play a game of "Old Maid." Deal the cards equally among a group of two to six players. Take turns pulling one card from the unseen hand of the player on your left, then discarding any pair, if possible, from your hand. Try not to let others know if you have the "old maid" or if they are about to pull it from your hand. Play continues until one player is left with the "old maid." What correlations can you draw between this card game and standard precaution procedures?

31. Conduct a campaign for clean hands to prevent the spread of infection at your school. Work with a group of up to five people to try to increase the number of students washing their hands before lunch at your school. Evaluate the results. How effective were your efforts?

What suggestions do you have to improve future efforts to increase hand washing?

THINK AND ACT LIKE A HEALTHCARE WORKER

32. What procedures and actions in the diagnostic pathway are controlled by federal laws? Why do you think the federal government has become involved in these areas? If you were a diagnostic worker, how would government involvement influence or affect your actions?

33. Suppose you have been asked to develop a training program that would teach new healthcare workers the basics of contact precautions, droplet precautions, and airborne precautions. What information would you need to include and how will you present the information in an interesting manner? Consider a demonstration, video, PowerPoint presentation, or other creative ways to share information. How will you assess the workers' knowledge of the material presented?

GO TO THE SOURCE

34. Visit the CDC website to read about the differences between masks and respirators. Search the CDC website for relevant articles and other information on this topic. Then write a brief essay explaining the differences between masks and respirators. Why are respirators required in some healthcare settings?

35. Watch the "STOP STICKS" video on the CDC website or interview a diagnostic worker who handles sharps as part of his or her job. What are the potential consequences for a healthcare worker who is stuck by sharps on the job?

36. Visit the CDC website to learn more about patient safety. Select and read an article or webpage that interests you. Highlight the important ideas in the article. Write a short essay on your findings and how the topic you chose relates to diagnostic healthcare workers or their guidelines.

37. Search the Merck Manuals online for one of the drug-resistant infections mentioned in this chapter. Read the section on diagnosis. Summarize the diagnostic procedures used to diagnose the infection you chose.

Chapter 13
Academic Knowledge: Body Systems for Transportation and Exchange

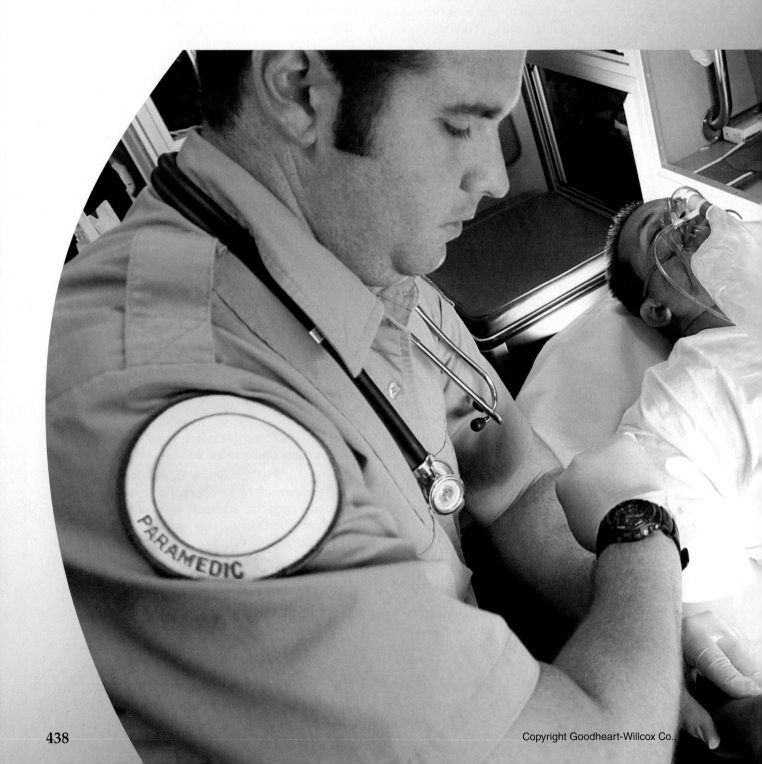

PROFESSIONAL VOCABULARY

 E-flash Cards

You will need to learn the essential terms listed below before you begin your reading. These terms will help you understand the main concepts of the chapter. These terms, which will be highlighted in yellow within the text, will become part of your professional vocabulary.

In addition to these essential terms, you will see bold terms throughout the chapter. The meanings of these terms are explained where the terms first appear. The bold terms, like the essential terms listed here, will become part of your professional vocabulary and deepen your understanding of the topics presented.

antibodies   proteins produced by leukocytes that bind with and disable antigens

antigen   a foreign substance that causes the body to make antibodies

artery   a major blood vessel that moves blood from the heart out to the body tissues

capillary bed   a network of very fine, thin-walled blood vessels (capillaries) located in body tissues

cardiovascular   related to the heart and blood vessels

erythrocyte   a red blood cell that transports oxygen and carbon dioxide to and from body tissues

learning style   an individual's preferred way of gaining or processing new information

leukocyte   a white blood cell that is involved in fighting infection

lymphatic   related to or containing the watery fluid (lymph) collected from body tissues

pulmonary loop   the flow of blood from the heart to the lungs and back to pick up oxygen and drop off carbon dioxide

respiratory   related to the act of, or organs involved in, breathing

systemic loop   the flow of blood from the heart to the body systems and back to drop off nutrients and pick up waste

vein   a main blood vessel that moves blood from body tissues toward the heart

CONNECT WITH YOUR READING

New Terms	Terms I've Heard Of	Terms I Know Well

There are many new terms to learn when you study the body systems. Some terms will require more effort to remember than others. Using the steps listed here, create a study aid to help you organize and remember these important terms. Be prepared to share your work with classmates and to learn from theirs.

1. Create a Vocabulary Sorting Organizer.

   a. Fold a piece of paper lengthwise to create three columns.

   b. Unfold the paper and label the three columns as *New Terms*, *Terms I've Heard Of*, and *Terms I Know Well*.

   c. Sort the terms in the Professional Vocabulary list into the columns you have created.

2. On the back of your organizer, write one of the new terms in the center of the page along with the definition given in the chapter.

3. Divide the page into four sections, and complete a "clinical diagnosis" of the new term.

How was the term used? What is the topic? What does the context tell you?	Opposites or non-examples of the term (what it isn't); don't use *not* or *un-*
(Term and Definition)	
Other words that relate to this term (shared word part, similar meaning)	Draw a picture to represent this term or use the word in a *meaningful* sentence.

   a. In one section of the page, explain how the word was used in the text. What topic is it related to? What does the context tell you about the meaning of the term?

   b. In the next section, list three or more related words that have a similar meaning or share a word part with this term.

   c. In the third section, use the word in a meaningful sentence or draw a picture of the concept described by the term.

   d. In the last section, explain the opposite of this term, or what it isn't. Avoid using the word *not* or the prefix *un-*.

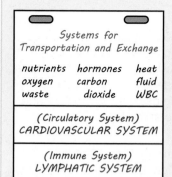

MAP YOUR READING

   Make a tablet organizer with two sheets of paper using the example shown here. Stack the sheets, keeping the edges even, but move the top sheet of paper up so that its bottom edge is ½ inch to 1 inch above the bottom edge of the sheet below it. Holding both sheets of paper, fold them down so the top edge of the top sheet is ½ inch to 1 inch above the bottom edge of the top sheet. Crease both layers and staple at the folded edge. Write *Systems for Transportation and Exchange* on the outside flap and list things that you know need to be moved around the body and in and out of cells. Label the edges of the flaps below it with the headings *Cardiovascular System*, *Lymphatic (Immune) System*, and *Respiratory System*. As you read, add visual cues, definitions of new terms, and notes on important concepts to each page of the booklet.

   The information involved in studying to be a healthcare worker can seem very overwhelming. There are many body systems to learn, terms to memorize, and diagrams to analyze. It is important to understand that everyone has his or her own way of learning. If you can figure out which style of learning works best for you, you will have an important tool for learning all of this new information.

   This chapter will help you identify whether you are a visual, auditory, or kinesthetic learner. Once you know your preferred learning style, you can refine it and practice others as you learn about the major systems that move and distribute substances within the body. These include the cardiovascular system, the lymphatic system, and the respiratory system.

Study Skills for Health Science Students: Finding Your Learning Style

   There is a lot of information to remember when you are learning about body systems. Paying attention to the way you learn can help you better understand this new information. Your **learning style** guides the way you take in, store, and recall information. Recognizing and understanding your own learning style allows you to use the method that's best for you.

learning style
an individual's preferred way of gaining or processing new information

   Learning styles can be grouped according to the way you prefer to take in information. **Visual learners** prefer pictures and have a good understanding of direction, spacing, and location. A visual-linguistic learner likes to see written words through reading and writing tasks. A visual-spatial learner may have a hard time with written activities but does better with charts, demonstrations, and videos. **Auditory learners** use sounds, rhythm, and music to store and recall information. They usually remember spoken words the best. **Kinesthetic learners** use their body, hands, and sense of touch to learn. Movement and touch help them pay attention.

   Do you recognize your preferred learning style from these descriptions? Although you will naturally use your preferred method of learning most often, you might find it helpful to practice using and building the skills for all of these styles. The more tools you have for learning and recalling information, the better off you are.

Some classes are not set up to appeal to all types of learners. What should you do when your learning style doesn't match the instructor's teaching style? The following are some changes you can make to tailor information to your learning style:

- If it's hard for you to pay attention to a lecture, try taking outline notes or creating a mental map of the information (Figure 13.1). Use symbols and pictures to represent the details. Visual learners benefit from seeing the words or pictures in this method, while kinesthetic learners benefit from the hands-on activity of doing the writing.

- If you get lost in the details of a lecture, ask for a brief outline before the lecture begins. If you're an auditory learner, you might like to tape the lecture to review with your notes after class.

- When wordy descriptions don't create a mental image for you, ask for a picture. Try searching for related video or image files on the Internet as part of your review.

- Building a model or drawing diagrams helps kinesthetic learners understand or remember new ideas.

- Both visual and auditory learners can remember details by creating their own mnemonic devices. You can learn more about mnemonic devices in chapter 4.

- Auditory learners can ask questions to clarify or confirm their ideas out loud.

- Form a study group as a fun support system. The practice of recalling and explaining new information to others is a great way to build your own memory and understanding.

Try to adapt your study habits based on your learning style. As you read this chapter, look for ways to connect with the cardiovascular, lymphatic, and respiratory systems through your preferred style.

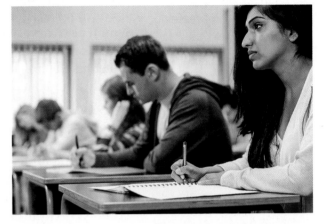

Figure 13.1   Creating visual notes such as an outline or a mental map can help visual learners better recall information presented in class. What are some study tips for auditory or kinesthetic learners?

RECALL YOUR READING

1. Identifying your _____ helps you understand how you take in, process and store new information.

2. _____ learners do best when they can see words and pictures associated with information.

3. _____ learners store and recall information through sounds and rhythm, like music.

4. _____ learners use movement and touch to help them remember information.

Complete the *Map Your Reading* graphic organizer for the section you just read.

Body Systems for Transportation and Exchange

cardiovascular
related to the heart and
blood vessels

respiratory
related to the act of or
organs involved in breathing

lymphatic
related to or containing
the watery fluid (lymph)
collected from body tissues

The **cardiovascular** [*cardi* = heart, *vas* = vessel, *ular* = pertaining to]
system is a transportation route within the body. When blood uses this
system to move through the body tissues, it brings many things to trade
with the body's cells. The **respiratory** system uses small blood vessels in
the lungs to transport and exchange carbon dioxide (CO_2) for oxygen (O_2).
White blood cells of the **lymphatic** system travel with the blood and extra
fluid from body tissues is returned through lymph vessels. Blood and
lymph also carry away waste so our cells don't die due to toxic buildup.
Transportation and exchange are so important that the cardiovascular
system is the first body system to begin functioning and death occurs
shortly after it stops.

The Cardiovascular System

Working with the cardiovascular system is a career option at all
levels of training. At the entry level, a phlebotomist (flih-BAHT-uh-mihst)
[*phleb* = vein, *otomy* = to cut into, *ist* = specialist] draws blood for medical
tests or donations. An emergency medical technician–basic
(EMT-B) receives 200 hours or more of classroom training in
basic life support. These workers handle cardiac, respiratory,
and trauma emergencies (Figure 13.2). Additional hours
of classroom training, hands-on practice, and testing are
required to move up to the level of a paramedic. Certification
requirements for paramedics vary in each state.

Paramedics provide more invasive medical support. They
may put in intravenous (IV) [*intra* = within, *ven* = vein, *ous* =
having] tubes for medications and endotracheal (ehn-doh-
TRAY-kee-uhl) [*endo* = within, *trach* = trachea, *eal* = pertaining
to] tubes for breathing. All of these healthcare workers need
a basic knowledge of the cardiovascular system's role in
transporting materials throughout the body.

If you are willing to put in 13 to 15 years of study, job
openings for cardiologists are increasing. Cardiologists make
life-or-death decisions, pay attention to details, have good
hand-eye coordination, and are sensitive to patient concerns.
They combine their knowledge of body system interactions
with information from other specialists to perform diagnostic
tests, transplants, and surgeries.

Modern technology can help solve many of the heart
and vascular problems of our aging population. An
electrocardiograph (EKG) [*electr* = electric, *cardi* = heart,
graph = instrument to record] technician uses an instrument to measure
electrical signals from the heart. The technician then provides the
cardiologist with this data about possible heart problems. A perfusionist
(per-FYU-zhuhn-ihst) operates the heart-lung machine during open-
heart surgeries. A hematologist (hee-muh-TAH-luh-jihst) [*hemat* =
blood, *ologist* = specialist] diagnoses blood-related diseases. All of these

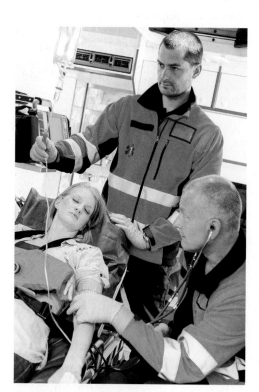

Figure 13.2   EMTs and
paramedics respond
to emergency health
situations. Who requires
more training—EMTs or
paramedics? What are the
certification requirements for
paramedics in your state?

professionals must communicate with each other to diagnose and treat cardiovascular illnesses.

The Role of Blood in the Cardiovascular System

Because of its role in circulating the blood and other materials throughout the body, this system is sometimes called the *circulatory system*. The heart, blood vessels, and blood are the key players in this delivery service provided by the cardiovascular system. The heart is the pump that keeps the blood flowing. Blood vessels are the route that blood follows from one place to another in the body. Different elements of the blood act together as a team of delivery people, carrying "packages" of water, oxygen, nutrients, hormones, and heat to all areas of the body. Each structure of the cardiovascular system has its own role and related diseases.

The average person's body contains about four to six liters of blood, depending on body size. Shock occurs when the volume of blood is decreased so much that major organs don't receive enough blood flow. Symptoms include tachycardia (ta-kee-KAHR-dee-uh) [*tachy* = fast, *cardi* = heart, *ia* = abnormal condition]; weak pulse; shallow breathing; blue lips; and cold, clammy skin. Shock can be life threatening and requires emergency medical attention.

More than half the volume of blood consists of yellowish liquid called **plasma**. Plasma is mostly water, but it also carries nutrients, hormones, and waste for other body systems.

Blood cells make up nearly half of blood's total volume (Figure 13.3). **Erythrocytes** (ih-RIHTH-ruh-slts) [*erythr* = red, *cyte* = cell], or *red blood cells* (RBCs), are shaped like donuts with dented centers. RBCs contain the protein **hemoglobin** (HEE-muh-gloh-bihn) [*hem* = blood], which helps them carry oxygen and gives them their red color. A hematocrit is a lab test that determines the percentage of RBCs in the total blood volume.

Anemia [*an* = without, *emia* = abnormal blood condition] is a condition characterized by a lower-than-normal level of red blood cells in the blood, or hemoglobin in the red blood cells. The result is a reduction in the ability of RBCs to carry oxygen. This condition causes a person to look pale, tire easily, have a rapid heartbeat, and feel faint. There are many different types of anemia. For example, in *sickle-cell anemia*, an inherited condition that is most common in African-Americans, the erythrocytes can become an abnormal crescent shape. These deformed red blood cells carry less oxygen and clot more easily in blood vessels. People with anemia may need to increase their iron intake to make more hemoglobin.

Some people with anemia receive a transfusion of donated blood to increase their RBC count. Although the life span of an erythrocyte is only four months, healthy people are able to donate blood every other month because 140 million new red blood cells are manufactured every minute in bone marrow.

erythrocyte
a red blood cell that transports oxygen and carbon dioxide to and from body tissues

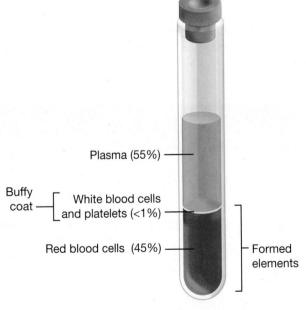

Plasma (55%)

Buffy coat — White blood cells and platelets (<1%)

Red blood cells (45%)

Formed elements

Figure 13.3   Blood consists of plasma and formed elements, which are red blood cells, white blood cells, and platelets.

Blood is categorized as type A, B, AB, or O according to the protein molecules present on the surface of the red blood cells (Figure 13.4). If the wrong blood types are mixed, blood cells stick together in clumps. This agglutination reaction can be fatal, so it is important to match blood types before a blood transfusion.

Type A red blood cells have **antigen** (AN-tih-juhn) [*anti* = against, *gen* = origin] A on their surface and produce **antibodies** in the blood plasma against antigen B. Antibodies attach themselves to invading antigens and disable or destroy them. Type A antibodies help the body destroy any type B blood cells that might enter the cardiovascular system. A person with type A blood can donate blood only to someone with type A or AB. A person with type A blood can receive blood only from someone with type A or O.

Similarly, type B red blood cells have antigen B on their surface and produce antibodies against antigen A. This means that people with type B blood can donate to those with type B or AB and receive blood from those with type B or O.

Type AB blood has both A and B antigens and no antibodies in the blood plasma. Type AB is known as a *universal receiver* because people with this blood type may receive type A, B, AB, or O blood without agglutination.

Type O blood is known as a *universal donor* because it does not have A or B antigens on the RBCs to cause agglutination and so can be donated to anyone. However, people with type O can receive only type O blood because their blood plasma contains both type A and type B antibodies to destroy the other blood types. In addition to the ABO blood types, other antigens such as the *Rh factor* also affect the success of blood transfusions.

Do you know your blood type? From what blood types can you receive blood? To which types can you donate blood?

Blood products don't have to be present in large quantities to be important. Just half of one percent of blood is composed of **leukocytes** (LOO-kuh-sIts) [*leuk* = white, *cyte* = cell], or *white blood cells* (WBCs). These blood cells are important to the function of the immune or lymphatic system, which will be discussed later in this chapter.

antigen
a foreign substance that causes the body to make antibodies

antibodies
proteins produced by leukocytes that bind with and disable antigens

leukocyte
a white blood cell that is involved in fighting infection

Figure 13.4 Blood Types

Blood Type	On the Blood Cell	In the Blood Plasma	Blood Donation Notes	US Prevalence
Type A	Antigen A	• Anti-B antibodies • Agglutinin B	• can donate to A or AB • can receive A or O	41%
Type B	Antigen B	• Anti-A antibodies • Agglutinin A	• can donate to B or AB • can receive B or O	9%
Type AB	Antigen A and B	• No agglutinins or antibodies	• can donate only to AB • universal receiver	3%
Type O	No antigens	• Anti-A and Anti-B antibodies • Agglutinin A and Agglutinin B	• universal donor • can receive only from O	47%

Another half of one percent of blood is composed of **thrombocytes** [*thromb* = clot, *cyte* = cell], also called *platelets*. These are cell fragments that form blood clots to repair injured blood vessels. A *thrombus* is a blood clot that forms in a blood vessel. If the clot breaks loose and travels to another part of the body, it is called an *embolus*. An embolus in one of the blood vessels of the heart can cause a heart attack. In the brain, it can cause a stroke. The blockage caused by an embolus cuts off the supply of nutrients and oxygen, which causes the tissues to die. Hemophilia is a condition that presents the opposite problem. Hemophiliacs can bleed to death from a small injury because their cells don't produce a protein that holds blood clots together.

The Role of Blood Vessels and the Heart in Controlling Blood Flow

Blood vessels are parallel networks of tubes that allow blood to flow from the heart out to every cell and then back to the heart (Figure 13.5). There are three types of blood vessels—arteries, capillaries, and veins.

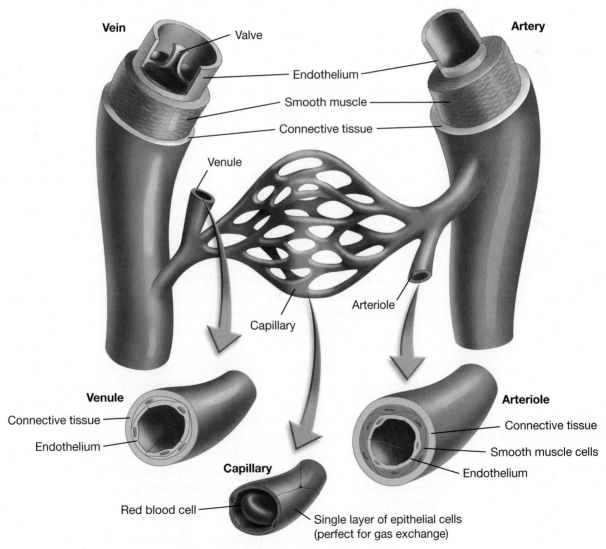

Figure 13.5   Networks of blood vessels—consisting of arteries, capillaries, and veins—transport blood throughout the body. What parts do these types of blood vessels have in common? What are their differences?

Label Art

artery
a major blood vessel that
moves blood from the heart
out to the body tissues

Arteries. **Arteries** usually carry oxygenated blood away from the heart. The layers of connective tissue, smooth muscle, and endothelium in the thick artery walls expand and contract as they receive blood under high pressure from the heart. Arterioles (ahr-TEER-ee-ohls) [*arteri* = artery, *ole* = small] are small arteries that branch out into capillaries.

capillary bed
a network of very small,
thin-walled blood vessels
(capillaries) located in body
tissues

Capillaries. **Capillary beds** contain many thin-walled blood vessels (capillaries) where gases, nutrients, wastes, hormones, and heat are able to move in and out of the blood vessels. Blood plasma soaks into tissues as interstitial (ihn-ter-STIH-shuhl) fluid—fluid located in the space between cells—from the capillaries and carries nutrients to the cells. Excess fluid returns to the capillaries, carrying waste products from the cells. As blood flows through capillaries close to the skin, it also gets rid of excess heat to help the body maintain a consistent temperature.

Veins. With the exception of blood in the pulmonary veins going to the lungs, the blood in veins is oxygen-poor, or *deoxygenated*. Blood leaves its nutrients in the capillary beds, picks up waste, and flows into gradually larger venules [*ven* = vein, *ule* = small]. Venules join to form **veins** (VAYNZ). The *vena cava* (vee-nuh KAH-vuh), which is the body's largest vein, carries deoxygenated blood back to the heart. Intravenous infusions take advantage of this pathway. A needle placed in a blood vessel of the hand or arm can deliver drugs and fluids to the body.

vein
a main blood vessel that
moves blood from body
tissues toward the heart

Veins have less smooth muscle than arteries and are farther from the pumping force of the heart. Veins use **valves** to prevent backflow as blood moves against gravity toward the heart. You can identify venous valves on your inner wrist or the back of your hand by running your finger against the flow of blood. Varicose veins have defective valves that allow blood to leak backward and collect in swollen blue "knots" near the skin surface. Veins also depend on nearby skeletal muscle contractions to help move blood along. When people with poor circulation are less active, elevating the legs and wearing elastic anti-embolism stockings helps to keep blood moving so that varicose veins and blood clots don't form.

The Heart. Like blood vessels, the heart is also formed from three layers of tissue. The endocardium [*endo* = within, *cardi* = heart] gives the inside of the heart a smooth surface that promotes blood flow. It also produces hormones that help with heart contractions. The epicardium [*epi* = upon, *cardi* = heart] forms the outside surface of the heart. The pericardium [*peri* = around, *cardi* = heart] is a second covering around the heart's surface. A small amount of fluid fills the space between the epicardium and pericardium to keep these two layers from sticking together. Congestive heart failure occurs when excess fluid builds up between these layers. This restricts the heart's ability to expand and fill with blood, reducing the amount of blood that is pushed out to the body.

pulmonary loop
the flow of blood from the
heart to the lungs and back
to pick up oxygen and drop
off carbon dioxide

systemic loop
the flow of blood from the
heart to the body systems
and back to drop off
nutrients and pick up waste

The heart is a four-chambered pump for the cardiovascular system. It consists of involuntary muscle that is *striated* for twitch contractions, not sustained contractions. Each short, hard squeeze pushes five liters of blood along a one-way path through the body. The blood travels through two loops to bring oxygen, nutrients, and hormones to the body's cells and remove waste. The short **pulmonary** (PUHL-muh-nair-ee) [*pulmon* = lung] **loop** carries deoxygenated blood from the heart to the lungs. The longer **systemic loop** takes the newly oxygenated blood from the heart

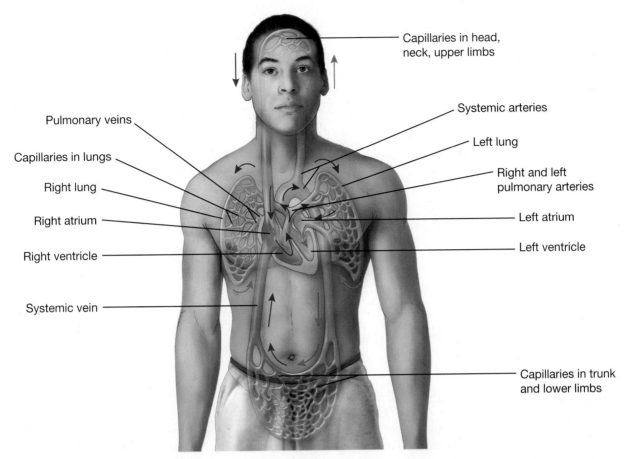

Figure 13.6   The heart pumps blood through two loops—the pulmonary loop and the systemic loop. Which loop transports oxygenated blood to the cells in the body? deoxygenated blood to the lungs?

out to cells in all areas of the body (Figure 13.6). The double loop system is an efficient way to keep oxygenated blood flowing through the body. This pumping action begins in the fifth week of embryonic development and continues throughout a person's life.

Just as valves prevent blood from flowing backward in veins, valves also prevent backward flow between the chambers of the heart. Deoxygenated blood from the vena cava enters the right **atrium**, the chamber at the top of the heart (Figure 13.7 on the next page). The blood then flows through the tricuspid atrioventricular (ay-tree-oh-vehn-TRIH-kyuh-luhr) valve, or *AV valve* and down to the right **ventricle**. When pressure in the right ventricle is higher than in the right atrium, the AV valve closes to prevent backward flow and the semilunar pulmonary valve opens.

The act of the valves closing when the heart contracts produces the characteristic "lubb-dupp" sound associated with a heartbeat. The first sound ("lubb") is the AV valves sweeping closed, and the second, louder sound ("dupp") is the semilunar valves snapping shut after the strong push of blood out of the heart. When a heart valve doesn't close properly, leaking blood flow can be heard with a stethoscope. This heart murmur may be caused by a structural problem present at birth or by other diseases. An artificial heart valve or pig's heart valve may be implanted to correct a heart murmur.

The heart ventricles are more muscular than the atria. Blood is squeezed out of the right ventricle to the lungs through the pulmonary

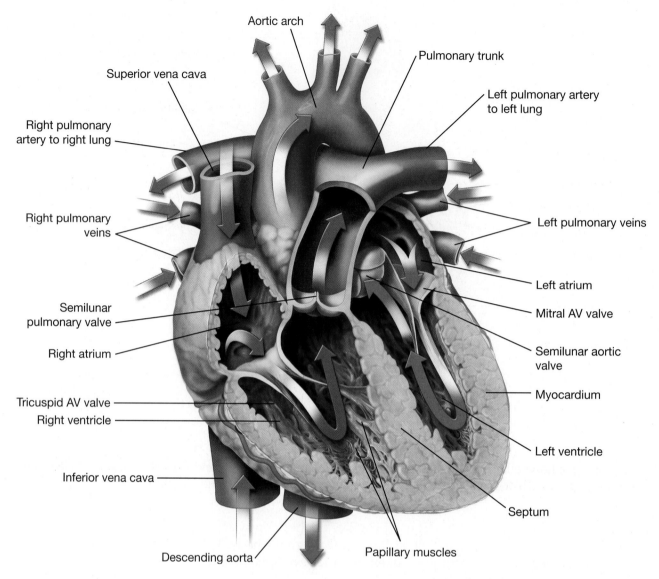

Figure 13.7   The arrows on this diagram of the heart show where blood travels with each heartbeat. Can you describe the flow of blood through the heart by naming the structures along the route?

Animation

artery. This is the only artery that carries deoxygenated blood away from the heart. In the pulmonary loop, the blood will release this carbon dioxide in exchange for oxygen. Oxygenated blood returns from the lungs through the pulmonary veins to the left atrium. These are the only veins that carry oxygenated blood to the heart. The left atrium of the heart, similar to the right, has little muscle tone for the short push down to the left ventricle. When the pressure in the ventricle is greater than that in the atrium, the mitral AV valve closes and the semilunar aortic valve opens. The left ventricle is even more muscular than the right ventricle, so it can pump the oxygenated blood out to the entire body. During heart surgery, blood flows through a heart-lung machine that temporarily takes over this work of warming, oxygenating, and circulating the blood.

Major Blood Vessels. Blood vessel locations and names follow a pattern (Figure 13.8). The systemic loop can be divided into deep and superficial

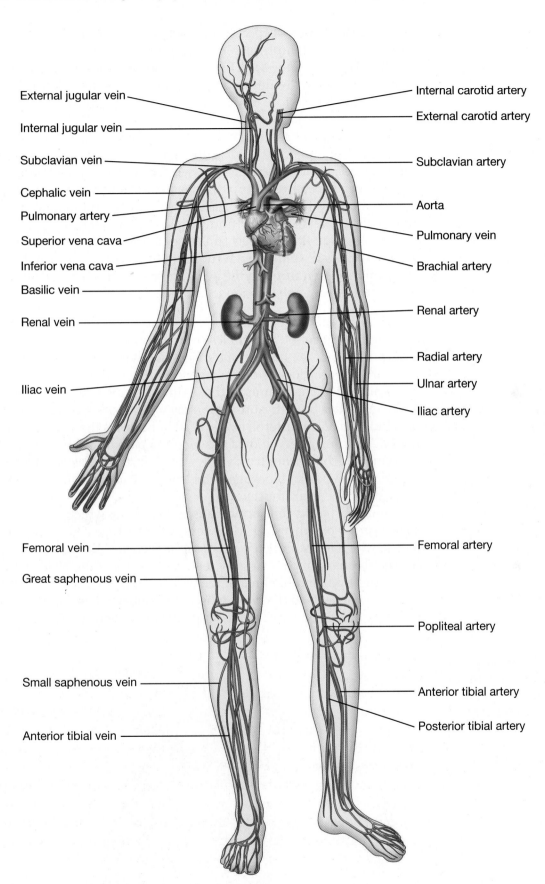

External jugular vein

Internal jugular vein

Subclavian vein

Cephalic vein

Pulmonary artery

Superior vena cava

Inferior vena cava

Basilic vein

Renal vein

Iliac vein

Femoral vein

Great saphenous vein

Small saphenous vein

Anterior tibial vein

Internal carotid artery

External carotid artery

Subclavian artery

Aorta

Pulmonary vein

Brachial artery

Renal artery

Radial artery

Ulnar artery

Iliac artery

Femoral artery

Popliteal artery

Anterior tibial artery

Posterior tibial artery

Figure 13.8   This figure shows both major arteries and major veins. What patterns do you see in the placement and naming of blood vessels?

blood vessels. Large, deep veins and arteries usually run parallel to the major nerves and lymph vessels. Their names change depending on their location. The *descending aorta* from the heart becomes the *abdominal aorta* in the belly. It then divides into the *left* and *right common iliac* (IH-lee-ak) *arteries* at the hips before running down each leg as the *femoral artery* and *popliteal* (pah-plih-TEE-uhl) *artery*.

The aortic arch has three branches that become the *subclavian artery* running under the clavicle, the *carotid artery* going to the neck, and the *brachiocephalic* (bray-kee-oh-seh-FA-lihk) *artery* leading to the arm and head. Deep veins typically have the same name as the artery they accompany. For example, the brachial, ulnar, and radial veins run alongside the brachial, ulnar, and radial arteries in the arm.

Smaller superficial vessels run closer to the surface of the skin. The *basilic* and *cephalic* veins, which run from the wrist to the armpit, can sometimes be seen through the skin. These superficial blood vessel names don't change from one location to another.

Coronary Blood Vessels. Heart muscle requires a constant supply of oxygen and nutrients. This tireless muscle is fed by coronary arteries on the outside of the heart, not by the blood within (Figure 13.9). If these arteries are blocked or damaged in some way, the heart cannot get nutrients and the heart muscle dies. Atherosclerosis (a-thuh-roh-skluh-ROH-suhs) [*ather* = fatty substance, *scler* = hard, *osis* = condition] is caused by a buildup of cholesterol, or *plaque*, that narrows the diameter of the artery. A narrow artery allows less blood to pass through. Think of this as trying to drink through a narrow stir stick straw instead of a regular sized straw. A partial blockage in the coronary arteries limits the flow of nutrients to the heart muscle.

Limiting the oxygen supply causes chest pain, which is known as *angina* [*angi* = blood vessel]. More complete blockage can cause a heart attack, which is also called a *myocardial infarction* (MI) [*my* = muscle, *cardi* = heart]. Coronary bypass surgery replaces arteries of the heart with veins or arteries from another area of the body to improve the blood supply bringing nutrients to the heart muscle. A double bypass replaces two coronary arteries, a triple bypass replaces three, and so on.

Figure 13.9 Coronary arteries are essential to the healthy functioning of the heart. What happens if these arteries are damaged?

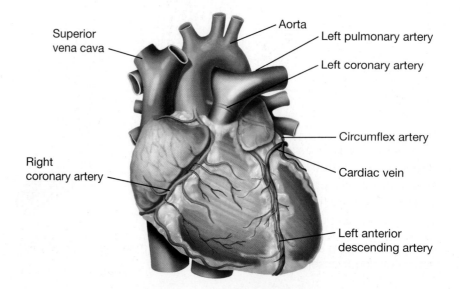

If the heart muscle is seriously damaged, a heart transplant may be required. Heart disease and coronary artery disease are the leading causes of death in the United States. These diseases currently begin as early as the teen years due to poor diet and exercise habits. You should have your cholesterol checked every five years, ideally starting at 20 years of age. The latest thinking is that even slightly high cholesterol should be treated with lifestyle changes or medication.

Monitoring Vital Signs

As you learned in chapter 10, vital signs measure temperature, pulse (heartbeat), respiration (breathing), and blood pressure. When you measure a person's pulse, you are feeling the cardiac cycle take place. The cardiac cycle has two parts—a contraction of the heart muscle followed by a relaxation of the heart muscle. Unlike skeletal muscle, which is voluntary, contractions of the heart muscle are involuntary. This means that the heart muscle contracts without you having to think about it.

Heart Rhythm. The cardiac cycle starts with an electrical signal from the sinoatrial (sI-noh-AY-tree-uhl) node (SA node) telling the left and right atria to contract. When the signal reaches the atrioventricular node (AV node), the electrical impulse spreads through the rest of the heart muscle, telling the ventricles to contract. Systole is the contraction of the heart's ventricles and diastole is the relaxation of the ventricles as they refill with blood. These terms are also used when measuring blood pressure.

An arrhythmia is an irregular heart rhythm that is treatable with a pacemaker or medication. An ineffective flutter of the atrium or ventricle means the heart is unable to rest and fill with blood or is too weak to pump blood. This fibrillation can lead to cardiac arrest, in which the heart stops. This may be corrected by an electrical shock from an automated external defibrillator (AED). This life-saving machine has become as common as fire extinguishers in public buildings.

Measuring Pulse. The pulse is felt as beats caused by the heart pumping waves of blood through the arteries. The heart beats an average of 60 to 100 times per minute in a healthy adult. The average heart rate for an infant or child is much faster because the heart is smaller. The pulse can be felt where the arteries run close to the body's surface (see Figure 10.18 in chapter 10). There are many different pulse points in the body. The carotid pulse at the neck is easy to locate in an emergency. The brachial pulse at the inner elbow is used when taking a person's blood pressure. The radial pulse at the thumb-side of the wrist is the site where a pulse is commonly measured.

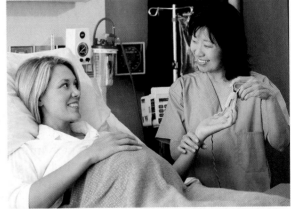

Figure 13.10 This nurse is using a pulse oximeter to measure her patient's pulse. How does a pulse oximeter work?

When recording a pulse, observe the rate, rhythm, and quality of the heartbeat for one minute. You can describe a pulse using terms such as *weak, thready, normal, full,* or *bounding.* A pulse oximeter measures the heart rate through an artery in the finger and estimates the amount of oxygen in the blood by analyzing changes in the color of the blood vessels behind the fingernail (Figure 13.10).

Heart rate is affected by sleep cycles, exercise, stress, fever, drug use, and heart disease. An unexplained change in heart rate may indicate a change in health status and should be closely monitored.

Blood Pressure. Blood pressure (BP) is the force of blood against the artery walls, measured in millimeters of mercury (mmHg). It is another vital sign that should be monitored for changes. Systolic pressure measures the force of blood against the artery walls when the heart is contracting. Diastolic pressure measures the force of blood against the artery walls when the heart relaxes. Healthy young adults usually have a systolic pressure of about 100 to 120 mmHg and a diastolic pressure of about 60 to 90 mmHg. As you learned in chapter 10, blood pressure is usually recorded as a fraction with the systolic pressure written over the diastolic pressure.

Hypertension, also called *high blood pressure*, is a condition in which blood pressure is consistently above 140/90 mmHg. This is an important predictor of strokes and aneurysms (AN-yuh-rih-zuhms). If the weak and bulging artery of an aneurysm bursts like a balloon, the affected person could quickly bleed to death. African-Americans are at a higher risk for hypertension than other groups. High blood pressure can be reduced through lifestyle changes such as exercise, stress reduction, and dietary changes (Figure 13.11).

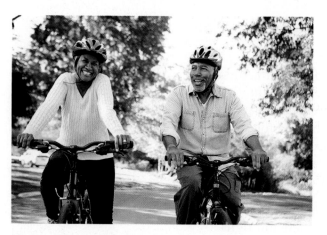

Figure 13.11   Hypertension is a preventable health condition. Regular exercise can lower your blood pressure and reduce your risk for hypertension.

Complete the *Map Your Reading* graphic organizer for the section you just read.

RECALL YOUR READING

1. Transportation and exchange of nutrients, fluid, gases, and waste in the body are done by the _____, _____, and respiratory systems.
2. _____ carry oxygen, the _____ pumps blood, and the _____ provide a transportation route.
3. The three types of blood vessels are the _____, _____, and _____.
4. Vital signs such as temperature, _____, respiration, and _____ are affected by the cardiovascular system.
5. High _____ can lead to a stroke or aneurysm.

The Lymphatic System

The lymphatic system provides another type of circulation in the body, but it is often involved with a different set of careers than the cardiovascular system. Immunologists are medical doctors who focus on infections and allergies that affect the body. Oncologists [*onc* = tumor, *ologist* = specialist in the study of] manage the diagnosis, treatment, and prevention of different types of cancer in the body. Both specialties are supported by biotechnology and pharmaceutical careers that research and develop new treatments, as well as medical imaging and laboratory technicians who help to diagnose and provide treatments.

Immunologists and oncologists treat a system made up of lymphatic vessels, specialized blood cells, and several lymphoid organs and tissues. This network of vessels and organs returns excess fluid from body tissues to the cardiovascular system, destroys invading microorganisms, and recycles dead blood cells. The lymphatic system is the body's main defense against infection, so it is important to the health of all other body systems.

Response to Pathogens

Many bacteria and fungi live on and in the human body. Some of these, called *normal body flora*, help the body digest food and maintain good health. Microorganisms that cause disease are called *pathogens* [*path* = disease, *gen* = producing]. An overgrowth of normal body flora, the growth of microorganisms in the wrong place, or the growth of pathogens can cause illness or infection.

There are several different types of pathogens (Figure 13.12). These include bacteria, viruses, fungi, protozoa, and rickettsiae. **Bacteria** are one-celled microorganisms that are so small they can only be seen

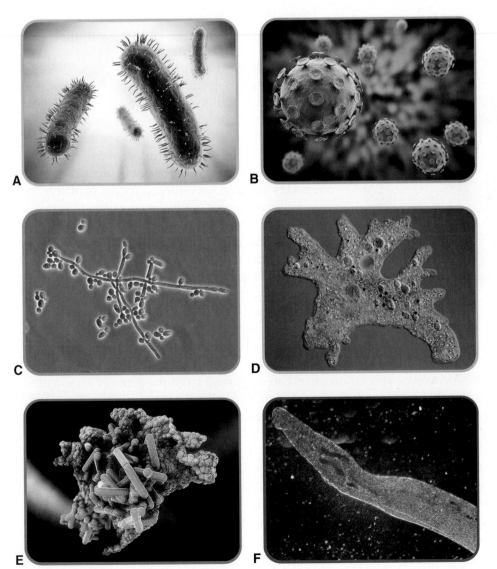

Figure 13.12   Types of pathogens include bacteria (A), viruses (B), fungi (C), protozoa (D), rickettsiae (E), and helminths (F). Can you name one disease caused by each of these types of pathogens?

under a microscope. Names of bacteria often describe their shape and arrangement. For example, *cocci* (KAHK-sI) are round, *bacilli* (buh-SIHL-I) are rod-shaped, and *spirochetes* (SPI-roh-kehts) are corkscrew-shaped. *Streptococci* (strehp-toh-KAHK-sI) are twisted chains of round bacteria that are responsible for strep throat, pneumonia, and a variety of other bacterial infections. **Antibiotics** [*anti* = against, *bio* = life, *tic* = pertaining to] are medications used to control bacterial infections.

A **virus** is a very small pathogen that invades and reproduces inside other cells. Viruses are usually spread through contact with body fluids. Chicken pox, herpes, hepatitis, mononucleosis (mono), influenza, HIV, and the common cold are all caused by viruses. *Latent viruses*, such as herpes, may lie dormant in the body for a long time and flare up later during times of stress. Immunizations can help prevent viral infections, and antiviral medications can help to reduce the effect of viruses that are identified early.

Most **fungi** are parasitic microbes that live in soil and on plants. A one-celled fungus called *yeast* commonly causes infections in the vagina or mouth. In addition, mold spores can cause lung infections. Antifungal medications and creams are used to control infections caused by these microbes.

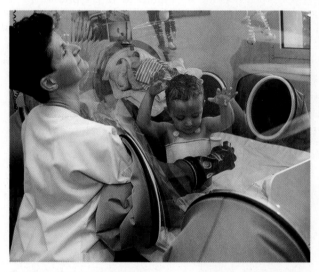

Figure 13.13   A condition known as *severe combined immune deficiency* (SCID) often requires those affected to be quarantined from others. A relatively minor infection could be fatal for a person with SCID.

Some people are more susceptible than others to infection by pathogens. The very young, for example, have an immune system not yet developed enough to fight off infections. Older adults take a longer time to produce an immune response to infections. Those who are already ill may be overwhelmed by an infection that would not be a problem for someone who is healthy (Figure 13.13). Early identification of the risks of infection helps healthcare providers take the necessary steps to keep their patients healthy.

Some pathogens are more common in less developed countries, where the conditions are right for these agents to grow and spread. *Protozoa* are one-celled microorganisms often found in dirty water and decaying material that cause malaria, dysentery, and trichomoniasis. *Rickettsiae* (rih-KEHT-see-ee) are parasites that live inside another organism called a *vector*, or *host*. When a mosquito, flea, or tick bites another animal or a human, it can pass on these parasites. *Helminths* are worms that live as parasites inside the body of a person or an animal. Roundworms and tapeworms can be spread from the feces of an infected animal to a food source or water supply. All pathogens require the right conditions for their growth and spread.

Infection Prevention

All pathogens are **infectious**, meaning they can live in a host and cause disease, but not all of them are virulent or contagious. A virulent pathogen is difficult to kill. A **contagious** disease is one that spreads easily from one person to another. A pathogen that is both virulent and contagious can cause an epidemic, in which many people become ill from the same disease. Some infections, such as athlete's foot, are localized and affect only a small area of the body. Others are systemic, like influenza or sepsis, with generalized body symptoms. Epidemiologists investigate the cause of diseases and other health conditions and develop ways to prevent and control them.

The chain of infection, as described in chapter 12, includes all of the conditions necessary for pathogens to grow and spread. Understanding this process can help you determine how to prevent that spread. Each step in the chain provides an opportunity to interrupt the process. It is the job of every healthcare worker to help prevent infection from spreading.

The immune system has several layers of defense against infections:

1. The skin and **mucous membranes** provide a natural barrier that acts as the body's first line of defense. Small hairs and mucus trap invading microbes so they can be coughed or sneezed out. Tears, saliva, urine, and stomach acid help to break down and flush out microbes that enter the body.

2. Once microbes are in the body, the immune system provides a second line of defense. Inflammation attracts white blood cells that trap and break down pathogens in the body.

3. As a third line of defense, the immune response causes the body to make antibodies. Antibodies disable the invading pathogens and mark them for destruction. Lymphatic tissue traps microbes that travel to the back of the throat, destroys them, and then produces antibody memory cells against future invasions.

People do not often catch the same disease more than once. This is because the memory cells created during the immune response allow for a faster response against that pathogen the second time it invades. The immune system is able to adapt its defense system to new invaders.

The Body's Defenders

The lymphatic system produces specialized blood cells to defend the body against pathogens. As stated earlier, leukocytes are white blood cells that fight infections and diseases. Several different types of leukocytes are made in bone marrow (Figure 13.14). These include lymphocytes, eosinophils, basophils, neutrophils, and monocytes.

Lymphocytes make antibodies to mark and destroy invading pathogens. Eosinophils (ee-oh-SIHN-uh-fihls) help destroy the marked invaders. Basophils release histamines that cause swelling to cushion an injury. High counts of eosinophils or basophils occur during allergic reactions, such as those caused by food allergies or asthma. Neutrophils are also called *phagocytes* [*phag* = to eat, *cyte* = cell]. They fight infection by attacking, surrounding, and eating bacteria. High numbers of neutrophils are common in a bacterial infection. Monocytes [*mono* = single] are phagocytes that surround and destroy foreign bodies and old red blood cells. High numbers of monocytes indicate a chronic infection.

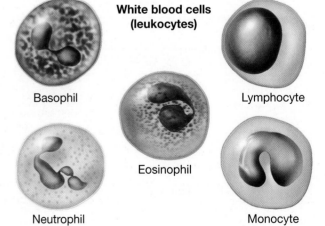

White blood cells (leukocytes)

Basophil

Neutrophil

Eosinophil

Lymphocyte

Monocyte

Figure 13.14   Each different type of leukocyte plays a unique role in fighting infections and diseases.

Animation

A complete blood count (CBC) is a diagnostic test that measures the number of each type of blood cell present.

Monocytes travel through the blood vessels to the lungs, liver, and other lymphatic tissue, where they develop into *macrophages*, which are large phagocytes. Many macrophages are found in the **spleen**. The spleen is a lymphatic organ just below the diaphragm (Figure 13.15). It makes lymphocytes, filters the blood, and removes old red blood cells. Because it is a storage site for blood cells, a ruptured spleen can cause uncontrolled internal bleeding.

A butterfly-shaped organ in the chest called the **thymus** grows during childhood as it helps program lymphocytes to respond to infection. The thymus shrinks after puberty when its T-cell lymphocytes have learned to tell the difference between body cells and invaders. T-cells mark foreign invaders in the body for destruction. This immune response must be suppressed with medications, such as cyclosporine, for an organ

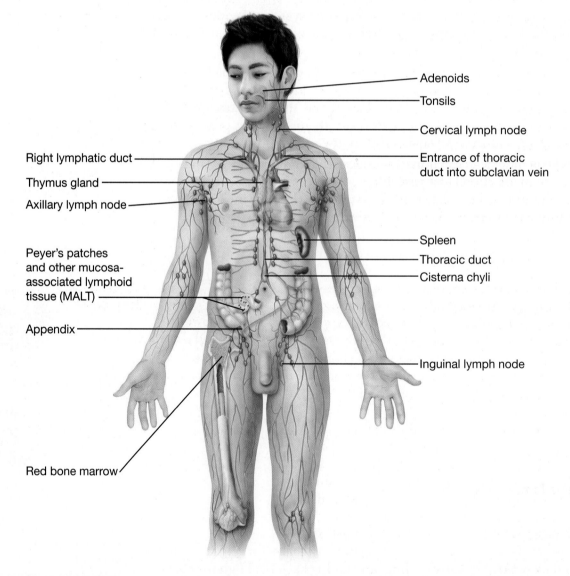

Figure 13.15   The organs of the lymphatic system. What are the functions of the tonsils, thymus gland, and spleen?

Label Art

transplant to be successful. Otherwise, T-cells will identify the antigens on the transplanted organ or tissue as foreign and direct the immune system to destroy these antigens. This leads to the body rejecting the new organ.

Immunizations take advantage of the immune system's ability to adapt. An immunization, or *vaccine*, contains a harmless form of a pathogen that is injected into the body to build protection against that disease. Leukocytes from the bone marrow, called *B-cells*, make antibodies to fight the pathogen. T-cells, trained by the thymus, create memory cells for the pathogen and its antibody. This allows the immune system to respond quickly to future infections by the same pathogen. Most children are vaccinated against many diseases before they reach school age. This immunity is used to prevent epidemics of serious infectious diseases such as polio.

Animation

Allergies and autoimmune [*auto* = self] diseases are caused by an overactive immune system that attacks the body's own healthy cells. Anaphylaxis (an-uh-fuh-LAK-suhs) is a severe allergic reaction that may cause death. The first exposure to an allergen sensitizes the body and creates memory cells for the allergen's antigen. A future exposure to the allergen triggers a hypersensitive allergic reaction. The body releases large amounts of histamines that can cause a sudden drop in blood pressure and difficulty breathing. The restricted airways caused by this response require advanced medical help. Death can occur within minutes or hours if left untreated. Common triggers for anaphylaxis include insect stings, foods such as peanuts, or medications like penicillin.

Epinephrine is a fast-acting prescription commonly used to treat anaphylactic shock (Figure 13.16). Immunologists can also treat this response by desensitizing the immune system. A series of shots provides limited exposure to an allergen so the body can build up a tolerance for it and reduce the hypersensitive allergic response.

The human immunodeficiency virus (HIV) attacks T-cells from the immune response and reprograms them to make new HIV cells. Acquired immunodeficiency syndrome (AIDS) is diagnosed when the number of T-cells in the body drops below 200 per microliter (µL) of blood. This low number of T-cells reduces the body's ability to fight infections. People with AIDS die from opportunistic infections, such as yeast and bacterial infections of the lungs. Opportunistic infections, which would not normally cause serious disease in a healthy person, take advantage of weakened immune systems.

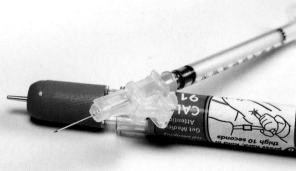

Figure 13.16   Epinephrine, which can be delivered through an *EpiPen*, stimulates the heart to beat strongly so blood pressure can be restored.

Fluid Collection

The lymphatic system also shares an important role with the cardiovascular system in transporting fluids. Blood plasma that remains between cells after delivering its oxygen, nutrients, and hormones is called **lymph**. Lymphatic vessels pick up this fluid from the body tissues and return it to the cardiovascular system to maintain fluid balance.

Lymphatic tissues filter and clean this interstitial fluid before it returns to the cardiovascular system. **Lymph nodes** are small capsules where lymphocytes collect to remove dead cells, destroy pathogens, and create antibodies against infection. These nodes occur in clusters around the body. Cervical lymph nodes are clustered along lymph vessels in the neck. Axillary lymph nodes can be felt in the armpits. Inguinal (ING-gwuhn-uhl) lymph nodes filter fluid from the legs and pubic region.

Some lymphatic tissues do not form capsules but serve a function similar to that of the lymph nodes. Mucosa-associated lymphoid tissue (MALT) occurs in patches along the intestines. The **tonsils** and **adenoids** are lymphatic tissues located in the back of the throat and behind the nose. When invaders are caught in these tissues, leukocytes rush in and the tissue becomes enlarged. Swollen lymph nodes are a common sign of infection (Figure 13.17). Lymph moves through one or more lymph nodes on its way back to the cardiovascular system.

Lymphatic vessels are similar to veins. Both have valves to prevent backflow. However, the lymphatic vessels form an open-ended, one-way system rather than a circular loop. The lymphatic system also lacks a pump like the heart. Instead, the skeletal muscles press against lymphatic vessels to squeeze the fluid along as the body moves. Surgery that removes lymph nodes, such as cancer treatment, cuts through lymphatic vessels and interrupts the flow of lymph. This can cause lymphedema [*lymph* = lymph, *edema* = swelling], or swelling with excess lymph fluid.

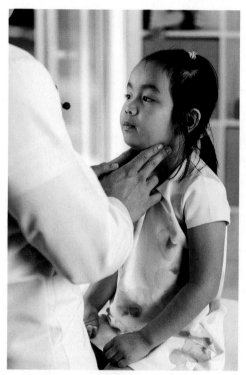

Figure 13.17   A doctor might examine your lymph nodes to determine whether you have an infection.

Lacteals are specialized lymphatic vessels that pick up digested fats and fat-soluble vitamins in the villi of the small intestine. When the fats are mixed with lymph, the resulting fluid is called *chyle*. Lymph from the lower body, left arm, and chest returns through the thoracic duct. The right lymphatic duct only collects fluid from the head and right side of the upper body. Both ducts empty lymph into the *subclavian veins*. In this way, the lymphatic system returns excess fluid to the cardiovascular system.

Cancer and the Lymphatic System

While the lymphatic system is designed to fight infection from invading pathogens, it may also cause some diseases to spread. Cancer cells often travel through the lymphatic system. **Cancer** is uncontrolled cell growth. It is the second leading cause of death in the United States. The early warning signs of cancer indicate a need for a more complete medical exam. You can remember these warning signs by using the acronym *CAUTION*:

- **C**hange in bowel or bladder habits

- **A** sore that does not heal

- **U**nusual bleeding or discharge

- **T**hickening or a lump in the breast or elsewhere

- **I**ndigestion or swallowing difficulties

- **O**bvious change in a wart or mole

- **N**agging cough or hoarseness

Types of cancer are named for the part of the body where they begin, although they may spread to other parts of the body. For instance, leukemia [*leuk* = white, *emia* = blood condition] is a cancer that causes an increased number of underdeveloped white blood cells. Lung cancer is a cancerous growth of cells in the lungs. If it spreads to the bones, it is still called lung cancer. Cancer can occur in any area of the body.

A benign growth is not cancerous. It may need to be removed if it is pressing on another organ, but it is not likely to spread or recur. A hemangioma [*hem* = blood, *angi* = vessel, *oma* = tumor] is a tumor of the blood vessels that grows during infancy but usually shrinks or disappears by 10 years of age without causing harm (Figure 13.18).

Malignant growths are cancerous. They are more harmful and tend to spread, or *metastasize* [*meta* = beyond, *stasis* = stopping, controlling] to new areas in the body. Breast cancer, for example, often spreads to the lymph nodes. From there, it can travel to other parts of the body. Breast self-exams (BSEs) and mammograms can help detect breast cancer before it metastasizes. Cancer is most likely to be curable if it is caught early.

A variety of treatments have been developed for different types of cancer. A mastectomy [*mast* = breast, *ectomy* = to cut out] is a surgical treatment for breast cancer that cuts out part of the breast and nearby lymph nodes. Some tumors are treated with controlled doses of radiation to damage the cancer cells' DNA. Chemotherapy uses chemicals to destroy fast-growing malignant cells and tissues. Unfortunately, healthy tissues are also destroyed in these processes. In addition to the search for a cure for cancer, research has focused on avoiding cancer through a healthy lifestyle and possible vaccinations to prevent some types of cancer.

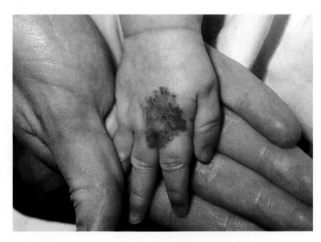

Figure 13.18   A hemangioma is one example of a benign growth. What are some other examples?

RECALL YOUR READING

1. The body is protected against infection by the _____ system.
2. Different types of pathogens include _____, _____, fungi, _____, rickettsiae, and helminths.
3. The body's three lines of defense against infection include natural barriers, _____ and leukocytes, and the _____ response.
4. Uncontrolled cell growth is known as _____.

Complete the *Map Your Reading* graphic organizer for the section you just read.

The Respiratory System

The respiratory system uses the cardiovascular system's network of blood vessels to exchange gases with cells all over the body. For this reason, medical professionals who focus on the respiratory system will often work closely with those in cardiovascular careers. A respiratory therapist provides education, treatment, and rehabilitation for patients with breathing problems caused by both heart and lung disorders. A thoracic surgeon, also called a *cardiothoracic surgeon*, is trained to diagnose and operate on conditions of the heart, lungs, and esophagus. Both jobs frequently involve consulting with pulmonologists and cardiologists about treatments.

The organs of the respiratory system are located in the head and chest. An otorhinolaryngologist (oht-oh-rI-noh-lair-uhn-GAHL-uh-jihst) [*ot* = ear, *rhin* = nose, *laryng* = voice box, *ologist* = specialist in the study of] is a physician who specializes in the diagnosis and treatment of diseases of the ears, nose, and throat (ENT). A pulmonologist [*pulmon* = lung] specializes in the diagnosis and treatment of lung disorders. Breathing difficulties can be life threatening, which makes their treatment stressful for both patients and caregivers.

Organs and Diseases of the Respiratory System

As oxygen moves through the respiratory system, it encounters many different organs (Figure 13.19). Oxygen moves from the nose and mouth, down the pharynx, passing the epiglottis, larynx, and trachea to get to the bronchi, then the bronchioles, and finally the alveoli that connect with the

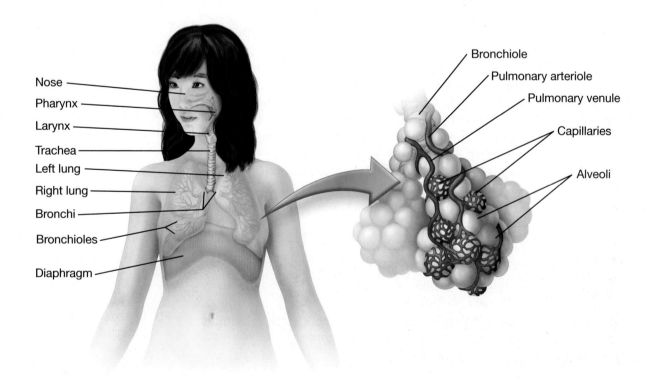

Figure 13.19   This is the basic route that oxygen takes through the respiratory system when you take a breath.

cardiovascular system to reach every cell in the body. This section will discuss each of these steps in more detail, but this is the basic route.

Air first enters the respiratory system through the mouth and nares, commonly known as the *nostrils* of the nose. The nasal septum [*sept* = wall] is a cartilage and bone structure that divides the nasal cavity into the right and left chambers of the nasal cavity. The air from the nasal cavity is funneled through nasal *conchae* (KAHN-kee), which are shaped like spiraled seashells, and into **sinus cavities** within the skull bones. The cavities' mucous membrane linings help to warm, filter, and moisten the air as we breathe in.

Sinus infections cause inflammation of these mucous membranes, which results in congestion, pressure, and pain. Tiny **cilia**, or *hairs*, in the mucous membranes filter out dirt and foreign material, sweeping it toward the throat. A cough or sneeze will eliminate small particles before they can enter the lungs. The common cold is a viral infection of the upper respiratory system that produces symptoms such as coughing, sneezing, and a runny nose.

The **pharynx**, commonly referred to as the *throat*, is divided into three sections (Figure 13.20). These include the nasopharynx, the oropharynx, and the laryngopharynx. The nasopharynx [*nas* = nose] is the section located behind the nose and above the uvula that dangles at the back of the throat. The oropharynx [*or* = mouth] is located at the back of the oral cavity, below the nasopharynx. The laryngopharynx [*laryng* = larynx, voice box] is the lower section of the pharynx, located behind the larynx. Lymphatic tissues trap and destroy microbes that make it to the pharynx. These tissues include the adenoids, located at the bottom of the nasopharynx, and the tonsils, located in the oropharynx. The adenoids and tonsils usually shrink by the time you reach your teens, but they may be removed during childhood if they become too enlarged.

The **larynx**, also known as the *voice box*, contains vocal cords that vibrate to create sounds. Since the laryngopharynx is located near the larynx, air moving through the laryngopharynx produces sound. The larynx connects the pharynx of the upper respiratory system with the trachea of the lower respiratory system. Laryngitis [*laryng* = larynx, voice box, *itis* = inflammation] is an inflammation of the larynx that causes hoarseness, coughing, and difficulty swallowing. An upper respiratory infection (URI) is any infection of the trachea, larynx, throat, or nose.

Air traveling down to the pharynx shares some of its route with food headed to the esophagus. Food should only use the oropharynx and laryngopharynx. The nasopharynx is intended for air. Sometimes, if you sneeze or laugh while drinking, it may come out your nose rather than go down your throat.

You may have experienced food going "down the wrong tube." Located at the bottom of the pharynx, the **epiglottis** [*epi* = upon, *glott* = tongue] is a flap of cartilage that helps direct food and air down the correct tubes. The **trachea** (TRAY-kee-uh), or *windpipe*, is the tube that leads to the lungs. The esophagus leads to the stomach and lies behind the trachea. The epiglottis

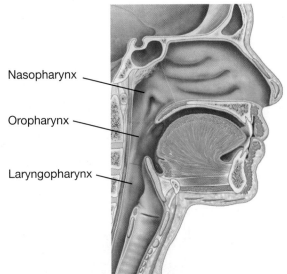

Nasopharynx

Oropharynx

Laryngopharynx

Figure 13.20   The pharynx is the third stop on oxygen's journey through the respiratory system.

covers the opening to the trachea when you swallow food. If you swallow too quickly, the epiglottis may not have time to close the airway, resulting in food going "down the wrong tube." *Aspiration*, which occurs when food or fluid enters the lungs, can be very serious. An involuntary cough will help to clear the trachea or lungs.

Air travels from the upper respiratory system through the trachea to reach the lungs. C-shaped cartilage rings in the trachea keep the airway open during pressure changes caused by breathing. The trachea is lined with mucous membranes similar to those of the nose and pharynx. Children younger than five years of age have a short, narrow trachea that makes them more susceptible to choking. When the throat swells or the trachea is blocked, a surgical opening can be created in the trachea to allow breathing. This operation is known as a *tracheotomy* (tray-kee-AHT-uh-mee) [*trache* = trachea, windpipe, *otomy* = cut into]. In a tracheotomy, a tube is inserted between the cartilage rings below the larynx and can be connected to a ventilator if breathing support is needed. Because air enters below the larynx and doesn't pass over the vocal cords, speech is not possible with a tracheotomy.

At the bottom of the trachea, tubes called **bronchi** (BRAHNG-kI) branch out to the left and right lungs. The bronchi divide into smaller **bronchioles** [*bronch* = bronchus, *ole* = small] that lead down to the air sacs in the lungs. A bronchoscope is a flexible, lighted tube that can be equipped with a camera, forceps, and other special tools to examine the inside of the bronchi. Bronchitis [*itis* = inflammation] is a sudden inflammation of the bronchi that can result from a URI or exposure to irritants in the air. *Asthma*, a chronic allergic disorder, involves a combination of smooth muscle contractions and mucous buildup in the bronchi (Figure 13.21). The narrowed airways that are characteristic of

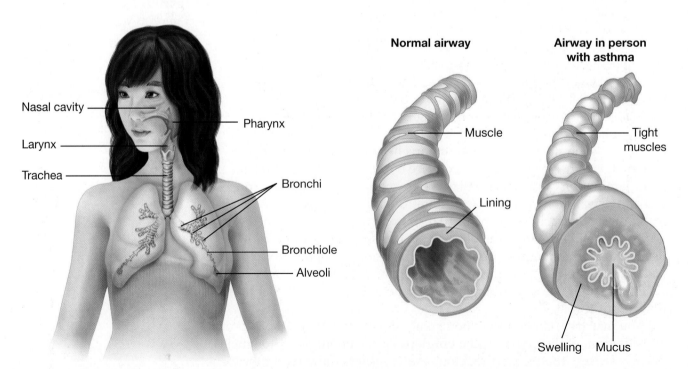

Figure 13.21   When a person has asthma, his or her bronchi become swollen and mucus builds up after contact with a trigger, causing an asthma attack.

asthma attacks cause coughing, wheezing, and breathlessness. Treatments include medications and avoiding triggers that cause flare-ups.

Oxygen and carbon dioxide are exchanged in capillaries surrounding the **alveoli** [*alveol* = cavity or socket]. These are tiny, hollow air sacs clustered like bunches of grapes at the ends of the bronchioles. The alveoli have elastic membranes that can expand and return to their regular size as air moves in and out. Infection and disease can destroy alveoli, making it difficult to exchange oxygen and carbon dioxide.

Smokers who suffer from emphysema are not able to push all of the used air out of their lungs because the alveoli have lost their elasticity. People with this condition take shallow breaths and have little room in their lungs for fresh air. Tuberculosis (TB) is a contagious disease caused by tiny, airborne bacteria that most often infect the lungs. It destroys alveoli and leaves scar tissue in their place. Chronic obstructive pulmonary disease (COPD) is a long-term lung disorder that reduces airflow. Two of the most common forms of COPD are emphysema and chronic bronchitis. Pressurized oxygen flowing from a tank can help to relieve the feeling of breathlessness for people with COPD (Figure 13.22).

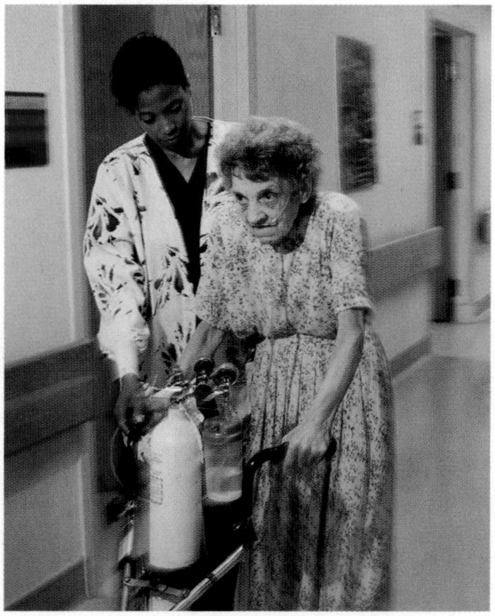

Alveoli provide more surface area for gas exchange than one large, hollow lung. If all the air sacs were spread out flat, they would cover an area the size of a tennis court! Infants have fewer and much smaller alveoli, resulting in a faster breathing rate and less lung volume than adults. Pneumonia (noo-MOH-nyuh) [*pneum* = lung, air, *ia* = abnormal condition] also causes a faster breathing rate, because a buildup of fluid in the lungs reduces the surface area available for air exchange. A bubbling or rattling sound in the lungs, called *rales*, can be heard with a stethoscope when fluid or secretions are present. Pneumonia can be life threatening in infants and the elderly.

Figure 13.22   Patients who have COPD sometimes use an oxygen tank to help them breathe.

The Two-Stage Process of Respiration

The movement of oxygen from air to the cells, or *respiration*, occurs in two stages. External respiration happens in the lungs. Capillaries surrounding the alveoli absorb oxygen from the air in the lungs and release carbon dioxide from the blood. The heart transports the oxygen from the lungs to other areas of the body. Internal respiration happens in capillary beds throughout the body. Carbon dioxide in the cells is released and exchanged for oxygen from the blood. External respiration happens during the pulmonary loop of the cardiovascular system. Internal respiration happens during the systemic loop of the cardiovascular system.

Oxygen and carbon dioxide are exchanged with the cardiovascular system during respiration. As discussed earlier, the thin walls of the capillaries allow gases to move in and out of the blood vessels. Carbon dioxide is released from the blood to the alveoli in the lungs and new oxygen is taken in through the alveoli to blood in the capillaries. Then, the cardiovascular system transports oxygen to the cells. Finally, the cardiovascular system removes carbon dioxide produced in the cells and sends it back to the lungs to be released from the body. A full cycle of respiration includes one inhalation and one exhalation (Figure 13.23).

During inhalation, oxygen-rich air is sucked into the lungs. The lungs are a pressurized system surrounded by membranes, or **pleura**. The visceral pleura [*viscer* = internal organ, *pleur* = side, rib] covers each lung's surface. The parietal pleura [*pariet* = wall, *pleur* = side, rib] lines the chest wall inside the pleural cavity. A lubricating fluid fills the pleural space between the two membranes to prevent friction as they slide against each other during respiration.

Contraction of the diaphragm, intercostal [*inter* = between, *cost* = rib, *al* = pertaining to] muscles, and abdominal muscles pull and expand the parietal pleurae. This pressure pulls and expands the visceral pleurae, which in turn pull and expand the alveoli to suck air into the lungs.

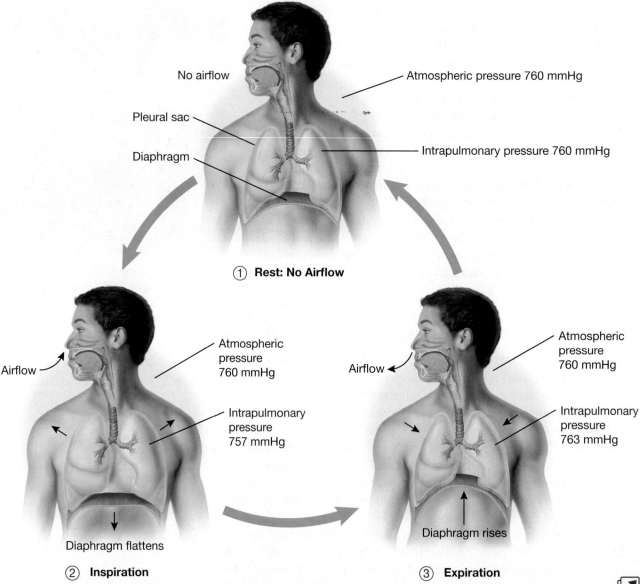

Figure 13.23   The respiratory cycle involves pressure changes inside the lungs and outside the body.

Animation

A hiccup is a sudden contraction of the diaphragm that causes you to suck air in quickly. During exhalation, the diaphragm relaxes, and the ribcage compresses to force carbon dioxide out of the alveoli and complete the respiratory cycle.

The lungs would collapse without the pressurized system created by the pleural membranes. A pneumothorax (noo-muh-THOR-aks), or *collapsed lung*, occurs when a pleural membrane is punctured or the space between the membranes is filled with fluid. Without the negative pressure in this lined pleural cavity, the inner surfaces of the lungs would stick to themselves and cause difficulty breathing, or *dyspnea* (DISP-nee-uh) [*dys* = difficult, painful, *pnea* = breathing]. Fluid in the pleural cavity presses on the lungs and takes up space that would have been filled by air. Thoracentesis (thoh-ruh-sehn-TEE-suhs) [*thorac* = chest, *centesis* = puncture] uses a needle or tube to drain the air or fluid from the pleural cavity so the collapsed lung can expand again.

Variation in Respiratory Rate and Volume

The respiratory rate is involuntarily controlled by the brain stem. Although we can consciously change our breathing rate, the body cannot store extra oxygen and requires a certain amount to continue functioning. We need to continue breathing an average of one pint of air about 10 to 20 times per minute. The respiratory rate naturally increases during exercise and illness and it may decrease slightly while sleeping.

Abnormal Breathing. Bradypnea [*brady* = slow, *pnea* = breathing], an abnormally slow breathing rate, may result from damage to the heart. Apnea [*a* = without, *pnea* = breathing], when breathing stops temporarily, is often present in premature babies and obese adults and near the end of life. Hypoxia [*hypo* = below normal, *ox* = oxygen, *ia* = abnormal condition] is a lack of oxygen. During hypoxia, a buildup of carbon dioxide in the blood triggers the brain to increase the respiratory rate and volume.

Lung Volume. Each breath moves air in and out of the lungs, but the lungs are never completely empty. **Total lung capacity** is the amount of air the lungs can hold when we take our deepest possible breath. This includes the *vital lung capacity* that can be exhaled after the deepest breath, plus the *residual volume* that remains in the lungs and airways after the strongest exhalation (Figure 13.24 on the next page). *Tidal volume* is the amount of air breathed in and out during light breathing while the body is at rest. This is a very small exchange of air in comparison to total lung volume, because resting doesn't require a lot of oxygen. A *spirometer* [*spir* = coil or winding, *meter* = measure] can be used to measure respiratory volumes.

Although residual volume can't be exhaled, that air is important to the function of the lungs. It helps to keep the inner surfaces of the lungs from sticking to each other, so it is easy for them to refill with the next breath. Just think how much easier it is to add air to a balloon that is half full than it is to blow that first breath into a brand-new balloon that is not yet inflated. Residual volume also provides enough air for the Heimlich maneuver to force an object out of the throat when a person is choking.

Figure 13.24 Lung Capacity

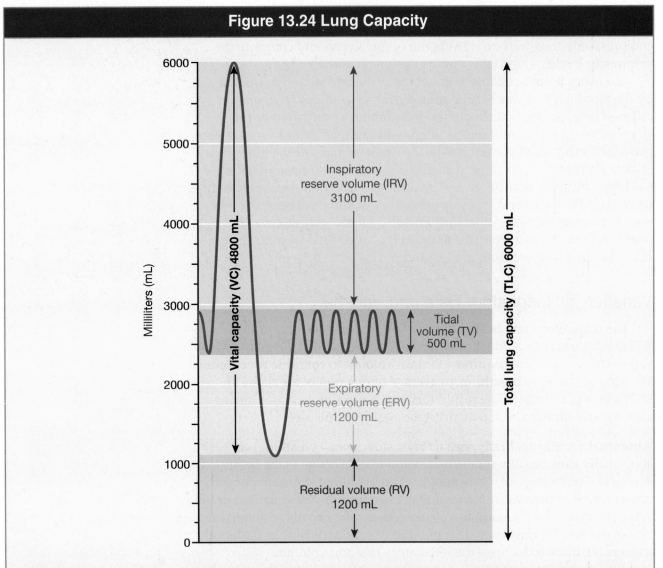

Lung capacities	Average Volumes	Definitions
total lung capacity (TLC) TLC = TV + IRV + ERV + RV	4,200–6,000 mL	maximum amount of air in the lungs after the deepest possible inhalation
tidal volume (TV)	500–600 mL	normal amount of air breathed in and out at rest
inspiratory reserve volume (IRV)	1,900–3,000 mL	maximum amount of air that can be taken in beyond a normal breath
expiratory reserve volume (ERV)	800–1,200 mL	additional amount of air that can be exhaled after a normal exhalation
residual volume (RV)	1,000–1,200 mL	amount of air that remains in the lungs after the deepest possible exhalation
vital capacity (VC) VC = TV + IRV + ERV	3,100–4,800 mL	maximum amount of air that can be breathed out after the deepest possible inhalation

Factors Affecting Lung Volume. Lung volume is affected by age, gender, body size, and physical condition. The right lung is shorter, broader, and has greater volume than the left. It is also divided into three lobes. The left lung has only two lobes to allow room for the heart. The surface area of the lungs decreases with age, which raises the respiratory rate in older adults. The number of cilia that protect the lungs from irritants declines with age at the same time that mucus production increases. These changes, in addition to reduced mobility and immune status, leave older adults more susceptible to respiratory infections and aspiration.

Adults and the physically fit will have greater lung volume than infants, older adults, or those who are out of shape. Regular exercise increases total lung capacity and vital capacity, but body size is the main factor in determining residual volume. In old age, the lungs become stiffer and respiratory muscle strength decreases (Figure 13.25). This decreases the vital capacity and expiratory reserve volume. Lungs usually reach their maximum capacity in early adulthood and then decline with age.

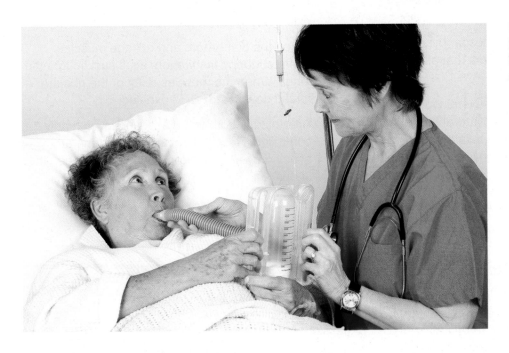

Figure 13.25   A manual incentive spirometer can be used to exercise and strengthen the lungs.

RECALL YOUR READING

1. The process of respiration exchanges _____ for _____.
2. The path that oxygen takes includes the nose, _____, _____, larynx, trachea, bronchi, _____, and alveoli.
3. _____ respiration occurs in the pulmonary loop and _____ respiration occurs in the systemic loop.
4. During _____, the diaphragm muscles contract to expand the lungs and pull air in.
5. Factors that affect respiratory rate include _____, gender, body size, and _____.

Complete the *Map Your Reading* graphic organizer for the section you just read.

SUMMARY

Assess your understanding with chapter tests

- Visual, auditory, and kinesthetic learners take in information in different ways. Knowing more about your learning style will help you adapt to different classroom situations and get the most from your education.

- The cardiovascular, respiratory, and lymphatic systems work with other body systems to transport and exchange materials in the body.

- The heart, blood vessels, and blood cells are the main organs of the cardiovascular system. Each has its own role in transporting materials in the body and removing body waste.

- The cardiovascular system affects the vital signs of temperature, pulse, respiration, and blood pressure.

- Bacteria, viruses, fungi, protozoa, rickettsiae, and helminthes are pathogens that all produce different types of disease.

- The lymphatic system has several types of defense against infections. Natural barriers are the first line of defense. Inflammation and leukocytes provide a second line of defense. The immune response helps the body adapt to fighting new infections as a third line of defense.

- Organs of the lymphatic system are closely related to the cardiovascular system. Lymphatic vessels return interstitial fluid to the cardiovascular system.

- Cancer is an uncontrolled cell growth. Malignant growths often spread through the lymph nodes to other parts of the body.

- The respiratory system exchanges carbon dioxide for oxygen in the lungs. These gases flow through the nose and mouth, pharynx, larynx, trachea, bronchi, bronchioles, and alveoli.

- Respiration and circulation occur in two stages—external respiration and internal respiration.

- When the diaphragm and ribcage muscles contract during inspiration, air is sucked into the lungs. When the muscles relax or the ribs are forced downward, air is exhaled.

- Breathing is both voluntarily and involuntarily controlled. Respiratory rate and volume are affected by age, gender, body size, and health status.

MAXIMIZE YOUR PROFESSIONAL VOCABULARY

Build vocabulary with e-flash cards, games, and audio glossary

Listed below are the essential, yellow-highlighted terms and the additional professional vocabulary that you encountered in this chapter. Complete the activities that follow the list to make all of these terms part of your everyday professional vocabulary.

adenoids	bronchioles	immunization
alveoli	cancer	infectious
antibiotics	capillary bed	kinesthetic learner
antibodies	cardiovascular	lacteal
antigen	cilia	larynx
artery	contagious	learning style
atrium	epiglottis	leukocyte
auditory learner	erythrocyte	lymph
bacteria	fungi	lymphatic
bronchi	hemoglobin	lymph node

lymphocyte	sinus cavities	trachea
mucous membranes	spleen	valve
pharynx	systemic loop	vein
plasma	thrombocyte	ventricle
pleura	thymus	virus
pulmonary loop	tonsils	visual learner
respiratory	total lung capacity	

VOCABULARY DEVELOPMENT

Matching. Match the essential terms from this chapter with the best descriptions below by writing the letter of the description next to the number of the essential term on your answer sheet.

1. antibodies
2. antigen
3. artery
4. capillary bed
5. cardiovascular
6. erythrocyte
7. learning style
8. leukocyte
9. lymphatic
10. pulmonary loop
11. respiratory
12. systemic loop
13. vein

a. related to the act of, or organs involved in, breathing

b. a red blood cell that transports oxygen and carbon dioxide to and from body tissues

c. a white blood cell that is involved in fighting infection

d. a foreign substance that causes the body to make antibodies

e. a main blood vessel that moves blood from body tissues toward the heart

f. a network of very fine, thin-walled blood vessels (capillaries) located in body tissues

g. the flow of blood from the heart to the lungs and back to pick up oxygen and drop off carbon dioxide

h. proteins produced by leukocytes that bind with and disable antigens

i. the flow of blood from the heart to the body systems and back to drop off nutrients and pick up waste

j. related to the heart and blood vessels

k. related to or containing the watery fluid (lymph) collected from body tissues

l. a major blood vessel that moves blood from the heart out to the body tissues

m. an individual's preferred way of gaining or processing new information

14. **Term Snap.** Make flash cards for each word part listed in the table on the next page. Sit in circles of 3 to 5 students and shuffle your cards, keeping them all facing in the same direction. The first player turns over a term card to reveal the definition and places it in the center, "term side" facing up. Other players go around the circle, taking turns to discard one card at a time with the definition side facing up. When the definition matching the term card in the center of the circle is discarded, the first to notice must slap the matching card. That player takes all the cards in the middle and draws the next term card. Play continues until the time is up or players run out of cards. The player with the most term cards at the end of play is the winner.

REFLECT ON YOUR READING

15. Review the vocabulary organizer you created for the *Connect with Your Reading* activity. Now that you have read the chapter, do you feel you better understand the terms in your *New Terms* column? Explain each of those terms in your own words and share with a classmate.

Medical Word Parts					
Prefixes	**Root Words**			**Suffixes**	
an-	alveoli/i	hem/o, hemat/o	phleb/o	-centesis	-ist
anti-	angi/o	laryng/o	pneum/o	-eal	-meter
auto-	arteri/o	leuk/o	pulmon/o	-ectomy	-ole
brady-	ather/o	lymph/o	sept/o	-edema	-oma
inter-	bi/o	nas/o	spir/o	-emia	-otomy
intra-	bronch/i	onc/o	thromb/o	-gram	-pnea
meta-	cost/o	or/o	trache/o	-graph	-tic
mono-	electr/o	ox/i	ven/o	-ia	-ular
sclera-	erythr/o	phag/o	viscer/o		
tachy-	gloss/o, glott/o				

BUILD CORE SKILLS

16. **Reading.** Search the Internet for a free online learning style inventory. Take the test to determine your learning style. Then search the Internet for more information on that particular style. Decide what you can do to enhance your learning experience. Summarize how you plan to improve your learning. Include something a teacher could do to help you learn in his or her classroom.

17. **Problem Solving.** On a separate sheet of paper, create a three-column chart. Label the columns with these headings: *Problem, Cause,* and *Effect.* Then research three diseases— one from the respiratory system, one from the cardiovascular system, and one from the lymphatic system—and fill in the chart with the information you find.

18. **Reading.** Search the Internet for the Disease Risk Index offered by the Harvard School of Public Health. Using this interactive tool, determine your risk of developing cancer. With this information, write a few paragraphs explaining what lifestyle changes you can make to decrease your risk of cancer.

19. **Problem Solving.** Search the Internet for Rice University's "MEDMYST" website. Play the interactive microbiology game to learn about infectious diseases. When you have played the game, write a brief summary of what you learned about pathogens, white blood cells, and how infectious diseases are spread.

20. **Writing.** Imagine that you are a lung. Write a letter of complaint to a cigarette that focuses on the effects of smoking.

21. **Math.** For every pound of fat gained, the body adds seven miles of additional arterioles, capillaries, and venules. The average American has gained 15 pounds in the last 15 years. If that weight gain is from fat, how many extra miles of blood vessels did the average American's body need to make? Morbid obesity is characterized by being 100 pounds over your ideal body weight. How many miles of additional blood vessels are created in the event of morbid obesity?

22. **Math.** Calculate your maximum heart rate during exercise by subtracting your age from 220. Then, calculate your target running heart rate by counting your pulse for one minute while your body is at rest and subtract that from your maximum heart rate. The next time you are exercising, stop and check your pulse to see if your workout is at an appropriate level of intensity.

23. **Critical Thinking.** Although one pound of fat doesn't look like much on the outside, it adds miles of new blood vessels. Explain why a morbidly obese person is more likely to die from a sudden heart attack. Why would you expect a morbidly obese person's heart to be enlarged when examined in an autopsy?

ACTIVATE YOUR LEARNING

24. To simulate what happens in an anemic person's body, create two lines of students— one to represent a person with anemia and one to represent a person with normal levels of hemoglobin. Each line will have a basket of tennis balls (oxygen) that must be carried from their baskets (lungs) on one side of the room to another set of baskets on the other side of the room (body cells). Students in the anemia line may carry one tennis ball at a time from the lungs to the cells. The students in the other line can each carry up to four tennis ball at once from the lungs to the cells. When all of the tennis balls have been transported, discuss your observations about the anemia line and the normal line. How much longer did it take the anemia line to get the oxygen to the cells? Which line was more tired at the end of the activity? Oxygen is used in the cellular process of creating energy. Discuss what is happening to a person with anemia and how it affects the body.

25. Use the following items to create a model of the lymphatic system, then explain what each item represents and why: straws, funnel, coffee filter, marshmallows, assorted candies or jelly beans.

26. Use these instructions to create a model of a lung that inflates through negative pressure. You will need a 2-liter soda bottle, an 8-inch piece of plastic wrap, a large rubber band, a small rubber band, a round balloon, and a 4-inch strip of tape.

    - Cut the soda bottle in half and keep the top half of the bottle.

    - Blow up the balloon and let the air out once or twice to stretch it out a little, then insert the bottom of the balloon into the mouth of the soda bottle and turn the balloon's lip over onto the top of the soda bottle opening.

    - Hold the balloon edge in place with the small rubber band. Place the saran wrap over the cut bottom of the soda bottle to cover the large opening and secure it in place with the large rubber band.

    - Fold the tape in half and stick the center together, but leave the two ends separated. Stick these two ends to the center of the saran wrap, allowing the center of the tape to stick out like a small handle.

    - Now, gently pull on the tape handle and watch the balloon expand. Release or press in and watch the balloon deflate. Label each part of the model with the respiratory system organ that it represents.

THINK AND ACT LIKE A HEALTHCARE WORKER

27. You are working at a healthcare clinic when a man walks in from the parking lot. He is pulling at the collar of his shirt and sweating. He says he can't catch his breath. He stumbles and grabs for the counter to steady himself. What are some logical assumptions about his health condition? What should you do?

28. You are working in a nursing home. A resident has taken his socks off because his foot was itchy. Now he wants help putting his socks and shoes back on. You notice that one foot has some odor and feels warmer to the touch than the other foot. It is also a little harder to fit the shoe on this foot. What are you suspecting may be wrong? What should you do?

GO TO THE SOURCE

29. Pick up a brochure about immunizations for children from your local clinic. Why is immunization recommended? At what ages are these childhood immunizations recommended? How many doses of each type of immunization are recommended? What are the most common side effects noted?

30. Check your nurse's office or search online for one of the CDC's "Get Smart" posters. Summarize the main message the poster is trying to get across. Explain how the poster's topic relates to the information in this chapter.

Unit 4
Support Services

Chapter 14

Career Skills in Support Services

Chapter 15

Fundamental Skills in Support Services

Chapter 16

Professional Knowledge in Support Services

Chapter 17

Academic Knowledge: Body Systems for Maintenance and Continuation

While studying, look for the online icon to:

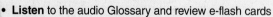

- **Listen** to the audio Glossary and review e-flash cards
- **Assess** learning with quizzes and online exercises
- **Expand** knowledge with animations and activities
- **Simulate** healthcare tasks and employability skills

www.g-wlearning.com/healthsciences

Study on the Go
Use your mobile device to practice vocabulary and assess learning
www.m.g-wlearning.com

Career Pathway

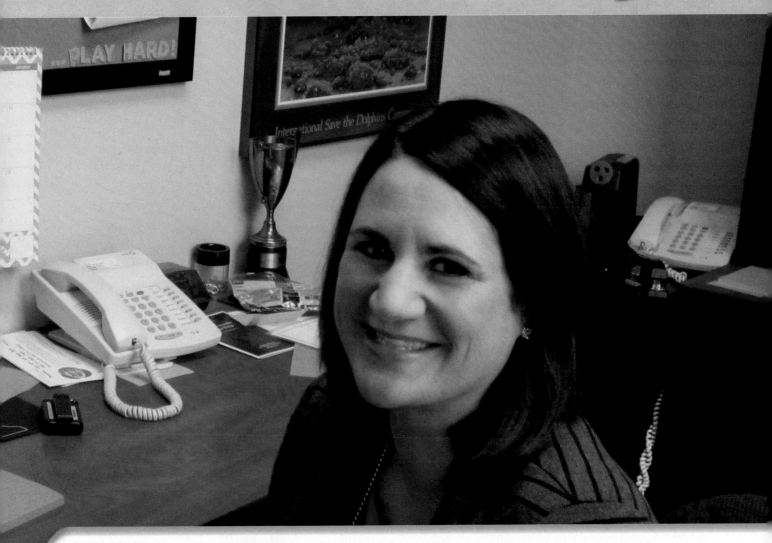

Healthcare Insider:

Lauren, BS Marketing
Director of Public and Community Relations

"I like my job because I have the opportunity to share success stories from the patients treated at Shriners Hospitals for Children. I work directly with news reporters and photographers to capture footage for stories, which has also allowed me to learn about pediatric orthopedics. My job duties include managing the Shriners Hospitals for Children brand, which means I have a hand in all advertising and marketing material. I have to make sure all of our brand requirements are met. It's fun to find new ways of sharing the amazing work that is done with pediatric orthopedics at Shriners Hospitals for Children. I feel lucky to be able to share that information every day."

Chapter 14
Career Skills in Support Services

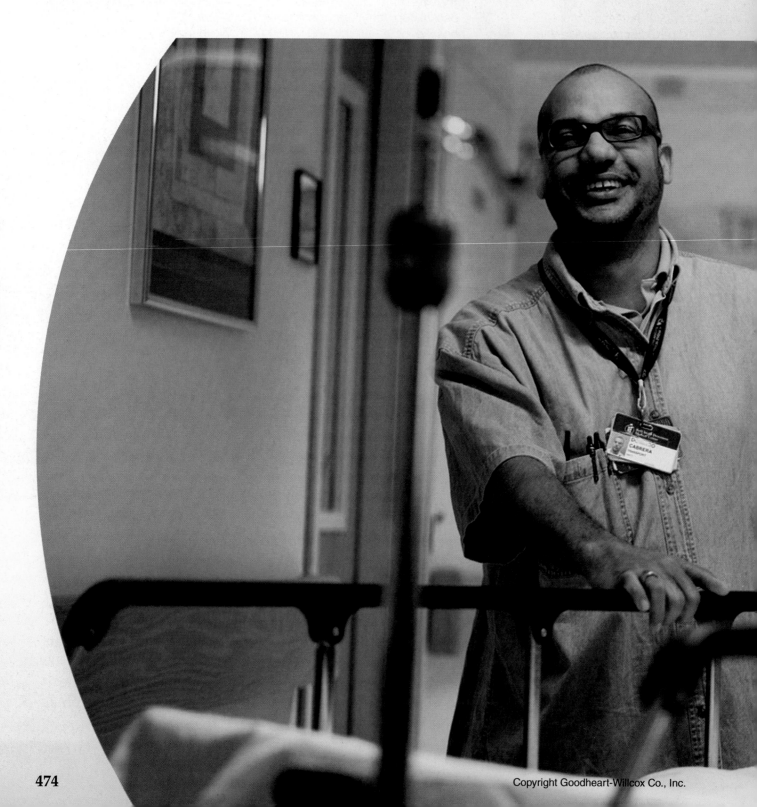

PROFESSIONAL VOCABULARY

E-flash Cards

You will need to learn the essential terms listed below before you begin your reading. These terms will help you understand the main concepts of the chapter. These terms, which will be highlighted in yellow within the text, will become part of your professional vocabulary.

In addition to these essential terms, you will see bold terms throughout the chapter. The meanings of these terms are explained where the terms first appear. The bold terms, like the essential terms listed here, will also become part of your professional vocabulary and deepen your understanding of the topics presented.

central services   the hospital department responsible for receiving, storing, cleaning, disinfecting, sterilizing, and distributing medical and surgical supplies and equipment

compassion   sympathy for the distress of others accompanied by a desire to help

contamination   the unwanted presence of harmful substances or microorganisms

disinfection   the use of chemicals to kill pathogens that are present on nonliving objects

environmental services   the hospital department responsible for housekeeping, laundry, and facility maintenance

initiative   the ability to decide independently what to do and when to do it

professional distance   term used to describe the act of showing a caring attitude toward patients without trying to become friends

sanitation   term that describes procedures and practices that maintain cleanliness and preserve public health

service learning   an educational experience that integrates academic achievement with community service

support services   the career pathway that focuses on creating a therapeutic environment for providing patient care

therapeutic diet   a special food plan ordered by a physician to help treat a disease

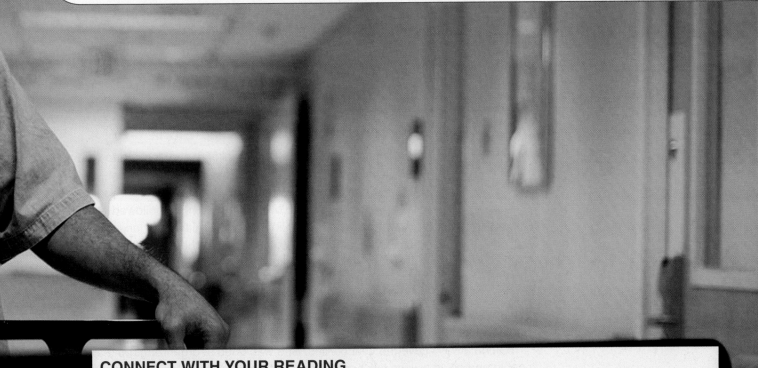

CONNECT WITH YOUR READING

While a wide variety of occupations focus on support services, these occupations are often invisible to patients. Connect the following items to a healthcare facility department or to a healthcare employee to help you envision healthcare support services occupations: a hospital bill, dinner, sterilized surgical equipment, a television ad for a hospital, an interview, a newsletter, a time study, a health club, and a group home. Share your responses with a classmate and discuss your results.

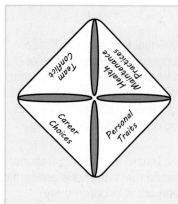

MAP YOUR READING

Create a visual summary of this chapter, just as you did in chapter 2. Begin with a square sheet of paper—an 8½-inch square works well. Fold each of the four points of the square to the center. Label each of the four resulting flaps with one of these topics: *Personal Traits*, *Career Choices*, *Team Conflict*, and *Health Maintenance Practices*. When you finish reading each of these sections in the chapter, open the corresponding flap and draw a picture or symbol to illustrate what you have read. Ask yourself what each topic looks like, how you could draw it, and what graphic or symbol best represents it. Finally, for each of the four topics, write two words that explain how the topic relates to you personally in the center square of your visual summary.

You may not always see them, but support services workers are important members of a healthcare facility's staff. This chapter introduces you to the tasks these workers perform to ensure the successful operation of a healthcare facility. These services focus on functions such as safety, sanitation, food preparation, equipment maintenance, counseling services, administration and management, and marketing. All of these functions support high-quality patient care.

In addition to learning more about support services, you will become acquainted with sources of conflict within teams and learn steps for resolving conflicts between team members. As you practice skills for disinfection, food handling, and wheelchair transport, consider the valuable roles that support services workers perform. Finally, you will learn ways to maintain your own health so you can model a healthy lifestyle as you carry out the tasks of your chosen healthcare occupation.

The Support Services Worker: Gloria

When Gloria headed off to college, she decided to study dietetics (dI-uh-TEH-tihks). Because she loved to cook, she thought a career working with menus and food would be a good fit. Her own family members followed a healthy diet to manage their health conditions and she wanted to help other people do the same thing. After a couple years of college, however, Gloria was bored and discouraged. She was a good student but did not enjoy all the chemistry-based science courses. She began to wonder if she would really like analyzing diets and planning menus. She was looking for something more creative.

Gloria always gave the best parties. She was good at organizing groups of people and could always talk her friends into following her plans. She thought business and marketing might be more exciting than dietetics, so she changed her major and finished her degree.

Two years later, Gloria had a job in business, but it was just a job. She was a good worker, but she didn't find organizing the sale and shipment of products satisfying. Around this time, Gloria volunteered to help a colleague organize a fundraiser to benefit AIDS patients. She planned an Oscar party event, which was a huge success. This was a project she really enjoyed, it was for a worthwhile cause, and it got her thinking.

Today, Gloria has a satisfying job in marketing at a nonprofit children's hospital. She is passionate about the care her organization provides for its patients. She loves planning children's fairs, annual proms for the teen patients, and other special events to enhance the experiences of children who spend so much of their young lives as hospital patients. Gloria is a healthcare worker. Her career is just one example of the wide variety of careers that make up the healthcare support services pathway.

Personal Traits

Do you like organizing people and events? Are you a natural leader? Then you might enjoy a career in healthcare administration, **marketing**, or **public relations**. People in these careers make sure that the business side of a healthcare facility is successful. They manage finances, plan for future growth, and make sure that potential patients know about their facility and its services. To succeed in these careers, you need a strong sense of **initiative** and self-motivation. You must be able to see the "big picture" for the future of your organization and be willing to set goals to achieve success.

Are you enthusiastic about improving the lives of others? Do you enjoy analyzing the challenges in their lives? Do you feel empathy and **compassion** for others? Then you might enjoy a career in social work or counseling. Healthcare professionals in these areas have strong communication skills. They use their problem-solving abilities to help people figure out their insurance coverage or locate community resources to meet individual needs. The work they perform allows patients to improve their personal relationships and live healthier lives.

Do you get satisfaction from doing a job the right way every time? Are you a responsible and reliable worker? Then you might find satisfaction in maintaining a healthcare facility. Building maintenance workers make sure that heat, water, and electricity are available even during a power outage. When you consider healthcare careers, maintenance engineer may not be the first one that comes to mind. However, patients who rely on ventilators to breathe know that this work is important.

Your attention to detail and commitment to doing things "the right way" may also lead to a career as an occupational health and safety expert or an environmental health practitioner. Occupational health and safety experts promote the development of safer, healthier, and more efficient ways of working. Environmental health practitioners identify and control health and safety hazards related to the work environment.

Do you like solving problems and working with your hands? If you are fascinated with understanding how things work, you might enjoy a career in maintaining and repairing medical equipment. From the simple tasks of calibrating scales and sphygmomanometers (blood pressure cuffs) to maintaining the most complex imaging equipment, these workers ensure the accuracy of diagnostic tests and the success of treatments that require sensitive equipment. Workers' attention to detail in this area supports a positive outcome for patients.

initiative
the ability to decide independently what to do and when to do it

compassion
sorrow for the distress of others accompanied by a desire to help

Support Services Career Choices

support services
term for the career pathway that focuses on creating a therapeutic environment for providing patient care

The **support services** career pathway encompasses a wide variety of healthcare occupations. All support services workers help create a therapeutic environment for providing patient care. This may be done by supporting the successful business operation of a healthcare facility or promoting a safe and healthy environment for patient care.

Social workers and counselors improve the personal lives of their patients through emotional support. Fitness instructors and nurse educators provide training in diet, exercise, and stress management. Workers in a mortuary or funeral home provide services to grieving families. All of these workers fall under the support services pathway.

The support services pathway offers a variety of entry-level positions, including dietary aide, housekeeper, transport technician, and central services technician. These positions can offer valuable work experience in the healthcare setting. Students can also use part-time jobs in these occupations to supplement their income while they complete their education and training for a chosen healthcare career.

Careers That Support Successful Business Operations

Successful businesses need capable leadership and efficient operating systems. Healthcare businesses are no different. Healthcare administrators and financial officers provide leadership and oversight for facility operations. Public relations workers and marketing specialists promote the services provided by the facility. Workers in human resources make sure the facility hires qualified workers.

Administration. Healthcare administrators or managers oversee the daily operation of a healthcare facility. In a small facility such as a nursing home, one administrator may manage personnel, finances, facility operations, and admissions. In a large hospital facility, however, several assistant administrators oversee daily operations in each clinical area, such as nursing, surgery, therapy, and medical records. Other assistants oversee human resources, finances, and facility operations. Each of these assistants reports to the top administrator in the facility.

Healthcare administrators may work in large hospitals, outpatient care centers, physicians' offices, nursing facilities, or for home health agencies. Since healthcare facilities often operate around the clock, administrators may be called on at all hours to address problems. They work long hours and may travel to attend meetings or oversee satellite facilities (Figure 14.1).

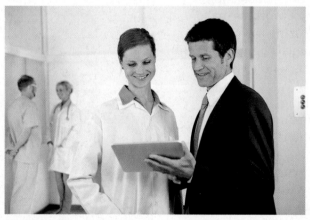

Figure 14.1   Both large and small facilities require the skills of a healthcare administrator. Some administrators oversee several facilities within the same healthcare system.

Successful healthcare managers and administrators possess strong leadership skills. They like to sell ideas or things and tend to be energetic and sociable. Regardless of their specific title, all managers must maintain positive communication between governing boards, medical staff, and department heads. They analyze and evaluate information to solve problems and monitor equipment and resources as they oversee spending. They also ensure that the facility complies with federal, state, and local regulations. Managers in charge of a specific department or function have unique job tasks (Figure 14.2).

Healthcare managers and administrators in entry-level positions need a bachelor's degree in healthcare administration, public health, or business administration. A master's degree is commonly required for positions in larger healthcare facilities. Becoming a clinical department head requires a degree in the department's field, a few years of work experience, and an advanced administration degree. For example, a hospital nursing supervisor is usually an experienced RN with a bachelor's degree in nursing. To become eligible for a nursing administrator position, the RN obtains a master's degree in administration. Nursing home administrators are licensed by each state. They complete a training program, an examination, and continuing education. Some states also require licensure for administrators of assisted living facilities. However, there is no license requirement for administrators in other areas of medical and health services management.

While the largest numbers of managers work in a hospital setting, the largest job growth will occur in the offices of health practitioners. Demand for managers in medical group practices will increase as these practices become larger and more complex. Job opportunities will be especially good for applicants with work experience in healthcare.

Marketing and Public Relations. Medical marketing professionals are responsible for planning and executing marketing initiatives. Directors of healthcare marketing work for regional medical centers, physicians' groups, private and public hospitals, and other healthcare organizations. They develop specific marketing plans to encourage future patients to use their organization's services. When you see advertising for a healthcare facility, for example, you are seeing the work of a marketing professional.

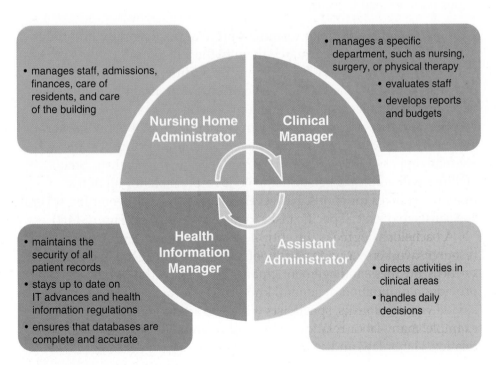

Figure 14.2   Specific types of healthcare managers have unique job tasks.

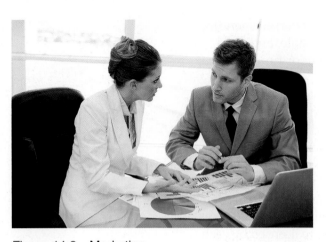

Figure 14.3 Marketing professionals use their creative and technical skills to promote healthcare. What information might be included in a marketing presentation for a healthcare facility?

Marketing positions usually require a bachelor's or master's degree. Courses in business law, management, economics, accounting, finance, mathematics, and statistics are required to provide important background knowledge for this career. The completion of an internship is also an advantage in the job market. Employers look for workers who are creative and can use new technologies to promote healthcare (Figure 14.3).

Individuals who specialize in healthcare public relations are in charge of the internal and external communications for a healthcare facility. They must have excellent communication skills because they interact with physicians, nurses, managers, administrators, and patients. Some responsibilities for those in healthcare public relations include writing for staff newsletters, handling calls from the media, and creating various materials that promote the services offered at their facility. The most important function of this position is handling all communication with the public. Public relations specialists must be highly organized and prepared to deal with a variety of situations.

Public relations professionals work in a variety of healthcare settings. In larger facilities, they may supervise several public relations assistants who help with daily operations. The majority of healthcare public relations positions require a bachelor's degree combined with a public relations internship. Employers usually prefer a degree in journalism, public relations, or advertising. Individuals may seek professional credentials through the Public Relations Society of America or the International Association of Business Communications. While the demand for marketing and public relations specialists is increasing, the job market is competitive because the number of qualified applicants is expected to exceed the number of job openings.

Human Resources. Human resources professionals work to find the most qualified employees, match them to the jobs for which they are best suited, and retain them at the company. In addition, these professionals oversee employee benefits such as healthcare and disability insurance, vacation and sick leave, and retirement benefits. Human resources workers also help their companies improve productivity and worker morale by providing training and development opportunities. There are many types of human resources managers and specialists. Small facilities will employ a generalist, who is responsible for all of the human resources functions. However, a large facility will employ several specialists to oversee specific tasks in human resources (Figure 14.4).

A bachelor's degree is the entry-level requirement for human resources workers. A wide variety of coursework in social and behavioral sciences, business management, finance, and industrial psychology provides a foundation of general knowledge. Because this field includes a wide variety of tasks, specialists will need additional training. For example, many labor relations jobs require graduate study in labor relations, labor law, and contract negotiations.

Figure 14.4 Tasks of Human Resources Specialists	
Specialists	**Duties**
Placement Specialists	• help set up interviews • match employers with qualified job seekers
Labor Relations Specialists	• interpret and administer labor contracts • handle grievance procedures
Employment Interviewers	• refer suitable candidates to employers • interview potential applicants for job openings
Recruitment Specialists	• find, screen, and interview applicants for job openings • test applicants, contact references, and extend job offers

Human resource assistants are entry-level workers who keep records of a company's employees. They update information in the records, complete reports for managers, and assist in the hiring of new employees. These assistants are usually high school graduates who are trained on the job.

Regardless of job title and training, all workers in human resources have to interact well with people and be able to keep employee information private (Figure 14.5). Since a wide variety of software is used to keep track of worker records and benefits, computer skills are essential. The ability to speak a foreign language is also an asset. As our workforce becomes increasingly diverse, human resources managers and specialists will work with or supervise people of various ages and cultural backgrounds.

Human resources workers can improve their knowledge and job opportunities by seeking training and certification from professional organizations. For example, the Society for Human Resource Management offers two levels of certification: Professional in Human Resources (PHR) and Senior Professional in Human Resources (SPHR). Certification usually requires completing coursework and passing certification exams along with demonstrated work experience. The field of human resources is growing. College graduates and those who have earned certification should have the best job opportunities.

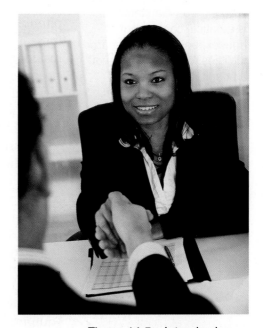

Figure 14.5   Interviewing potential job candidates is a major function of the human resources specialist. What skills are needed for this particular job task?

Careers That Support a Safe and Healthy Facility Environment

Facility maintenance is a large task that requires many types of workers. Engineers and equipment repair technicians make sure that heating, air, and ventilation systems are maintained at healthy levels. They also oversee special systems for preventing the spread of airborne pathogens that transmit diseases such as tuberculosis (too-ber-kyuh-LOH-sihs). These workers keep all of the facility's diagnostic and therapeutic equipment functioning accurately so that patients can receive high-quality care.

Housekeeping and central services workers make sure the facility and its equipment are sanitary to prevent the spread of infection, while dietary workers support the ongoing health of patients by carefully preparing foods that follow their individualized therapeutic diet guidelines. Finally, transport technicians move patients to different areas of the facility and move specimens to the laboratory.

Engineering and Maintenance. A variety of engineering professionals support the work of a healthcare facility. Most positions require a bachelor's degree in a specific type of engineering. Healthcare engineering and maintenance managers are responsible for all aspects of facility management for the organization's physical plant, including repairs to the facility and its equipment. The plant includes the building and all its heating, ventilation, electrical, and air conditioning systems. In addition, the engineering manager makes sure that the facility complies with all regulatory agency rules. Managers typically have several years of work experience in a healthcare facility in addition to their bachelor's degree.

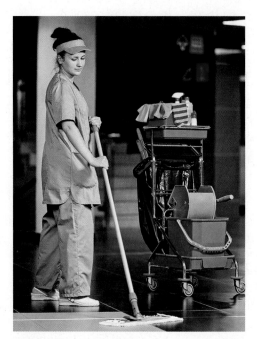

Figure 14.6   Sanitation is a critical component of housekeeping in healthcare facilities. What is the role of a hospital housekeeper?

environmental services
term for the hospital department responsible for housekeeping, laundry, and facility maintenance

Maintenance technicians and housekeepers also work in this department. Technicians are responsible for routine plumbing and electrical repairs and may need technical training in these areas. Housekeepers clean and stock areas such as patient or resident rooms, bathrooms, offices, lounges, and hallways using proper cleaning techniques. They usually receive on-the-job training and must be familiar with healthcare sanitation standards. Some facilities refer to this department as **environmental services** and include the combined functions of housekeeping and laundry (Figure 14.6).

Environmental engineers are concerned with safe drinking water, air quality, and other issues affecting the health of the public. They work for universities, public health agencies, research agencies, and various commercial industries as compliance officers. Other positions include county public health directors, hazardous waste specialists, and water quality scientists.

Clinical engineers have a college degree in biomedical engineering. Their primary job is to use medical technology to improve healthcare delivery. They consult with physicians and medical equipment companies and provide advice about design improvements for specialized medical equipment. They also train and supervise biomedical equipment technicians. These technicians usually have an associate's degree. They are responsible for equipment installation, routine inspections, and calibration of diagnostic instruments. They may earn a national certification and go through specialized training to understand laboratory and radiology equipment.

Industrial engineers work primarily with people and processes rather than machines and products. They identify the most efficient ways to use space, time, workers, and other resources. For example, they may forecast the number of hospital patients to be treated in future years so that human resources can plan for adequate staff hiring. The results of industrial engineers' work improve patient care and reduce the costs of providing care.

The **central services**, or *central supply* department in a hospital receives, stores, and distributes medical and surgical supplies and equipment. Central services technicians provide important support to the patient care services in a healthcare facility by helping prevent infections. These technicians must know all of the tools used in an operating room and be proficient in sterilizing and packaging surgical instruments.

Technicians may be trained on the job, but many complete a technical training program. Employers prefer workers who are certified by the Certification Board for Sterile Processing and Distribution or by the International Association of Healthcare Central Service Materials Management. Through these agencies, technicians receive continuing education and can complete coursework for job specialties such as instrumentation specialist, central supply manager, or ambulatory surgery technician.

central services
term for the hospital department responsible for receiving, storing, cleaning, disinfecting, sterilizing, and distributing medical and surgical supplies and equipment

Food Services. If you have recently been a hospital patient, you know that hospital food service has changed dramatically from what you may have expected. Instead of standardized menus delivered at scheduled times, patients now order room service meals from a restaurant-style menu at whatever times they choose to eat. Customized menus meet special dietary needs, such as those for patients with heart problems. In addition to a traditional cafeteria, visitors and employees may eat at the hospital bistro or even at a commercial restaurant located within the medical center. Large facilities may employ an executive chef as well as the more traditional cooks and kitchen aides (Figure 14.7).

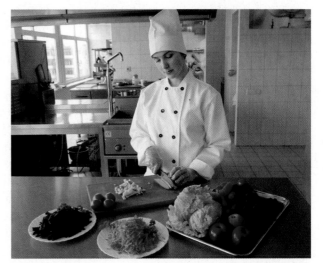

Figure 14.7   Hospital chefs use their talents to prepare appealing, healthy meals for patients and staff. *What are some dietary specifications chefs must consider when preparing meals for patients?*

Dietitians (dI-uh-TIH-shuhns) are food and nutrition experts. They are therapeutic workers who advise patients about what foods to eat to improve their particular health condition. They are also support workers who develop meal plans for patients and residents in healthcare facilities. Many dietitians educate the public on topics related to food and nutrition (Figure 14.8).

Dietitians earn a bachelor's or a master's degree in dietetics, food service management, or food and nutrition. Students must complete a supervised internship and pass an exam to become licensed as registered

Figure 14.8 Specializations within the Field of Dietetics		
Clinical Dietitian	Management Dietitian	Community Dietitian
• provides medical nutrition therapy • creates nutritional programs for patients or residents	• plans meal programs • oversees kitchen staff or other dietitians	• educates the public about food and nutritional issues • works in public health or nonprofit agencies

dietitians (RDs). The job market for dietitians is expected to grow due to increased awareness of the role that diet plays in preventing and treating illnesses such as diabetes and heart disease. An aging population and an increase in newly-diagnosed diabetics of all ages will fuel the need for more dietitians and nutritionists.

A **dietetic technician** holds an associate's degree and works under the supervision of a dietitian or food services manager. Technicians plan and produce meals based on established guidelines, teach principles of food and nutrition, or help clients make healthy food choices. These workers are often employed in hospitals, nursing homes, and long-term care facilities. Schools, day care centers, and government agencies such as prisons also hire them.

A sense of creativity combined with a strong knowledge of food and nutrition help dietetic technicians prepare food that patients will enjoy. Employment for dietetic technicians is expected to grow, with the largest number of positions located in nursing homes, residential care facilities, and physician clinics. Dietary services departments also employ cooks, dishwashers, cafeteria attendants, and dietary aides. Regardless of their job title, all dietary workers must meet high standards for safety and cleanliness to avoid contamination and injury.

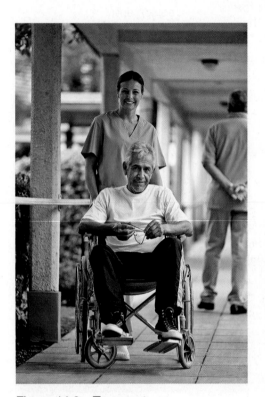

Figure 14.9 Transport technicians may use a wheelchair to take hospital patients to and from imaging and surgery appointments.

Patient Transport. **Transport technicians** take patients to and from diagnostic imaging appointments (Figure 14.9). They may also be asked to transport specimens for laboratory analysis. These technicians maintain transportation devices such as wheelchairs and gurneys and perform general cleaning and storage of patient-related equipment. Technicians are trained on the job. They need strong customer service and interpersonal skills for communicating with a variety of patients. They must also work efficiently under stress, such as when they are transporting trauma patients.

Careers That Improve the Personal Lives of Patients, Residents, and Clients

Supportive healthcare services are provided by marriage and family counselors and social workers who work with children, hospital patients, or individuals with mental health needs. Support workers may also provide diet and exercise training to improve patient health. Mortuary and funeral service workers provide support by providing meaningful end-of-life observances for families.

Counseling and Social Work. Counselors and social workers help community members who are facing challenges in their everyday lives. These careers require an advanced degree such as a master's or a PhD. Direct-service social workers help people solve and cope with problems, while clinical social workers diagnose and treat patients with mental, behavioral, or emotional issues. Social workers are employed in mental health clinics, schools, hospitals, and private practices. They generally work full time and may need to work evenings and weekends.

Counselors specialize in the specific needs of a patient population such as marriage and family therapy, substance abuse counseling, or career counseling. Counselors have at least a master's degree and usually must be certified or licensed to work (Figure 14.10). They work in private practice, mental health centers, hospitals, and colleges. They generally work full time and may work evenings and weekends since counseling sessions are scheduled to accommodate clients who may have job or family responsibilities.

Employment is expected to grow in all areas of counseling because this form of treatment is becoming an accepted part of healthcare. Increasingly, insurance companies are providing reimbursement for mental health counselors and marriage and family therapists as a less costly alternative to psychiatrists and psychologists.

Social and human services assistants support the work of counselors and social workers. They might work directly with clients to help them find benefits and access community resources such as food stamps or Medicaid health coverage (Figure 14.11 on the next page). They may supervise homes for clients recovering from alcohol or drug abuse, or they may support developmentally disabled individuals living in a group home setting. They monitor and keep case records on clients and report progress to supervisors and case managers.

These assistants often have technical college training. They work for nonprofit organizations, private for-profit social services agencies, and state and local governments. Employment is expected to grow for social and human services assistants due to an increase in the elderly population and

Figure 14.10 Specific Types of Counselors	
Counselors	**Duties**
Rehabilitation Counselor	• helps people with emotional and physical disabilities to live independently • helps clients overcome the effects of disabilities as they relate to employment
Marriage and Family Therapist	• helps people manage or overcome problems with their family and relationships • helps clients develop strategies to improve their lives
Mental Health Counselor	• helps people manage or overcome mental and emotional disorders • helps clients develop strategies to improve their lives
Substance Abuse and Behavioral Disorders Counselor	• advises people who have alcoholism or other types of addiction • provides treatment and support to help clients recover from addiction
School and Career Counselor	• helps students develop social skills and succeed in school • helps people choose a career or educational program

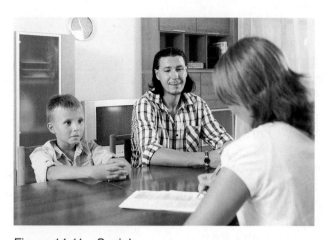

Figure 14.11   Social service workers help clients locate and access community resources. What are some examples of these resources?

an increase in the number of drug offenders who are sent to treatment programs rather than to jail.

Fitness Training. A national trend toward adopting healthy lifestyles is driving an increase in the need for fitness trainers and instructors. These healthcare workers are employed by health clubs, community recreation departments, and large businesses that want to maintain a healthy workforce.

Fitness instructors receive training in specific exercise methods such as Pilates or yoga. They complete certification programs to teach a specific type of class. CPR certification is also a requirement. An increasing number of employers require fitness workers to have an associate's or bachelor's degree related to a health or fitness field, such as exercise science, kinesiology, or physical education. Programs often include courses in nutrition, exercise techniques, and stress reduction.

Employment for fitness instructors is expected to grow in the coming years. Aging baby boomers will be encouraged to remain active to help prevent injuries and illnesses associated with aging, so instructors will be needed in retirement communities and residential care facilities (Figure 14.12). Businesses and insurance organizations continue to recognize the benefits of health and fitness programs for employees, so incentives to join gyms or other types of health clubs are expected to increase the need for fitness trainers and instructors.

Mortuary Science. While you might not associate death with healthcare support services, the funeral home director provides an important service for grieving families. Funeral directors, also called **morticians** (mor-TIH-shuhns) and *undertakers*, manage funeral homes and arrange

Figure 14.12   Fitness instructors may be employed at a residential care facility, where they will lead programs and classes for older adults.

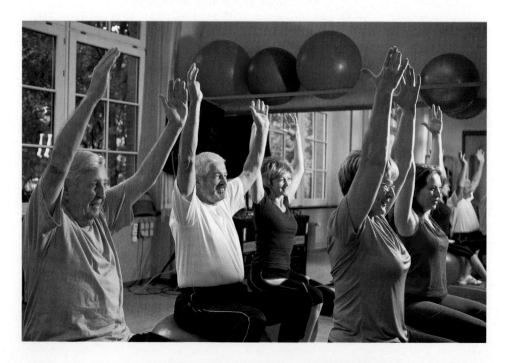

the details of a funeral. They provide for transportation of the deceased and submit paperwork and legal documents. They assist the family in planning wakes, memorial services, and burials. Because funeral practices vary among cultures and religions, morticians must be sensitive to the needs of the family when determining whether a body will be entombed, cremated, or buried.

Funeral directors complete an associate's or bachelor's degree in mortuary science. Following an apprenticeship of one to three years, they must pass a qualifying exam to become licensed. Because the mood is consistently somber, the work of a mortician can be stressful. Funeral directors have to arrange all of the details of a funeral within 24 to 72 hours of death and may be responsible for multiple funerals on the same day. Employment opportunities in this field are more favorable for those who are willing to relocate for available job openings.

RECALL YOUR READING

1. The _____ pathway includes a variety of healthcare occupations and has a very important role in supporting quality patient care.

2. Medical _____ professionals create plans that _____ their organizations and the services they provide.

3. _____ professionals manage training opportunities, oversee _____, and hire new employees.

4. Healthcare facilities depend on _____ professionals to keep many aspects of a healthcare building and equipment safe, clean, and working properly.

5. Food service professionals include _____ who counsel patients and develop meal plans for patients and _____ who plan and prepare meals for residents.

Complete the *Map Your Reading* graphic organizer for the section you just read.

Team Conflict and Conflict Resolution

Conflicts between healthcare team members cause problems for both patients and employees. Because ineffective teamwork reduces the quality of healthcare, team members must be aware of the factors that lead to conflict. They must also be committed to resolving conflicts quickly so that quality of care is not compromised.

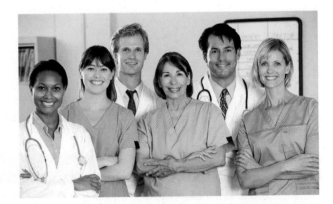

Figure 14.13   Team members are individuals, so they will bring unique opinions and work styles to a project. Explain how this is a benefit to the team and why it might also cause problems.

Identifying Factors That Lead to Team Conflict

Team members are unique individuals with differing viewpoints and work habits (Figure 14.13). This is generally a good thing because team functions can be better completed with a variety of talents. A team needs practical workers and creative thinkers, detailed people and "big picture" people, reserved workers and outgoing workers. However, these differences can also lead to conflict. Team conflict is an interpersonal problem that occurs between two or more members of a team. As a result, the whole team works less effectively.

Many conflicts arise from differences in individual viewpoints and in the ways that people like to work. It's easy to think that other team members should "see things your way." However, there is more than one right way to accomplish most tasks, and you can learn a lot by observing other team members. They may obtain great results by using a different method than what you're used to. The "my way is right" mindset will only cause more conflict.

Team members often attempt to analyze each other's behavior by using their own personal viewpoint. For example, if you are naturally talkative, do you assume a quiet person is angry or upset? Another person's behavior does not necessarily mean what you think it does. Using your own viewpoint to interpret the behavior of others is often the root of misunderstandings between team members and can lead to conflict.

When a team member wants to do something in a new or different way, try not to be judgmental. It's easy to label this person as a troublemaker and begin to gossip or complain about his or her ideas. However, these "troublemakers" are actually good for us. When they challenge us, we tend to reevaluate, consider, and maybe even learn a new and better way to accomplish a task.

Just as individuals have different learning styles, team members have different **work styles** (Figure 14.14). When you identify the work preferences of fellow team members, you can take advantage of style differences to allow all members to contribute and to avoid misunderstandings. Ignoring work styles leads to ineffective teamwork and frustrated team members. Do you see your own preferences in the following list of contrasting work styles?

Avoiding potential conflicts begins with each team member. Analyze your own behavior and avoid the patterns that lead to serious conflict with other members. Learn to recognize the work style preferences of each team member and use them to provide positive results.

Managing Team Conflict

People are imperfect communicators, so problems that lead to conflict can occur at various times. Your first goal when managing conflict is to recognize and correct simple misunderstandings. Begin by checking your

Figure 14.14 Work Preferences

complete one task before starting a new one	or	work on several projects at once
work alone	or	work with others
work with details	or	create ideas
know exactly what to do	or	figure it out along the way
receive lots of direction	or	work with little supervision
prefer quiet and order	or	thrive on noise and activity

own motivation and attitude. Are you trying to prove you're right, or are you trying to make things right? Successful team members focus on resolving problems and working toward achieving the common goals of the team.

Now look at how your team is functioning. When you see these behaviors, your team needs to focus on conflict resolution:

- gossip, blaming, and complaining

- hoarding of information that should be shared

- late work, poor quality work, and absenteeism

Resolving conflict begins with setting up clear goals for the team. What are we supposed to accomplish as a team? What are our individual roles and responsibilities? How will we share information, and how can we get help when we need it? As you work to resolve a conflict, remember to listen to other points of view (Figure 14.15). You can certainly speak up and share your ideas and opinions, but always state your view positively. Blaming or ridiculing another team member only increases conflict.

Finally, be willing to accept the team's decision even if it's not your first choice. As you move forward, do not allow disagreements to become personal. Instead, focus on doing your part as a team member. Complete your work to the best of your ability. Ask for help when you need it and volunteer to help others as well. Practice using the key skills shown in Figure 14.16 for managing and resolving conflict.

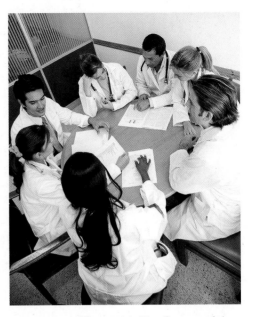

Figure 14.15 Successful teams resolve conflicts and move onto more important tasks. What are some signs that your team needs to focus on conflict resolution?

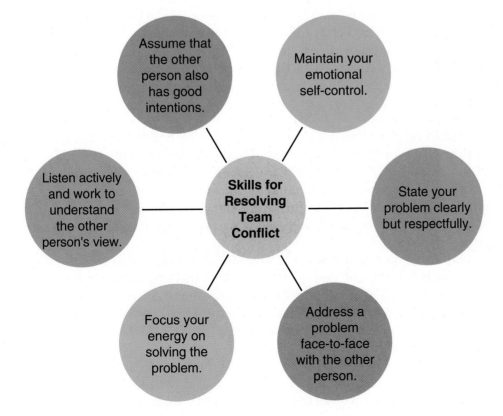

Figure 14.16 The behaviors described here will help team members resolve conflicts and keep a positive working relationship in the process.

Assume that the other person also has good intentions.

Maintain your emotional self-control.

Listen actively and work to understand the other person's view.

Skills for Resolving Team Conflict

State your problem clearly but respectfully.

Focus your energy on solving the problem.

Address a problem face-to-face with the other person.

Complete the
Map Your Reading
graphic organizer for the
section you just read.

Technical Skills for Support Services Workers

The tasks of support services workers are as varied as the departments and positions in which they work. Environmental workers are particularly focused on maintaining facility safety. Preventing the spread of infection is critical as more bacteria become resistant to antibiotics. In this section, you will practice skills for cleaning and disinfecting healthcare facilities and learn safe food handling techniques. You will also learn safe wheelchair transport techniques and see how therapeutic diets are used to improve patient health.

Cleaning and Disinfecting the Healthcare Environment

Patients, employees, and visitors bring viruses, bacteria, and other microbes with them when they enter a healthcare facility (Figure 14.17). These organisms are a source of infection for anyone who enters the facility, but infection is a significant concern for patients whose immune systems are stressed by illness. Improved cleaning and **disinfection** of the healthcare environment decreases healthcare-associated infection (HAI) rates. Because of this, cleaning and disinfecting are two of the most important methods used to prevent the spread of infectious disease in healthcare facilities.

The Centers for Disease Control and Prevention (CDC) ranks various healthcare environments as *noncritical*, *semicritical*, or *critical* based on classifications developed by Dr. Earle Spaulding (Figure 14.18). These rankings are based on the potential for infectious disease to spread via equipment, instruments, and furniture. They also consider the level of sterility normally required for the body part coming into contact with the surface.

Typically, waiting areas need only general cleaning. This involves dirt and dust removal using detergents, scouring powders, and toilet bowl and glass cleaners. This part of hospital cleaning is similar to that of an office building or hotel. However, patient rooms need both general cleaning and low-level disinfecting. Surgical suites require high-level disinfecting as well as sterilization of instruments.

Using disinfectants limits the spread of infection. Disinfection means reducing the number of microbes on a surface to very low levels. Disinfection involves the use of chemicals that can be toxic, or

disinfection
the use of chemicals to kill pathogens that are present on nonliving objects

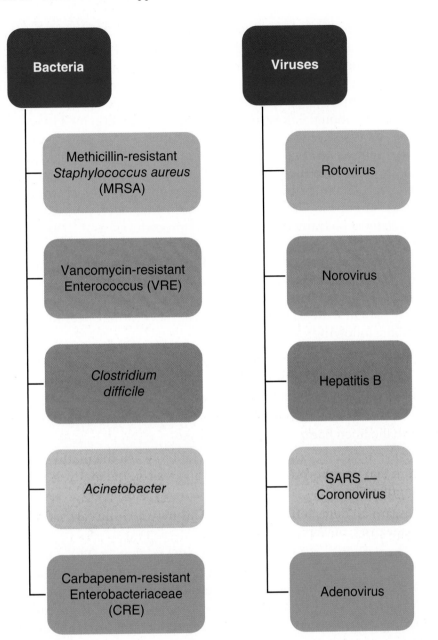

Figure 14.17   Surface contamination by these pathogens can lead to healthcare-associated infections.

Figure 14.18 Spaulding's Classifications				
Level	**Definition**	**Procedure**	**Goal**	**Example**
Critical	objects that enter sterile tissue or vascular system	sterilization	kill all organisms, including spores	sterilization of surgical instruments
Semicritical	objects that touch mucous membranes or non-intact skin	high-level disinfection	kill all vegetative organisms; spores not killed	high-level disinfection of endoscopes
Noncritical	objects that touch only intact skin	low-level disinfection or cleaning	removal of pathogenic organisms	cleaning patient room

poisonous. The **Environmental Protection Agency (EPA)** recommends the appropriate chemicals for reducing the spread of infection while minimizing the risks to the environment. Cleaning and disinfecting in an appropriate and organized manner ensures adequate infection protection but also minimizes patient and staff exposure to toxic chemicals.

The Occupational Safety and Health Administration (OSHA) protects patients and employees by providing guidelines for the safe disposal of sharps such as needles used in vaccinations and insulin injections. OSHA also regulates the safe disposal of hazardous medical waste and provides specific guidelines for employee training to protect workers from exposure to bloodborne pathogens. An entry-level housekeeping employee must be trained in these safety procedures, as well as in the steps for cleaning a patient hospital room.

Certain steps are used to clean and disinfect a patient hospital room in preparation for a newly admitted patient. This procedure is called **terminal cleaning** and is especially important in preventing the infection of a new patient with an HAI. The steps in the terminal cleaning process include the following:

1. Wash your hands and put on gloves.

2. Strip all linens, including pillows, by folding them in on themselves. Some facilities use disposable pillows.

3. Hold linens away from your uniform as you deposit them directly into the linen hamper or laundry bag.

4. Use your facility-approved disinfectant to wash the mattress, making sure that you thoroughly disinfect all areas on the mattress slide handles.

5. Discard all items left in the room. This may include cards, flowers, magazines, newspapers, and more.

6. Disinfect all surfaces that are likely to be touched (Figure 14.19). This includes tabletops, faceplates of medical equipment, countertops, bed controls, and side rails. Remember that door handles, computer keyboards and screens, and television controls are frequently touched. While less common now because of cell phone use, some rooms still have telephones. They need disinfection as well.

7. Mop the floor using a disinfectant solution.

8. Clean, disinfect, and store the commode (portable toilet).

9. Clean the bathroom's toilet, sink, and shower. Mop the floor.

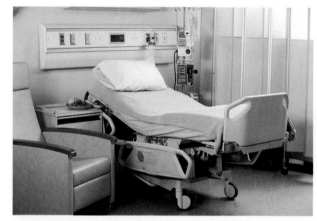

Figure 14.19   Disinfect all surfaces that are likely to be touched. What are some items you see in this photo that would need to be disinfected?

10. Discard your gloves and wash your hands.

11. Make the bed (Figure 14.20).

   • Wear gloves if required by your facility. Select clean linens, including a bottom sheet, top sheet, pillow, pillowcase, and bedspread. Place them on the clean over-bed table.

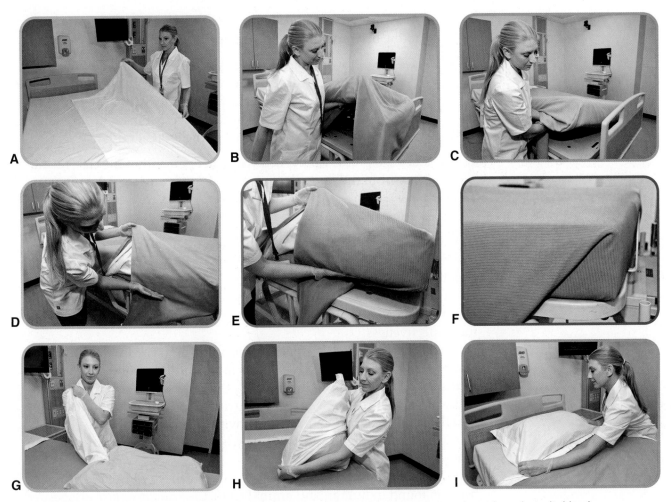

Figure 14.20   Follow the steps listed in the chapter and these images to properly make a hospital bed.

- Raise the bed to a comfortable working height and lower the side rails.

- Place the bottom sheet on the bed and pull the corners of the nearest side over the corners of the mattress. Smooth down the sides.

- Move to the other side of the bed and repeat the previous step to secure the bottom sheet, if you are using a fitted bottom sheet. When using a flat bottom sheet, you will save time and energy by finishing all steps on one side of the bed before moving to the other side.

- Place the top sheet with the centerfold at the middle of the bed and the wide hem at the top of the mattress. Open the sheet, keeping it centered, and place the bottom edge over the foot of the bed. (A)

- Repeat the previous step with the bedspread.

- Tuck the bedspread and top sheet together under the foot of the mattress. Make a **mitered corner** on both sides. (B through F)

- Fold the top of the bedspread and sheet back to make a cuff at the head of the bed. Check to make sure the linens are smooth, with no visible wrinkles, and that seams will face away from the patient's skin. Usually, the top sheet is placed right side down, and the bedspread is right side up.

- Place the pillow on the bed and grasp the closed end of the pillowcase. Turn the case inside out over your hand and grasp the pillow with the same hand. Pull the case down over the pillow. Avoid shaking the pillow or sheets when making a bed to reduce surface contamination from dust particles. (G and H)

- Place the pillow on the bed with the open end of the case facing away from the door. (I)

12. Remove and properly store all cleaning equipment. Remove gloves, if worn. Wash your hands.

Observing the length of time a disinfectant needs to work is vital. If the disinfectant is removed too quickly, pathogens will remain. Pay close attention to your facility's policies, which are designed for the specific chemicals you are using. Healthcare facilities must also make sure that disinfectant levels are maintained by replacing chemicals that have lost their effectiveness.

Some organisms create special concerns. The presence of **multidrug-resistant organisms** (MDROs) such as methicillin-resistant *Staphylococcus aureus* (MRSA) (meh-thuh-SIH-luhn; staf-uh-loh-KAHK-uhs; MER-suh) and vancomycin-resistant *enterococcus* (van-kuh-MIS-uhn; ehn-ter-oh-KAHK-uhs) (VRE) may require that environmental surfaces be cleaned and disinfected more frequently. MDROs are difficult to control and can cause serious infections.

Clostridium difficile (klah-STRIH-dee-uhm dee-fih-SEEL) is a strain of bacteria found in human and animal feces. *Clostridium difficile*-associated diarrhea (CDAD) is the most common cause of healthcare-associated diarrhea. The symptoms of this disease can range from mild diarrhea to colitis and death. Specific disinfectants recommended by the CDC are used when CDAD is present in the environment.

Type A influenza requires specialized precautions as well as disinfection with specific products reviewed by the EPA. Guidelines have recently been developed for disinfection during an outbreak of the highly contagious norovirus (NOR-oh-vI-ruhs). Better known as the *cruise ship virus*, it requires a high frequency of disinfection during outbreaks.

Guidelines for infection control change as new chemicals and treatment procedures are developed. Environmental services workers play an important role in controlling infection. The actions of a healthcare facility's housekeeper can influence whether infections are kept under control or are spread to patients and fellow employees.

Using Proper Food Handling Techniques

Dietary workers are also concerned with preventing the spread of pathogens. Improper food handling can result in *foodborne illness*, meaning any illness caused by eating contaminated food. An outbreak of foodborne illness occurs when two or more people eat the same food and get the same sickness. Because patients in a healthcare facility already have compromised health, an outbreak of foodborne illness may have even more serious outcomes than it would in a healthy population. Therefore, all dietary workers must know how to safely handle and serve food.

Dietary workers practice proper **sanitation** by using clean and healthy food handling habits that prevent **contamination**. Food that does not have dangerous levels of contamination is considered safe. However, food that contains harmful substances or dangerous levels of microorganisms is contaminated and not fit for human consumption. The mnemonic *FAT TOM* can help you understand how to limit the growth of pathogens in food as a first step in preventing foodborne illness (Figure 14.21).

Proper food handling begins with clean surfaces and clean hands. Food preparation surfaces are cleaned by using hot water and detergent to remove all visible dirt or food particles. Equipment and utensils are cleaned in the same manner.

sanitation
term that describes procedures and practices that maintain cleanliness and preserve public health

contamination
the unwanted presence of harmful substances or microorganisms

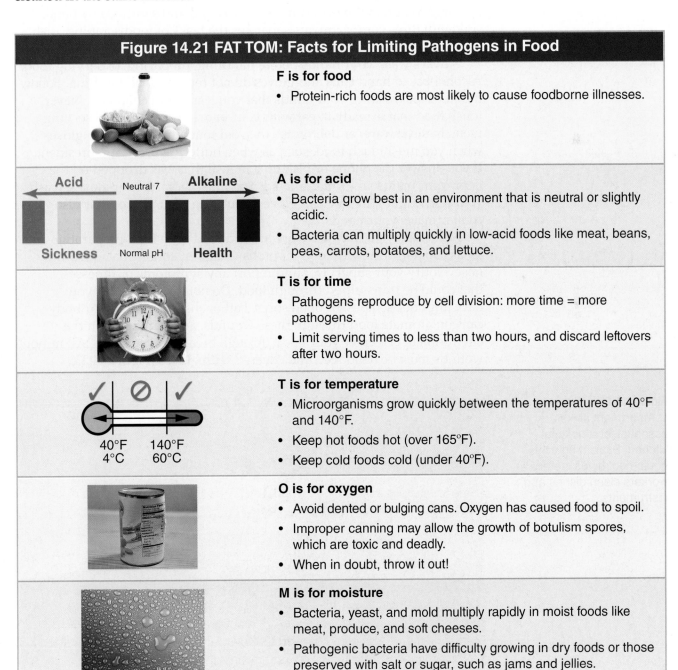

Figure 14.21 FAT TOM: Facts for Limiting Pathogens in Food

F is for food
- Protein-rich foods are most likely to cause foodborne illnesses.

A is for acid
- Bacteria grow best in an environment that is neutral or slightly acidic.
- Bacteria can multiply quickly in low-acid foods like meat, beans, peas, carrots, potatoes, and lettuce.

T is for time
- Pathogens reproduce by cell division: more time = more pathogens.
- Limit serving times to less than two hours, and discard leftovers after two hours.

T is for temperature
- Microorganisms grow quickly between the temperatures of 40°F and 140°F.
- Keep hot foods hot (over 165°F).
- Keep cold foods cold (under 40°F).

O is for oxygen
- Avoid dented or bulging cans. Oxygen has caused food to spoil.
- Improper canning may allow the growth of botulism spores, which are toxic and deadly.
- When in doubt, throw it out!

M is for moisture
- Bacteria, yeast, and mold multiply rapidly in moist foods like meat, produce, and soft cheeses.
- Pathogenic bacteria have difficulty growing in dry foods or those preserved with salt or sugar, such as jams and jellies.

Next, the surfaces are sanitized using a chemical sanitizer that is diluted to the correct strength. Allow the surfaces to air-dry after using the sanitizer. This gives the chemical enough time to destroy pathogens and prevents recontamination from a drying cloth. Clean and sanitize surfaces after completing one food preparation task and before starting a new one. Surfaces that are in continuous use must be sanitized at least every four hours. Take care when using cleaning and sanitizing chemicals to ensure effectiveness but avoid harming patients or workers.

Small equipment is sanitized using heat. Sanitizing or dish machines clean and sanitize dishes and utensils by using a water temperature that is higher than 180°F. Some machines apply a chemical sanitizer during their final cycle. Since there are many types of machines, you will need training to use the specific machine at your facility. Equipment that is too large to fit into the dish sanitizer is cleaned and sanitized by hand. A sink with three compartments separates the tasks of food scraping, dish cleaning, and dish sanitizing (Figure 14.22).

Always wash your hands before handling, preparing, or serving food. Alcohol-based hand rubs and gloves do not replace hand washing! Follow the steps for washing your hands that you learned in chapter 6. Never touch food that is ready to eat with your bare hands. Use food serving utensils, silverware, or deli wraps to avoid touching food. Wear gloves when you must touch food, such as when buttering bread for a resident. If you answer the phone or pick up a utensil that was dropped on the floor, your hands are contaminated. You must discard your gloves, wash your hands, and put on clean gloves. Touching your face or hair also contaminates your hands.

Sick employees may not work around food or in food preparation areas. Do not work with food if you have a fever, sore throat, or runny nose. Notify your supervisor and report any symptoms or illnesses that could be transmitted through food. Do not handle food if you have any cuts, scrapes, or open sores. Pathogens present in your body can contaminate food through these wounds, and pathogens in the environment can enter your body through breaks in your skin. All minor wounds must be bandaged and covered with gloves (Figure 14.23).

Figure 14.22 Three-compartment sinks are essential for a hospital kitchen. Explain how this equipment helps dietary workers clean dishes and instruments.

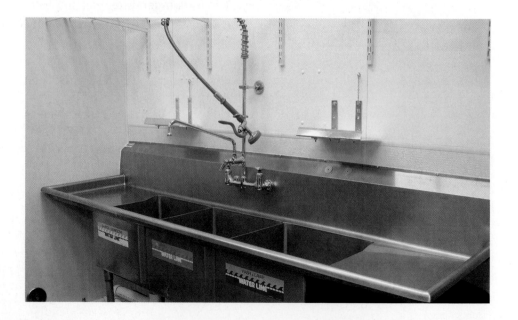

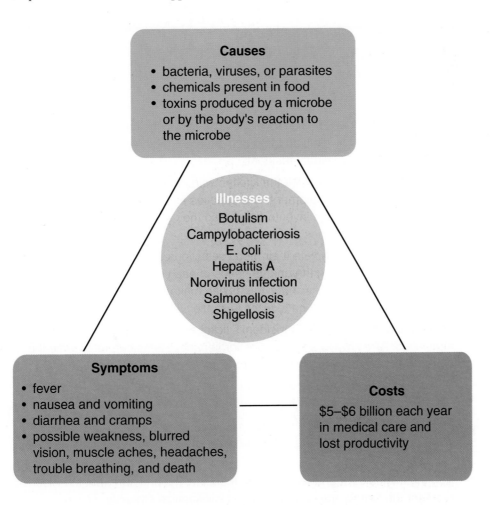

Figure 14.23   Infectious diseases that spread through food or beverages are a common and sometimes life-threatening problem for millions of Americans.

Handle dishes and utensils without touching any surface that will come into contact with the patient's mouth directly or indirectly. Touch only the handles of forks, knives, and spoons. Keep your thumbs off the top surface of plates. Hold cups and glasses at the bottom rather than around the rim. Never carry glasses with your fingers inside the rim.

Cross-contamination transfers harmful substances from one food or food preparation surface to another. You can prevent cross-contamination by following these guidelines:

- Wash foods, hands, utensils, and surfaces properly. Use sanitary wipes, disinfectants, and sanitizers as required.

- Use separate utensils for each food item.

- Wash your hands after contact with food, patients or residents, or contaminated surfaces.

Contaminated food may not look, smell, or taste spoiled. Dietary workers keep track of food freshness by following the *first in, first out* (FIFO) rule. Rotate foods by placing new stock behind older stock. Check expiration dates regularly to make sure food supplies are fresh.

Discard foods that have been left out of refrigeration for more than two hours or have been mishandled. Do not keep any leftovers. If you are uncertain about the safety of any food, follow the guideline that states, *when in doubt, throw it out.* It is better to be overly cautious than to risk food contamination and illness.

The Support Services Worker: Allie

Allie works as a dietary aide in an assisted living healthcare facility. She follows these steps to serve a meal to 20 residents:

- Make coffee and set out meal tickets for each resident. The tickets display the menu choices prepared by the dietitian to meet the dietary requirements of each individual resident.

- Restock the kitchen with additional beverages, snacks, equipment, and supplies as needed. Record items on the inventory sheet so they will be reordered when supplies run low.

- Assist residents to complete their menu selections on the meal tickets. According to Allie, learning the unique needs of each resident is important. Low vision, hearing loss, and arthritic hands can make this task challenging for some people. Your assistance reduces frustration and keeps mealtime pleasant.

- Plate food according to each resident's ticket selections. To prevent food contamination, Allie always wears gloves for serving. She is careful to ladle the correct amounts as well as the correct foods for each resident's tray.

- Serve each resident. Assist with slicing meats as requested by the resident. Alert residents if the food is hot. Observe residents and be alert for any eating problems, such as choking on meat.

- Clear tables when residents have finished eating. Scrape all dishes and discard leftover food.

- Run the dishes through the sanitation machine, making sure that the machine is set for the temperatures and time that will sanitize correctly.

- Clean and sanitize tables, then set the tables in preparation for the next meal (Figure 14.24).

Figure 14.24   This is the proper layout for a basic table setting.

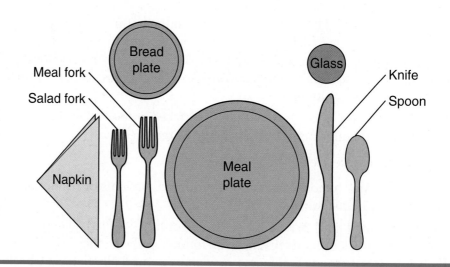

Providing Therapeutic Diets

Your diet includes the food and fluids you regularly consume as a part of daily living. Healthy diets follow guidelines recommended by the **United States Department of Agriculture (USDA)** and provide the nutrients needed to maintain or improve your general health. Most residents in healthcare facilities follow the general diet, or *house diet*. There are no food restrictions in this diet, but the facility may follow NAS (no added salt) or NCS (no concentrated sweets) guidelines in meal planning and preparation. In addition to the house diet, there are three standard diets: clear liquid, full liquid, and texture modified (Figure 14.25).

Physicians order a **therapeutic diet** to help treat a disease or medical condition. In a therapeutic diet, some food amounts may be increased, some foods may be omitted as in the case of a food allergy, and some foods may be restricted to carefully measured amounts. A dietitian plans and manages all therapeutic diets. However, following therapeutic diet guidelines is the responsibility of all dietary workers. When a dietary aide serves a resident his or her meal, the tray must be correct with the right meal for the right resident. For example, the aide must know whether a resident's request for sugar in her coffee can be met or if a sugar substitute should be used. Correct diets are essential to maintaining good health, so take care to serve only the foods that are permitted (Figure 14.26).

Clear liquid diet	• tea, broth, gelatin, soda, and some fruit juices • for residents experiencing stomach or intestinal distress
Full liquid diet	• clear liquids plus milk, ice cream, sherbet, custards, and other foods that are liquid at room temperature • for residents with digestive disorders or difficulty chewing, and for recovery from illness
Texture modified diet	• same as a regular diet, but food has been chopped fine, ground, or puréed • for residents having difficulty chewing or swallowing

Figure 14.25   These diets, along with the house diet, are considered standard diets. What is the house diet?

therapeutic diet
a special food plan ordered by a physician to help treat a disease

Figure 14.26 Therapeutic Diets		
Type of Diet	**Description**	**Function**
high calorie, high protein	encourages small but frequent intake of high-protein and high-calorie foods; may include nutritional supplements	provides extra energy; promotes weight gain; helps wounds heal
reduced sodium	restricts the use of table salt and omits processed foods that are high in sodium	reduces excess fluid retention in body tissues
low fat, low cholesterol	restricts the type of fats or the total amount of fats per day	helps patients with liver, gallbladder, or heart disease; promotes weight loss
carbohydrate controlled	limits total intake of carbohydrates and/or calories, limits intake of refined carbohydrates, or balances carbohydrate intake throughout the day	promotes weight loss; helps patients manage diabetes

Residents who have difficulty swallowing may drink thickened liquids. This helps to prevent **aspiration**, or the inhalation of a liquid into the lungs. A special thickening product is added to bring liquids to the required **consistency**, which is the way the liquid flows. Dietary workers must recognize the following consistencies and may be asked to prepare thickened liquids according to a resident's care plan:

- **Nectar-like or nectar-thick liquids.** These fluids can be sipped from a cup or through a straw. They will slowly fall off a spoon that is tipped. Examples include buttermilk, cold tomato juice, and eggnog.

- **Honey-like or honey-thick liquids.** These fluids can be eaten with a spoon but do not hold their shape on a spoon. They can be sipped from a cup but are too thick for a straw. Examples include thick yogurt, tomato sauce, and honey.

- **Spoon-thick, pudding-thick, or pudding-like liquids.** These very thick fluids must be eaten with a spoon. They hold their own shape on a spoon and can't be sipped from a cup. Examples include thickened applesauce and thick milk pudding.

Residents' dietary guidelines may also be influenced by culture, religious beliefs, or other food preferences. For example, vegetarians do not eat meat, fish, or poultry, and some do not eat eggs or dairy products. Muslims do not eat pork, Mormons do not drink beverages that contain caffeine, and Roman Catholics have meat restrictions on Fridays during Lent and on some religious holidays. According to the Omnibus Budget Reconciliation Act (OBRA), these preferences must be accommodated.

The passage of OBRA shifted the focus of long-term care from "rules and routines" to resident-centered care. The dining experience offers a significant opportunity to focus on residents' preferences. Making healthy food choices, socializing with friends, interacting with attentive staff, and enjoying a tasty meal are powerful elements in maintaining the quality of a patient or resident's everyday life. The following aspects of the resident's dining experience are included in OBRA:

- Meals must meet the individual nutritional requirements of each resident.

- Dining with other residents is recommended.

- Residents who are relearning independent eating skills must have a private eating area available.

- Food must be served at the proper temperature.

- Food must be appealing to look at and seasoned according to the resident's preference.

Feeding Residents

Independent eating is always encouraged, but when residents can't maintain good nutrition through self-feeding, feeding assistants or nursing assistants provide support (Figure 14.27). Both types of assistants receive training in the complete dining experience. They know the elements of good nutrition and learn to recognize signs of malnutrition and fluid imbalance. They use adaptive equipment and techniques to encourage healthy eating. They understand that positive social interaction enhances the dining experience and improves dietary outcomes.

Watch for signs of fluid imbalance as you assist residents. The amount of fluid consumed should be equal to the amount eliminated through urine output, stool, perspiration, and respiration. Too much fluid in body tissues results in **edema** (eh-DEE-muh) and too little fluid causes **dehydration**. Since fluid balance regulates body functions such as temperature maintenance and digestion, you must be alert to signs of dehydration or edema (Figure 14.28).

Preventing dehydration is challenging for elderly residents because a person's sense of thirst declines with age. First, check the resident's care plan for information on fluids to be encouraged and fluids to be restricted. Then offer fluids frequently, especially when the weather is hot or the resident has a fever. Keep fresh water within reach to encourage drinking water throughout the day. Pay attention to the resident's preferences and offer the beverages that appeal to him or her.

Making the dining experience pleasant and relaxed is an important goal when assisting with feeding. Provide for the resident's comfort by asking the nurse's aide to toilet and transfer the person before mealtime. Check to see that the resident is neatly dressed and has eyeglasses, dentures, and hearing aids if necessary. Wash the resident's hands and position the eating utensils within easy reach. Make sure the resident's head is upright to make swallowing easier. If permitted, raise the head of the bed to high Fowler's position for residents eating in bed. Use clothing protectors to keep clothing clean but ask for the resident's preference before using one. Remember that a clothing protector is not a bib. Since infants wear bibs, the term is considered demeaning for an adult.

Provide companionship as well as assistance during feeding. Checking your cell phone, talking with other aides about your weekend plans, or complaining about personal problems during a resident's meal is poor etiquette at the very least. It is also not consistent with high-quality

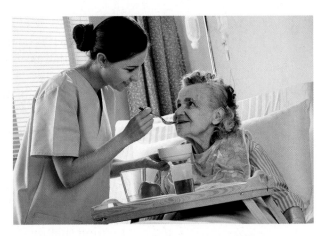

Figure 14.27 When independent eating is not possible, a feeding assistant will help a patient with his or her meal.

Expand

Figure 14.28 Signs of Fluid Imbalance

Edema (too much fluid)	Dehydration (too little fluid)
• swelling or puffiness in feet, ankles, and hands • congestion or wheezing • weight increase • decrease in urine output because the body is retaining fluid	• dry mouth and lips, trouble swallowing, and appetite loss • tongue that is thick and coated • skin that is dry and itchy • decrease in urine output because there is not enough fluid (urine is concentrated, darker in color, and has a strong odor) • unusual fatigue and weakness • onset of confusion • weak or rapid pulse

care and may lead to neglect of the resident. Focus on talking to your resident even if he or she doesn't answer you. The sound of your caring voice will increase the resident's appetite and improve digestion.

Providing Wheelchair Transport

Many different healthcare workers transport patients in the course of a day. Clinic nurses, radiology technicians, therapy aides, nursing assistants, and even hospital volunteers may be asked to transport a patient in a wheelchair. In large facilities, the transport technician takes patients in wheelchairs and on gurneys from one part of the hospital to another for diagnostic tests, medical appointments, and surgeries. In any situation that involves wheelchair transport, safety is the number one priority.

Become familiar with the parts and operation of the wheelchair before you try to transport a person (Figure 14.29). Practice opening and folding the chair, adjusting and removing the footrests, and setting the brake. Drive cautiously through doorways and down hallways, being especially

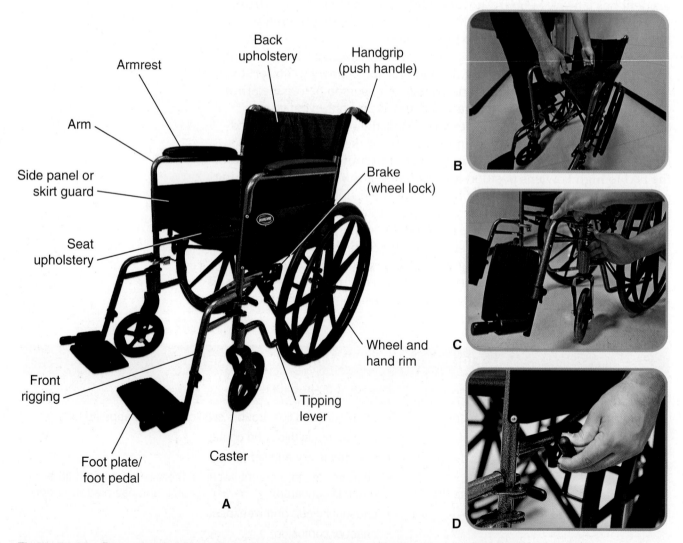

Figure 14.29   Becoming familiar with a wheelchair means learning its parts (A) as well as practicing opening and folding it (B), adjusting the footrests (C), and setting the brake (D).

careful at intersections. Bend your knees and keep your back straight as you begin to push the chair. These good body mechanics help to prevent back injury. Allow plenty of turning room to avoid smashing a footrest against the wall.

Learn how to turn and reverse the wheelchair smoothly (Figure 14.30). Wheelchairs need to be moved in reverse when entering elevators, traveling down steep ramps, and rolling over bumps to avoid throwing the patient out of the chair. If you need to move up onto a curb, use the wheelchair's tipping lever. Step on the lever to raise the front casters onto the curb. Then roll the wheels up and over the curb.

The following steps for transporting a patient in a wheelchair assume that the patient can transfer independently. Patients who need help to stand and move to the wheelchair will need the assistance of one or two aides who are trained in the use of transfer belts and techniques for transferring to and from a wheelchair.

1. Follow standard precautions by washing your hands.
2. Rotate the footrests to the side of the chair.
3. Position the chair close to the patient.
4. Set the brakes. For safety reasons, this is the single most important step in using a wheelchair. Set the brakes during any transfer.

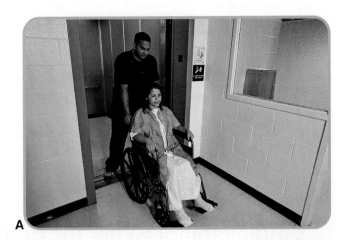

A

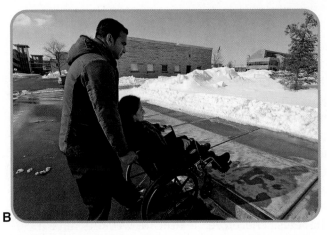

B

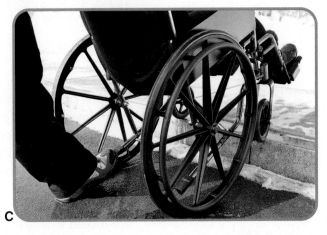

C

Figure 14.30 Wheelchairs must be backed into elevators (A) and in several other situations. You should practice moving a wheelchair up onto a curb using the tipping lever (B and C).

5. Make sure the patient is wearing nonskid shoes or slippers. Ask the patient to sit in the chair and check to see that he or she is seated comfortably. Tuck loose clothing away from the wheels.

6. Adjust the footrests and ask the patient to keep his or her arms close to his or her body. This will avoid injury from bumping into walls or furniture in narrow spaces.

7. Release the brakes and push forward, keeping your knees bent and your back straight.

8. Remember to turn and back into elevators, over bumps, and down ramps. For the comfort of your passenger, the chair should never tilt forward.

9. When you reach your destination, set the brakes again. Move the footrests out of the way and allow the patient to stand and move away from the chair.

10. Make sure your patient is comfortable and notify the appropriate person that the patient has arrived.

11. Wash your hands.

Complete the *Map Your Reading* graphic organizer for the section you just read.

RECALL YOUR READING

1. Improved _____ and _____ reduce the rate of _____ infections.

2. The mnemonic _____ helps you understand how to prevent foodborne illness.

3. A _____ may include _____ food amounts, omitted foods in case of _____, and carefully _____ amounts of food.

4. Providing _____ during feeding is just as important as providing assistance.

5. Practice _____ and folding a wheelchair, adjusting and _____ the footrests, and setting the _____.

Employability Skills for Healthcare Workers

Are you actively working to stay healthy? Personal health may not be your main focus as you prepare for your future career, but it is an important one for healthcare workers. Those who work directly with patients can't risk transmitting pathogens to people with compromised immune systems. If healthcare workers aren't healthy, they can't work.

Healthcare workers have an additional obligation to wellness. Besides understanding the fundamentals of wellness and prevention of disease, they are expected to practice and promote healthy behaviors with their clients. Lifestyle choices play a role in the development of many of the diseases affecting patients today. For example, obesity and poor diet are linked to a rise in diabetes. Therefore, healthcare workers have a responsibility to practice healthy behaviors to set a good example for clients.

Health Maintenance Practices

Many healthcare workers are helpers by nature. Perhaps your desire to help others drew you to this field. However, that focus on helping others can keep you from maintaining your own health. Do you skip meals or eat fast food simply because it's convenient? Are you just too busy to exercise regularly? Do you get by on a few hours of sleep each night because 24 hours is just not enough time in one day? Are you so busy focusing on the problems in your friends' lives that you avoid your own problems until they reach a crisis point? If you answered *yes* to any of these questions, you should consider taking a closer look at your personal health maintenance practices.

The holistic view of wellness promotes a balanced relationship between the mind, body, and spirit throughout the life span. You probably already know that maintaining physical wellness includes diet, exercise, sleep, and routine medical care. Figure 14.31 lists the elements of mental and intellectual wellness, as well as social, emotional, and spiritual wellness. Good health means that all three of the main components are balanced. When too much emphasis is put on one area of wellness, the other areas become unbalanced and good health suffers. Have you ever stayed up late to study for a test? You focused on learning, which is part of mental wellness, but neglected sleep, which is part of physical wellness.

Physical Wellness

Staying healthy is the subject of more websites, documentaries, advertisements, and magazine and newspaper articles than ever before. Some of the information is reliable, while some of it is not. Maintaining your physical health includes several basic components: diet, exercise, adequate sleep, personal hygiene, and medical care.

Diet. The food we eat provides our bodies with the nutrients needed for proper health and body development. Scientists have identified six main nutrients that are essential for maintaining good health (Figure 14.32 on the next page). When our diet lacks any of these nutrients, optimal body functioning is interrupted and signs of malnutrition may appear over time. Malnutrition leads to the development of disease conditions such as goiter, which is caused by a lack of iodine; rickets, caused by a vitamin D deficiency; and pellagra, which develops from a deficiency of vitamin B. When specific vitamins are not represented in the available food supply, they can be added to foods in which they don't naturally occur. These fortified foods help to prevent deficiency diseases. For this reason, salt is fortified with iodine, milk is fortified with vitamin D, and grains are fortified with B vitamins.

The USDA, in combination with the Department of Health and Human Services (HHS), sets guidelines for healthy eating and develops consumer materials for teaching the components of a healthy diet. The guidelines reflect the public's current dietary needs. They apply to

MIND
stress management
goal setting
time management
problem solving

BODY
healthy diet
physical activity
adequate sleep
preventive
medical care

SPIRIT
supportive social relationships
concern for community
emotional self-control
personal values
spiritual practices

WELLNESS

Figure 14.31   Holistic wellness promotes a balanced relationship between mind, body, and spirit.

Carbohydrates

- major source of human energy
- easily digested

- dietary sources: bread, pasta, crackers, cereals, potatoes, corn, peas, fruits, sugar, and syrups

Fats (Lipids)

- concentrated form of energy
- aid in the absorption of fat-soluble vitamins
- give food flavor

- dietary sources: butter, margarine, oils, cream, fatty meats, cheeses, and egg yolks

Protein

- builds and repairs body tissue
- provides heat and energy

- dietary sources: complete proteins — meats, fish, milk, cheese, and eggs incomplete proteins— cereal, nuts, and dried beans

Vitamins

- important for metabolism, tissue building, and regulating body processes

- dietary sources: fruits, vegetables, some grains, meat, and dairy

Minerals

- regulate body fluids
- contribute to growth
- aid in building tissues

- dietary sources: meat, fish, poultry, dairy, whole grains, and some fruits and vegetables

Water

- essential for the digestion of food
- makes up the majority of blood plasma
- helps body tissues absorb nutrients
- helps move waste material through the body

- dietary sources: 6 to 8 cups of water each day and water present in foods

Figure 14.32 These six essential nutrients are necessary to maintain health and proper body function.

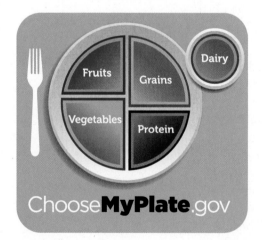

Figure 14.33 The MyPlate diagram shows what proportions of the food groups we should eat. Why do you think the USDA chose to display this information on a plate?

individuals two years of age and older, and they are not considered therapeutic. In other words, they are not intended for the treatment of a medical condition.

The MyPlate graphic, developed by the USDA, is a visual guide for a healthy eating pattern that provides the correct balance of nutrients (Figure 14.33). It shows the proportion of foods to eat from each of the five food groups. Following the 10 tips that appear on the MyPlate website will result in a healthier diet while addressing the public's dietary concerns. The 10 tips emphasize reducing total food consumption; increasing intake of fruits and vegetables; and reducing intake of sodium, solid fats, and added sugars. If all citizens followed these guidelines, what improvements would you expect to see in the health of the general population?

The **Food and Drug Administration (FDA)** developed the nutrition facts label to help consumers make informed food choices that contribute to a healthier diet. Reading labels when you shop or plan meals makes it easy to figure out the amount of nutrients you are getting. You can also use the label to compare foods. This allows you to make the healthiest choice possible. Watch for upcoming changes in the nutrition facts label.

The FDA has proposed updates to align serving size listings with the amounts people typically eat today and to highlight calories and serving sizes. The proposed updates reflect new public health and scientific information. Because of the link to obesity and heart disease, for example, information about added sugars may be included.

Reading food labels also allows you to review the ingredients list found near the nutrition label. A product's ingredients are listed in descending order of predominance. This means that the ingredient that weighs the most is listed first, and the ingredient that weighs the least is listed last. Use this feature to limit your intake of fats, sugars, and sodium. Beware of foods whose ingredients lists begin with sugars (sugar, corn syrups, and sucrose), fats and oils (vegetable oil, soybean oil, partially hydrogenated oils), and salt. If these ingredients appear early in the ingredient list, the food is probably a less healthy choice.

A long ingredient list may also signal a less healthy food choice. In many cases, a long list indicates fewer natural ingredients and more processing. Look for foods with a short ingredient list and ingredient names that you recognize (Figure 14.34).

Maintaining a healthy body weight improves your overall health and well-being. Being overweight or obese, however, increases your risk of developing many diseases, including type 2 diabetes, heart disease, and

Ingredients: Roasted Peanuts, High Maltose Corn Syrup, Sugar, Whole Grain Oats, Tapioca Syrup, Palm Kernel Oil, Rice Flour, Cashews Roasted in Safflower Oil, Almonds, Fructose, Whole Grain Wheat, Canola Oil, Maltodextrin, Salt, Soy Lecithin, Reduced Minerals Whey, Nonfat Milk, Partially Defatted Peanut Flour, Honey Roasted Almond Butter (almonds, honey, maltodextrin, palm oil, mixed tocopherols), Barley Malt Extract, Cashew Butter (cashew nuts, safflower oil), Baking Soda, Natural Flavor. Mixed Tocopherols Added to Retain Freshness.
CONTAINS PEANUT, CASHEW, ALMOND, WHEAT, MILK, SOY; MAY CONTAIN PECAN AND MACADAMIA INGREDIENTS.

A

INGREDIENTS: SUGAR, CORN SYRUP, NONFAT **MILK**, HIGH FRUCTOSE CORN SYRUP, SOYBEAN OIL, CONTAINS 2% OR LESS OF: FULLY HYDROGENATED COTTONSEED OIL, MOLASSES, CORN STARCH-MODIFIED, NATURAL FLAVOR (WITH **MILK** AND **SOYBEAN**), CARAMEL COLOR, MONOGLYCERIDES, SODIUM PHOSPHATE, SODIUM CITRATE, SALT, XANTHAN GUM, VANILLIN (ARTIFICIAL FLAVOR), YELLOW 6, TBHQ (ANTIOXIDANT), RED 40.

B

INGREDIENTS: UNBLEACHED ENRICHED FLOUR (WHEAT FLOUR, NIACIN, REDUCED IRON, THIAMINE MONONITRATE (VITAMIN B1), RIBOFLAVIN (VITAMIN B2), FOLIC ACID), SOYBEAN OIL*, SALT, PARTIALLY HYDROGENATED COTTONSEED OIL*, YEAST, BAKING SODA.
CONTAINS: WHEAT.
*ADDS A TRIVIAL AMOUNT OF SATURATED FAT

C

INGREDIENTS: TOMATO PUREE (WATER, TOMATO PASTE), WATER, LESS THAN 2% OF: DEXTROSE, TOMATO FIBER, CITRIC ACID, SPICE, NATURAL FLAVORS.

D

Figure 14.34   Review these ingredient labels. Which shows the most highly processed food? Which shows the least processed food? Which shows the food with the highest level of sugar? Why are ingredient labels important to people with food allergies?

some types of cancer. In addition, maintaining a healthy weight makes you feel better, while excess weight puts extra strain on your joints and can increase the risk of joint pain and osteoarthritis as you grow older. Dropping below a healthy weight range also has negative health effects. It weakens your immune system and increases your risk of infection. Dangerously low weight reduces your body's ability to absorb nutrients, leading to a variety of harmful conditions such as osteoporosis, anemia, fatigue, and exhaustion.

Weight management begins with healthy food choices based on the individual needs of your body. Maintaining a healthy weight is not really about weight loss or weight gain diets. It is about learning how much food and which foods your body needs, then making healthy changes to your diet and sticking with them over time.

Exercise. Physical activity is another important component of managing weight, but it can also improve your overall health. Regular exercise helps you sleep better and decreases your chances of becoming depressed. We have become a sedentary society. We sit too long at desks in school, in office chairs at work, and in front of screens at home. The use of technology contributes to a sedentary lifestyle. How much time do you spend sitting in front of your "screens," including your computer, smartphone, tablet, television, or game console?

Because many individuals no longer have a job that provides regular physical activity, we need to choose physical activities that will keep our bodies healthy. The best physical activity is the one you will actually do. Make plans to be physically active on a daily basis. Work toward 30 to 60 minutes of moderate or vigorous physical activity each day. You can break this into shorter intervals or do it all at once. You don't need to run a marathon to have a healthy level of physical activity. The following are all examples of healthy options for moderate physical activity:

- walking two miles in 30 minutes
- bicycling five miles in 30 minutes
- dancing quickly for 30 minutes
- playing basketball for 15 to 20 minutes

If necessary, you can work toward increasing your physical activity by using the suggestions in Figure 14.35.

Sleep. Many people don't recognize that sleep is a component of healthy weight management and physical wellness. Because so many things seem more interesting or more important, we often choose to give up on getting more sleep. However, sleep is just as essential as nutrition and physical activity for achieving health and happiness. The quality and amount of sleep you get directly affects your mental alertness and productivity, your emotional stability and creativity, your physical energy, and even your weight.

The amount of sleep you need depends primarily on your age. For example, infants and children require 10 to 18 hours of sleep each night, while teens need 8½ to 9¼ hours. The average adult sleeps less than seven

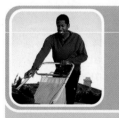

Tips for Staying Active

- Choose activities that fit your schedule and your personality.
- Team up with a friend and motivate each other.
- Get active during the time of day when you have the most energy.
- Use routine chores such as walking the dog or mowing the lawn to increase your exercise levels.
- Walk up the stairs instead of taking the elevator.
- When you care for young children, join them in playing tag or kickball.
- Just get yourself moving every day!

Figure 14.35   The best exercise for you is any exercise that you will actually do! Consider these techniques for increasing your physical activity.

hours each night even though most adults need seven and a half to nine hours each night for optimal functioning.

Many teens know that they need even more sleep than adults do, but typical school schedules present a challenge. Teens' circadian rhythm, or internal biological clock, tells them to fall asleep later and wake up later. They may naturally fall asleep after midnight but still need to wake up early for school. This limits sleep to six or seven hours per night on a regular basis and creates a **sleep deficit**.

Sleep deficit affects everything from paying attention in class to everyday mood. Teens with sleep deficits experience lower grades, reduced athletic performance, increased feelings of sadness and depression, and an elevated risk of car crashes caused by driving when drowsy.

Even if you think you're getting enough sleep, the following signs will tell you otherwise:

- difficulty waking up in the morning

- an inability to concentrate

- a tendency to fall asleep during class

- feelings of moodiness and even depression

Your commitment to good health includes paying attention to sleep deficits. Try some of the tips listed in Figure 14.36 to help you improve the quantity and quality of your sleep.

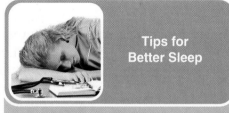

Tips for Better Sleep

- exercise each day
- set a regular bedtime
- no caffeine after 4:00 p.m.
- turn off all technology one hour before bedtime
- avoid all-nighters
- wake up with a bright light in the morning

Figure 14.36   **Try these techniques for improving your sleep if you feel tired during the day.**

Personal Hygiene and Medical Care. Other techniques for maintaining physical health include attention to personal hygiene and routine preventive medical care. Good hygiene benefits your general health, but it is also part of the professional appearance standards expected of healthcare workers. Begin with personal cleanliness, including your hair, hands, fingernails, clothing, and shoes. Keep your nails short and avoid wearing artificial nails. This reduces the risk of healthcare-associated infections.

Obviously, you will want to use deodorant, but you should avoid using perfumes and other strong-smelling personal products. Patients who are ill may find them nauseating or may be allergic to the fragrance. Asthmatic patients can experience attacks triggered by strong fragrances.

Practice good oral hygiene and seek regular dental care. Getting regular medical check-ups will promote good health and provide early treatment for identified health conditions. Keep up with recommended vaccinations for your own safety and your patients' safety.

Social, Emotional, and Spiritual Wellness

Social wellness is the ability to interact with the people around you. It requires positive communication skills and includes meaningful relationships with a support system of family members and friends. Social wellness has a positive effect on physical, as well as emotional, health. For example, social wellness appears to strengthen the immune system. People with strong social connections have been known to get fewer colds and fewer cavities.

Socially skilled individuals develop healthy relationships that are interdependent, not dependent. Rather than limiting contact with other people, a healthy relationship lets you develop your own interests (Figure 14.37).

Social wellness usually includes a sense of care and concern for communities. A desire to improve your community can lead to volunteering. Both community service and **service learning** provide excellent opportunities for health science students to improve their communities while learning about the field of healthcare and the needs of patients. Because of concerns about patient privacy, you may have difficulty securing a meaningful healthcare job shadowing experience. However, as a volunteer, you learn the guidelines for protecting patient privacy through training provided by the healthcare facility. As a result, you may have more opportunities to interact with both patients and healthcare professionals as a volunteer at a healthcare facility (Figure 14.38).

While they are striving to maintain social wellness, healthcare workers must also develop the skill of maintaining **professional distance**. This means that healthcare workers are caring toward their patients but

service learning
term for an educational experience that integrates academic achievement with community service

professional distance
term used to describe the act of showing a caring attitude toward patients without trying to become friends

Figure 14.37   As you develop new social relationships, be alert for these signs.

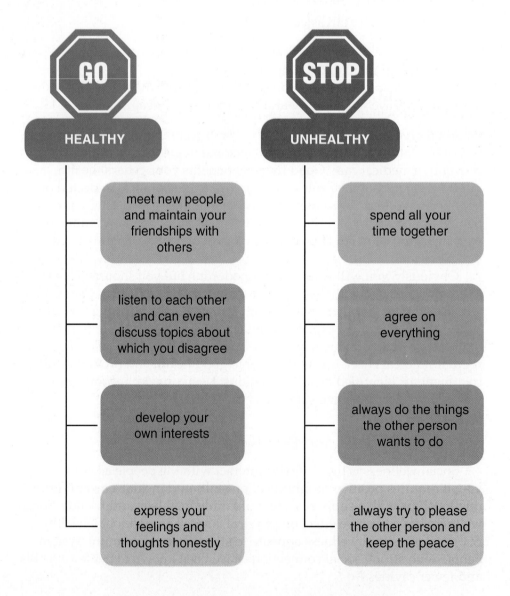

GO

HEALTHY

- meet new people and maintain your friendships with others
- listen to each other and can even discuss topics about which you disagree
- develop your own interests
- express your feelings and thoughts honestly

STOP

UNHEALTHY

- spend all your time together
- agree on everything
- always do the things the other person wants to do
- always try to please the other person and keep the peace

Figure 14.38 Knowledge and Skills Gained from Volunteering

Volunteer Position	Knowledge and Skills Learned
hospital volunteer	wheelchair transport and information on a wide range of hospital departments
food pantry volunteer	an understanding of the number of community families who cannot meet basic needs for food and clothing
long-term care volunteer	an understanding of the needs and interests of the geriatric population; communication skills with residents
hospice volunteer	an understanding of palliative care and issues surrounding death and dying
Special Olympics volunteer	communication skills and an appreciation of people with developmental delays
American Red Cross volunteer	an appreciation for the field of disaster response planning
Salvation Army volunteer	an understanding of homelessness and the healthcare needs of homeless clients

do not try to become friends with them. Ideally, healthcare workers get satisfaction from helping others become healthy, but they don't need to have the approval or friendship of the people they serve. You demonstrate an appropriate worker-patient relationship when you focus on the patient's health-related goals and not on how much the patient likes you.

Emotional wellness begins with the ability to identify and name your own feelings and emotions. Feelings come and go. It is in their nature to change, and they often do so quickly. When you pay attention to your body's signals, you can better identify your feelings. For example, a tight jaw and clenched teeth along with a pounding heart may signal anger.

Emotions can last longer than feelings. Think about the love of a parent for a child. The parent can feel frustrated by the child's actions but will continue to love her and work to support her needs. Emotions can also affect your physical wellness.

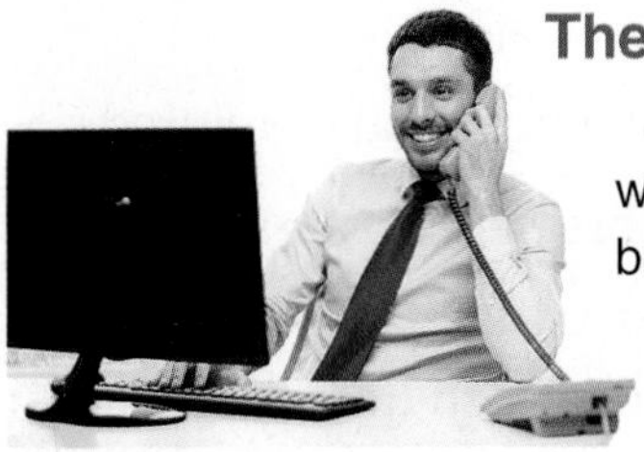

The Support Services Worker: Marco

Marco was a social worker who couldn't figure out what was wrong. He had no energy and no ambition, but he didn't know why he felt this way. His social life was fine. He had a solid group of friends in his biking club and often went home to spend time with his family. He wasn't experiencing problems at work and usually enjoyed his counseling groups and working with the students and families at his school. He wasn't feeling angry, frustrated, or sad, and he wasn't facing any unusually stressful situations. What could be wrong?

Marco finally decided to see his doctor and learned that he had a double ear infection. After a course of antibiotics, Marco was back to normal and enjoying life again.

Emotional Wellness

If you answer *no* to any of the questions below, you can improve your emotional wellness.

- Do I maintain a balance of work, family, friends, and school?
- Do I use methods to reduce stress?
- Can I make decisions with a minimum of stress and worry?
- Do I set priorities?

Figure 14.39 These are guidelines for judging your emotional wellness. What improvements can you make?

Marco knew that our emotions, values, and relationships also affect our wellness (Figure 14.39). Unlike most people, he was so attuned to his social and emotional wellness that he missed the signs of physical illness. When he didn't feel well, he checked his feelings (emotional), his relationships (social), and his personal values (spiritual) for any areas that were out of balance or under stress. Keeping our social, emotional, and spiritual lives in balance maintains our energy and enthusiasm for life. It pays big dividends as we work toward accomplishing our goals, and it provides a sense of satisfaction when we achieve them.

Spiritual wellness involves our inner motivations. Sometimes called the *soul*, the inner spirit is the place where our strongest beliefs live. This is the place where we look for answers to life's mysterious questions, such as *Why am I here?* or *What will happen to me when I die?* From these strong beliefs, we develop our values. Our values tell us what is important and what is right in terms of moral and ethical behavior. We use our values to make important life decisions and to guide our interactions with other people.

When our decisions and behaviors are consistent with our values, we feel a sense of inner peace and spiritual wellness. People use prayer, meditation, or specific spiritual practices to foster spiritual balance and maintain their connection to a higher power or belief system. Your religious faith, values, beliefs, ethical principles, and morals all define your spirituality.

Mental and Intellectual Wellness

When our lives are in balance, we are curious, we look forward to learning new skills, and we can easily solve the problems of everyday life. However, when stress wears us down, we lose interest in life and become more prone to physical illness.

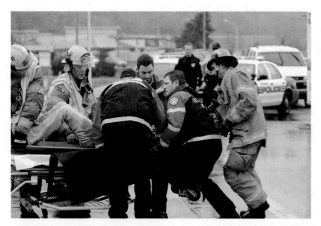

Figure 14.40 Emergency workers must remain calm even in life-threatening situations. What are some other stressful healthcare occupations?

Managing Stress. **Stress** is your body's attempt to adjust to a change. All of us face stressful situations, such as dealing with illness, taking an important test, or even getting married. While everyone feels some form of pressure, healthcare workers face a unique set of stressors:

- working with people who are ill or injured
- staying calm in life-threatening situations (Figure 14.40)
- performing tasks with a high degree of accuracy
- remaining vigilant at all times

Since we can't avoid stress, we must learn to recognize its signs and practice methods to manage it effectively.

The Support Services Worker: Jean

Jean was sailing through her workday. Her schedule was light and she was catching up on tasks that needed to be finished. Then came the news: her hospital was experiencing low occupancy due to the poor economy and was planning to cut back on staff hours. Suddenly, Jean's mood changed dramatically. A knot formed in her stomach, her heart began to pound, and her back started to hurt—all common signs and symptoms of stress. Jean was paying off school loans and her budget was tight. She couldn't afford to lose any income.

Will Jean choose positive or negative methods for coping with her stress? Too many of us choose overeating, not eating enough, smoking, or using drugs or alcohol as a way to relax. The problem is that, over time, all of these behaviors put us at risk for serious health problems. The following methods for coping with stress will actually have a beneficial effect on your health:

- Physical exercise increases endorphin production and improves mood and sleep.

- Prayer can inhibit the release of cortisol, thereby reducing the negative impact of stress on the immune system.

- Meditation provides a sense of calm that enhances emotional and physical well-being.

- Positive relationships with family and friends help you recover more quickly from illness and may actually help you live longer.

- Spending time on a hobby you enjoy may reduce blood pressure and alleviate the symptoms of depression.

Individuals who maintain mental and intellectual wellness also practice skills that help them limit the impact of stressful situations. These people are good planners and managers of their own lives. They begin by identifying personal priorities, then rank their responsibilities in order of importance according to these priorities. When conflict between responsibilities arises, they look at the long-term impact of each choice.

Stress and Students: Jake

Jake claimed that he had a serious case of "senioritis." With one month of school left, he lacked the ambition to do homework and even to get out of bed on time each morning. He was ready to give up on his plan for graduation and college. Maybe he'd take the GED and enter the military instead. That wasn't really what he wanted, but it seemed easier somehow.

(Continued on the next page)

Jake was working about 30 hours a week at a local restaurant and his shift ended at midnight. He got home by 1:00 a.m. and crashed on the couch. When the alarm went off in the morning, he was too tired to get up and head to school. He claimed that he needed his job to pay for everyday expenses and future college costs.

Jake's part-time job was taking priority over his high school graduation and future college education. Why do you think he was so set on keeping a late work schedule? Couldn't he have compromised and worked fewer hours during school and more hours during the summer? This would have been a logical choice, but Jake had a serious sleep deficit. Do you recognize the signs of sleep deprivation in his mood and mental focus?

Setting Goals. While your priorities identify your thoughts and beliefs, your goals put them into action. Setting goals and working toward achieving them provides a sense of satisfaction that helps you maintain your intellectual wellness. It's not enough to just set a goal; you also have to take action to achieve it. Roxie was always talking about going back to school someday. "I know I could do that job if I could just get myself back to school," she would say. However, she never did go back. While school was her spoken priority, she didn't make a plan or take the steps needed to make her goal a reality.

Setting goals means breaking down the steps to achieving them into manageable pieces (Figure 14.41). First, make a list of steps for the long term. These will be completed over the next few months or years. Then break the first long-term step into short-term steps and complete these in the next few days or weeks. Continue in this pattern until you accomplish your ultimate goal. As you work toward achieving a goal, keep track of your progress in a visible way. Cross steps off a list or post signs where you can see them so that you keep your goal in mind. Celebrate each milestone on the way to reaching your goal. It's easy to say that you want to be a doctor, but a long list of goals and accomplishments actually makes you an MD.

Be realistic about your goals. Do you really want to reach a specific goal, or are you setting it based on someone else's expectations? Are you willing to spend your time, energy, and money to achieve your goal? Does your goal match your personal priorities rather than the priorities of other people in your life?

Managing Your Time. Effective time management also contributes to mental wellness by helping us reach our goals and reducing stress. No one gets more than 24 hours a day, but an organized person can accomplish more in four hours than a disorganized person completes in a whole day.

Effective time management begins with priorities. Make a list of tasks and obligations. List your most important items first. Are there items you can remove because they aren't important enough to demand your time? Effective time managers know how to say no when a request doesn't match their personal priorities.

Organize your work into long-term and short-term tasks in much the same way you set your personal goals. A long-term task, such as writing a term paper, needs to be broken down into smaller steps so that sections of

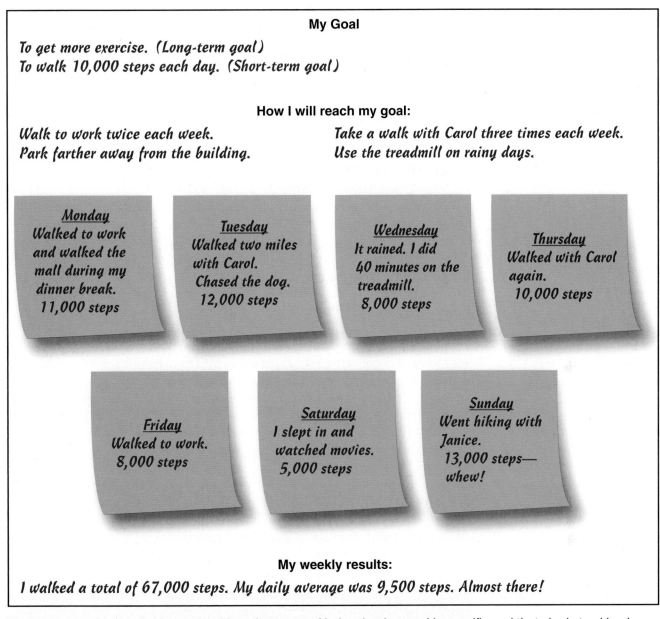

My Goal

To get more exercise. (Long-term goal)
To walk 10,000 steps each day. (Short-term goal)

How I will reach my goal:

Walk to work twice each week.
Park farther away from the building.

Take a walk with Carol three times each week.
Use the treadmill on rainy days.

Monday
Walked to work and walked the mall during my dinner break.
11,000 steps

Tuesday
Walked two miles with Carol.
Chased the dog.
12,000 steps

Wednesday
It rained. I did 40 minutes on the treadmill.
8,000 steps

Thursday
Walked with Carol again.
10,000 steps

Friday
Walked to work.
8,000 steps

Saturday
I slept in and watched movies.
5,000 steps

Sunday
Went hiking with Janice.
13,000 steps— whew!

My weekly results:

I walked a total of 67,000 steps. My daily average was 9,500 steps. Almost there!

Figure 14.41 Sue is working on health maintenance. Notice that her goal is specific and that she is tracking her progress each day. These are important factors in achieving any goal.

the project are completed over several days. Start with your due date and work backward to schedule the smaller steps. Make your to-do list for the day and you are ready to begin working.

Once you have your to-do list, you can schedule a time to work each day. Pick the time when you are most alert and energetic and begin with your most difficult tasks first. Avoid interruptions at all costs. Checking messages, replying to texts, and posting or checking status updates all interfere with your focus and delay your work. Once you have completed the difficult tasks, cross them off your list. You will feel a big sense of accomplishment and finishing the remaining tasks will seem easier.

Consider this daily schedule developed by a first-year medical student:

- **6:00 to 6:30:** breakfast/shower

- **6:30 to 8:30:** study

- **8:30 to 10:30:** class

- **10:30 to 11:30:** study

- **11:30 to 12:30:** lunch

- **12:30 to 1:30:** class

- **1:30 to 2:30:** class

- **2:30 to 6:00:** study

- **6:00 to 11:00:** relax

Notice that this student finishes studying by 6:00 each evening and has several hours of free time. He is earning excellent grades. He is successful because he is committed to getting up early every day and he makes it a priority to dedicate time to studying (Figure 14.42). He goes to a remote corner of the library where he won't see anyone he knows. He studies for 50 minutes, does a few minutes of physical exercises to refresh his focus, then gets right back to work. While his schedule is not magical, this student's time management skills are. He has taken control of his time and is focused on his primary goal of graduating from medical school.

A practical system for organizing the tasks in your life will go a long way toward conquering procrastination. You may be putting off work because it seems overwhelming, but procrastination actually increases your stress. It will take trial and error to develop a time management system, but a system will pay big dividends in improved school and work performance.

First, you will need a place to store the dates, tasks, appointments, and details of the projects that make up your life. This is a good opportunity to put technology to work. Capture this information in a device that you carry with you each day, such as a smartphone or tablet (Figure 14.43). That way, you will have all of the information in one place. You won't have to remember it and you won't worry about trying to find it later. If you store this information online, you can access it later from any device, in any location, at any time.

Figure 14.42 A disciplined study schedule is important if you want to succeed in school.

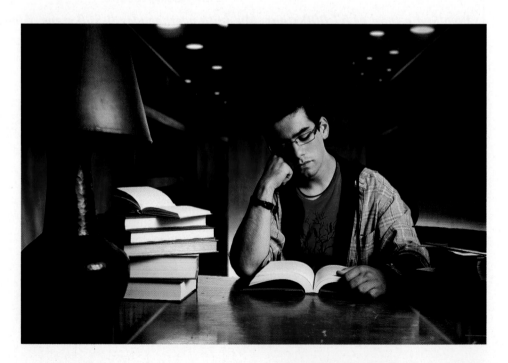

While technology is helpful, you might consider a low-tech option when you plan and organize. The plan is more important than the use of technology to make it pretty. A simple piece of notebook paper can outperform a detailed scheduling system that requires time to input and update information. Use paper to make a plan for the week. List your priorities for each day and note specific appointment times. You can break larger projects into smaller steps by working backward from the due date as shown for the case study assignment in Figure 14.44. You'll get the satisfaction of crossing off completed items and can easily revise the list if your plans change. If you have trouble keeping track of paper, snap a photo of your plan with your phone, and your list will travel with you.

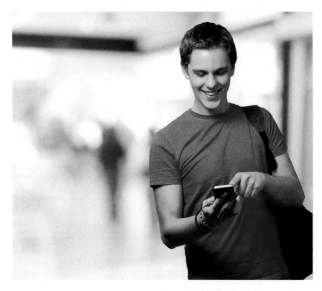

Figure 14.43   Load information about appointments, projects, and assignments you need to study onto your smartphone or tablet so that you can access it wherever you are.

Expand

Solving Problems. Organized workers take the routine problems and conflicts of life in stride. They use their priorities and time management skills to handle a variety of decisions and problems automatically. Sometimes, however, you will encounter a problem that creates an obstacle on the path to reaching your goals. When the right choice is not obvious, problem-solving skills can help you overcome this obstacle (Figure 14.45 on the next page). These skills allow you to make the best decision available for a given situation. You can use problem-solving skills throughout life to improve both your personal and career decisions.

When the mind, body, and spirit are in balance, a person is healthy or well. Promoting wellness can actually reduce the incidence of illness. For this reason, healthcare facilities offer classes in nutrition, exercise, meditation, and other wellness components to their patients and employees. Health insurance companies may reimburse the cost of these classes to motivate their customers to improve personal health practices. As a future healthcare worker, you will benefit personally from practices that maintain your own wellness. In addition, your knowledge

Figure 14.44 Weekly Plan						
Sun	**Mon**	**Tues**	**Wed**	**Thurs**	**Fri**	**Sat**
1-lunch at Scott's; bring salad	Work on med terms 8-1 field trip; meet in 2705 5-9 work	Ask teacher about case study questions Finish med terms homework	Med terms homework is due Ch. 14-16 3:15 haircut 5-9 work	Practice case study reading Study for micro 6- HOSA fund-raiser at Bariosos	Present case study Microbiology test Ch. 12	Get cash for the week 12-6 work

Figure 14.45 Continue to cycle through the problem-solving steps until you find a workable solution.

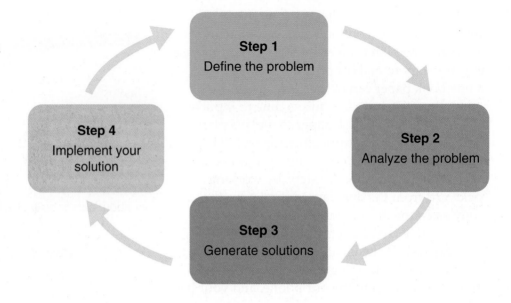

of wellness will benefit your patients as you work with them to improve their habits and lifestyle choices.

HOSA Connections

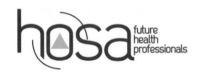

HOSA is a great place to experience healthcare through service to your community. Look for service learning opportunities as you acquire new healthcare skills. When you learn how to test vision and hearing and then use your skills to assist your school nurse in completing vision and hearing screening, you have a great service learning experience. Remember that your community can include your school, city, state, country, or the world.

Is there a healthcare concern of special importance to you—providing healthy drinking water, ensuring vaccinations for children, increasing exercise levels, reducing obesity, or increasing social occasions for seniors? Take your health science knowledge and create a service learning activity to address your concern. This will give you the satisfaction of improving your community while strengthening your own healthcare work skills.

Keep a log of your service activities in your career portfolio (Figure 14.46). This list will help you identify the healthcare skills you

Build Portfolio

Figure 14.46 Volunteering and Community Service Log					
NAME			Teacher		
Date	Hrs.	Type of Service	Place	Supervisor's Signature & Phone #	Skills Acquired

have learned and serve as a record of service hours completed. You may refer to this list as you write college entrance essays or complete scholarship applications.

Several HOSA competitive events will strengthen your support services skills. Read about them in the competitive events section of the HOSA website (Figure 14.47).

Figure 14.47 HOSA Events	
Event Name	**Event Description**
Public Service Announcement	PSA to inform the community about an important healthcare issue
Parliamentary Procedure	written test and simulated business meeting
Community Awareness	portfolio and presentation of activities conducted to raise awareness of a health-related issue
Researched Persuasive Speaking	oral presentation based on researching a health issue
Medical Photography	using digital photography to analyze a health career
Extemporaneous Health Poster	illustration of a health issue or HOSA topic
Prepared Speaking	speech related to the National Conference theme
National Service Project	service projects to support a healthcare organization selected by national HOSA
Medical Reserve Corps Volunteer Recognition	joint MRC/HOSA activities that support a strong and healthy community
Healthy Lifestyles	written test assessing knowledge of health literacy topics and documentation of a personal healthy lifestyle goal
HOSA Happenings	sharing HOSA activities in a newsletter format
Nutrition	written test

RECALL YOUR READING

1. Maintaining your health means maintaining _____ wellness; mental and _____ wellness; and _____, emotional, and _____ wellness.
2. The best kind of _____ is the kind that you will actually do because it fits into your schedule.
3. Social wellness for healthcare workers includes developing _____ with their patients.
4. _____ can help you practice healthcare job skills as you work to improve your community.
5. Maintaining intellectual wellness means setting _____, _____ your time, and learning to solve _____.

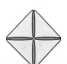

Complete the
Map Your Reading
graphic organizer for the
section you just read.

Chapter 14 Review

SUMMARY

 Assess your understanding with chapter tests

- Support services careers encompass a wide variety of healthcare occupations, but all support service workers help create a therapeutic environment for providing patient care.

- Self-motivation and a sense of initiative will lead to success in marketing, public relations, and healthcare administrative careers.

- Counseling and social work careers need workers who are empathetic and compassionate.

- Responsible and reliable workers support patient well-being in central services, occupational health and safety, and environmental health careers.

- A variety of engineering professionals including maintenance, environmental, clinical, and industrial engineers support the work of a healthcare facility.

- The roles of dietary workers are changing as healthcare food service options expand to meet the individual needs of patients, employees, and visitors.

- Employment for fitness instructors is increasing to support a national trend toward adopting healthy lifestyles.

- Team conflict is an interpersonal problem that occurs between two or more members of a team.

- The work style preferences of each team member can be used to provide positive teamwork results.

- Resolving team conflict requires positive communication and commitment to accomplishing the goals of the team.

- Cleaning and disinfecting are important steps in preventing the spread of infectious disease in healthcare facilities.

- Government agencies such as the CDC, EPA, and OSHA provide guidelines for maintaining safety in healthcare facilities.

- Following proper sanitation techniques when handling food prevents contamination and reduces the occurrence of foodborne illness.

- Physicians might order a therapeutic diet to help treat a disease or medical condition.

- Making the dining experience pleasant and relaxed is an important goal when assisting with feeding.

- Setting the brake is the single most important step when using a wheelchair to transport patients.

- Healthcare workers must maintain their own personal health to work with patients.

- Healthcare workers practice and promote healthy behaviors with their clients.

- Wellness refers to a balanced relationship between the mind, body, and spirit.

- Healthcare workers must learn to establish professional distance in their relationships with patients, clients, and residents.

- Service learning provides opportunities to use the skills you have learned in health science classes while providing a beneficial service to your community.

MAXIMIZE YOUR PROFESSIONAL VOCABULARY

 Build vocabulary with e-flash cards, games, and audio glossary

Listed below are the essential, yellow-highlighted terms and the additional professional vocabulary that you encountered in this chapter. Complete the activities that follow the list to make all of these terms part of your everyday professional vocabulary.

aspiration	consistency	dietetic technician
central services	contamination	dietitians
clinical engineer	cross-contamination	disinfection
compassion	dehydration	edema

environmental engineer	marketing	sleep deficit
environmental services	mitered corner	stress
Environmental Protection Agency (EPA)	morticians	support services
	multidrug-resistant organisms	terminal cleaning
Food and Drug Administration (FDA)	professional distance	therapeutic diet
		transport technicians
human resources	public relations	United States Department of Agriculture (USDA)
industrial engineer	sanitation	
initiative	service learning	work styles

VOCABULARY DEVELOPMENT

Matching. Match the essential terms from this chapter with the best descriptions below by writing the letter of the description next to the number of the essential term on your answer sheet.

1. central services
2. compassion
3. contamination
4. disinfection
5. environmental services
6. initiative
7. professional distance
8. sanitation
9. service learning
10. support services
11. therapeutic diet

a. term that describes procedures and practices that maintain cleanliness and preserve public health

b. term used to describe the act of showing a caring attitude toward patients without trying to become friends

c. the unwanted presence of harmful substances or microorganisms

d. a special food plan ordered by a physician to help treat a disease

e. the ability to decide independently what to do and when to do it

f. the hospital department responsible for receiving, storing, cleaning, disinfecting, sterilizing, and distributing medical and surgical supplies and equipment

g. an educational experience that integrates academic achievement with community service

h. the hospital department responsible for housekeeping, laundry, and facility maintenance

i. sympathy for the distress of others accompanied by a desire to help

j. the career pathway that focuses on creating a therapeutic environment for providing patient care

k. the use of chemicals to kill pathogens that are present on nonliving objects

12. Vocabulary Sorting. Sort each of the professional vocabulary terms under one of these headings: *skills and techniques, careers, conditions/diagnosis, departments,* and *regulatory agencies.* Be able to explain your choices. Use any remaining words in a sentence to see if they might fit under or connect with any of the headings.

REFLECT ON YOUR READING

13. Consider the occupations you came up with in the *Connect with Your Reading* activity.

Most of these occupations were located in a healthcare facility. However, many support services occupations exist in businesses other than healthcare. List five of these occupations. What do you think motivates these support services employees to work in the field of healthcare?

BUILD CORE SKILLS

14. Writing. Create a newsletter, marketing ad, or brochure promoting a healthcare facility such as a nursing home, hospital, clinic, or assisted

living facility. Make your writing clear, but brief, and include graphics to appeal to the public.

15. **Critical Thinking.** Describe a disagreement or conflict you have experienced recently. Using each guideline in Figure 14.16, rate your conflict-resolution behaviors on a scale of one to five. Five indicates that you followed the guideline and one indicates that you did not. Draw conclusions about your conflict-resolution skills.

16. **Critical Thinking.** Review the section in this chapter that discusses safe food handling procedures. Identify three situations that could result in contamination or cross-contamination of foods. Then identify methods that could be used to prevent unsafe food handling or storage. Use this information to create a poster that promotes safe food handling practices.

17. **Reading.** Use the Internet to research NAS (no added salt) and NCS (no concentrated sweets) diets. Determine the specific guidelines for each of these commonly used diets. Compare and contrast the guidelines for and health benefits of these diets across the life span. Discuss your findings with a classmate.

18. **Critical Thinking.** Imagine that you observe the following conditions in residents or patients. Place an "E" for *edema* in front of the signs typical of fluid retention. Place a "D" for *dehydration* in front of the signs of too little fluid.

   a. unusual fatigue or weakness
   b. wheezing or congestion
   c. coated, thick tongue
   d. rapid pulse
   e. puffy feet, ankles, and hands
   f. dry, itchy skin
   g. onset of confusion
   h. trouble swallowing and loss of appetite

19. **Problem Solving.** Who would you go to for help in a healthcare facility to solve the following problems? For each situation, identify the support services worker who can address it.

   a. a patient needs help paying for healthcare
   b. a patient wants to participate in a program to prevent falls

   c. a resident's call light is not working
   d. a patient needs a ride to the imaging department
   e. the medical clinic needs to expand
   f. a diabetic patient needs nutritious snacks
   g. you need an ad campaign to promote your healthcare facility
   h. there are no paper towels in a patient's room
   i. you need suggestions for streamlining average time for each patient encounter in a new ER addition
   j. surgical tools needed for an appendectomy must be sterilized
   k. you want the public to know that your hospital received the highest rating for patient safety
   l. a potential employee needs to be interviewed
   m. the bone density machine needs recalibration

20. **Speaking and Listening.** Work in a group to create a video that illustrates a poor atmosphere in a healthcare facility's resident dining area. Each person in the group should have a role such as playing a resident or healthcare worker, writing the video, or working behind-the-scenes with the camera. Be sure to show examples of healthcare workers who act or speak inappropriately. Show your video to the class and explain how the examples you chose could influence the resident's quality of care.

21. **Problem Solving.** Locate and read three articles that explain how to manage stress. What information did you find was most helpful to you personally? How might you use this information as a worker in a healthcare setting?

ACTIVATE YOUR LEARNING

22. Plan a meal that follows a specific therapeutic diet. Using a paper plate, create a visual that shows the meal's components. Identify the specific diet that you followed and include a description of health conditions that are improved with this diet. Analyze the meal's visual appeal based on variety of color, texture, temperature, shape, and flavor.

23. Review the steps for completing terminal cleaning of the patient environment and for making a bed. Assemble the necessary supplies and practice these procedures.

24. Determine a time period during which you will chart one or more of the following components for maintaining wellness: sleep, exercise, or relationships. Decide what data is most important to record. Develop low- and high-tech systems to use simultaneously for tracking your data. After your determined time period is up, analyze the data you collected and determine the positive and negative effects on your physical and emotional wellness. What further steps will you take to improve your wellness? Which tracking system seemed to meet your recording needs the best? Compare your systems and discuss their effectiveness with your classmates.

25. Review the steps for wheelchair transport. Then take turns practicing this skill with a classmate.

THINK AND ACT LIKE A HEALTHCARE WORKER

26. Analyze the following scenario to identify the lack of professional distance between this patient and healthcare worker. How would you handle this situation if you were the healthcare worker involved?

    Julio is an RN who is taking care of a patient named Georgia. Georgia is 80 years of age and is having difficulty breathing. She expressed concern to Julio about maintaining her home and being able to care for her lawn while in the hospital. Julio told her not to worry. He said that he and his brother, Juan, could stop over at her house and mow her lawn. He called his brother immediately to ask for his help. Georgia was hesitant to agree to this because she lived alone and wasn't sure how long she needed to stay in the hospital.

GO TO THE SOURCE

27. Use the Internet to research the CDC, EPA, or OSHA. Learn more about your chosen agency's functions or purposes related to safety in healthcare facilities. What types of guidelines does the agency create for healthcare facilities? What types of healthcare-related issues does the agency focus on? Write a short response to these questions and share your findings with your classmates.

28. Use the Internet to learn more about support services careers. Select two careers of interest to you and complete a career profile for each one. Use at least one site that ends in .gov and one site that ends in .org. Record the following information for each career:

    - name of the career
    - tasks involved in this career
    - personal traits and abilities
    - educational requirements
    - type of credential needed and how it is obtained
    - work conditions
    - wages and benefits
    - job outlook for the future
    - the websites you accessed

    How do the two careers compare? Why might you prefer one to the other?

DEVELOP YOUR HEALTH SCIENCE CAREER PORTFOLIO

29. Create a community service log using the example shown in Figure 14.46. Chart your service during a time period designated by your instructor. Add the log to your career portfolio.

30. Use the HOSA website to research the competitive events listed in this chapter. Select and note which event is your top choice and list reasons for your choice.

31. Review the section in this chapter that discusses personal work styles. Assess your personal work style. How well does your work style mesh with the job duties of the two support services occupations that you researched for question 28? Explain why these two occupations would or would not be a good fit for you.

Chapter 15
Fundamental Skills in Support Services

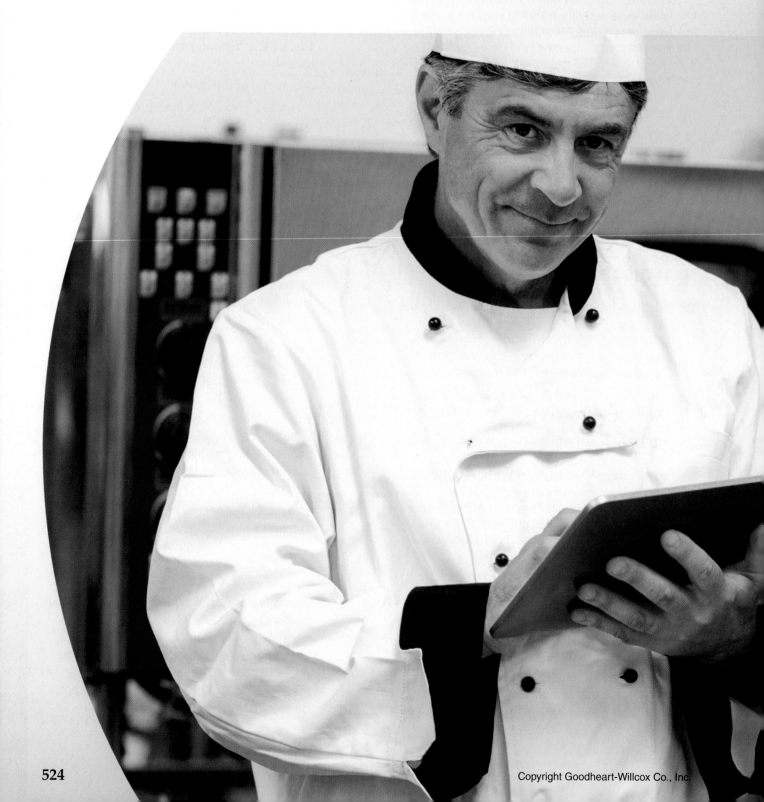

PROFESSIONAL VOCABULARY

 E-flash Cards

You will need to learn the essential terms listed below before you begin your reading. These terms will help you understand the main concepts of the chapter. These terms, which will be highlighted in yellow within the text, will become part of your professional vocabulary.

In addition to these essential terms, you will see bold terms throughout the chapter. The meanings of these terms are explained where the terms first appear. The bold terms, like the essential terms listed here, will become part of your professional vocabulary and deepen your understanding of the topics presented.

bar code scanner a device that captures a printed series of numbered black bars and spaces, translates them into numbers and letters, and sends the data to a computer to access information about a patient or product

fluid balance term for a state in which the amount of fluid taken into the body equals the amount of fluid that leaves the body

intake and output (I&O) term for measurements of all the fluids that enter and leave the body

interoperability the ability to exchange and use computer information within and across networks

portion the amount of food in one serving

quick response (QR) code a two-dimensional bar code that is used to provide easy access to information through a smartphone; also known as *quick read code*

radio frequency identification (RFID) a data collection technology that uses electronic tags for storing data

solutions uniform mixtures of two or more substances, which may be solids, liquids, gases, or a combination of these

tare weight the weight of an empty container

technical reading a skill used to comprehend science, business, or technology publications

technical writing a type of writing used in the workplace to inform or persuade a specific audience

unit cost the price of one measurable unit of a food item, such as 1 pound, 1 ounce, or 1 piece

yield the number of portions a recipe will produce

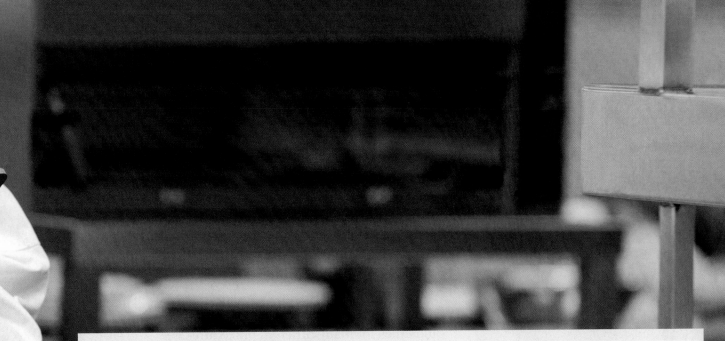

CONNECT WITH YOUR READING

Recall a recent challenging reading assignment. This could be a chapter in your science textbook, an instruction manual for a new phone, or a sales contract for a new purchase. How did you accomplish the purpose of your reading? What techniques did you use to improve your understanding of the technical information? List the steps you took and consider them as you read this chapter.

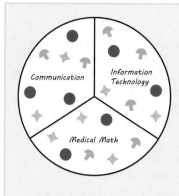

MAP YOUR READING

Create a visual summary by drawing a large circle on a blank sheet of paper. Divide the circle into three pizza slices. Label one slice *Communication*, another *Information Technology*, and the last one *Medical Math*. As you finish reading each section of the chapter, place these following "toppings" on your pizza:

- Draw "pepperoni" circles containing the main ideas, or the "meat" of the information.
- Draw "mushroom" shapes containing bits of information that are new or interesting for you and kept you from "vegging out" as you read.
- Draw "mystery" toppings (you create the shapes) that contain questions you still have about your reading.

As you learned in chapter 14, support services workers contribute to the successful operation of a healthcare facility. This means generating promotional materials for the facility, preparing food for patients or residents, and ensuring that equipment is running smoothly. All of these tasks rely on the important skills of technical reading and technical writing. Without these skills, as well as a strong knowledge of math applications, support services workers would not be able to do their jobs.

This chapter explains and demonstrates the steps for reading and writing technical documents, which help healthcare workers accomplish job tasks. You will learn about technology applications used by support services workers, as well as math applications used in food measurement and recipe costing. You will practice the skills for measuring intake and output that help patients maintain adequate nutrition and support fluid balance. Finally, you will learn the mathematical calculations needed to prepare the solutions used in a wide variety of healthcare applications.

Technical Communication Skills

While the majority of literature classes in high school focus on reading and interpreting novels, short stories, drama, and poetry, the world of work requires the ability to read technical materials. Workplace reading includes various technical documents including correspondence, instruction manuals, government regulations, professional journals, product labels, records, reports, and proposals (Figure 15.1). Workplace writing can involve all of these as well as marketing materials, patient education brochures, and the guidelines for many different procedures.

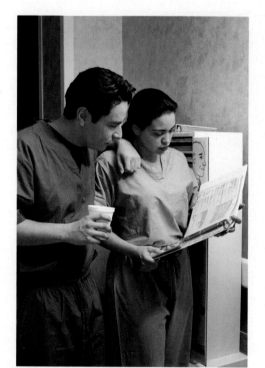

Figure 15.1   Healthcare workers use technical reading skills to understand and interpret manuals, procedures, and other materials.

Technical communication helps workers accomplish tasks. Chapter 2 introduced you to some of the business elements of technical communication that are used in healthcare. These include business correspondence, résumés, and patient information forms.

However, technical communication also focuses on new technologies. Documents explain technological advances to workers so they can use new equipment and new procedures to improve healthcare. Technical communication also provides information on new developments in the field of healthcare and the progress of experiments related to the diagnosis and treatment of disease.

The Support Services Worker: Salina

Salina was feeling desperate. As the dietary manager at a long-term care facility, her job duties included reading the newly published nutrition guidelines. Once she read the guidelines, Salina would have to write a set of instructions for her staff to follow as they prepared healthy snacks, or **nourishments**, for the residents. There was so much information to read! How could she put all that information into a single set of instructions?

She realized that she required some help to complete this task. Salina needed to learn the skills for technical reading and technical writing.

Reading Technical Documents

When you read literature, you must use your imagination and read between the lines. You develop an emotional connection with the characters and interpret their actions based on your own feelings and experiences. However, when you read technical documents, you must focus on understanding the facts and the logic presented. Technical documents require a different reading strategy because they are filled with detailed information, and they use technical terms specific to their topic. Taking the time to learn **technical reading** skills allows you to keep up with the latest advances in healthcare. These skills also improve patient and worker safety as you handle hazardous chemicals, administer patient medications, and operate new equipment.

technical reading
a skill used to comprehend science, business, or technology publications

Think back to chapter 3. When Manny read the instruction manual for a new imaging machine, he followed these steps:

1. Read with a purpose.
2. Scan the entire document and read the overview of the document, called the **executive summary**.
3. Use the table of contents, headings, or index to locate specific information.
4. Take notes about important ideas, steps in a process, or warnings and tips about the process.
5. Use the glossary to learn the meanings of new words.
6. **Paraphrase** by writing important information in your own words or saying the information aloud.

Technical reading requires attention and concentration. To read successfully, select the time of day when you are most alert. Pick a location with few distractions, such as a quiet conference room at work or a quiet corner of the library (Figure 15.2). Silence your cell phone to avoid interruptions. Your own bedroom may offer peace and quiet, but don't get too comfortable. Relaxing on your bed to read technical material usually leads to falling asleep! Know your preferences regarding background music—does it distract you or help you focus?

Read technical documents slowly. They are packed with information, and you will miss the details if you read quickly. When you lose your concentration, you can continue to read, but you won't remember the content. You may need to pace yourself and take short breaks from your reading about every 15 minutes. Summarize what you have just read before continuing.

As you read technical documents, don't skip the graphics. Tables, charts, graphs, and even photographs provide detailed information that you will need to accomplish your task or solve your problem. Once you have finished reading a document, consider doing some additional reading from other sources to clarify your understanding.

Let's look more closely at Salina's task. Remember that she needs to read the revised dietary guidelines. She located the guidelines on the United States Department of Agriculture (USDA) website. The full document is available online, but it's 112 pages long! Salina followed the steps for reading a technical document:

1. Her purpose was to develop a set of instructions for her staff to follow when preparing healthy snacks for residents. She needed to know what foods and beverages would promote good health and what foods and beverages needed to be restricted or omitted from the residents' diets.

2. Salina began the scanning process by reviewing the table of contents and reading the executive summary. The executive summary is helpful because it makes key recommendations that include foods to reduce in the diet and foods and nutrients to increase in the diet. She took notes on the key recommendations that affected her residents.

3. Returning to the table of contents, Salina selected three chapters for focused reading (Figure 15.3).

Figure 15.2   When reading a technical document, finding an area without distractions is important. What is a distraction-free area you could use for technical reading?

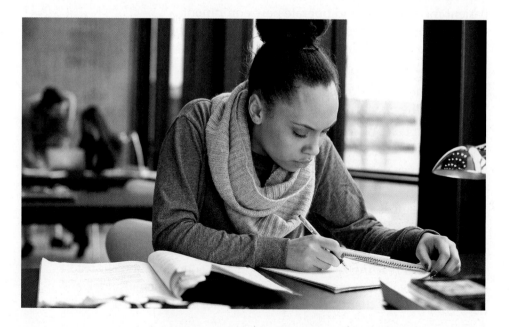

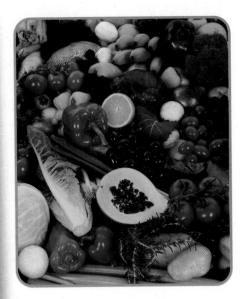

Contents

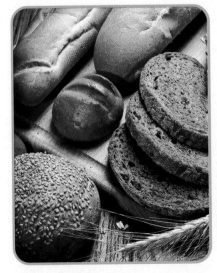

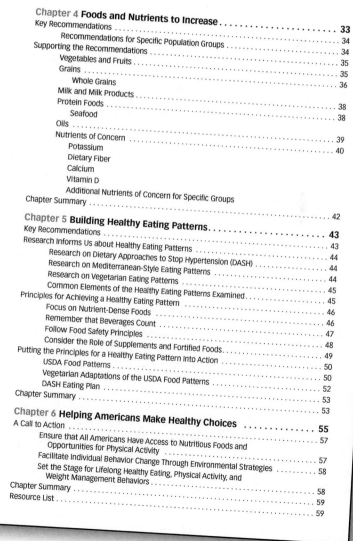

Figure 15.3 The table of contents from the USDA guidelines that Salina reviewed. If you were Salina, which three chapters would you choose for focused reading?

4. Salina carefully read each chapter. She took frequent breaks and summarized important information in her own words as she took notes.

5. Salina made a list of unfamiliar terms and used the glossary at the end of the document to learn the meaning of each term.

6. Finally, Salina reviewed her notes and selected the main information that her staff would need to know (Figure 15.4).

Salina followed several links on the USDA website to find additional resources. Since most of her residents are senior citizens, she read a report about older Americans' fruit and vegetable consumption and another about the quality of older Americans' diets.

In the material Salina read, charts provided information about specific foods to include and avoid in her residents' diets (Figure 15.5).

Technical documents will rarely entertain you. However, when you use technical reading skills along with a desire to learn, these documents will inform you. In this way, technical reading skills lead to improved care for patients and improved job performance for you.

Dietary Guidelines

Chapter 3	Terms to clarify
Reduce sodium because it raises blood pressure.	nutrient-dense
Avoid salted snack foods.	chronic disease
Avoid processed foods containing salt.	cholesterol
Don't add salt to foods.	solid fats
Stay below 2,300 mg/day.	saturated fats
Residents with diabetes, kidney disease,	trans-fatty acids
hypertension and those over age 51 stay	DASH diet
below 1,500 mg/day.	AI
Reduce saturated fats because they increase	UL
the risk of cardiovascular disease.	added sugars
Choose low-fat dairy products and lean meats.	
Use unsaturated fats in food preparation.	
Consume the smallest possible amount of trans fatty acids.	
Limit cholesterol to less than 300 mg/day.	
Restrict intake of solid fats, added sugars, and refined grains.	

Figure 15.4   As Salina read chapters 3, 4, and 5 of the dietary guidelines, she took notes, listed and clarified the meanings of unfamiliar terms, highlighted the most important information, and underlined the main points in the chapter.

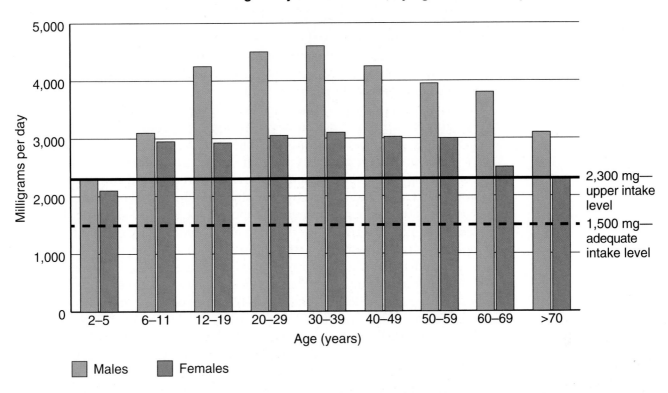

Estimated Average Daily Sodium Intake, by Age-Gender Group

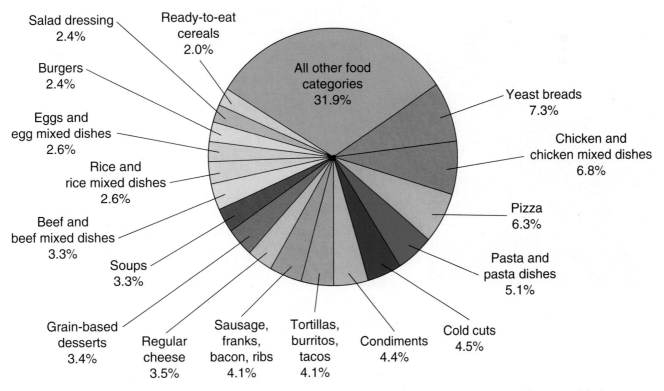

Sources of Sodium in the Diets of the US Population Ages 2 Years and Older

Figure 15.5   Salina reviewed the data in each of the charts found in the USDA guidelines. They provided important details about food choices for her residents. What do these graphics tell you about sodium consumption in American diets?

Writing Technical Documents

technical writing
a type of writing used in the workplace to inform or persuade a specific audience

Technical writing meets a specific need. Rather than expressing the writer's thoughts or experiences, a technical document informs or persuades a specific audience. Salina's technical writing informed her staff about dietary guidelines so the staff could prepare nourishments for residents of their healthcare facility. When a medical equipment manufacturer prepares a brochure explaining the benefits of a new imaging machine, the technical writer hopes to persuade healthcare facilities to purchase that machine (Figure 15.6).

Technical writing targets a specific group. Frequently, the writer must compile expert-level information and then translate and summarize it into language easily understood by the intended audience. For example, when writing patient education materials about hyperlipidemia (hI-per-lih-puh-DEE-mee-uh), you could say that it involves abnormally elevated levels of lipids, such as cholesterol or triglycerides. However, most patients would better understand that hyperlipidemia is too much fat in your blood.

Technical writing is clear and concise. A physician writes a prescription for "125 mg amoxicillin (uh-mahk-suh-SIH-lihn) po q 8h," not "The patient needs some of that pink liquid that treats bacterial infections." Technical documents use headings, lists, and graphics to direct the reader to specific information. When replacing a filter in the heating system, a technician can quickly locate the directions by finding the maintenance section in the table of contents. She can simply scan the headings, looking for "Replacing a Filter." She doesn't need to read the entire manual to complete her task.

Technical writers follow these basic steps:

- **Plan.** During the planning stage, clearly define the purpose of the document and identify the characteristics of the specific group known as your **target audience**. Then gather the information needed to write the document. Gathering information may involve reading, doing research and surveys, and even conducting interviews.

- **Draft and Revise.** First, select a format that fits the purpose of the document. For example, instructions will use numbered lists, reports may need a summary or an abstract, and a proposal will include a request for a plan of action or the purchase of goods or services. Keep the purpose and audience in mind while writing your first draft. During the revision process, verify that the information is accurate, well organized, and written clearly. Finally, focus on the document design. Are the headings easy to spot? Do bulleted or numbered lists highlight important information? Do the graphics make the data easy to understand?

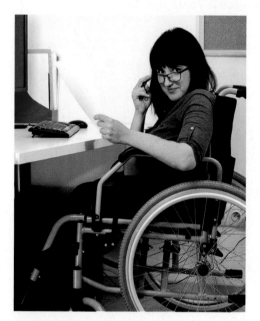

Figure 15.6 Technical writers create materials meant to inform or persuade an audience.

- **Edit and Publish.** Editing removes errors in spelling and grammar. It produces a professional document that represents your company. Having another person edit your work will catch errors that your brain automatically corrects. Reading aloud may help you hear awkward phrases or incomplete sentences. Remember to cite your sources. Submit your document before the deadline so there is adequate time for publishing.

Salina already knew the purpose for her writing. Before beginning to write, she considered her audience, the dietary aides who worked in her facility. They would need to know some background information about why there were new guidelines for nourishments. They would also need a set of instructions to follow for selecting appropriate snacks for residents. Finally, they would need to be aware of foods to avoid so that residents' health conditions were not made worse by poor food choices. Using the information in her notes, Salina prepared a first draft (Figure 15.7).

FIRST DRAFT

Revised Guidelines for Preparing Nourishments

The USDA recently revised the dietary guidelines, which we follow in planning menus for our residents. The changes in the new guidelines are focusing on improving the health of US citizens by achieving the following dietary goals:

- reducing sodium intake because it increases hypertension
- reducing intake of saturated fats, which contribute to cardiovascular disease
- reducing intake of added sugars often found in baked products and beverages
- increasing consumption of fruits and vegetables, whole grains, seafood, and low-fat dairy products
- improving food sources of fiber, potassium, calcium, vitamin D, and vitamin B_{12}

As you prepare nourishments for our residents, follow these guidelines:

Check the resident's food plan and note restrictions based on current health conditions.

Use water, coffee, low-fat milk, or other low-calorie beverages to maintain hydration.

Serve 100% juice beverages.

Choose fresh fruit with low-fat yogurt or vegetables with low-fat dressings for residents without chewing difficulty.

Use fruits canned in natural juices.

Crackers, toast, or other bread items should be whole-grain.

Limit serving cakes, cookies, or other sweets to special occasions if they are not restricted foods in the patient's diet.

Do not use salt to season foods.

These guidelines may represent significant changes from the snacking habits our residents have followed for many years. Be patient and encouraging. Offer snacks that are healthy but also visually appealing as we work to promote healthy snacking for our residents.

Figure 15.7   After doing her focused reading, Salina created the first draft of the document she would eventually give to her staff.

During the revision process, Salina followed a checklist of tips for technical writing and made changes to her document (Figure 15.8). She then asked one of her dietitians to proofread it for readability and

---

FIRST DRAFT

Revised Guidelines for Preparing Nourishments

The **USDA** *(United States Department of Agriculture)* recently revised the

dietary guidelines. We use these in planning menus for our residents.

The new guidelines aim to improve the health of citizens by achieving

the following dietary goals:

- Reducing sodium intake because it increases blood pressure
- Reducing intake of saturated fats, which contribute to heart disease
- Reducing intake of added sugars often found in bakery products and beverages
- Increasing consumption of fruits and vegetables, whole grains, seafood, and low-fat dairy products
- Improving food sources of fiber, potassium, calcium, vitamin D, and vitamin B_{12}

Follow these guidelines when preparing nourishments:

1. Check the resident's food plan and note restrictions based on current health conditions.
2. Use water, coffee, low-fat milk, or other low-calorie beverages to maintain hydration.
3. Serve 100% juice beverages.
4. Choose fresh fruit with low-fat yogurt or vegetables with low-fat dressings for residents without chewing difficulty.
5. Use fruits canned in natural juices.
6. Use whole-grain crackers, toast, and other bread products.
7. Serve cakes, cookies, and other sweets only on special occasions and only when permitted in the resident's diet.
8. Do not use salt to season foods.

These guidelines may represent significant changes from the snacking habits our residents have followed for many years. Be patient and encouraging. Offer snacks that are not only healthy but also visually appealing as we work to promote healthy snacking for our residents.

Annotations (right margin):
- Explain acronyms by writing out the words when first used.
- Keep sentences short.
- Write using the active voice; subject-verb-object.
- Use common rather than complex words.
- Use concise terms rather than wordy phrases.
- Use bulleted or numbered lists for detailed information.

Figure 15.8   Note the changes (in red text) that Salina made to her first draft and the corresponding technical writing tips she used. Following the revision process, Salina asked a colleague to read her document and made the changes shown in green.

typographical errors. She made a few corrections and improvements based on her colleague's suggestions. After completing the final draft, Salina considered other changes to make the document easier to read. She increased the size of the headings to show the different sections of the document. She also added color blocks to make the numbered steps stand out from the rest of the document. Then she determined how many posters and what sizes would work best before ordering copies of her document.

When you are familiar with a subject, you can easily become engrossed in the topic and use technical terms in your document. That's fine if you are writing for colleagues with similar knowledge and career experience. However, technical writing is most successful when complex information is put into simple language that a specific audience is able to understand. Your purpose and your audience should always remain the focus of your technical writing.

RECALL YOUR READING

1. In addition to job-related reading and writing tasks, technical communication can also focus on new _____.
2. Technical _____ skills improve patient and worker _____.
3. Technical writing seeks to _____ or _____ a specific audience.
4. Having another person _____ your writing can help catch mistakes you missed.

Complete the *Map Your Reading* graphic organizer for the section you just read.

Information Technology

Considering the rapid advances in computer technology, why has the implementation of a fully functioning electronic health record system taken so long? This section details the reasons for the delay and explains steps being taken to improve EHR systems. You will learn how support services workers use technology to keep track of equipment, inventory, and even patients themselves, as well as their special diet and exercise requirements.

Electronic Health Records: Standards and Credentialing

As many medical record software programs were being developed and put into use in the 1990s, three core issues delayed the development of full-scale EHR systems:

- **Functionality.** Many systems had limited functions. Oftentimes, one system could record patient care but a separate system was required for patient billing. In some cases, scheduling and e-mail software were separate programs, so the same data had to be entered many times in the patient care process. Some programs could not perform specific functions such as e-prescribing or providing alerts about allergies and adverse reactions to medications.

- **Interoperability.** Proprietary systems could not communicate with each other. For example, a hospital and clinic that shared

interoperability
the ability to exchange and use computer information within and across networks

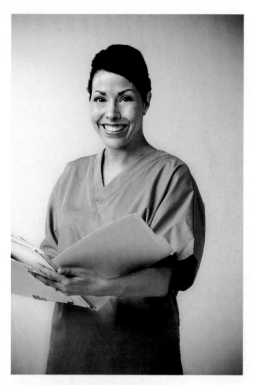

Figure 15.9 A lack of interoperability between early electronic health records systems meant paper records were still used in some circumstances.

patients but used different records systems had to transfer records using paper copies. Different clinic locations within the same healthcare system sometimes had different records systems. If patients went from the urology department to the surgery department, for example, they had to carry paper records with them (Figure 15.9). Because records could not be shared easily or quickly, diagnostic tests were unnecessarily repeated when a patient saw a new provider.

- **Security.** There were no system-wide standards for the privacy and security of electronic health information until 1996. At that point, HIPAA began to establish accountability standards and criteria affecting practice management software systems used for office functions such as patient scheduling and billing. That was the starting point for the development of uniform standards and a credentialing system for electronic health records.

Today, EHR systems go through a certification process to verify that they have met the current requirements for functionality, interoperability, and security. The Office of the National Coordinator for Health Information Technology Health IT Certification Program helps to ensure that electronic health record programs comply with the standards and certification criteria adopted by the Secretary of Health and Human Services. Since new criteria and test steps are added to the certification requirements each year, software companies list the year of their certification in their product specifications. That tells the customer exactly which criteria an EHR program meets and encourages frequent software updates. Certified programs must include categories such as

- access to scheduling;

- test results handling;

- prescriptions;

- patient medical history;

- patient instructions;

- allergy lists;

- medication lists; and

- wellness and prevention criteria.

While the certification is voluntary, only certified programs may interact with government healthcare programs such as Medicare or Medicaid. Electronic health record companies use certification agencies approved by the **Office of the National Coordinator as Authorized Testing and Certification Bodies (ONC-ATCB)**. Because of the certification process, all EHR programs perform similar functions and have similar capabilities. However, each program varies in the way it displays data, in its level of complexity, and in the number of functions available to each user.

Support Services Applications

Support services workers interact with technology on a daily basis. From programming mannequins to bar coding supplies, they are responsible for maintaining the equipment and operating the software that supports a therapeutic environment for patient care. Some of this new technology may seem complicated, but learning more about it can help prepare you to use it in a healthcare setting.

The Support Services Worker: Beth

Beth was raising the hospital bed before changing the linens when the bed's alarm began to beep. She tried several buttons on the keypad with no luck. The constant beeping continued. She phoned maintenance and a technician came in a few minutes to reprogram the bed controls. This made Beth consider how technology is transforming even simple pieces of equipment like hospital beds.

bar code scanner
a device that captures a printed series of numbered black bars and spaces, translates them into numbers and letters, and sends the data to a computer to access information about a patient or product

Computerized clinical simulators used in healthcare facilities and educational programs provide hands-on care training for healthcare workers (Figure 15.10). These highly sophisticated mannequins can be programmed to **simulate**, or *imitate*, medical emergencies. They include speech capabilities and adjustable vital sign readings to lend realism to training. The clinical simulator technician sets up simulation events and preprograms the mannequin for care scenarios. Following a training session, the technician conducts technical debriefings and is responsible for maintaining and updating simulation software.

The central services department employs technology to improve inventory functions. **Bar code scanners** read the line codes on patient supplies and track inventory while assessing charges for supplies used in patient care. Check-in and check-out procedures track the location of reusable diagnostic tools and medical equipment. Fixed inventory items such as chairs, televisions, and computers are found throughout a healthcare facility. Using a handheld computer, a worker can walk around scanning the bar codes on these objects. The worker can then run a report of all items in the facility to show which items are missing or have been moved.

Bar codes also play a role in patient identification. For example, nurses will scan a patient's barcoded wristband and the bar code on the patient's chart to verify that they are talking to the right patient. Then they can view the patient's medical record on a computer screen and update charts by entering current vital signs and progress notes. Before administering medication, a nurse scans the patient's wristband, the medical record bar code, and the bar code on the medication to verify he or she is with the right patient and has the right medication. Using bar code technology for

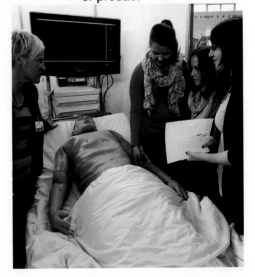

Figure 15.10 Programmable mannequins simulate care situations and provide excellent training opportunities for healthcare workers. Which healthcare worker maintains and facilitates use of these mannequins?

lab specimens, radiology reports, and pharmacy labels reduces medical record errors and improves patient care.

Radio frequency identification (RFID) is a more sophisticated tracking technology. It uses electronic tags for storing data. Like bar codes, RFID tags identify items. However, they don't require "line of sight" for reading because antennas on the RFID tag and on the reader use radio waves to exchange data. The tags on clothing and library books that prevent theft are common uses of RFID technology.

radio frequency identification (RFID)
a data collection technology that uses electronic tags for storing data

Another benefit of RFID technology is that each individual item can be tracked. For example, the Universal Product Code (UPC), a common example of a bar code, identifies a *type of item* such as a 16-ounce jar of peanut butter. However, an RFID code tracks *a specific jar* of peanut butter and can show which jars in your inventory have passed their expiration dates.

Hospitals use RFID systems to track their inventory of medical devices such as stents and catheters. An employee's RFID tagged identification card must be scanned before the system can allow authorized workers to remove implants or other devices from a locked cabinet. The system automatically creates a digital record showing which items have been removed and who removed them. In addition, the system will use bar code scanning to track which items are actually used. Therefore, when a worker selects three of the same implant but in different sizes, the scanner can track which item is used and indicate the need for reordering. It can also track the return of the unused items and note which worker is responsible for their return (Figure 15.11). Once the surgery has concluded, the worker returns to the locked storage unit, scans his or her ID badge, and places any unused items back on the shelves. The system will automatically indicate that those products were unused and returned.

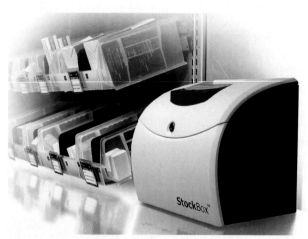

Figure 15.11   When an RFID stock tag is inserted into this inventory system, the correct item is automatically ordered. What are some advantages of using an RFID system?

quick response (QR) code
a two-dimensional bar code that is used to provide easy access to information through a smartphone; also known as *quick read code*

Quick response (QR) codes, or *quick read codes*, are two-dimensional bar codes that can be displayed almost anywhere, such as on a sign, in a book, or on a computer or TV screen. You can use your smartphone to take a picture of the code, which takes you to a website or video with more information—no typing is needed, you just point and click. In healthcare settings, this technology can replace patient care videos and printed instructions. Instead of sending a heart disease patient home with a DVD and a binder of information, the patient can scan QR codes in a brochure to view videos with instructions, diet and exercise recommendations, and postsurgical care guidelines (Figure 15.12). In addition, the QR codes can connect with smartphone apps to help patients monitor their vital signs, exercise, and food intake.

Healthcare marketing and public relations departments can use QR codes on brochures and in magazines to provide information about healthcare services and clinic locations. Potential patients can scan physician QR codes to view the physicians talking about their background, specialty, and willingness to accept new patients.

QR codes can connect you to your mobile pharmacy. By scanning the bar code on your prescription, you can quickly order a refill. You can also access an app that lets you manage prescriptions by showing you expiration dates and remaining refills, providing a pharmacy locator, and sending dosage reminders to your phone.

A healthcare facility's dietary staff relies on technology to track and manage inventory and may employ bar code or RFID systems for that purpose. In addition, computers are essential for managing recipes, menus, and individual patient diets. When was the last time you used a cookbook? Even for home use, online recipe access is commonplace. In a healthcare facility, software programs manage recipes and specify ingredients and amounts.

Dietitians and nutritionists use diet analysis programs to manage diseases and conditions that require special diets. Using unique factors such as the patient's gender, age, height, and weight, computer software programs analyze food intake and exercise. The results will show caloric needs and nutrient deficiencies or excesses. Then the program will make recommendations for changes that will improve the patient's health. The USDA offers a "SuperTracker" program that lets you develop a personalized nutrition and fitness plan (Figure 15.13). You can track your food intake and fitness activities and compare them to your plan. The program will analyze your results and offer tips for making healthier choices.

Figure 15.12   QR codes provide quick access to information online. Follow this QR code with your smartphone. Where does it lead?

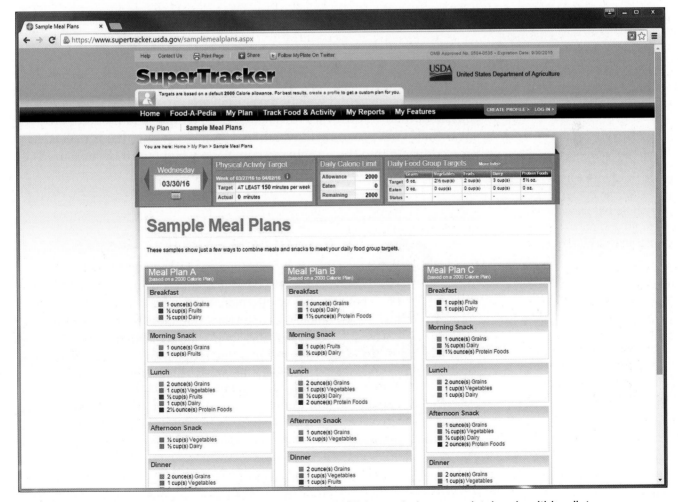

Figure 15.13   SuperTracker, a website provided by the USDA, can help you maintain a healthier diet.

Complete the
Map Your Reading
graphic organizer for the
section you just read.

Medical Math

Support service workers use measurement mathematics as they portion food servings and adjust recipe yields. They use budgeting mathematics by keeping a close watch on inventory and carefully costing each item to stay within budget expectations. Skills for estimating and for using ratios and proportions to prepare solutions are also part of healthcare mathematics.

Measuring Food

Whenever possible, food service workers measure food by weight, using a food scale. Food weight measurements are more accurate and consistent than volume measurements. For example, a half cup of brown sugar that is not packed will weigh less than a half cup that is packed or pressed firmly into the measuring cup. Food weights can be measured using ounces and pounds or grams and kilograms.

The Support Services Worker: Gerry

Gerry is the dietary manager for a small hospital. Of course, he is responsible for meeting the dietary needs of patients, but he also manages the hospital cafeteria used by employees and visitors. To meet budget expectations, Gerry carefully tracks the costs of the foods purchased by the hospital and uses recipe costing to monitor the prices charged for cafeteria meals. Food portions are carefully measured to meet patients' dietary requirements, but also to manage the cost of foods served in the hospital.

---

tare weight
the weight of an empty
container

Workers must consider **tare weight** when using a food scale. This is the weight of the container that holds the food being measured. Place the empty container on the food scale and reset the weight indicator to zero. Then place the food in the container for an accurate reading of food weight. Most scales can be reset to account for tare weight. If your scale cannot be reset, simply subtract the weight of the empty container from the total weight of the food and the container. If the container weighs 1 ounce and the total weight of the food and the container is 8 ounces, the weight of the food alone is 7 ounces.

A fluid ounce is the basic unit of volume in the US system. Smaller units include the teaspoon, which is ⅙ ounce, and the tablespoon, which is ½ ounce. Larger units of volume include the cup, pint, quart, and gallon. The metric system uses a liter as the basic unit of volume. The milliliter, which is ⅟₁,₀₀₀ liter, is also commonly used for volume measurements.

Knowing the correlation between the weight and volume of certain liquids can save measuring time. For water or other liquids such as broth, milk, or juice that have a similar density, 1 fluid ounce is equal to 1 ounce in weight. Similarly, in the metric system, 1 milliliter is equal to 1 gram, and 1 liter is equal to 1 kilogram. If your recipe calls for "16 oz milk," that will be the same as 16 fluid ounces. Since 1 cup equals 8 fluid ounces, you can simply measure 2 cups for 16 oz of milk. Using the metric system, 480 grams of milk is the same as 480 milliliters and can be measured using a liquid measuring cup with mL markings.

Two additional measuring steps will ensure that your individual measurements are accurate. When measuring dry ingredients, always level the measuring container. Begin by overfilling the cup or spoon and then use a spatula to scrape off ingredients that are above the rim of the measuring container. For liquid ingredients, set the container on a level surface, bend if necessary, and read the container at eye level (Figure 15.14).

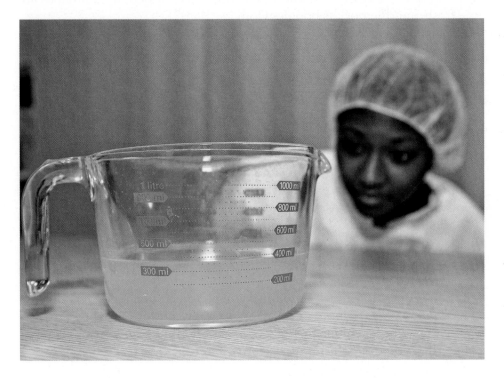

Figure 15.14 For accurate liquid measurements, place the measuring cup on a level surface and read the measurement at eye level.

Using Standardized Recipes

In a standardized recipe, the list of ingredients, the amount of each ingredient, and the preparation methods allow you to make the food item the same way each time. Standardization of food items is important to customers who expect the same food product each time they order it. For patients, standardization can be critical when a health condition depends on including or avoiding particular food items or ingredients. For this reason, healthcare food service workers carefully follow standardized recipes without making changes. Ingredient substitutions must be approved so that therapeutic diets remain accurate and wholesome for each patient.

A standardized recipe has several distinct parts and features more details than the typical home recipe (Figure 15.15):

1. The name of the recipe matches its listing on the hospital menu.

2. The **yield** section describes the quantity or number of servings the recipe will make. Yield can be adjusted to make more or fewer servings.

3. **Portion** size indicates the amount for each serving. Portion size can be listed by weight, volume, or count. For example, one portion could be 8 ounces, 1 cup, or 3 pieces of a food item such as chicken strips. Food service workers use specific ladles and scoops to serve individual portions. These tools have been selected because they will scoop an accurate portion of the food being served each time. Food scales may also be used to weigh individual portions. Accurate food portioning is important to the health of patients on specialized diets. In addition, it satisfies customers who expect the same amount as the next person with the same order. Portioning also controls food costs.

4. The recipe lists ingredients with descriptions or specifications. For example, the carrots are diced, the onion is chopped, the tomatoes are fresh, and the pork is boneless loin.

5. The quantity or amount of each ingredient is listed by weight. For small amounts of food items such as seasonings, teaspoon or tablespoon units are given.

6. The list of directions includes cooking times and temperatures to ensure food safety.

7. Plating instructions may indicate which dish to use when serving and the specific method for garnishing.

8. A marketing guide lists the amount of food to purchase for ingredients that are prepared before adding them to the recipe. For example, how many ounces of red peppers do you need to purchase to equal the 1 cup of diced peppers in a recipe?

9. Nutrition information is often listed to show amounts of major nutrients provided by the food item.

Adjusting Recipe Yields. Sometimes you will need to change the yield of a recipe to prepare more or fewer servings. To do this, you need to know how many portions the recipe makes and how many portions you need. Then you can determine the **conversion factor**. The conversion

yield
the number of portions a recipe will produce

portion
the amount of food in one serving

Name of the recipe

Quantity/amount
of ingredients

List of directions

Description of
ingredients

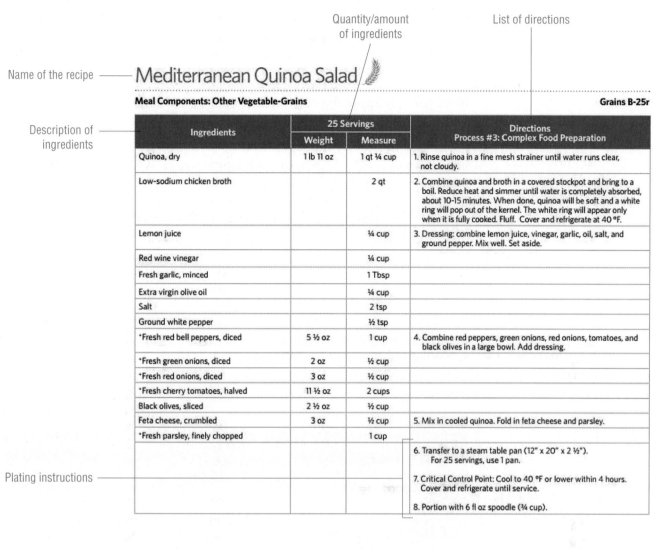

Mediterranean Quinoa Salad

Meal Components: Other Vegetable-Grains

Grains B-25r

Ingredients	25 Servings		Directions Process #3: Complex Food Preparation
	Weight	Measure	
Quinoa, dry	1 lb 11 oz	1 qt ¼ cup	1. Rinse quinoa in a fine mesh strainer until water runs clear, not cloudy.
Low-sodium chicken broth		2 qt	2. Combine quinoa and broth in a covered stockpot and bring to a boil. Reduce heat and simmer until water is completely absorbed, about 10-15 minutes. When done, quinoa will be soft and a white ring will pop out of the kernel. The white ring will appear only when it is fully cooked. Fluff. Cover and refrigerate at 40 °F.
Lemon juice		¼ cup	3. Dressing: combine lemon juice, vinegar, garlic, oil, salt, and ground pepper. Mix well. Set aside.
Red wine vinegar		¼ cup	
Fresh garlic, minced		1 Tbsp	
Extra virgin olive oil		¼ cup	
Salt		2 tsp	
Ground white pepper		½ tsp	
*Fresh red bell peppers, diced	5 ½ oz	1 cup	4. Combine red peppers, green onions, red onions, tomatoes, and black olives in a large bowl. Add dressing.
*Fresh green onions, diced	2 oz	½ cup	
*Fresh red onions, diced	3 oz	½ cup	
*Fresh cherry tomatoes, halved	11 ½ oz	2 cups	
Black olives, sliced	2 ½ oz	½ cup	
Feta cheese, crumbled	3 oz	½ cup	5. Mix in cooled quinoa. Fold in feta cheese and parsley.
*Fresh parsley, finely chopped		1 cup	
			6. Transfer to a steam table pan (12" x 20" x 2 ½"). For 25 servings, use 1 pan.
			7. Critical Control Point: Cool to 40 °F or lower within 4 hours. Cover and refrigerate until service.
			8. Portion with 6 fl oz spoodle (¾ cup).

Plating instructions

Notes

Marketing
guide

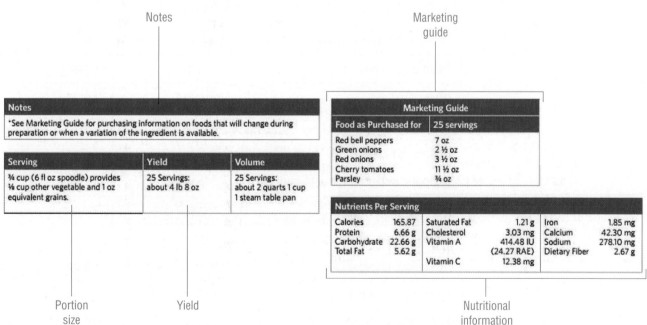

Notes

*See Marketing Guide for purchasing information on foods that will change during preparation or when a variation of the ingredient is available.

Serving	Yield	Volume
¾ cup (6 fl oz spoodle) provides ¼ cup other vegetable and 1 oz equivalent grains.	25 Servings: about 4 lb 8 oz	25 Servings: about 2 quarts 1 cup 1 steam table pan

Marketing Guide	
Food as Purchased for	25 servings
Red bell peppers	7 oz
Green onions	2 ½ oz
Red onions	3 ½ oz
Cherry tomatoes	11 ½ oz
Parsley	¾ oz

Nutrients Per Serving					
Calories	165.87	Saturated Fat	1.21 g	Iron	1.85 mg
Protein	6.66 g	Cholesterol	3.03 mg	Calcium	42.30 mg
Carbohydrate	22.66 g	Vitamin A	414.48 IU	Sodium	278.10 mg
Total Fat	5.62 g		(24.27 RAE)	Dietary Fiber	2.67 g
		Vitamin C	12.38 mg		

Portion
size

Yield

Nutritional
information

Figure 15.15   The distinct parts of a standard recipe, which was found at the USDA website.

factor adjusts the amount of each ingredient from the original recipe to determine how much is needed in the revised recipe. Calculate a conversion factor using this formula:

$$\text{new yield} \div \text{old yield} = \text{conversion factor}$$

Now you can apply the conversion factor to each ingredient in the recipe.

$$\text{original quantity} \times \text{conversion factor} = \text{new quantity}$$

Gerry, the dietary manager, would like to sample a new recipe to see if it would be a good addition to the hospital menu. While the standardized recipe for Mediterranean Quinoa Salad (see Figure 15.15) makes 25 portions, he will need only five portions for sampling. He adjusts the yield by determining the conversion factor. For Gerry's recipe, the formula looks like this:

$$5 \text{ portions} \div 25 \text{ portions} = 0.2 \text{ conversion factor}$$

Gerry now converts the ingredient measurements using the conversion factor.

Note that for calculations of smaller amounts of an ingredient, the nearest measurable amount is used. For example, the measurement for salt in Figure 15.16 is 2 tsp. When multiplied by the conversion factor of .2, the result is .4 tsp. The nearest measurable amount is ½ tsp because measuring spoons do not have markings in 1/10 increments.

Figure 15.16 Recipe Ingredient Conversions		
Ingredient	25 servings	5 servings
quinoa	1 lb, 10 ½ oz	5.3 oz
chicken broth, low-salt	2 quarts	12.8 oz
lemon juice	¼ cup	0.4 oz
vinegar, red wine	¼ cup	0.4 oz
fresh garlic, minced	1 tbsp	½ tsp
olive oil	¼ cup	0.4 oz
salt	2 tsp	½ tsp
pepper, white ground	½ tsp	1/10 tsp
peppers, sweet red, fresh, chopped	5 ½ oz	1.1 oz
parsley, raw, chopped	1 cup	0.2 cup
green onions, diced	2 oz	0.4 oz
red onion, chopped	3 oz	0.6 oz
cherry tomatoes, halved	11 ½ oz	2.3 oz
black olives, sliced	2 ½ oz	0.5 oz
feta cheese, crumbled	3 oz	0.6 oz

Costing Recipes. Like most food service establishments, healthcare facilities purchase food in bulk amounts such as a case, bushel, or flat. However, to stay within budget guidelines, the manager must figure out how much money is needed to make each food item. This process is called *costing*. To cost a recipe, you must convert the bulk purchase units into the units used in the recipe, such as pounds, ounces, or pieces. When you know the **unit cost** of each item, you can calculate the total cost for each ingredient in a recipe. Use the following formulas to determine the unit cost of food items.

unit cost
the price of one measurable unit of a food item, such as one pound, one ounce, or one piece

- **Per pound unit cost:** divide the unit cost by the number of pounds in the unit

  Example: $73.00 (per case of apples) ÷ 40 (pounds per case) = $1.83/pound

- **Per ounce unit cost:** divide the price per pound by 16 to get the price per ounce

  Example: $14.00 (per pound of feta cheese) ÷ 16 = $0.88/ounce

- **Per piece unit cost:** divide the cost of the unit by the number of pieces in the unit

  Example: $40.00 (per box of oranges) ÷ 75 (oranges in each box) = $0.53/orange

When you know the unit cost of each ingredient, you can easily multiply the unit cost by the number of units used in the recipe to determine the **ingredient cost** of each item. For example, Gerry's recipe calls for feta cheese: 5 oz (in the recipe) × $0.88 (unit cost per ounce) = $4.40 (cost for feta cheese used in the recipe).

Add the cost for each ingredient to determine the total food costs for a recipe, or the **recipe cost**. Since recipe costing is repeated regularly to reflect changing food costs, most organizations purchase a software program that will automatically cost a recipe as new food prices are entered into the program.

Gerry follows a budget for the hospital food services department, so he tracks the costs of all foods purchased for hospital use. In addition, he routinely costs the recipes used in food preparation. By knowing the cost of each recipe, Gerry can make appropriate substitutions to save money. For example, he can save money by substituting canned tomatoes for fresh tomatoes in a chili recipe. In addition, he uses the cost of a recipe as a guide for pricing menu items sold in the hospital cafeteria. Figure 15.17 on the next page shows how Gerry determines the recipe cost for his new recipe.

Note that standard equivalents such as 1 cup equaling 8 ounces work only for liquid ingredients. Measurements of dry ingredients like the parsley used in this recipe must be calculated based on the actual weight of each ingredient. For example, 1 cup of parsley does not weigh nearly as much as 1 cup of butter.

Measuring and Recording Food Intake

Because healthcare workers use therapeutic diets to improve patients' medical conditions, workers are concerned not only with food service but also with food intake. Serving the healthiest foods will not improve

Figure 15.17 Recipe Cost Sheet

Recipe	Yield		Portion	
Mediterranean Quinoa Salad	25 servings		¾ cup	
Ingredient	**Amount**	**Unit Cost**	**Total Cost**	
quinoa	1 lb, 10 ½ oz	$0.43/oz	$11.40	
chicken broth, low-salt	2 quarts = 64 oz	$0.10/oz	$6.40	
lemon juice	¼ cup = 2 oz	$0.07/oz	$0.14	
vinegar, red wine	¼ cup = 2 oz	$0.22/oz	$0.44	
olive oil	¼ cup = 2 oz	$0.31/oz	$0.62	
salt	2 tsp = .4 oz	$0.03/oz	$0.01	
pepper, white ground	½ tsp = .08 oz	$3.51/oz	$0.28	
peppers, sweet red, fresh, chopped	5 ½ oz	$0.16/oz	$0.88	
parsley, raw, chopped	1 cup = .9 oz	$0.35/oz	$0.32	
green onions, diced	2 oz	$0.30/oz	$0.60	
red onion, chopped	3 oz	$0.09/oz	$0.27	
cherry tomatoes, halved	11 ½ oz	$0.29/oz	$3.34	
black olives, sliced	2 ½ oz	$0.45/oz	$1.13	
feta cheese, crumbled	3 oz	$1.00/oz	$3.00	
Total Recipe Cost	**Date Costed**		**Portion Cost**	
$28.83	11/19/2015		$1.15	

Simulate
EHR

a patient's condition if the patient does not consume the food. For this reason, healthcare workers estimate and record food intake for residents in most long-term care facilities and some patients in hospitals. Sometimes you will estimate the total percentage of a meal that was consumed, such as *ate 70% of breakfast, 80% of lunch, and 50% of dinner* . If a person eats less than 70 percent of a meal, report that information to the nurse as well as recording it.

In some facilities, you will record the percentage of each food eaten, such as *for dinner—ate 100% of rice, 50% of chicken breast, 80% of salad, and 100% of bread* (Figure 15.18). The dietitian converts these percentages into total calories consumed and records this information in the patient's chart. Using standardized recipes that include nutritional information simplifies this calculation.

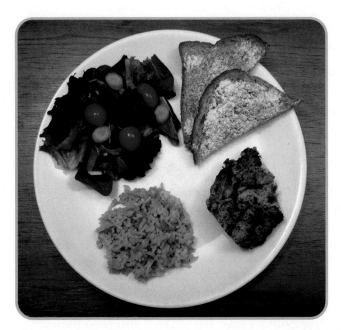
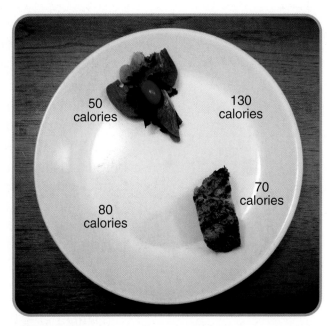

Figure 15.18 Using the nutritional information for each food item, a dietitian converts the percentages of each food eaten into total calories consumed. In this instance, the patient ate 100 percent of the rice, 50 percent of the chicken breast, 80 percent of the salad, and 100 percent of the bread.

Measuring and Recording Intake and Output

Fluid balance is important to the healthy functioning of your body. It prevents heatstroke and helps maintain proper kidney and heart functions. A drop in fluid levels can result in hypotension and reduced kidney function. Healthcare workers must be alert for signs of fluid imbalance in all of their patients because it can result in dehydration or edema. However, patients with medical conditions such as heart or kidney disease, severe burns, or hemorrhaging require particular attention regarding fluid balance.

When the physician writes an order to "maintain intake and output measurements," all of the fluids that enter and leave the body are measured and recorded using an **intake and output (I&O)** sheet. In healthcare facilities, fluids are measured in milliliters (mL) or cubic centimeters (cc). One fluid ounce equals 30 mL or 30 cc. At the end of each shift and at the end of each 24-hour period, the amounts are totaled. Ideally, the intake amount will roughly equal the output amount to maintain fluid balance. Healthy adults consume 48 to 96 ounces (1,440 to 2,880 mL) of liquid each day to keep up with the fluids that normally leave the body as urine, feces, sweat, and the air we exhale.

Fluid intake includes all of the fluids we drink as well as foods that are liquid at room temperature. Gelatin, broth, ice cream, and sherbet are part of fluid intake. If a patient receives IV fluids or enteral (tube) nutrition, the nurse will record the amounts given.

Follow these steps to record fluid intake:

1. Begin by learning the amount of fluid held by the cups, glasses, and bowls used in your facility.

fluid balance
term for a state in which the amount of fluid taken into the body equals the amount of fluid that leaves the body

intake and output (I&O)
term for measurements of all the fluids that enter and leave the body

2. Be prepared to convert ounces to milliliters.

   Example: 8 oz glass × 30 mL = 240 mL

3. Remember to record the amount consumed rather than the amount that remains.

   Example: if a patient leaves an 8 oz glass ¾ full, he has consumed ¼ of the 8 oz (¼ × 8), which equals 2 oz. Multiply by 30 and record (2 oz × 30 mL = 60 mL).

4. Estimate the amount consumed unless the patient requires an exact intake measurement.

   Example: about ¼ (25%) of an 8 oz glass of juice remains when the patient is finished. That means the patient has consumed ¾, or 75%, of the 8 oz (¾ *or* .75 × 8 oz = 6 oz). Multiply by 30 to convert and record (6 oz × 30 mL = 180 mL).

5. When an exact measurement of fluid intake is ordered, collect all remaining liquids at the end of a meal in a **graduated cylinder** (Figure 15.19). Place the cylinder on a flat surface and read the amount at eye level. Subtract this amount from the total amount of liquids offered at the meal to arrive at the accurate fluid intake measurement.

   Example: the patient receives 4 oz of juice, 6 oz of coffee, and 8 oz of milk for a total of 18 oz or 540 mL (18 × 30) of liquid offered with breakfast. At the end of the meal, leftover liquids are poured into the graduated cylinder. They measure 120 mL (540 mL offered – 120 mL not consumed = 420 mL of fluid intake).

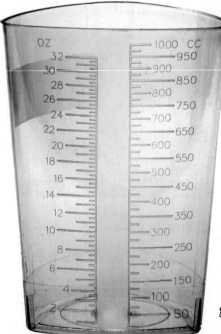

Figure 15.19 Liquid intake is measured in a graduated cylinder and recorded in milliliters.

Measure fluid output in the same way you measured fluid intake. Urine, vomit, blood, wound drainage, and diarrhea are all considered fluid output. Always wear gloves when measuring fluid output. A patient who uses the toilet will need to urinate into a measuring device called a **commode hat**. This container is placed under the toilet seat before the patient urinates. Commode hats and **urinals**, which are used by males confined to bed, have measurements marked on the container for easy reading (Figure 15.20). However, urine from a bedpan or urinary catheter drainage bag must be emptied into a graduated cylinder for measuring.

Vomit is measured using the markings on an emesis (EH-meh-sihs) basin. However, amounts are estimated by the nurse when a patient vomits on the floor or the bedsheets. Amounts for diarrhea, blood, and wound drainage are also estimated unless there is a drainage device to collect wound fluids. Remember to record all output and tally the total amounts at the end of each shift and at the end of each 24-hour period (Figure 15.21 on page 550). The physician will compare fluid intake and output numbers to assess the patient's fluid balance.

Preparing Solutions

Sam needs a 1:10 bleach solution for disinfecting surfaces in patient rooms. Gwen needs to mix frozen juice concentrate with water in a ratio of one part concentrate to four parts water. A dermatologist wants his patient's wound treated with a 10 percent vinegar solution. From

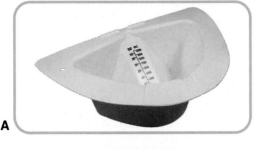

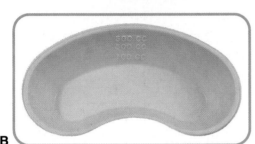

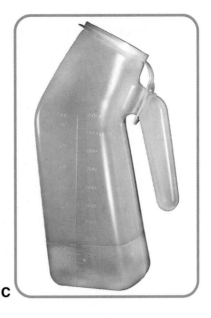

Figure 15.20 Liquid output is frequently measured using a commode hat (A), emesis basin (B), or urinal (C).

housekeeping to food service, from nursing to the medical laboratory and pharmacy, healthcare workers prepare solutions for a wide variety of uses.

Solutions are liquid mixtures that contain two or more chemicals. The liquid used to dissolve a chemical is called the **solvent**. The chemical is the **solute** (SAHL-yoot). All of the preceding examples use water, which is a common solvent. A 1:10 proportion, called the **dilution ratio**, for bleach solution uses one part bleach and nine parts water. A recipe for making bleach solution calls for ¼ cup of bleach and 2¼ cups of water. This represents the measurable amounts for a 1:10 solution.

solutions
uniform mixtures of two or more substances, which may be solids, liquids, gases, or a combination of these

What if you need a larger quantity of bleach solution? Follow these steps to calculate specific amounts of a solution:

1. Begin with the total volume; for example, 1 gallon of bleach solution.

2. Divide this total volume by the second number in your dilution ratio. This second number tells you how many total parts are in the dilution, so the answer will tell you the size of each part.
   Example: 1 gallon (16 cups) ÷ 10 = 1.6 cups

3. Multiply your answer by the first number in your dilution ratio to learn the amount of solute you will need to measure. Since the first number is often one, this calculation is easy. You will need 1.6 cups of bleach.

4. Subtract the amount of solute from the total volume of the solution to learn how much solvent will be needed (16 cups – 1.6 cups = 14.4 cups of water).

5. Note that 0.6 of a cup and 0.4 of a cup are difficult to measure. These amounts must be converted to a combination of tablespoons, teaspoons, and fractions of a cup for accurate measurements because measuring cups aren't calibrated for tenths of a cup.

Working in metric numbers makes calculations and measurements easier. For instance, follow these steps to make 4 liters of 1:10 bleach solution:

- 4 L ÷ 10 = 0.4 L

- 0.4 L × 1 = 0.4 L of bleach (0.4 L can be measured as 400 mL)

- 4 L – 0.4 L = 3.6 L of water (0.6 L can be measured as 600 mL)

Intake and Output Record

Patient's Name: Ben Jones

Water glass 180 mL   Cup 120 mL
Juice glass 100 mL   Soup bowl 200 mL
Small bowl 120 mL   Mug 240 mL

Time	Oral	IV	Irrigation	Remarks	BM	Emesis	Urine	Suction	Remarks
0715	50 mL						550 mL		
0800	240 mL								
0945	120 mL								
1000									
1115	80 mL								
1200 (noon)									
1300									
1430							400 mL		
1500									
TOTAL	490 mL			8 Hr Intake 490 mL			950 mL		8 Hr Output 950 mL
1600	240 mL								
1730	180 mL								
1800	300 mL						375 mL		
1900									
2000									
2130	50 mL					400 mL			
2200									
2300									
TOTAL	770 mL			8 Hr Intake 770 mL		400 mL	375 mL		8 Hr Output 775 mL
2400 (midnight)						200 mL			
0115						150 mL			
0230						80 mL			
0300									
0400									
0530		500 mL					300 mL		
0600									
TOTAL		500 mL		8 Hr Intake 500 mL		430 mL	300 mL		8 Hr Output 730 mL
TOTALS	1260 mL	500 mL		24 Hr Intake 1760 mL		830 mL	1625 mL		24 Hr Output 2455 mL

Figure 15.21   A patient's intake and output should be recorded in a chart like this one.

Simulate EHR

Mixing juice using one part juice concentrate and four parts water means that you are making a 1:5 solution (1 + 4 = 5 total parts in the solution). You can calculate the amounts to make 1 liter of grape juice using the same steps you used for the bleach solution:

- 1 L ÷ 5 = 0.2 L

- 0.2 L × 1 = 0.2 L (200 mL) of juice concentrate

- 1 L − 0.2 L = 0.8 L (800 mL) of water

Solutions are often expressed as percentages. Percent means *per hundred,* so a solution expressed as a percentage tells you how much of the solute is found in every 100 mL of the solution. For example, a 10% vinegar solution contains 10 mL of vinegar in 100 mL of solution; 10% represents the ratio 10:100, which can also be expressed as 1:10 (Figure 15.22). Therefore, the vinegar solution uses the same dilution formula as the bleach solution. You can use the same steps to calculate the amounts of vinegar and water for the total volume of solution you will mix.

Because solutions contain chemicals, always be alert for possible hazards. Consult safety data sheets (SDS) and never mix solutions until you have verified that the chemicals are compatible. Follow all safety guidelines for handling, storing, disposing of, and removing spills of chemical solutions.

Consider the effectiveness of the solutions you prepare and use. They may have a limited life. For example, bleach solutions begin to lose their disinfectant power quickly when exposed to heat, sunlight, and evaporation. To be certain that a bleach solution is still strong enough to kill germs, mix a fresh solution each day and discard unused amounts at the end of the day.

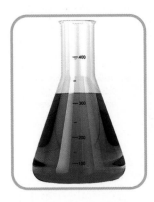
1:10
solution

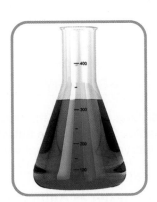
10%
solution

Figure 15.22 Solutions can be expressed as percentages or ratios. Which solution is stronger?

RECALL YOUR READING

1. Food _____ measurements are more accurate and consistent than _____ measurements.

2. _____ of recipes is critical when a health condition depends on _____ or _____ certain foods or ingredients.

3. Recipes can be adjusted by calculating the _____ factor.

4. Healthcare workers measure and record _____ and _____ to monitor fluid balance.

5. Solutions have two parts, the _____ and the _____.

Complete the
Map Your Reading
graphic organizer for the
section you just read.

SUMMARY

 Assess your understanding with chapter tests

- Technical communication helps workers accomplish job tasks.

- Technical reading requires attention and concentration because technical documents are filled with detailed information.

- The graphics found in a technical document, such as charts and tables, may provide important information needed to accomplish your task.

- Technical writing is clear and concise and informs or persuades a specific audience.

- Successful technical writing expresses complex information in language that the target audience can understand.

- Electronic health record systems go through a certification process to verify that they have met the current requirements for functionality, interoperability, and security.

- Clinical simulation technicians set up simulation events and program care scenarios that are used to train healthcare workers.

- Technologies such as bar code scanning and radio frequency identification (RFID) tracking are streamlining healthcare inventory functions and medical chart access.

- QR codes provide quick access to websites that provide healthcare information and instructions for patients.

- Dietitians and nutritionists use diet analysis programs to manage diseases and conditions that require special diets.

- Food weight measurements are more accurate and consistent than volume measurements.

- Healthcare workers follow standardized recipes because standardization can be critical for patients whose health condition depends on regulating or avoiding particular food items or ingredients.

- Healthcare workers measure and record intake and output for the purpose of monitoring fluid balance.

- When estimating fluid intake, make sure you record the amount consumed rather than the amount left in the container.

- Healthcare workers prepare solutions for a wide variety of uses. Because some solutions contain chemicals, workers must be alert to potential dangers and follow safe handling procedures.

MAXIMIZE YOUR PROFESSIONAL VOCABULARY

 Build vocabulary with e-flash cards, games, and audio glossary

Listed below are the essential, yellow-highlighted terms and the additional professional vocabulary that you encountered in this chapter. Complete the activities that follow the list to make all of these terms part of your everyday professional vocabulary.

bar code scanner
commode hat
conversion factor
dilution ratio
executive summary
fluid balance
graduated cylinder
ingredient cost
intake and output (I&O)
interoperability
nourishments

Office of the National Coordinator as Authorized Testing and Certification Body (ONC-ATCB)
paraphrase
portion
quick response (QR) code
radio frequency identification (RFID)
recipe cost
simulate

solute
solutions
solvent
tare weight
target audience
technical reading
technical writing
unit cost
urinals
yield

VOCABULARY DEVELOPMENT

Matching. Match the essential terms from this chapter with the best descriptions below by writing the letter of the description next to the number of the essential term on your answer sheet.

1. bar code scanner
2. fluid balance
3. intake and output (I&O)
4. interoperability
5. portion
6. quick response (QR) code
7. radio frequency identification (RFID)
8. solutions
9. tare weight
10. technical reading
11. technical writing
12. unit cost
13. yield

a. uniform mixtures of two or more substances, which may be solids, liquids, gases, or a combination of these

b. term for a state in which the amount of fluid taken into the body equals the amount of fluid that leaves the body

c. the number of portions a recipe will produce

d. a device that captures a printed series of numbered black bars and spaces, translates them into numbers and letters, and sends the data to a computer to access information about a patient or product

e. term for measurements of all the fluids that enter and leave the body

f. a data collection technology that uses electronic tags for storing data

g. a type of writing used in the workplace to inform or persuade a specific audience

h. the price of one measurable unit of a food item, such as 1 pound, 1 ounce, or 1 piece

i. the ability to exchange and use computer information within and across networks

j. the amount of food in one serving

k. the weight of an empty container

l. a two-dimensional bar code that is used to provide easy access to information through a smartphone; also known as *quick read code*

m. a skill used to comprehend science, business, or technology publications

14. **Write It, Define It.** Select one or more of the professional vocabulary terms from the chapter. Write the terms you chose on slips of paper. Put the slips of paper in a basket or bowl with all of your classmates' terms. Pass the bowl or basket around the class, each student selecting a term at random. When you select a term, define the term on your slip of paper, explain how it applies as a fundamental skill, or connect it to healthcare support services. Keep passing the bowl or basket of words around until they have all been taken.

15. **That's My Term.** The instructor will distribute one professional vocabulary term card or definition card to each student. Students will take turns reading a definition card. The student with the term card that matches the definition being read will stand up and say, "That's My Term."

REFLECT ON YOUR READING

16. Review the *Reading Technical Documents* section in this chapter. Compare and contrast

the list of techniques you developed in the *Connect with Your Reading* activity with the information suggested in the text. Discuss your findings with a classmate and develop a final list of steps you will take to improve your technical reading skills.

BUILD CORE SKILLS

17. **Reading.** Identify which of the following are excerpts from technical documents. Explain your answers.

- A simple technique has been developed to encapsulate lidocaine, a common painkiller, in the tiny needles attached to an adhesive patch.

- I believe arthritis can be managed and treated so that people afflicted can live productively and comfortably.

- The class about stem cells is the best course this school offers because Dr. Smith has so much experience working in this field.

- Healthy lifestyles include a wide variety of fruits and vegetables. Individuals who consistently eat five or more servings per day see improvements in skin health, brain health, and vitality.

- This new machine features the fastest imaging rate available on the market.

- Sun exposure rapidly reduces plasmacytoid dendritic cells and inflammatory dermal dendritic cells in psoriatic skin.

18. Writing. Work with a partner to compile and organize information and then write a technical report that would be used in a healthcare setting. This might be a hospital menu, patient brochure, or set of instructions for a piece of equipment. Once you have your document, exchange it with another group's document. Edit and evaluate the other team's document. What criteria did you use? Share your findings with the class.

19. Reading. Search the Internet sites for PubMed Health or Cochrane reviews. Select an executive summary or research report related to healthcare. Read the document and use the technical reading techniques mentioned in this chapter to ensure your understanding of the material. Record which techniques you use and discuss your process with a classmate.

20. Writing. Rewrite the technical document that you read for the previous activity. Use simpler terms so that the document is easier for a patient to understand. Ask a family member to read your simplified document. Explain any information they did not understand and use your explanations to clarify your writing.

21. Math. Display the data listed below in a graph that makes the data easier to visualize and compare. Numbers indicate procedures performed in one year.

Inpatient Surgeries Performed in the US
- coronary artery bypass graft: 395,000
- total knee replacement: 719,000
- total hip replacement: 332,000
- Cesarean section: 1,300,000
- cardiac catheterizations: 1,000,000
- diagnostic ultrasound: 1,100,000
- reduction of fracture: 671,000

Total number of procedures performed: 51,400,000

22. Critical Thinking. Think about what you do when you need to read and comprehend a difficult document for class or for work. Analyze and describe your ideal technical reading environment. What do you think is the best setting for reading a difficult document? Do you listen to music or prefer silence? Compare your criteria for a technical reading environment with a classmate's criteria.

23. Speaking and Listening. Survey a healthcare worker about the records system used in the facility where he or she works. Focus on the functionality, interoperability, and security of the system. Share your findings with the class.

24. Critical Thinking. Identify QR codes that you or your family currently use. How or why are they useful?

25. Critical Thinking. Relate the use of QR codes to healthcare. How are QR codes used in the following healthcare areas?
- patient care
- healthcare marketing and public relations
- pharmacy

26. Problem Solving. Use the USDA's SuperTracker to analyze your personal diet and exercise habits. Apply the results to create personal goals for developing a healthier lifestyle.

27. Problem Solving. Develop and write a one-day menu plan for a patient with a specific chronic health condition using the USDA SuperTracker. Organize your ideas and compile them into a summary that includes recommendations regarding calories and nutrients that may need to be limited. Analyze your menu to verify that it meets the dietary recommendations. Present your menu plan to the class and explain how it will improve your patient's condition.

28. Math. For dinner, each patient in your care receives the following meal: a 4-oz. chicken breast (186 calories), a cup of green beans (44 calories), a small dinner roll (87 calories), and a cup of apple juice (110 calories). Calculate the total number of calories consumed by each patient using the percentages below.
- Mabel ate 50% of chicken breast, 90% of green beans, 100% of dinner roll, and 100% of apple juice.
- Saul ate 80% of chicken breast, 20% of green beans, 100% of dinner roll, and 100% of apple juice.

29. **Critical Thinking.** Answer the following questions related to intake and output (I&O).

   a. Why or how is fluid balance critical to body functioning?

   b. Which items are considered intake and which are included in output?

   c. Why are gelatins, ice cream, and sherbet considered part of fluid intake?

   d. How are I&O measurements taken and recorded?

   e. How does the physician use I&O data?

30. **Math.** Use the following information to answer the questions below: Kris needs to mix three gallons of sports drink to keep his physical therapy patients properly hydrated. The sports drink solution should be one part concentrate and five parts water.

   a. What is the dilution ratio of concentrate in the sports drink solution?

   b. How much concentrate does Kris need to make three gallons of sports drink?

   c. How much water should Kris use to make three gallons of sports drink?

31. **Math.** Calculate the specific amounts of solute and solvent for solutions based on the percentages or dilution ratios listed here. Refer to the *Preparing Solutions* section in this chapter and, if needed, use the equivalents information in Figure 7.22 to convert your calculations to measurable amounts.

   a. 1 liter of a 10% solution

   b. 100 mL of a 25% solution

   c. 5 mL of a 15% solution

   d. 2 gallons of a 50:100 solution

   e. 1 cup of a 1:12 solution

ACTIVATE YOUR LEARNING

32. Find a low-fat recipe that has at least six ingredients. Convert the recipe by doubling the yield. Then, visit a local grocery store or use the Internet to find prices of the various ingredients. Cost the original recipe. Complete a recipe cost sheet using Figure 15.17 as a guide.

33. For each measurement listed here, calculate the weight of the product using two different containers. The tare weight of the containers are 1 oz and 5 oz respectively.

- 1 lb
- 6 oz
- 2.5 lbs
- 30 oz
- 1¼ lbs

Assemble equipment and supplies provided by your instructor and practice weighing food items. Record the food weights, taking into account the tare weight of the container used.

34. Assemble supplies and equipment provided by your instructor. Prepare 500 mL of a 1:10 solution.

THINK AND ACT LIKE A HEALTHCARE WORKER

35. Work in groups of three to prepare a technical document that will be used in the following scenario: Your group is part of the public health department and you're writing a one-page proposal explaining your plan for advising the public about environmental hazards and household toxins. Collaborate as a team to develop a clear and convincing document. In your group, one person should plan the document, one should draft and revise the document, and one should edit the document into a final draft.

36. The central services department has requested an inventory of equipment for a resident's room at your worksite. Imagine that your classroom is that room. Identify and make a list of equipment and items that would have bar codes for tracking inventory. Then list 10 consumable items that could have bar codes for billing purposes. Compare your list with the lists your classmates created to see what bar codes you may have missed.

GO TO THE SOURCE

37. Visit a simulation lab to observe a simulation mannequin. How does the technician use this technology to create a realistic simulation? What are the advantages and disadvantages of this type of technology for someone training to be a healthcare worker?

38. Locate a healthcare-related QR code on a billboard, in a magazine, or in some other type of advertisement. How might you use this information in your role as a healthcare worker?

Chapter 16
Professional Knowledge in Support Services

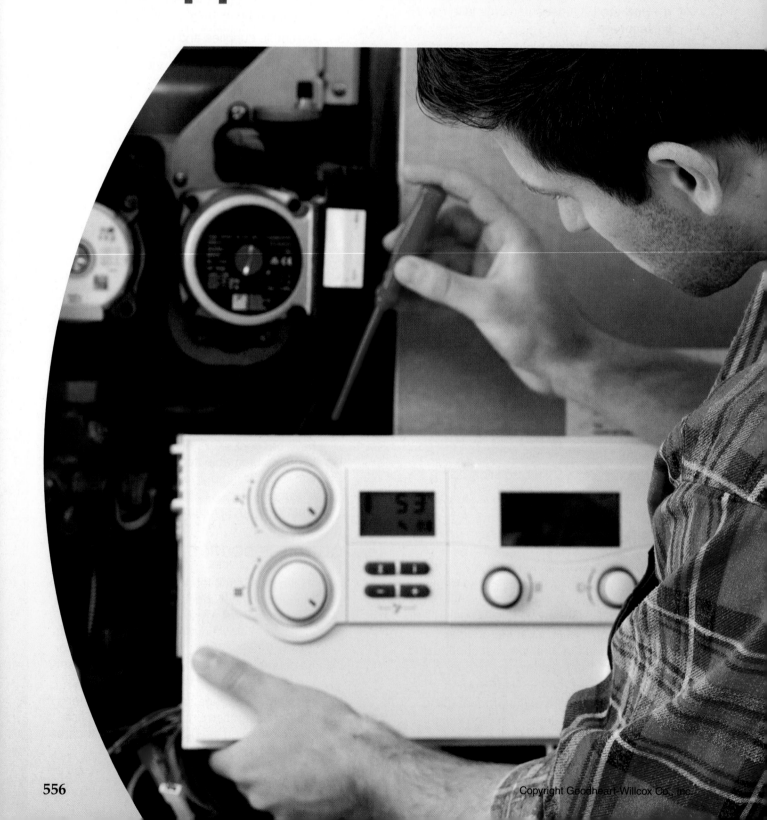

PROFESSIONAL VOCABULARY

 E-flash Cards

You will need to learn the essential terms listed below before you begin your reading. These terms will help you understand the main concepts of the chapter. These terms, which will be highlighted in yellow within the text, will become part of your professional vocabulary.

In addition to these essential terms, you will see bold terms throughout the chapter. The meanings of these terms are explained where the terms first appear. The bold terms, like the essential terms listed here, will also become part of your professional vocabulary and deepen your understanding of the topics presented.

calibration   the adjustment of a piece of equipment so that it operates within its intended standards of performance

danger zone   the range of temperature from 40°F to 140°F at which bacteria grow most rapidly to the levels that cause food poisoning

discrimination   unfair treatment of individuals on the basis of their membership in a specific group, such as age, ethnicity, gender, nationality, or religion

fire triangle   term that describes the three elements of a fire, which include oxygen, fuel, and a heat source

grounding   the act of carrying current safely away from an electrical circuit to prevent shocks from occurring in the event of a problem with the circuit

harassment   unwelcome, offensive, and repeated language or actions based on race, color, religion, sex, national origin, age, disability, or genetic information that affect an employee's job performance or advancement opportunities or create an uncomfortable working environment

infrastructure   term that describes the internal systems that a facility needs to operate, such as power supplies; electrical, plumbing, and heating and cooling systems; water; waste management; and phones and computer systems

minimum wage   the lowest hourly earnings that an employer can legally pay a worker

overtime pay   payment at one and a half times the regular wage for each hour an employee works beyond 40 hours in a week

soft skills   employability skills related to communication, attitude, teamwork, and problem solving that are difficult to teach but critical to workplace success

work ethic   a belief in the benefits of working hard, demonstrating initiative, and being personally accountable for the work you do

CONNECT WITH YOUR READING

Are support workers really important to the healthcare system? Rolando Santiago works in an urban hospital as a transport technician. His job is to help move patients from their rooms to other areas of the hospital, such as the imaging center, other labs, surgery, and the front lobby when they are discharged.

Rolando understands that many patients feel anxious in the hospital and does his best to ease their fears. He always introduces himself when he appears in their room. He explains what he will be doing and where he is taking them before he begins. He tells them to let him know when they are ready to move, though he also finds ways to coax those who are reluctant to move because they are tired, worried, or in pain. When Rolando sees children who have cancer, or older patients who are frail and mentally confused, his heart aches. Nevertheless, he always has a smile and a hopeful word for them as he tries to make them feel at ease.

Rolando's work supports the healthcare team. He is happy not to have the life-and-death stress that doctors and nurses face when diagnosing and curing disease. At the same time, he believes that a patient in good spirits is more likely to respond to treatment. "And," he says, "if there's anything I can do to help someone feel good, or feel a little hope, you can bet I'll do it."

Rolando plays a support services role in moving patients from one place to another. How do his attitude and actions make a difference to those patients?

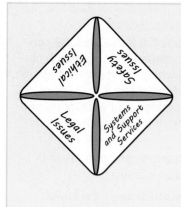

MAP YOUR READING

Can you identify the important role of support services workers in healthcare? Create a visual summary to record your ideas. Begin with a square sheet of paper—an 8½-inch square works well. Fold each of the four points of the square to the center. Label each of the four resulting flaps with one of these topics: *Systems and Support Services*, *Legal Issues*, *Ethical Issues*, and *Safety Issues*. When you finish reading each of these sections in the chapter, open the corresponding flap and draw a picture or symbol to illustrate Rolando's role in this situation. Ask yourself how support services workers impact the healthcare system, legal issues, ethical issues, and safety. Finally, write three or four keywords below each drawing that help highlight these important topics.

As you have learned in this unit, support services workers play an important role in the function and safety of a healthcare facility. Much of their job relies on certain professional knowledge, such as safety guidelines and employment laws. In this chapter, you will learn what support services workers need to know to help keep the healthcare system running smoothly.

Support services provide the processes for the throughput and feedback functions of that system. An overview of basic employment laws will help you, as an entry-level worker, to know your rights and responsibilities. Knowing safety guidelines will help you protect patients, yourself, and other workers from falls, fire, electrocution, foodborne illness, and other disasters.

Systems and the Support Services Pathway

People who work in support services careers do not generally deal directly with patients or provide healthcare. Nevertheless, they are vital to a healthcare facility's ability to provide efficient, high-quality care. Remember what you learned about systems in chapter 4. Every system consists of input, throughput, output, feedback, and its internal and external environment. Healthcare providers rely on the work of those in the support services pathway to create a smooth flow in the throughput and feedback mechanisms of the healthcare system.

A physician who speaks only English may need an interpreter to gather information from a patient or communicate a diagnosis to a patient who speaks Hmong. A pathologist depends on biomedical equipment technicians to ensure that the diagnostic equipment in the lab is working properly. A nurse requires workers in the central services department to ensure that all supplies are on hand when they are needed. Every healthcare employee participates in some aspect of quality improvement feedback for the betterment of the system (Figure 16.1). These functions are provided through support services.

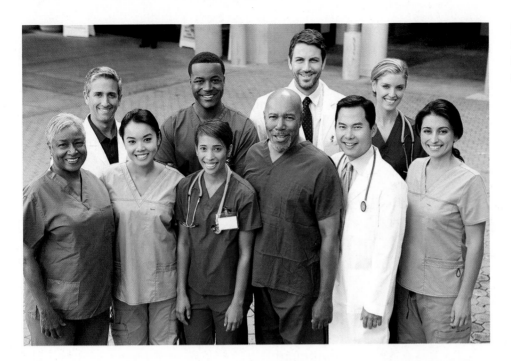

Figure 16.1   All of the employees in a healthcare setting help the facility run smoothly.

Maintaining the Healthcare Environment

As you can see from these examples, support services are essential to maintaining the healthcare environment. Without this system throughput, the healthcare system would break down. Support services include several different areas of work.

Facilities Management. Facilities managers have the overall responsibility of ensuring that a healthcare facility operates smoothly. They address issues concerning the facility's **infrastructure**, which includes all of the internal systems that a facility needs to function day-to-day. The facilities manager is responsible for regular operations, such as maintaining parking facilities and other areas used by outpatients and visitors. This person must plan for emergencies, making sure that there is a backup power supply in case of a power outage. He or she is also concerned with controlling costs and avoiding waste in all facility operations.

infrastructure
term that describes the internal systems that a facility needs to operate, such as power supplies; electrical, plumbing, and heating and cooling systems; water; waste management; and phones and computer systems

Health and Safety. Health and safety workers ensure that healthcare facilities follow all occupational health and safety laws and regulations. This is, of course, a vital function of healthcare facilities. Ensuring that a health care facility complies with Occupational Safety and Health Administration (OSHA) regulations is a full-time job for occupational health and safety specialists. They examine conditions and equipment for potential hazards, conduct safety trainings, and investigate accidents. Their goal is to increase employee productivity and save money by reducing fines, insurance premiums, and workers' compensation costs. They may use an **Illness and Injury Prevention Program (I2P2)** as a proactive, systemic approach to finding and fixing hazards before people are injured. Industrial hygienists ensure that patients and visitors are not exposed to biological or chemical hazards that could cause illness or injury or worsen existing conditions.

Housekeeping. The housekeeping department supports the healthcare system by complying with OSHA standards for cleanliness and safety. Workers perform general cleaning, sanitization, and disinfection of patient care areas and workspaces. Housekeeping staff may be called on to clean up spills or perform terminal cleaning when a patient is transferred out of a room. Housekeepers' work helps prevent the spread of communicable diseases and assists the healthcare facility in presenting its best appearance to its customers.

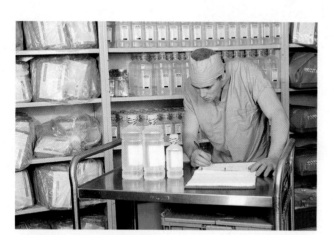

Figure 16.2   Employees in the central services department help maintain a healthcare facility's inventory of equipment, instruments, linens, and uniforms.

Central Services. The central services, or *central supply*, area of a healthcare facility is vitally important. Workers in this area provide the supplies and equipment used by healthcare providers throughout the facility. They maintain the **inventory**, or *count*, of both disposable and durable medical equipment (Figure 16.2). In a large healthcare facility, central supply is responsible for a huge amount of materials and equipment.

These workers ensure that instruments, equipment, linens, and uniforms are clean and germ-free. They sort, inspect, and use specialized equipment and chemicals to clean, disinfect, or sterilize them. The healthcare industry averages 15.5 pounds of linen per day per patient. Some facilities rent their linens and uniforms from a contracted linen service that provides laundry disinfection and delivery.

Pharmacy. Healthcare facilities such as hospitals maintain their own pharmacies so they can provide both inpatients and outpatients with necessary medications. Pharmacy managers control the ordering and dispensing of these medications. They must maintain an inventory of the medications to ensure that there is an adequate stock on hand at all times. They also have to follow rules when giving out medications to prevent errors that could jeopardize patients' health or allow healthcare personnel to obtain drugs for personal or other use. It is important to check the drug label carefully against the prescription name and dosage (Figure 16.3).

Some powerful medications are called **controlled substances**, which means the government has strict rules about dispensing them for medical use. Pharmacy managers must be sure that these medications are given only to authorized people for legitimate medical reasons. Managers must maintain careful records regarding who received a drug, when the drug was received, how much was received, and for whom it was intended. Even with other medications, pharmacy managers need to maintain careful records.

Pharmacy staff must check medication orders against patient records to make sure that each medication is appropriate for a patient's condition. A medication that is contraindicated may cause an allergic reaction, have a negative impact on another medical condition, or interact with another medication the patient is taking. In this case, the medication should not be given without further consultation with the medical professional who prescribed it. This medication check is an important safeguard against medical errors.

Biomedical Equipment. Engineers design and evaluate the performance of medical devices and machines used for diagnostic and therapeutic purposes. They also teach other healthcare workers how to use this equipment. A biomedical technician installs these machines, calibrates them, and maintains and repairs them to ensure that they function properly. **Calibration** is an important step that ensures a piece of equipment works as intended. Workers in this area affect the work of professionals in the diagnostic and therapeutic pathways. Those workers use the machines and equipment biomedical engineers design and maintain them.

Transport Services. Workers in transport services move patients from one area of a healthcare facility to another or from one facility to another. Transport technicians interact directly with patients, making them unlike most other workers in support services. While they do not provide healthcare, their work facilitates the work of healthcare providers and helps patients have a comfortable and satisfactory experience.

Transport technicians may take patients from their rooms to testing rooms or to the exit when they are discharged from the hospital. Patients are moved on **gurneys**, which are wheeled stretchers, or in wheelchairs. Transport technicians may have to manage drainage bags, IV poles, and oxygen tanks that are part of a patient's treatment.

Technicians also move equipment from storage areas to other areas of the facility so it is available when needed. Some transport technicians drive transport vehicles to move patients between healthcare facilities or to their home. Transport staff must know how to operate the wheelchair lift and properly secure their patient for transport. These services may also be contracted out through transportation service companies.

Dietary Services. Dietary services workers support patients by following the diet prescribed in their healthcare plans (Figure 16.4). They also serve employees and visitors through the cafeteria food service. Dietary workers need to manage their inventory and pay attention to special food handling procedures so that food is not wasted or allowed to spoil. Careful food handling also prevents problems created by food allergies or special diets.

Dietary workers check prepared meal trays carefully against the patients' choices and any prescribed diets to ensure that they match before delivering trays to the patient. The timely and appetizing presentation of food helps encourage patients to eat an adequate supply of healthful nutrients, which is an important part of the healing process.

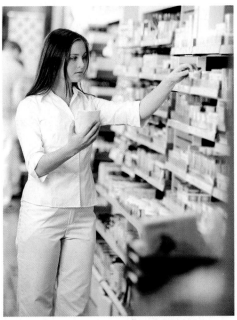

Figure 16.3   Pharmacy workers must check each medication carefully before it is dispensed. What is the purpose of these checks?

calibration
the adjustment of a piece of equipment so that it operates within its intended standards of performance

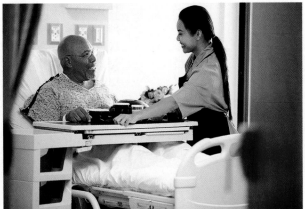

Figure 16.4   Dietary services workers serve patients meals created especially for them. Why would servers need to practice good food handling procedures?

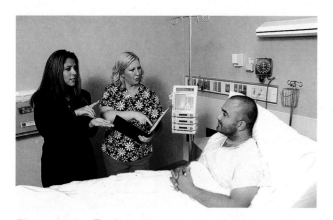

Figure 16.5   Each state has its own requirements for certification or licensure of interpreters. The training for sign language interpreters is different from training for foreign language interpreters.

Interpreting Services. Interpreter is another support services career that brings workers into direct contact with patients. An interpreter bridges the language gap between provider and patient so they can communicate effectively with patients or family members who have limited or no ability to speak English. Interpreters usually specialize in one or more languages, including American Sign Language (Figure 16.5).

While they are not directly involved in providing care, interpreters enable providers to give care and patients to receive care. These workers ensure that information is communicated in a way that patients can understand before they consent to medical procedures. Interpreters also assist healthcare providers in gathering essential information to diagnose conditions, make treatment decisions, and avoid medical errors.

Mortuary and Bereavement. Morgues may be located in hospitals, care centers, hospices, or nursing homes. They preserve dead bodies in refrigerated compartments until viewing, identification, or autopsy can be completed, or until the bodies are transported to funeral homes. A morgue cart may be used to move the body, often using freight elevators and separate entrances from those used by visitors and staff. This separation reduces anxiety for family and other patients who don't want to be reminded of death. Funeral homes support the family with embalming, cremation, funeral, and burial services. Hospitals, nursing homes, hospice facilities, and funeral homes have bereavement staff who are specially trained to support patients, family, and staff in dealing with end-of-life issues.

Staff Management and Training

Medical and health services managers oversee and coordinate the functions of a healthcare system to provide efficient, quality care. They are supported by human resources staff who hire and train new employees, manage employee relations, and monitor continuing education for staff. Managers provide regular training on harassment, diversity, and violence prevention that support the well-being of both staff and patients.

Employee Assistance Programs. **Employee assistance programs (EAPs)** are intended to help employees who are facing problems in their personal lives. The goal is to minimize the effect these personal issues have on employees' job performance. Employees with mental health, addiction, anger, relationship, financial, or legal concerns may self-report, or their employer may refer them for help. This benefit may extend to other members of the employee's household, because whatever is going on at home may affect the worker on the job.

EAP counselors assess each situation and offer support through counseling or connections to additional resources. These confidential services and resources are usually free or paid for by the employer and are available 24 hours a day, seven days a week. The employer benefits because these services mean employees are more focused and effective on the job.

Quality Improvement. Healthcare systems must be able to show quantitative, objective evidence that they are providing high-quality services. Both consumers and licensing or accrediting bodies, such as CMS, state boards, and The Joint Commission, will use this data to monitor performance and make decisions about the quality of an organization and its services.

Quality improvement (QI) involves the continuous focus of the healthcare team on productive and efficient care. The process of determining what care is required and how it is done is tied to **standards of care**. These best practice guidelines are based on past clinical experience. Opportunities for improving the process of healthcare are visualized by mapping out a diagram of who performs each step in the healthcare process. A process map shows how all of the people involved are connected and who may be affected by changes to the system (Figure 16.6). It may also reveal gaps, inefficiencies, or overlaps in service.

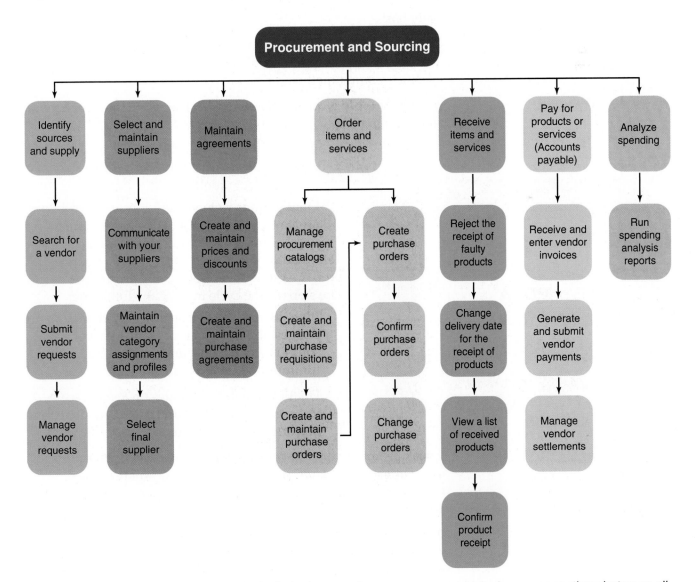

Figure 16.6   Quality improvement might include the use of a process map, which shows connections between all people involved in a process or procedure. How does a process map help with the task of quality improvement?

Quality improvement uses data to describe how the healthcare system is working and analyze what happens when changes are applied. **Quantitative** data, or *statistics*, may include the number of medication errors or length of wait times. This data comes from lab reports, waiting room logs, and admissions forms. **Qualitative** data, or descriptions of things that can't be measured, may include patient or employee satisfaction. This data comes from satisfaction surveys, interviews, or observations. Quantitative and qualitative data are analyzed and the results are used to make decisions about healthcare services and opportunities for improvement.

The coordinated efforts of an interdisciplinary QI team are most effective when they take into account how changes will impact the larger healthcare system. QI teams usually include someone who works with the process in question, someone who is affected by the process, and someone in authority who can assign resources and give permission to try various actions.

For example, if central services wanted to review cleaning procedures of diagnostic equipment, their QI team might include the following:

- a medical laboratory technician who uses the equipment on a daily basis

- a biomedical technician who evaluates the durability of equipment and identifies problems that might be caused by specific cleaning methods

- a central supply worker who performs cleaning, disinfection, and sterilization tasks

- the central supply manager who oversees the cleaning procedures and ensures that they meet OSHA guidelines

Quality improvement activities usually follow a Plan-Do-Check-Act (PDCA) model (Figure 16.7). This cycle can be *reactive* in response to an identified problem or *proactive* when a study of processes shows an opportunity for improvement. The steps in the cycle include the following:

- **Plan.** Identify an opportunity for change. Suggest the root causes and design a possible solution. Gather baseline data and set a goal for improvement in performance measures.

- **Do.** Begin making changes on a small scale in a controlled setting and collecting data on performance and outcomes.

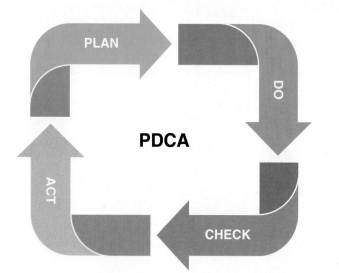

Figure 16.7 When performing Quality Improvement, try following the PDCA cycle to determine changes you may need to make to a procedure or system.

- **Check.** Compare data to your own baseline and to **benchmarks**, or *performance standards*, set by other facilities. Analyze the data, including customer satisfaction, looking for successes and additional problems.

- **Act.** Integrate and standardize successful solutions as everyday practices. Monitor data as evidence of continued improvement, or use the data to identify further changes that may be needed. Seek solutions to any new problems identified by beginning the process again.

This PDCA model teaches groups of employees to monitor their own performance and take corrective action. The focus of QI is always on fixing the system processes that allowed a problem to occur, not on blaming people who made mistakes. Solutions may include building in safeguards, retraining staff, replacing equipment, or streamlining a procedure to reduce waste.

The QI team members are important to the successful adoption of new practices. When they share their satisfaction with a change, others are more likely to accept it. The support of management also tells employees that QI is an organization-wide priority and that everyone is expected to participate.

Larger healthcare systems and facilities have dedicated staff to coordinate the overall QI process and help individual teams work on specific projects. Benefits of implementing QI include improved patient health outcomes, reduced costs, increased efficiency, and higher patient and staff satisfaction.

Marketing and public relations are alerted when the organization meets or surpasses industry standards. These departments make sure that consumers know about the facility's involvement in special programs and receipt of awards for healthcare quality. These accomplishments can be highlighted in brochures and press releases as well as on websites and billboards.

RECALL YOUR READING

1. Facilities managers monitor and address issues with a facility's _____.
2. Proper food handling is key to preventing problems created by food _____ or _____.
3. Healthcare providers are able to communicate across language gaps and obtain essential _____ through the use of _____.
4. _____ programs support employees with personal problems and seek to minimize the effect of these problems on _____.
5. Quality improvement tasks might include setting a(n) _____ for improvement, collecting and and analyzing _____, and integrating successful _____.

Complete the
Map Your Reading
graphic organizer for the
section you just read.

Legal and Ethical Issues for Support Services Workers

Many jobs in the support services pathway are entry level, meaning they do not require a degree or advanced training. While facilities managers, dietary managers, and central services managers are all highly trained and experienced professionals, dietary aides, transport technicians, and central services technicians may just be starting their careers. This may even be their first job. As a result, you may benefit from reviewing the basics of employment laws that apply to these careers. This section discusses the fundamental laws concerning the employer-employee relationship and the various protections granted to workers by law.

The employer-employee relationship is affected by many state and federal laws. These laws cover a wide range of considerations, from how old you need to be before you can be legally employed, to how workers interact with one another. Some federal laws apply to all workplaces and involve workers' fundamental rights. Other laws apply only to workplaces with a minimum number of workers or those with employees who work a minimum number of hours a week. Laws may be stricter at the state level. It is important for both employers and employees to know how state laws apply to them.

Employment Laws

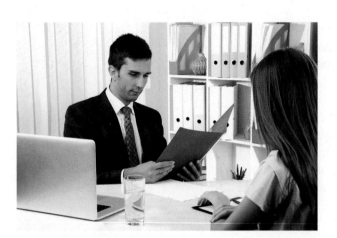

Figure 16.8   When employees are hired for a job, they must understand that an agreement has been created between them and their new employers. What are the terms of this agreement?

The fundamental principle underlying employment law is **employment at will**. Under this principle, employment is a mutual agreement between employer and employee that either party can end whenever they wish (Figure 16.8). An employee can choose to quit a job in favor of taking a new one. An organization can fire or lay off an employee. Generally, employers who end a worker's employment must have a valid reason for their action. They must be able to show that they haven't violated a contract or broken any discrimination laws in deciding to fire someone.

While employment at will is the basic premise of the workplace, various other considerations affect the employer-employee relationship. Some organizations have work contracts with their employees. In these cases, both the organization and the worker must follow the terms of the contract. Some labor unions have collectively bargained contracts that apply to an entire group of workers. These agreements usually specify the terms and conditions of employment for those workers, including grounds for dismissal. This generally requires the employer to document steps that were taken to fix the situation. The worker should be informed that his or her performance was not up to the desired standard. The worker may be given training or suggestions for improvement and an opportunity to fix the situation. If an organization fires a contracted worker without just cause, the worker may bring legal action. He or she might claim to be the victim of **wrongful discharge**, or dismissal without cause.

Laws That Affect Hiring. The US Department of Labor monitors child labor to protect young people's health, safety, and educational opportunities. The federal **Fair Labor Standards Act (FLSA)** restricts work settings and hours for workers younger than 18 years of age. Sixteen is the minimum age for employment in healthcare. Some cashiering, cleaning, lifeguarding, cafeteria, and office jobs are available to 14- and 15-year-olds (Figure 16.9). Workers younger than 16 years of age may not be employed during school hours, more than three hours on school days, or between the hours of 7:00 p.m. and 7:00 a.m.

Some jobs are considered hazardous and require workers to be at least 18 years of age. Jobs using power-driven lifting or mixing machines are among these hazardous occupations, so work for minors in kitchens, as nursing assistants, or as transport technicians may be restricted. State laws may also require a minor to obtain a work permit. Child labor laws no longer apply once a person reaches 18 years of age.

The Immigration Reform and Control Act of 1986 also set employment restrictions. Employers may not knowingly hire an undocumented immigrant. This law was passed to discourage illegal immigration into the United States. Employers must verify the identity and employment authorization of all new employees within three days of their hire. You may be asked to show your US birth certificate, passport, driver's license, Social Security card, permanent resident (green) card, or other form of verification. A green card grants an immigrant legal authorization to live and work in the United States.

Although it is not a law, many professional associations require proof of identity and a Social Security number from anyone taking their certification exams. This helps organizations avoid certifying an undocumented immigrant for work that they could not be legally hired to perform. Employers who violate immigration reform laws may have to pay a fine or face other criminal penalties.

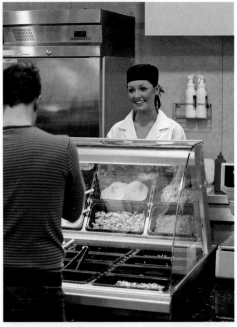

Figure 16.9   Workers who are 14 or 15 years of age can be hired for jobs such as food service in a hospital cafeteria.

Laws That Affect Wages and Hours. In addition to regulating child labor, the FLSA also establishes minimum wage and overtime rules. **Minimum wage** is the lowest hourly wage permitted by law. That minimum was set at $7.25 per hour in July 2009, but it has been raised at various times over the years and could go up again. Some states have their own minimum wage laws. When state and federal laws conflict, the employer must pay the higher of the two amounts. In 2014, for instance, the minimum wage for California workers was $9.00 per hour.

The FLSA also sets rules for payment of regular and overtime wages. Break times of less than 20 minutes are included as part of the hours worked. Meal periods of 30 minutes or longer, during which no work duties are required, are not counted in hours worked. Under federal law, employees who work more than 40 hours a week must be paid one and a half times their regular hourly rate for those additional hours. This is known as *time-and-a-half* pay. The FLSA does not specify a maximum number of hours that may be worked in one day.

These **overtime pay** rules do not apply to all workers. Salaried professionals who earn at least $455 a week ($23,660 per year), outside sales employees who travel to make sales, and some computer employees may be exempt from the minimum wage and overtime provisions of the FLSA. First responders, paramedics, licensed practical nurses, and other similar healthcare professionals are generally protected by the FLSA because an advanced degree is not a standard requirement for employment, and their salary may be less than the $23,660 per year. Nurses and doctors, however, are considered exempt and are not entitled to overtime pay unless it is part of their employment contract.

The healthcare industry has some additional exceptions to the normal overtime rules. Hospitals, nursing homes, and other healthcare facilities can form an agreement with their employees to calculate overtime based

minimum wage
the lowest hourly earnings that an employer can legally pay a worker

overtime pay
payment at one and a half times the regular wage for each hour an employee works beyond 40 hours in a week

on work exceeding 8 hours in a day or 80 hours in two weeks. This **8 and 80 system** allows an employee to work more than five 8-hour days in one week and fewer days the following week without receiving overtime.

Some emergency medical services (EMS) workers use *Garcia cycles* when calculating their standard pay and overtime (Figure 16.10). Some people call these *7K cycles* because they follow a maximum hour standard chart in statute 207(k) of the FLSA regulations. The chart is based on a repeating work schedule between 7 and 28 days in length.

It is common for EMS workers to have a repeating shift of 24 hours on duty and 48 hours off duty. If sleep accommodations are provided and employees sleep more than five hours during the 24 hours worked, their pay may be reduced for sleep time. Over a 28-day cycle, this could be as many as 240 hours. According to the FLSA schedule, anything over 212 hours is considered overtime.

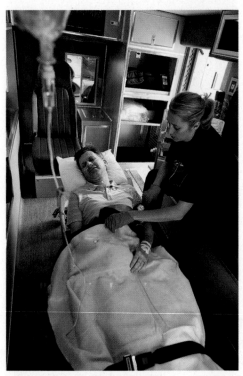

Figure 16.10   EMS workers often need to work overtime. What kind of shift do EMS workers commonly have?

Mandatory overtime is common in healthcare careers such as nursing. Refusing to work overtime hours when requested can result in penalties or termination unless those requests are in violation of a contract, are unpaid, or would result in a health hazard. The federal law does not restrict the total number of hours that an employee may be required to work as long as that employee is properly compensated for the overtime hours, and the additional hours do not create a safety risk. This helps employers cover patient care needs when an employee calls in sick and a replacement has not been found to cover the shift.

OSHA recognizes the risk that tired workers pose to themselves, their coworkers, and their patients. The agency recommends that employers provide extra breaks for workers whose shifts exceed eight hours per day, but these are just guidelines and are not legally enforceable. Some union contracts and some states restrict the amount of overtime that can be requested of an employee.

On-call pay is also regulated by the FLSA. Workers who are required to remain on-site while waiting for a call summoning them to their next job must be paid their regular on-call wage for those hours. There are various other requirements for those who carry a phone or beeper and must respond to emergency calls within a short time frame. Doctors or EMS employees who work on-call may receive a weekly bonus for carrying a beeper. If they respond to a call outside of their regular 40-hour workweek, they may be compensated by overtime pay in addition to their regular wage and bonus. If an employee is a professional exempted by the FLSA, the employer may negotiate compensation other than time-and-a-half pay. They may agree on **compensation time**, allowing the employee to take an equivalent number of hours off instead of receiving additional pay.

discrimination
unfair treatment of individuals on the basis of their membership in a specific group, such as age, ethnicity, gender, nationality, or religion

Antidiscrimination Laws. Discrimination, in legal terms, is the unfair treatment of individuals based on their membership in a specific group. In terms of employment, the main antidiscrimination law is the **Civil Rights Act** of 1964. This law bans employment discrimination based on a person's race, color, religion, gender, or national origin. The law applies to workplace decisions such as hiring, starting salary, promotion, and firing.

The **Age Discrimination in Employment Act (ADEA)** of 1967 extended civil rights protection to workers 40 years of age or older. The **Rehabilitation Act** of 1973 and the **Americans with Disabilities Act (ADA)** of 1990 gave similar protections to workers with physical or mental disabilities. Under these laws, discrimination includes an employer's refusal to make reasonable accommodations for a job applicant with a disability if the applicant is otherwise qualified for employment.

Modifications may be requested to remove barriers created by rules or physical obstacles so that a person with a disability may perform his or her job duties and access the same benefits of employment as nondisabled workers. For example, a person with a visual impairment may require his or her employer to provide computer applications and equipment that allow him or her to listen as text on the computer screen is read aloud. A person with diabetes may request specific break and meal times to take insulin and eat on a regular schedule. An employee in a wheelchair may request that break room appliances be moved to accessible heights so he or she can use them at lunch (Figure 16.11).

If you are protected by the ADA or Rehabilitation Act, your employer may be required to modify your mandatory overtime schedule to accommodate a disability that causes fatigue, the need to change positions, or an inability to concentrate for long periods of time. The only limitation to reasonable accommodations is that they should not cause significant hardship for the employer.

Under the **Genetic Information Nondiscrimination Act (GINA)** of 2008, employers cannot discriminate against a job applicant or an employee based on genetic information obtained about the individual or a family member. This act puts strict limits on employers' ability to gather or disclose genetic information. It protects individuals from suffering discrimination such as being rejected for a job because of information about a known inherited health condition that could affect their job performance or the employer's health insurance costs.

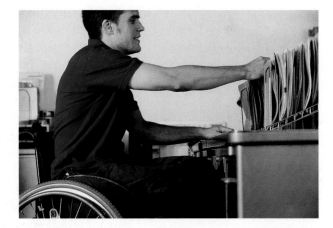

Figure 16.11   Disabled workers may make requests to modify their workplaces so they can better access files or other items necessary for their jobs.

Another important antidiscrimination law is the **Equal Pay Act** of 1963. This law requires employers to pay men and women equally for performing the same job under the same conditions. If two maintenance engineers, one male and one female, have the same level of skill, responsibility, and effort required in their jobs, they should receive equal pay. However, if one job requires additional training and supervisory responsibilities, that employee may receive a higher rate of pay whether male or female.

In addition to banning discrimination, all of these laws prohibit an employer from taking any negative action against a worker who has filed complaints against that employer for violating the worker's rights. For instance, an employee who has filed a lawsuit regarding age discrimination cannot be punished by being fired, having pay cut, or being sanctioned by the employer in any way.

These acts are enforced by a federal agency known as the **Equal Employment Opportunity Commission (EEOC)**. The EEOC has the power to bring lawsuits on behalf of workers who believe they have been discriminated against. Individuals can also file their own lawsuits. Under the Lilly Ledbetter Fair Pay Act of 2009, each paycheck that reflects discriminatory practices is subject to legal action. In other words, a female worker who wins a discrimination lawsuit based on unequal pay due to gender is compensated for all the wages she lost, even if the difference stretches back several years. While these antidiscrimination laws are meant to protect workers' rights, they do not necessarily apply to all workplaces. Figure 16.12 shows which employers are covered by the different laws.

Antiharassment Laws. Workers are also protected from all types of **harassment**, including sexual harassment, by Title VII of the Civil Rights Act. The EEOC defines harassment as "unwelcome conduct that is based on race, color, religion, sex (including pregnancy), national origin, age (40 or older), disability, or genetic information." Sexual harassment is defined as "unwelcome sexual advances; requests for sexual favors; and other verbal, nonverbal, or physical conduct of a sexual nature." Both male and female workers can be subjected to sexual harassment. You do not have to be the direct recipient of harassment to be a victim; the law applies to anyone affected by the offensive conduct.

Harassment does not include simple teasing or single off-hand comments, but it can include unintentional actions, such as repeated off-color jokes or pictures displayed in a work locker. Harassment is illegal if (1) enduring the harassment is a condition for continued employment; (2) a benefit or detriment, such as a raise or job loss, is directly linked to complying with the harassment; or (3) the harassment creates an intimidating or hostile environment.

If you are a victim of harassment, tell the harasser to stop. If the behavior continues, make a formal complaint to your supervisor or the human resources office. Documenting the instances of harassment in a journal will help you make your case. Individuals may be tried under civil law for harassment. In organizations with 15 or more employees,

harassment
unwelcome, offensive, and repeated language or actions based on race, color, religion, sex, national origin, age, disability, or genetic information that affect an employee's job performance or advancement opportunities or create an uncomfortable working environment

Figure 16.12 Employers Covered by Federal Antidiscrimination Laws	
Law	**Type of Employer Covered**
Equal Pay Act of 1963	all employers
Civil Rights Act of 1964	employers with 15 or more employees who work at least 20 weeks a year
Age Discrimination in Employment Act of 1967	employers with 20 or more employees who work at least 20 weeks a year
Rehabilitation Act of 1973	employers who have contracts with the federal government worth $2,500 or more
Americans with Disabilities Act of 1990	employers with 15 or more employees who work at least 20 weeks a year

employers are liable if they know about harassment and fail to take immediate corrective action to prevent it. Employers should work to prevent harassment through training and zero-tolerance policies.

Other Workplace Laws. The **National Labor Relations Act (NLRA)** of 1935 gives workers the right to join together, with or without a union, to discuss ways of improving their working conditions. **Unions** bring together workers from the same company or region to bargain collectively. The collective voice of many employees is used to negotiate with an employer for specific terms of employment, such as wages, hours, working conditions, or benefits. Employers are prevented from banning such discussions or punishing workers who take part in them.

Workers do not have to form a union to enjoy the benefits of collective bargaining, but if they do form a union, the employer cannot refuse to bargain in good faith with the union's elected representative. The Service Employees International Union (SEIU) is the fastest-growing union in the United States and the largest healthcare union in North America. In 2007, healthcare, property services, and public services workers from 29 states (including Puerto Rico) and Canada joined together to improve the lives of working families. Worker safety, wages, and overtime compensation have been important topics of their negotiations. Some professional organizations, such as the American Nurses Association (ANA), function in similar ways to unions. These organizations also provide a collective voice and advocate for the needs and concerns of their members.

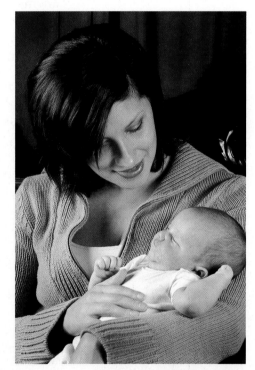

Figure 16.13   The Family and Medical Leave Act allows workers time away from work to care for a newborn child. What other circumstances are covered under this law?

The **Family and Medical Leave Act (FMLA)** of 1991 grants workers the right to up to 12 weeks off work in a 12-month period to give birth to a child, care for a newborn or newly adopted child, care for a seriously ill family member, or recover from a personal illness or injury (Figure 16.13). This time off is taken as *leave*, meaning it is unpaid. While the employer is not required to pay the worker, the employee has a right to his or her job when he or she is able to return to work. The FMLA applies only to workers hired by employers with 50 or more employees who work 20 or more workweeks in a year.

The federal government also prevents employers from enforcing English-only rules in the workplace. Employees are allowed to speak a foreign language in situations unrelated to work, if they wish. Sometimes, problems occur when other employees assume the non-English language speakers are talking about them. Employers have only a limited ability to require that English be spoken in work situations. For example, English may be required when communicating with customers, coworkers, or supervisors who only speak English. In emergencies, English may be required as a common language to promote safety. It is not legal to require English for casual conversations between employees.

Ethical Standards of Conduct

In addition to complying with laws, healthcare workers need to behave ethically. Professional codes of ethics, as discussed in chapter 4, typically call on healthcare workers to put patients above all other interests and maintain standards of professional competence. Workers in entry-level jobs, such as dietary aides or transport technicians, are often required to follow codes of ethics developed by their employer. These codes typically emphasize patient care and comfort, professional competence, and personal responsibility.

Many studies have focused on generational differences in work-related characteristics and expectations. Generally, older generations value hard work and demonstrate respect for authority figures. Today's youth are characterized as placing more importance on the end results rather than the process used to complete their work. They also feel that respect must be earned. They do not expect to "pay their dues" by working in entry-level jobs to get to the management level of the career ladder.

These shifts in attitude have created a negative stereotype toward young people in the workforce. The *Wall Street Journal* noted that unemployment rates for Americans younger than 25 years of age were more than two and a half times higher than rates for people 25 years of age and older. A character reference from a teacher or past employer can make an important difference in whether or not a young person gets a job.

Soft Skills. *Forbes* magazine, a leader in business and financial information, says that young workers don't understand the importance of **soft skills**. Employers want workers to dress appropriately, show up on time, solve problems through critical thinking, and demonstrate good customer service and communication skills. These nontechnical skills are subjective and difficult to teach, but they can be more important than technical skills that can be retaught.

Flexibility, attention to detail, and problem solving are important soft skills for healthcare workers who must make quick decisions. Healthcare workers must be on time, follow procedures rather than take shortcuts, be honest in admitting their mistakes, and demonstrate integrity by sticking to their principles about what is right and wrong. Employers look for people who can demonstrate empathy and emotional stability when working under stress. Evidence of these soft skills is observed in the way you present yourself during an interview and what your references say about your past conduct at school or on the job.

Work ethic is commonly mentioned when employers ask about an applicant's soft skills. This is described as your own value for working hard, being self-reliant and dependable, and not wasting time (Figure 16.14). Employers value a strong work ethic. This demonstration of professionalism is an important contributor to success in the workplace. It takes self-discipline and determination to choose work over social distractions. An employee who looks for more to do when his or her regular duties are completed is an asset to an employer. Those who meet these high standards can feel a sense of accomplishment and pride in their work. They must also be careful to balance their work and personal lives so they don't burn out. At the end

soft skills
employability skills related to communication, attitude, teamwork, and problem solving that are difficult to teach but critical to workplace success

work ethic
a belief in the benefits of working hard, taking the initiative, and being personally accountable for the work you do

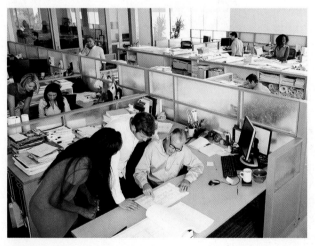

Figure 16.14   Part of a good work ethic is avoiding distractions even in a busy work environment. What are some distractions you've had to deal with on the job?

of an important project, take time to relax and remember to acknowledge those around you who were involved in your success.

Avoiding Misconduct. Providing high-quality care is the ultimate goal of all healthcare workers. The relationship between the healthcare worker and the patient is based on trust. Behavior that violates that trust or deviates from recognized standards of care can be considered misconduct.

For example, transport technicians should treat patients with respect and show concern for their well-being. When moving patients from a bed to a chair or piece of transport equipment, technicians need to respect their privacy and avoid touching them anywhere that would make them feel uncomfortable (Figure 16.15). Technicians should use clear and open communication about what they are doing. This can reduce stress for patients, allow them to anticipate what is needed of them, and help prevent the perception that the worker is doing something wrong.

A special concern for misconduct in the support services pathway is **misappropriation** by employees. Workers in central supply, housekeeping, or the pharmacy, among others, have access to patient belongings, expensive medical supplies, and controlled medications. Taking these items is theft, whether they belong to a patient, a visitor, or the facility. This is obviously more than just an ethical concern—theft is a crime.

In addition to the legal issue, misappropriation also represents a betrayal of trust to the facility and its patients. The misappropriation of goods meant for patient care could leave some patients without the supplies or medications they need. It also drives up the cost of healthcare.

You can avoid charges of misappropriation by conducting yourself properly. You should never touch patients' belongings without their permission. Never reach inside their bags, drawers, or pockets. If you must move a patient's belongings to clean around them, be sure the patient knows what you are doing. If you are asked to remove a patient's

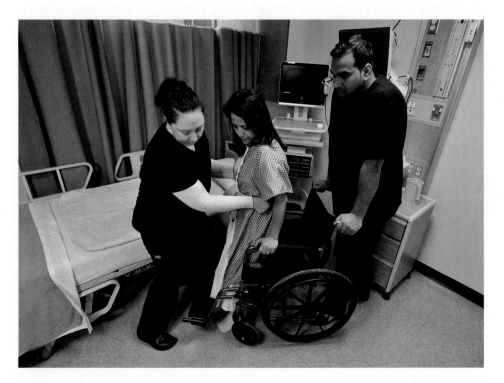

Figure 16.15 Transport technicians must avoid inappropriate contact and use clear communication to prevent problems.

jewelry before transporting him or her to surgery or the morgue, have another employee witness your actions and fill out an inventory of the patient's belongings. If you are aware of another worker's illegal or unethical behavior, you should report those actions to your supervisor or a higher-level authority.

Complete the *Map Your Reading* graphic organizer for the section you just read.

RECALL YOUR READING

1. Under the principle of _____, employment is a mutual _____ between employer and _____ that may be ended at any time.
2. Workers younger than _____ may have limits on the number of _____ they may work in a day or settings where they are allowed to work.
3. The _____ Act of 1964 applies to workplace decisions such as _____, starting _____, _____, and _____.
4. _____ is unacceptable in the workplace and can be prevented through training and zero-tolerance policies.
5. Employers prefer to hire workers who demonstrate good _____ in their conduct at the interview and in past experiences.

Health and Safety in Support Services

Workers in the support services pathway are exposed to many hazards. They have a responsibility to perform their work in ways that promote their own safety and the safety of others, including patients, visitors, and coworkers.

The key areas of health and safety concerns in the support services pathway are falls, fire safety, safe handling of oxygen, electrical safety, transportation safety, and food safety. In addition, healthcare facilities must have disaster plans and procedures in place. Your first day on the job should include an orientation to the specific safety guidelines and procedures for your facility. You will see how these basic safety principles are applied in context.

Falls

Accidents often occur when workers are tired, distracted, or rushed. Falls are among the most common accidents that cause occupational injuries. Healthcare workers must protect their own safety in this area as well as the safety of the facility at large. A worker's fall may cause another accident, such as a patient fall or hazardous material spill (Figure 16.16). Following these precautions can prevent falls from occurring:

- **Always walk.** Running in the hallway of a healthcare facility is dangerous. Hallways are full of workers, patients, visitors, and equipment. Running increases the risk of colliding with one of these individuals or objects and causing a fall.

- **Stay to the right.** Walk on the right side of hallways and stairwells, leaving the other side for people moving in the opposite direction.

- **Use corner mirrors to look ahead where corridors meet.** Healthcare facilities typically mount mirrors high on the walls where corridors intersect. These mirrors allow people walking in either corridor to see oncoming traffic in the other corridor. This is especially important when you are pushing a wheelchair or gurney because you cannot stop or move out of the way as quickly. Use mirrors to help identify and avoid potential collisions.

- **Be alert around doorways.** A door that suddenly opens in your path can cause a fall. Revolving doors pose potential hazards as well. Always be alert when using or moving past a doorway, and be prepared to stop if necessary to avoid a collision.

- **Hold on to handrails when climbing stairs.** Using the handrail helps you maintain your balance and prevents falls or slips.

- **Clean hallways by halves and post warning signs.** By cleaning one half of a hallway at a time, you leave space for others to use the opposite side where it is dry. When washing floors, be sure to post signs warning people that the floor is wet and there is a danger of slipping.

- **Clean up spills as soon as possible after they occur.** If a liquid spills, place caution signs around the area and have the spill mopped up as quickly as possible.

- **Keep walkways clear.** Remove excess equipment, push in chairs, and avoid cluttering up hallways and other thoroughfares. Monitor fire exits and be sure to remove anything that prevents easy access to the exit during an emergency.

- **Avoid the use of throw rugs.** Rugs without nonslip backings can slide out of position for a person walking with a cane or crutches. Any ridge or uneven floor surface presents a tripping hazard, particularly to those who have difficulty lifting a leg or walker to avoid the hazard. If you see a rug that presents a hazard, notify your supervisor immediately so it can be removed or replaced.

- **Control the fall.** Further injury can result from trying to keep a falling person upright. You can control the fall of a patient by grasping the sides of the transfer belt or wrapping your arms around the patient's chest, bringing him close to your center of gravity, lowering him safely to the floor, and protecting his head. Protect yourself by keeping your back straight, chin up, and using your leg muscles to slow the fall. Call for help so the patient's condition and the cause of the incident can be assessed before getting him up.

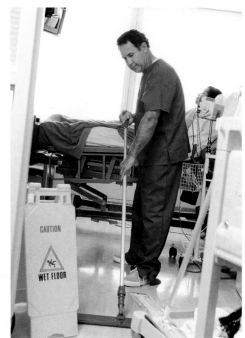

Figure 16.16   Spills should be cleaned up immediately to prevent falls.

Fire Safety

In a healthcare setting, fires are often caused by carelessness while smoking, or electrical sparks resulting from frayed wires or

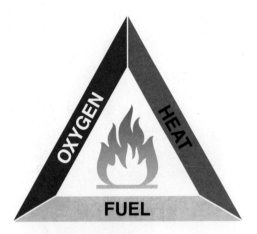

Figure 16.17   The fire triangle shows the three elements needed for a fire to occur—fuel, heat, and oxygen.

fire triangle
term that describes the three elements of a fire, which include oxygen, fuel, and a heat source

overloaded circuits. A fire must have oxygen, fuel, and a heat source. These three elements are called the **fire triangle** (Figure 16.17). Removing any of these three components from a situation will prevent a fire or stop a fire in progress.

Every healthcare facility has a fire plan and it is every employee's responsibility to know that plan. It should be practiced once a month so that everything goes smoothly when there is a real fire. Healthcare workers need to know emergency evacuation routes and the location of fire doors and fire extinguishers in the areas where they work.

Handling a Fire Emergency. The acronym **RACE** will help you remember the steps to take when there is a fire. RACE stands for **r**escue, **a**larm, **c**ontain, and **e**xtinguish/**e**vacuate. Each of these can be explained as actions you should take during a fire:

- Remove or **rescue** patients who are in the same room as the fire and in immediate danger from it.

- As you remove patients from the room, alert others to the fire by pulling the safety **alarm** and calling for help.

- **Contain** the fire by closing all the doors and windows. This limits the amount of oxygen available. Fire doors may be triggered electronically to close when the fire alarm is pulled. Shut off electrical equipment and oxygen tanks that may fuel the fire.

- If the fire is small, **extinguish** it using a fire extinguisher, a fire blanket, or another means of smothering the flame. In a kitchen, put the lid on a burning pan.

- Begin **evacuating** the rooms directly above, below, and next door to the area if the fire cannot be contained or is too large to be extinguished. If a full evacuation is required, patients who are unable to walk or cannot be transferred to a wheelchair may need extra help. An entire bed may be wheeled out of the facility. A mattress can also be dragged to transport a patient. Elevators should never be used during a fire.

Types of Fire Extinguishers. Fire extinguishers work by using certain substances to smother the fire. By cutting the oxygen supply to the flames, they eliminate one corner of the fire triangle and thus stop the fire. Different types of fires require specific types of fire extinguishers (Figure 16.18). Using the wrong type of extinguisher can cause injury to the user and increase the fire rather than put it out. Six types of extinguishers are commonly found in healthcare facilities:

- **Class A** extinguishers use pressurized water to put out fires in which paper, wood, or other ordinary combustibles are the fuel. These silver canisters are marked by a green triangle containing the letter *A* and a drawing of a burning trash can and a burning wood pile.

- **Class B** extinguishers use carbon dioxide to smother flames from grease fires and fires caused by flammable liquids. These cylinders

Figure 16.18 Types of Fire Extinguishers

Pressurized Water	Carbon Dioxide (CO_2)	Dry Chemical	Dry Chemical	Dry Chemical or Wet Chemical	Multi-Purpose Dry Chemical
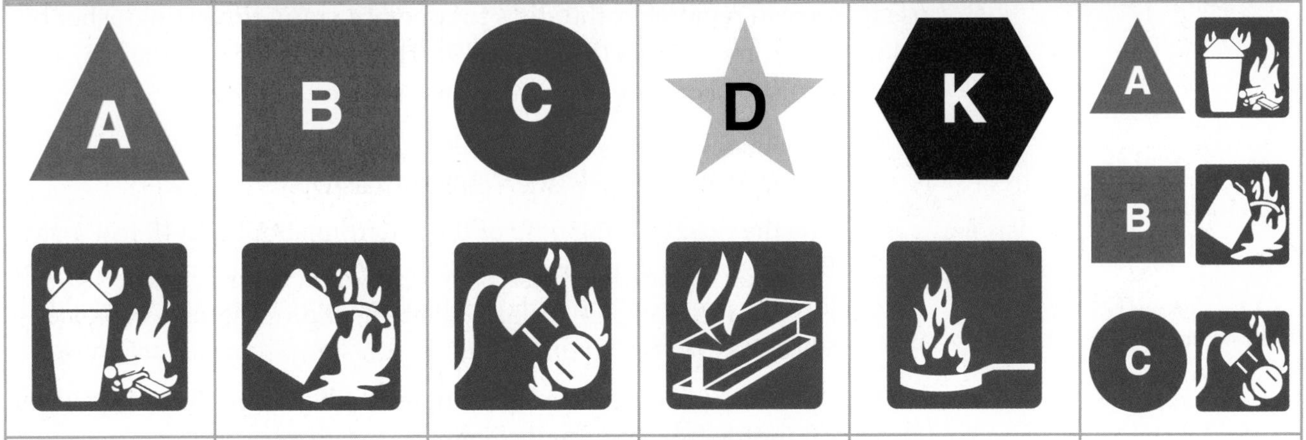 **A**	**B**	**C**	**D**	**K**	**A** **B** **C**
Ordinary combustibles (wood, paper, or textiles)	**Flammable liquids** (grease, gasoline, oils, and paints)	**Electrical equipment** (wiring, computers, and any other energized electrical devices)	**Combustible metals** (magnesium, potassium, titanium, and sodium)	**Kitchen fires** (grease fires in commercial kitchens)	Labeled for use on ordinary combustibles, flammable liquids, and electrical equipment fires

are marked with the letter *B* in a red square and a picture of a puddle near a burning gasoline can.

- **Class C** fire extinguishers use potassium bicarbonate or potassium chloride to put out electrical fires. These cylinders are marked with the letter *C* in a blue circle and an image of an electrical plug and outlet on fire. Never use water on an electrical fire!

- **Class D** extinguishers are used to put out burning metals, such as aluminum, lithium, zinc, and potassium that may be present in labs and pharmacies. They use pressurized nitrogen gas combined with either sodium chloride or powdered copper. The cylinders are marked with the letter *D* within a yellow star.

- **Class K** extinguishers use potassium bicarbonate or a fine chemical mist to put out grease fires in industrial kitchens. The electrical power must be turned off before you use them. These large, silver canisters are labeled with the words *Class K* in a hexagon and a frying pan full of flames.

- **ABC** extinguishers can be used for paper and wood fires, flammable liquid fires, or electrical fires. They use either carbon dioxide or a dry chemical to smother the flames. The cylinders are red, marked by the letters *ABC*, and display pictures showing the types of fires for which they are appropriate.

Operating a Fire Extinguisher. In the event of a fire, you will need to make a quick decision about whether to try to extinguish the fire or evacuate. Before you attempt to use a fire extinguisher, be sure the fire is small, you have the right type of extinguisher, and you know how to use it. You can remember the steps for operating any fire extinguisher by using the acronym **PASS** (Figure 16.19). This stands for **p**ull the pin, **a**im the extinguisher, **s**queeze the handle, and **s**weep the nozzle:

- *Pull* the pin at the bottom of the trigger. Removing this safety pin allows you to operate the trigger.

- *Aim* the nozzle at the base of the fire from about 6 to 10 feet away. Be sure to aim at the base of the flames. If you aim too high or too low, the fire won't be extinguished and may be blown around to start more fires.

- *Squeeze* the trigger with your fingers to discharge the extinguisher solution while holding the extinguisher firmly.

- *Sweep* the fire extinguisher from side to side to smother the fire.

Fire extinguishers must be kept in good working order. OSHA requires a monthly visual inspection, annual maintenance, and testing every 5 to 12 years, depending on the type of extinguisher. Once a fire extinguisher has been used, it must be recharged or replaced. A trained, qualified individual should do the inspection and recharging.

Figure 16.19   The PASS acronym can help you learn how to use a fire extinguisher properly and effectively.

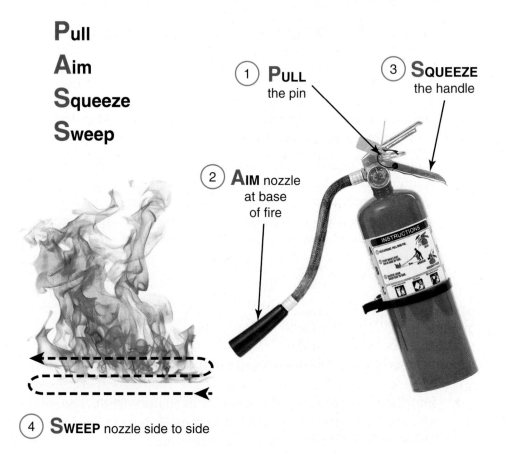

Pull
Aim
Squeeze
Sweep

(1) **P**ULL the pin

(3) **S**QUEEZE the handle

(2) **A**IM nozzle at base of fire

(4) **S**WEEP nozzle side to side

Oxygen Safety

Some patients with respiratory problems require constant delivery of oxygen so they can breathe and function (Figure 16.20). This oxygen may be delivered from a large metal tank or a concentrator that pulls oxygen from the air. As you know, oxygen is one of the components of the fire triangle. As a result, fire is a very serious threat when an oxygen tank is present. To prevent hazards associated with oxygen use, follow these rules:

- **Secure the oxygen tank.** Make sure the tank is stable and unlikely to fall or tip over.

- **Post warning signs when oxygen is in use.** Signs that read "No Smoking—Oxygen in Use" should be placed near patients who are receiving oxygen.

- **Keep sparks and flames away from oxygen.** Oxygen helps fires burn, so extra precautions must be taken to keep any heat source, such as cigarettes and electric razors, away from oxygen supplies or tubing.

- **Use cotton clothing and blankets for patients receiving oxygen.** Avoid wool and synthetics that may create static electricity, which could spark a fire.

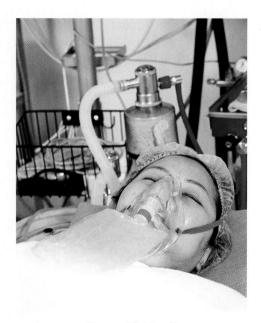

Figure 16.20 Because oxygen is one element in the fire triangle, you should take extra precautions around patients using oxygen equipment.

Electrical Safety

Healthcare facilities use a wide variety of electrical equipment, including electric-powered beds, MRI and X-ray machines, and mobile computer workstations. This equipment requires a huge investment of resources, and maintaining it is important to the facility's ability to function smoothly. An abundance of electrical equipment also poses certain hazards, including electrical shock, fires, and explosions. The chief causes of electrical hazards are faulty equipment or wiring, damage to receptacles or connectors, and unsafe work practices. The need for electrical safety is heightened in a hospital setting because patients may be connected to several electronic devices, increasing the chances that something could go wrong (Figure 16.21 on the next page).

Electrical current is very dangerous. Three to five milliamperes (mA) of current can produce a shock that forces a person to pull away. Six mA of current or more cause painful shocks, and 9 to 15 mA can cause muscle contractions that make it impossible for a person to let go. One hundred to three hundred mA can interrupt the heart rhythm and, if the contact lasts for three minutes, cause death. Because of this danger, electrical equipment in a healthcare facility must be checked regularly to ensure that it is in good working order.

Support service workers often come into contact with electrical equipment. OSHA recommends several practices to ensure electrical safety:

- Install and use equipment according to the instructions provided. Make sure that electrical equipment is kept free from hazards noted on the label.

Figure 16.21 Electronic equipment in a patient's room can pose a threat of electrical shock. How can you ensure electrical safety?

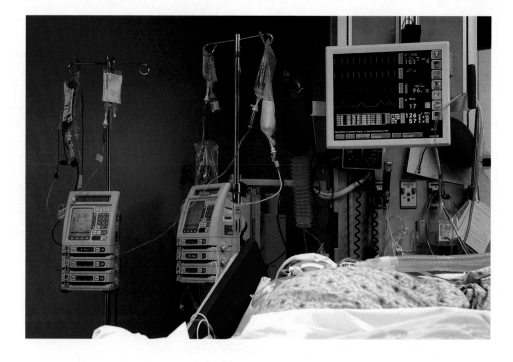

grounding
the act of carrying current safely away from an electrical circuit to prevent shocks from occurring in the event of a problem with the circuit

- Provide sufficient working space around electrical equipment to allow for safe access, operation, and maintenance.

- Make sure that all electrical equipment near water is properly grounded. **Grounding** carries current safely away from an electrical circuit to prevent shocks or electrical fires when there is a problem with the circuit. A *ground-fault circuit interrupter* (GFCI) will break the circuit at the outlet when an imbalance is caused by unexpected grounding. Circuit breakers and fuses cut the flow of electricity at the power box.

- Inspect electrical cords, plugs, and equipment regularly. Remove from service any receptacles or equipment that show damage, report them, and repair them before putting them back in service.

- Follow safe procedures when using electrical equipment, including making sure that employees are trained not to plug in or unplug equipment when they have wet hands.

Transportation Safety

Transport workers need to follow certain precautions to ensure that they move patients through a facility safely. Chapter 14 discusses wheelchair transport procedures. In addition, use the following safety guidelines when transporting patients in wheelchairs or on gurneys:

- **Lock the wheels before transferring.** Wheelchairs and gurneys have lockable wheels. Be sure to lock those wheels during the transfer of a patient to or from the equipment. Accidental rolling can lead to a dangerous fall. After a transfer is complete, wheelchair locks are considered a restraint if the patient isn't able to undo the lock independently.

- **Be sure the patient is secure.** After placing a patient on a gurney, secure him or her by fastening straps over the legs, waist, and upper torso. Leave the patient's arms free, however. You should also raise the side rails on the gurney before moving it. When securing a patient in a wheelchair transport vehicle, use the seatbelt and shoulder harness provided. Be certain that the patient's feet are off the ground and resting on the footrests before moving the wheelchair.

- **Recognize situations that require backward movement.** Generally, patients should not be moved backward in transportation equipment because it is disorienting. However, when moving up stairs, down ramps, or over gaps such as at an elevator door, backward movement is appropriate to prevent the patient from tipping forward out of the device (Figure 16.22). Always warn the patient before moving backward.

Food Safety

Dietary workers provide for patients' nutritional needs. These workers must follow safety procedures prescribed by the FDA and OSHA to prevent foodborne illnesses. Chapter 14 presents sanitation practices for dietary workers and safe food handling guidelines. Foodborne illnesses can arise because microorganisms in food are not killed during food preparation. Bacteria are the most common cause of foodborne illness. This problem can be prevented by cleaning, cooking, and storing food properly. For example, bacteria can sometimes be found on fresh produce, so food safety rules call for washing produce before serving it (Figure 16.23 on the next page).

The following are important food safety procedures for anyone who handles food:

- Wash your hands before handling food. This is especially important after going to the bathroom; coughing, sneezing, or blowing your nose; and touching uncooked meat or produce.

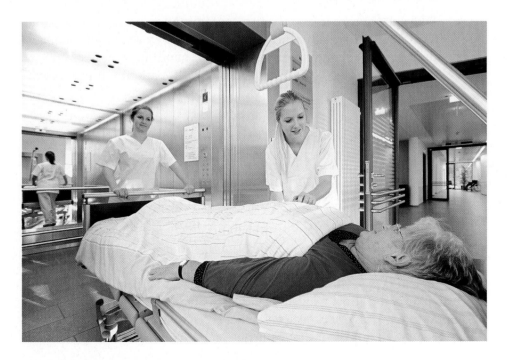

Figure 16.22 When moving patients over the gap at an elevator door, transport technicians should always move backward.

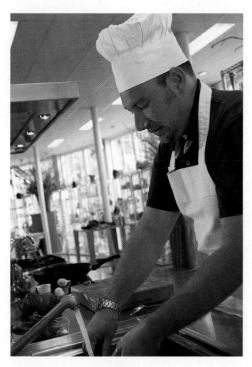

Figure 16.23   Dietary workers must practice safe food handling procedures to prevent the spread of foodborne illness.

danger zone
the range of temperature from 40°F to 140°F at which bacteria grow most rapidly to the levels that cause food poisoning

- Wash fresh produce before serving. Bacteria can be found on fresh fruits and vegetables. If produce will not be cooked to kill the bacteria, it must be washed under running water. Scrub firm produce, such as apples, with a produce brush while washing.

- Keep raw meat, poultry, and seafood away from already cooked foods and fresh food such as fruits and vegetables that will not be cooked. Different colored cutting boards and knives are used for raw meat, cooked meat, unwashed vegetables, salads, and bakery items to help keep them separate. This prevents cross-contamination, which is the transfer of harmful bacteria that may be in the raw foods. Thoroughly clean any utensils and cutting boards used to cut meat, poultry, or seafood in hot, soapy water before using them again.

- Clean and sanitize all utensils, equipment, and food preparation surfaces. The heat of a dishwasher helps to kill bacteria. Special sanitizing solutions for use in kitchens are also effective.

- Keep food out of the temperature **danger zone**. Between the temperatures of 40°F to 140°F, bacteria multiply quickly and may cause food poisoning. Refrigerate food to below 40°F for storage within two hours. At this temperature, bacteria can only grow slowly. Freeze food to 0°F for long-term storage. Defrost frozen food in the refrigerator to reduce the time food spends in the danger zone.

- Cook food to an appropriately high internal temperature. Heat kills bacteria, reducing the risk of foodborne illness. Cook roasts and steaks to at least 145°F, ground beef to 160°F, and poultry or leftovers to 165°F.

- Take special care to avoid cross-contamination between foods that will trigger allergic reactions and those that won't. Something as simple as not changing gloves between handling a cookie with nuts and a cookie without nuts can cause a patient with allergies to have a severe reaction.

- Use gloves, utensils, or tissues to handle ready-to-eat foods. Do not touch food with your bare hands, which may carry germs picked up from other surfaces.

Disaster Plans

Healthcare facilities have a responsibility to ensure the safety of the patients in their care. For that reason, organizations must have well-developed plans for responding to emergency situations such as disasters. A disaster can be a severe weather event such as a tornado or hurricane, a fire, or a terrorist attack. Severe weather can cause power outages. The loss of power can have serious, even fatal, consequences for patients who depend on equipment that runs on electricity. Healthcare facilities have backup power generators so equipment will continue to operate in the event of a power outage (Figure 16.24).

In addition, healthcare facilities must maintain an emergency water supply so that water is available for hand washing, bathing patients, providing drinking water to staff and patients, laundering soiled linens, and other needs. The Centers for Disease Control and Prevention (CDC) states that developing an emergency water supply plan can help organizations assess their water usage, response capabilities, and alternative water supplies.

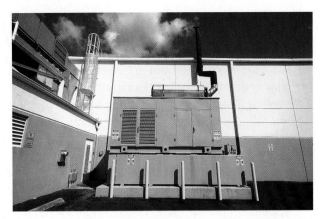

Figure 16.24   A backup generator is one important component of a healthcare facility's disaster plan. What are some other components of a typical disaster plan?

Healthcare facilities must also have an evacuation plan in place for some types of emergencies. You already know that fires can require the evacuation of staff and patients, but other extreme situations can create the same need. For instance, when Hurricane Sandy hit the East Coast in October 2012, some hospitals were forced to evacuate. They could not run on emergency power because generators were in low-lying areas that were flooded by heavy rain and high seas. Facilities managers should make sure that staff members are well trained in the proper procedures so that, should an emergency arise, the evacuation will proceed smoothly.

In the event of a disaster, healthcare workers should follow these rules:

- Remain calm for your own sake and to project a sense of calm to patients and others. Patients take their emotional cues from a facility's staff. Maintaining your own calm will help reassure patients and prevent them from panicking, which will also make them easier to manage.

- Remember your facility's evacuation procedure and do a quick mental review of any emergency training you have received.

- Keep yourself out of danger so you can help others.

- Move anyone who is in danger out of the threatening situation, if that can be done safely.

- Use stairways rather than elevators and make use of emergency exits in addition to normal exit routes.

RECALL YOUR READING

1. _____, the most common cause of occupational injuries, often occur when workers are _____, distracted, or _____.

2. When there is a fire, you must remove one of the three elements of the _____, which includes _____, _____, and _____.

3. Basic precautions for transporting patients include _____ the wheels before transfers and _____ the patient before moving.

4. _____ practices and safe food handling guidelines can prevent _____ illness caused by _____.

5. When preparing for _____ situations, a backup _____, a(n) _____ supply, and a(n) _____ plan are essential.

Complete the *Map Your Reading* graphic organizer for the section you just read.

Chapter 16 Review

SUMMARY

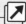 Assess your understanding with chapter tests

- The work of the support services pathway provides the throughput and feedback that are vital to the smooth functioning of the healthcare system. They support facility operations by adhering to health and safety regulations, sterilizing and maintaining equipment, and monitoring the inventory of supplies and medications.

- Dietary services support patient health through appetizing presentation of prescribed diets and prevent foodborne illnesses and allergies through proper food handling.

- Interpreters ensure that patients who don't speak English or cannot hear are able to give informed consent to procedures and that healthcare providers are able to obtain and communicate essential information.

- Human resources supports employees through training, managing employee relations, and providing an employee assistance program.

- Aspects of quality improvement include setting goals for improvement, collecting quantitative or qualitative data, analyzing results, and sharing results among team members.

- Under the principle of employment at will, employment is a mutual agreement between employer and worker that may be ended at any time, though employers must have a legitimate reason for firing or laying off workers.

- Minors have limits on the number of hours they may work and the types of jobs they may do.

- Employers must pay a federal- or state-set minimum wage to all employees, as well as overtime wages to some employees.

- Employers may not discriminate in employment decisions on the basis of race, color, religion, gender, national origin, age, or physical or mental disability.

- Workers have a right to form unions and to have as many as 12 weeks of leave in a year for medical reasons related to themselves or a family member.

- If workers are being harassed, they should tell the person to stop and to let their supervisors know there is a problem.

- Healthcare workers follow the code of ethics of their particular occupation or of the institution that employs them.

- Employers look for workers with good soft skills and a strong work ethic because these skills are more difficult to teach than technical job skills.

- Following basic precautions when moving through hallways and doorways and cleaning up spills can help prevent falls.

- Removing one of the three elements of the fire triangle— fuel, heat source, or oxygen—can put out a fire. It is important to use the correct type of fire extinguisher for the type of fire.

- Safety around oxygen equipment is very important because of the potential fire hazard.

- Proper grounding, maintenance, and use of electrical equipment can help prevent electrical hazards, including shock and electrical fires.

- Transport workers need to take basic precautions to ensure the safety of patients they move on gurneys or wheelchairs.

- Food service workers can reduce the growth of bacteria that causes foodborne illness by using proper food preparation, food storage, and hygiene procedures.

- Healthcare institutions need to be prepared for emergencies, which includes having backup energy, an emergency water supply, and an evacuation plan.

MAXIMIZE YOUR PROFESSIONAL VOCABULARY

 Build vocabulary with e-flash cards, games, and audio glossary

Listed below are the essential, yellow-highlighted terms and the additional professional vocabulary that you encountered in this chapter. Complete the activities that follow the list to make all of these terms part of your everyday professional vocabulary.

8 and 80 system

Age Discrimination in
   Employment Act (ADEA)

Americans with Disabilities
   Act (ADA)

benchmark

calibration

Civil Rights Act

compensation time

controlled substance

danger zone

discrimination

Employee Assistance Programs (EAPs)

employment at will

Equal Employment Opportunity Commission (EEOC)

Equal Pay Act

Fair Labor Standards Act (FLSA)

Family and Medical Leave Act (FMLA)

fire triangle

Genetic Information Nondiscrimination Act (GINA)

grounding

gurney

harassment

Illness and Injury Prevention Program (I2P2)

infrastructure

inventory

mandatory overtime

minimum wage

misappropriation

National Labor Relations Act (NLRA)

overtime pay

Pull, Aim, Squeeze, Sweep (PASS)

qualitative

quality improvement (QI)

quantitative

Rehabilitation Act

Rescue, Alarm, Contain, Extinguish/Evacuate (RACE)

soft skills

standards of care

unions

work ethic

wrongful discharge

VOCABULARY DEVELOPMENT

Matching. Match the essential terms from this chapter with the best descriptions below by writing the letter of the description next to the number of the essential term on your answer sheet.

1. calibration

2. danger zone

3. discrimination

4. fire triangle

5. grounding

6. harassment

7. infrastructure

8. minimum wage

9. overtime pay

10. soft skills

11. work ethic

a. term that describes the three elements of fire, which include oxygen, fuel, and a heat source

b. the range of temperature from 40°F to 140°F at which bacteria grow most rapidly to the levels that cause food poisoning

c. payment at one and a half times the regular wage for each hour an employee works beyond 40 hours in a week

d. the act of carrying current safely away from an electrical circuit to prevent shocks from occurring in the event of a problem with the circuit

e. the adjustment of a piece of equipment so that it operates within its intended standards of performance

f. a belief in the benefits of working hard, demonstrating initiative, and being personally accountable for the work you do

g. term that describes the internal systems that a facility needs to operate, such as power supplies; electrical, plumbing, and heating and cooling systems; water; waste management; and phones and computer systems

h. unfair treatment of individuals on the basis of their membership in a specific group, such as age, ethnicity, gender, nationality, or religion

i. the lowest hourly earnings that an employer can legally pay a worker

j. unwelcome, offensive, and repeated language or actions based on race, color, religion, sex, national origin, age, disability, or genetic information that affect an employee's job performance or advancement opportunities or that create an uncomfortable working environment

k. employability skills related to communication, attitude, teamwork, and problem solving that are difficult to teach but critical to workplace success

12. **Creating Sentences.** Select six to ten of the professional vocabulary terms in this chapter. Without using the actual term, create a sentence or two that explains the term and your understanding of the concept.

    Example: *mandatory overtime*—This term is used when people, especially in healthcare, are asked to work longer shifts or more hours than they're scheduled for. The person being asked to do this cannot refuse without a penalty or termination of employment unless the hours are not stated in the contract, the hours are unpaid, or the person is being asked to do something hazardous.

REFLECT ON YOUR READING

13. Review the story about Rolando Santiago at the beginning of the chapter. Using the notes in your *Map Your Reading* visual summary, identify what actions Rolando takes that contribute to patients' well-being and what questions his behavior raises. Try to use your professional vocabulary as you support your answer.

BUILD CORE SKILLS

14. **Critical Thinking.** Identify the laws governing working hours and wages. Which groups of workers are exempt from overtime pay provisions? Why do you think mandatory overtime is common in the field of healthcare?

15. **Critical Thinking.** Choose one of the careers in the support services pathway. Write a brief code of ethics and a scope of practice for workers in that career. Compare the two documents. How should these workers go about performing their jobs? What ethical dilemmas might arise for workers in that career?

16. **Math.** Use the Internet to search for "Medical Errors Statistics." Copy a chart or graph of particular interest to you. Write a summary of what the statistics reveal. What are your personal reactions to the quantitative data? Share your findings with the class.

17. **Writing.** Customer service is an important soft skill that employers look for in employees. Work with a partner to write an invented conversation between a healthcare worker and a patient that demonstrates poor customer service and communication skills. Then rewrite the dialogue to show how the conversation should have gone if the worker was demonstrating good customer service and communication skills.

18. **Problem Solving.** Imagine you work as a supervisor in a hospital's operating room. What are three potential situations or actions of employees that would be valid and legal reasons for dismissal? For each one listed, answer the following questions:
    - What documentation is needed?
    - What steps, training, or suggestions would you offer for improvement to remedy each situation?

19. **Problem Solving.** For the situations you listed in the previous activity, determine how you would incorporate the PDCA process.

20. **Speaking and Listening.** Create a response you could use during an interview when asked to give an example of how you have demonstrated a good work ethic. Practice the response with a partner until it comes out smoothly and sounds confident.

21. **Critical Thinking.** Why is employee theft a particular concern with workers in the support services pathway? What are the consequences to both the patient and the worker involved? What steps can be taken to minimize employee theft in this area?

22. **Math.** Ana is a support services worker. Last week, she worked 16 hours overtime in addition to her scheduled 40 hours. Calculate how much pre-tax money Ana earned last week if her regular hourly rate is $14.50/hour. Assume her overtime rate is time-and-a-half pay.

23. **Critical Thinking.** Which employment law applies to each of the following workplace scenarios?
    - Jessa and Karl started working as central services technicians at the same time. They both earn the same hourly wage.
    - Andrew and his wife just adopted a child. He will be taking 12 weeks off work to stay home and care for his new child.
    - The housekeepers at Cara's hospital belong to a union.

- Luca's father has Huntington's disease, an inherited disease that affects the brain.

24. **Problem Solving.** Imagine that you work in a hospital kitchen. While moving a pot of boiling soup off the gas stove, you drop a towel on the burner and it catches fire. By the time you can set down the soup without scalding yourself, the blaze is a foot high. What should you do?

25. **Critical Thinking.** What are the different types of fire extinguishers? Identify healthcare-related situations in which you might need to use each of the different types of extinguishers.

26. **Reading.** Go to the website for the Occupational Safety and Health Administration. Read their regulations for food preparation in healthcare settings. Pay particular attention to the actions workers should take to ensure food safety.

27. **Writing.** After reading OSHA's food preparation regulations, list food handling procedures that reflect the OSHA guidelines for preparing a particular food that might be served in a hospital cafeteria. Explain why these guidelines are important for healthcare workers to follow.

ACTIVATE YOUR LEARNING

28. Practice controlling a patient's fall so that you are prepared when it happens on the job. Create a safe space by clearing away tables and chairs. Place a large gym mat on the floor or provide a "spotter" to help, if needed. Use a transfer belt if it is available. Have a pair of students act as the healthcare workers walking behind their patient. After the patient takes a few steps, he or she will say, "I am feeling weak." The workers will reach around their patient's chest or tighten their underhand grasp on the transfer belt, pull the patient in toward their chest, step back with one leg to broaden their base, then support the patient to slide safely down their other leg to the ground. Keep the chin up and back straight to prevent back injuries.

29. Ask your local fire department to demonstrate proper use of a fire extinguisher. If allowed, practice the PASS procedure so that you can experience the feel of using a fire extinguisher.

THINK AND ACT LIKE A HEALTHCARE WORKER

30. Imagine that you work in a hospital. A fellow employee has been making comments about your ability to do your job because of your age and gender. You feel like you are being harassed. What will you do to handle this situation appropriately?

31. Take the role of a department supervisor in support services. Write a memo to your staff explaining how important it is that they follow set procedures. Include any health and safety consequences that could occur if these procedures are not followed.

32. What safety rules should transport technicians follow? Develop a one page, eye-catching "reminder" list of these rules that could be posted in a healthcare setting.

GO TO THE SOURCE

33. Visit the CDC website. Find statistics on foodborne illnesses in the United States. Answer the following questions:
    - What is the estimated number of Americans who get sick due to foodborne illnesses each year?
    - What is the number of hospitalizations due to foodborne illness per year?
    - How many deaths occur from foodborne illness?
    - What is the number of outbreaks due to a single confirmed pathogen?
    - What are the most common causes of foodborne illnesses?

34. Go to the website for the Equal Employment Opportunity Commission. Read about one aspect of employment that the EEOC addresses. Write a paragraph describing the issue and explaining why the EEOC becomes involved with it.

35. Visit the American Nurses Association website. Find information on their code of ethics. Investigate additional information on the framework, provisions, interpretive statements, ethics challenges, application of ethics keywords, and definitions of ethical principles and theories. How helpful is the site for you as a future healthcare worker? Support your answer with specific examples.

Chapter 17
Academic Knowledge: Body Systems for Maintenance and Continuation

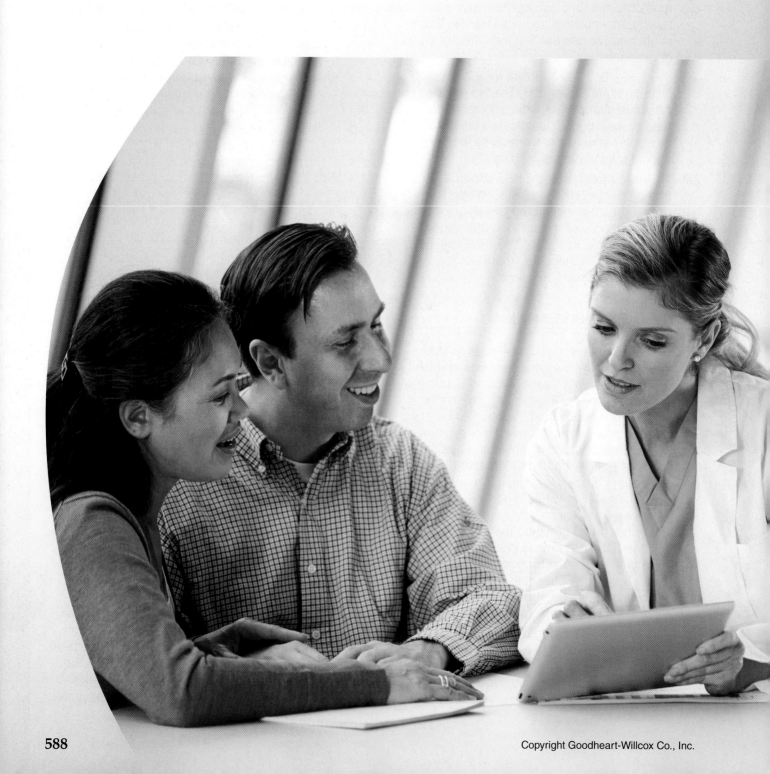

PROFESSIONAL VOCABULARY

 E-flash Cards

You will need to learn the essential terms listed below before you begin your reading. These terms will help you understand the main concepts of the chapter. These terms, which will be highlighted in yellow within the text, will become part of your professional vocabulary.

In addition to these essential terms, you will see bold terms throughout the chapter. The meanings of these terms are explained where the terms first appear. The bold terms, like the essential terms listed here, will become part of your professional vocabulary and deepen your understanding of the topics presented.

absorption the act of taking up a substance into a tissue, such as the movement of nutrients from the small intestines into the bloodstream

digestion term for the mechanical and chemical breakdown of food into nutrients that can be absorbed and used by the body

excretion the removal of waste products from the body

filtration the process of separating substances, such as solid from liquid, large from small, or impure from pure

gametes reproductive cells that have half the normal number of chromosomes and unite during fertilization; sperm in males and ova in females

heredity the passing of traits (such as eye color, height, and some diseases) from parent or ancestor to offspring through chromosomes

ingestion the stage of digestion in which food is taken into the body through the mouth

meiosis the sexual process of cell division that produces four new haploid cells, each with a unique combination of 23 chromosomes

mitosis the asexual process of cellular reproduction that creates two identical copies of a cell, each with a full set of 46 chromosomes

nutrients molecules such as carbohydrates, proteins, fats, vitamins, and minerals used by the body to grow and maintain body processes

reabsorption the act of returning a substance to the part of the body from which it was previously filtered out

secretion the release of a liquid substance from blood, cells, or tissues

CONNECT WITH YOUR READING

New Terms	Terms I've Heard Of	Terms I Know Well

How was the term used? What is the topic? What does the context tell you?	Opposites or non-examples of the term (what it isn't); don't use *not* or *un-*
Term and Definition	
Other words that relate to this term (shared word part, similar meaning)	Draw a picture to represent this term or use the word in a *meaningful* sentence.

There are many new terms to learn when you study the body systems. Some terms will require more effort to remember than others. Using the steps listed here, create a study aid to help you organize and remember these important terms.

1. Create a Vocabulary Sorting Organizer.
   a. Fold a piece of paper lengthwise to create three columns.
   b. Unfold the paper and label the three columns as *New Terms*, *Terms I've Heard Of*, and *Terms I Know Well*.
   c. Sort the terms in the Professional Vocabulary list into the columns you have created.
2. On the back of your organizer, write one of the new terms in the center of the page, along with the definition given in the chapter.
3. Divide the page into four sections, and complete a "clinical diagnosis" of the new term.
   a. In one section of the page, explain how the word was used in the text. What topic is it related to? What does the context tell you about the meaning of the term?
   b. In the next section of the page, list three or more related words that have a similar meaning or share a word part with this term.
   c. In the third section, use the word in a meaningful sentence or draw a picture of the concept described by the term.
   d. In the last section, explain the opposite of this term, or what it isn't. Avoid using the word *not* or the word part *un-*.

MAP YOUR READING

> **Systems for Maintenance and Continuation**
> food   reproduction
> growth   energy
> elimination   nutrients
> water   homeostasis
>
> DIGESTIVE SYSTEM
>
> (Urinary System)
> DIGESTIVE SYSTEM
>
> Male and Female
> REPRODUCTIVE SYSTEM

Make a tablet organizer with two sheets of paper using the example shown here. Stack the sheets, keeping the edges even, but move the top sheet of paper up so that its bottom edge is ½ inch to 1 inch above the bottom edge of the sheet below it. Holding both sheets of paper, fold them down so the top edge of the top sheet is ½ inch to 1 inch above the bottom edge of the top sheet. Crease both layers and staple at the folded edge. Write *Systems for Maintenance and Continuation* on the outside flap and list things that you know need to happen in our bodies for us to continue living and things we can do to keep our bodies healthy. Label the edges of the flaps below it with the headings *Digestive System*, *Excretory (Urinary) System*, and *Reproductive System*. As you read, add visual cues, definitions of new terms, and notes on the main functions of and careers and diseases related to each system.

As you know by now, learning about health science topics requires a lot of reading. For health science students, the most important aspect of reading is comprehension. There's a lot of information in your required reading and you're expected to take it in and understand all of it. You may be worried that you won't be able to understand your coursework, or that you won't have time to read everything assigned to you.

This chapter will show you how to improve your reading efficiency so you can remember more information. You can practice your reading skills in this chapter as you learn about the major body systems that maintain and continue life. These systems involve digestion, excretion, and reproduction.

Study Skills for Health Science Students: Reading Strategies

As you continue your studies in health science occupations, you may begin to feel overwhelmed by the amount of reading required. You can avoid this feeling by using specific strategies to read more efficiently. Just as your body sorts the materials coming in and decides how to use them, your brain needs to sort information to help digest the large quantities of reading that you do in school.

Begin by surveying the material. What is its source and why are you reading it? Skim the chapter title, headings, and subtitles. What is the main topic? How is the text organized? How much time will you need to read and understand this information? Are there natural divisions so you can break the reading into manageable segments?

Next, preview the introduction and summary sections for a shortened version of what you will be reading. What do you already know about this topic? What do you expect to read about in each of the sections? What questions do you have? How will the figures and bold terms be important to understanding this topic? Your preview will help you organize your thoughts before you read and take notes (Figure 17.1).

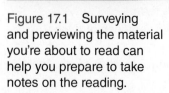

Figure 17.1 Surveying and previewing the material you're about to read can help you prepare to take notes on the reading.

After your preview, set your brain up to look for information as you read. Turn the title of each section of material into a question. As you read, look for information to help you answer that question. For example, this section is titled *Study Skills for Health Science Students: Reading Strategies.* You might ask yourself, "What skills will help me read more efficiently?" The details that answer this question are what you should highlight or include in your notes. How does information from any figures in the material help to explain the topic? What new questions occur to you as you read? Be sure to include any new terms, but write the information in your own words rather than copying straight from the text. This active involvement in your reading will help you develop your understanding of the new information and remember it.

Stop to take notes as you read. After each section, build an outline of the chapter in your notes. Be sure to leave room around each heading. If you read and outline a chapter before it is discussed in class, you can use this space to add more information. If the material will not be discussed, you should return to your notes in the next day or two to do your own review. Circle key terms. Divide the information into logical sections. Take time to answer the questions you've developed. Underline key points in your notes that may be important for future reference. Highlight terms that you are still working to remember.

Digesting your reading in this manner is the most efficient way to absorb the information. Stopping to process information in small segments prevents your mind from straying or becoming overwhelmed. Previewing and questioning will help you pay attention to the most important information. Taking notes in your own words will help you actively process the information. Summarizing and reviewing that information will make sure it remains in your memory. Try these techniques as you read the remainder of this chapter.

RECALL YOUR READING

1. When reading, first _____ the material, then _____ the introduction and summary sections.
2. Information is easier to absorb when you work with small _____ at a time.
3. Taking _____ in your own words helps you _____ the information.
4. _____ and _____ information to ensure it remains in your memory.

Complete the *Map Your Reading* graphic organizer for the section you just read.

Body Systems for Maintenance and Continuation

At all organizational levels of life, from cells and tissues to complete organisms, growth, repair, regeneration and new life are dependent on the processes of the digestive, excretory and reproductive systems. The digestive system extracts nutrients from food that are needed for energy, growth and processes that maintain the body. The excretory system removes waste products and helps to maintain homeostasis for a healthy environment within the body. The reproductive system is responsible for producing, protecting, and sustaining new life from conception to birth. This provides a means for continuing the species.

The Digestive System

The food services department plays an important role in maintaining the health of patients through their digestive system. Many careers are available in the area of food service. Dietitians plan and prepare therapeutic diets to meet the unique dietary or nutritional needs of their patients. Food service managers oversee the day-to-day operations of food preparation and service in healthcare kitchens and cafeterias. They ensure that the portion sizes, meal requirements, and presentation are correct. They also assign work tasks to the food service staff, manage financial transactions, and handle customer complaints. Feeding assistants encourage and support residents in eating a well-balanced diet (Figure 17.2).

These careers may be found in large hospitals as well as smaller long-term care facilities. Staff typically work regular hours, from early morning to evening, and have limited contact with patients. Dietary workers require knowledge of nutrients, digestion, and dietary principles to protect the health of their patients. They all play a role in analyzing information and investigating solutions so that digestive disorders don't deprive the body of the nutrients it needs.

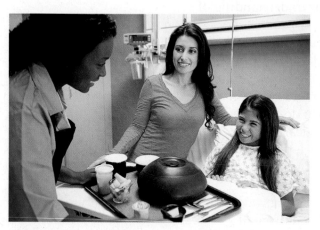

Figure 17.2   A feeding assistant is one member of a hospital's food services department.

The Support Services Worker: Tyler

As a food safety specialist, Tyler is in a unique position to protect the health of many people. More than 76 million Americans suffer from a foodborne illness each year. These days, fewer people prepare their own meals, relying instead on restaurants and commercially prepared foods. Tyler inspects food service operations in hospitals, restaurants, and production facilities. He helps educate staff about food safety regulations and seeks to enforce those regulations. He has a good understanding of infection control and the way body systems react to foods and foodborne illness. He is part of healthcare support services, but his role does not give him a lot of interaction with patients.

---

nutrients
molecules such as carbohydrates, proteins, fats, vitamins, and minerals used by the body to grow and maintain body processes

Food as a Source of Energy and Nutrition

Nutrients are used for energy, structure building, and chemical reactions taking place in the body. Carbohydrates, such as bread, are a source of energy and fiber. Meat and eggs are common sources of protein, which is important for the growth and repair of cells. Fat stores energy and carries fat-soluble vitamins. Without a variety of foods, patients will not have all of the vitamins and minerals required for good health. Dietary careers play a vital role in supporting and protecting the health of patients.

The digestive system is important to the maintenance and health of all body systems. **Calories** are the units used to measure energy gained from digestion. Although we can survive without food for as long as two months, the body lacks more than just calories during that time. The macronutrients [*macro* = large] of carbohydrates, proteins, and fats are needed in larger quantities to provide energy and nutrition. The micronutrients [*micro* = small] of vitamins and minerals are needed in smaller amounts for chemical reactions within the body. A healthy diet provides both energy and nutrition for the body on a daily basis. This also reduces the risk of many diseases such as diabetes, heart disease, cancer, and osteoporosis.

Carbohydrates. Different foods provide the body with different nutrients (Figure 17.3). Carbohydrates make glucose [*gluc* = sugar] and are the body's first source of energy. Whole grains are the best source of

Figure 17.3 Macronutrient Values			
Food	Carbohydrates (g)	Protein (g)	Fat (g)
apple, small (100 g)	11.1	1.0	0.4
banana, medium	21.7	1.1	0.3
beef patty, 3½ oz	0.0	21.6	15.5
carrots, 1 cup	12.3	1.3	0.3
cheese, cheddar, 1 slice (28 g)	0.0	7.0	9.0
chicken, roasted, 3½ oz	0.0	29.0	3.0
cola, 12 oz	35.2	0.3	0.1
cottage cheese, low-fat (1%), 1 cup	6.0	28.0	2.0
milk, nonfat, 1 cup	12.0	8.0	0.0
milk, reduced fat (2%), 1 cup	11.0	8.0	5.0
oatmeal, plain, 1 cup	22.4	5.4	2.1
pizza, cheese, 1 slice	20.5	7.7	3.2
potato, baked with skin, 7 oz	58.1	7.0	0.4
salmon, canned, 3½ oz	23.1	4.8	0.8
spaghetti, no meat, canned, 100 g	14.6	2.5	0.8
spinach, ½ cup	3.2	2.6	0.3

carbohydrates. These complex carbohydrates, or *starches*, must be broken down into sugar to be used for energy. They also contain dietary fiber. Starch, sugar, and fiber are found in most grains, as well as in fruits and vegetables. Fiber does not produce energy, but it is important for moving food through the bowels, lowering cholesterol, and preventing some cancers. Excess carbohydrates are stored as fat in the body.

Fats. Everyone must have some fat in their diet to build insulation, pad the vital organs, transport fat-soluble vitamins, and store energy. Fats are found in different amounts in most foods. Look for foods that get less than 30 percent of their total calories from fat and less than 10 percent from saturated fats or trans fats. Saturated and trans fats are often called *bad fats* because they raise cholesterol levels and increase your risk for developing heart disease and cancer.

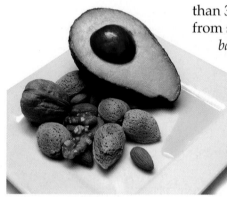

Figure 17.4   Good fats can be found in avocados and nuts like almonds and walnuts.

Good fats, such as unsaturated fat and omega-3 fatty acids, protect your heart and support good health. Good fats are usually liquid at room temperature and are often found in nuts and fish (Figure 17.4). Bad fats are typically solid at room temperature and are found in processed foods that contain hydrogenated or partially hydrogenated vegetable oils.

Meat, fish, poultry, nuts, dry beans, and dairy foods are major sources of protein. The **amino acids** in protein provide the building blocks for the body to repair and make new cells. The body requires about 20 different amino acids. Different sources of protein provide different combinations of these amino acids. Nine of them are considered *essential amino acids* because they are not made by the body and must come from the diet. Protein deficiency is a serious medical condition in developing nations with limited food sources. This deficiency can also be a problem for people who follow "crash diets" or are recovering from illness.

Vitamins and Minerals. Vitamins and minerals have no energy value, but they are important to body processes. For example, calcium helps build strong bones and is important for nerve and cell functions. Iron helps the body's red blood cells carry oxygen. Vitamin A is important for good eyesight and healthy skin, while vitamin C helps fight infection, repair wounds, and build healthy connective tissues. The vitamins and minerals listed here are required information on food labels in the United States because many people do not get enough of them in their diets.

Managing Your Weight. The US Food and Drug Administration (FDA) requires that most packaged foods carry specific ingredients and nutrition facts on their labels. The nutrition facts label lists the number of calories, amount of nutrients, and serving size for a food item. This label is an easy way to compare foods to make healthy choices.

The phrase *empty calories* is used to describe the calories added to the diet by foods that don't have much nutritional value. Alcohol and snack foods such as candy, soda, and chips have empty calories. These snacks are usually high in solid fats and added sugar, and the empty calories add up quickly. At seven calories per gram, alcohol adds up faster than carbohydrates or proteins.

Excess carbohydrates and fat are stored in the body as fat. There are only two ways to remove this fat—exercise or liposuction [*lip* = fat] surgery! The best strategy is to watch your serving sizes and choose a diet that's low in fat, sodium, and sugar. Eating a variety of food types and colors helps provide your body with all the nutrients it needs.

Weight can be controlled by balancing the amount of food energy taken in and the amount of body energy used. The US Department of Health and Human Services recommends an average of two and a half hours of moderate aerobic activity or one and a quarter hours of vigorous aerobic activity per week to maintain a steady weight (Figure 17.5). Moderate activities such as jogging or riding a bike burn about 550 calories per hour. Thirty-five hundred calories of energy burned during activity are equivalent to one pound of food energy taken in. Recommended energy intake is based on the energy needs for your body size, level of activity, growth, and pregnancy or lactation needs.

Food energy can be calculated based on the energy values shown in Figure 17.6. Adult women who are not pregnant or lactating need approximately 2,000 calories per day. The average adult male has more muscle mass to support than a woman, so he requires approximately 2,500 calories per day. These calories and nutrients should come from a variety of different food groups.

The MyPlate graphic, shown on page 506, is a visual guide for balancing the proportions of food from each of the five food groups. This helps you achieve the correct balance of nutrients needed for a healthy diet. Vegetables should be the focus of the meal, with two to three cups taken in per day. Fruits are also a good source of carbohydrates, vitamins, and minerals, but they are higher in calories than vegetables. Grains, particularly whole grains, should form the next largest portion of your diet. An average adult male needs six to eight ounces of grains per day. About six ounces of protein per day should come from a variety of lean meats, seafood, and nonmeat sources. The proportions are different for various ages, body sizes, and activity levels. The US Department of Agriculture (USDA) produces materials to help you find the right proportions of nutrients for your unique needs. You can find this information at the MyPlate website.

Figure 17.5 Calories Burned per Hour of Exercise

Exercise	Calories Burned per Hour
playing volleyball	250
walking	300
dancing fast	380
bicycling	550
running	650
jumping rope	680
playing basketball	700

Figure 17.6 Food Energy Values by Macronutrients

Macronutrients	Energy Content
protein	4.0 calories/g
carbohydrates	4.0 calories/g
fat	9.0 calories/g

The Process of Digestion

The process of breaking down food for use by the body occurs in four stages: ingestion, digestion, absorption, and excretion. During **ingestion**, food is taken into the **alimentary canal** at the mouth. This long, hollow tube made up of digestive organs runs from the mouth to the anus. Digestion takes place in the alimentary canal.

The mouth contains different types of teeth that are used to chew food for ingestion (Figure 17.7 on the next page). The milk teeth, or *baby teeth*, that emerge first are temporary and are pushed out by permanent

ingestion
the stage of digestion in which food is taken into the body through the mouth

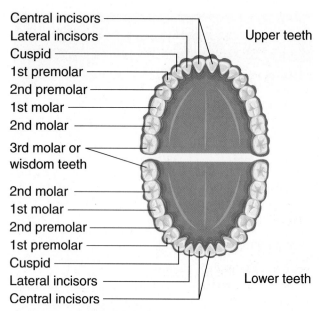

Central incisors
Lateral incisors
Cuspid
1st premolar
2nd premolar
1st molar
2nd molar
3rd molar or
wisdom teeth

2nd molar
1st molar
2nd premolar
1st premolar
Cuspid
Lateral incisors
Central incisors

Upper teeth

Lower teeth

Figure 17.7 Different types
of teeth help break down food
for ingestion. Choose one
type of tooth and describe its
role in chewing food.

digestion
term for the mechanical and
chemical breakdown of food
into nutrients that can be
absorbed and used by the
body

Figure 17.8 Each tooth
consists of a crown that is
visible in the mouth and a
root that extends downward.
What part of the tooth do
you clean when you brush
your teeth?

Label Art

teeth that come in behind them. Incisors have
a thin, flat edge for cutting into soft and crispy
foods. Canines and bicuspids are pointed for
piercing and tearing through foods, such as meat
on a bone. Molars are shaped for crushing and
grinding food into small pieces.

Each tooth is covered with a hard layer of
enamel over a softer layer of dentin (Figure 17.8).
The pulp in the center of a tooth carries the nerves
and blood supply to the root. Although the use
of fluoride and sealants to protect tooth enamel
has reduced the rate of dental caries, or *cavities*,
since the 1970s, cavities remain the most common
problem found by dentists.

The **digestion** stage uses a combination of
chemical and mechanical activities to break
food down into usable molecules of nutrients.
Chemical digestion uses enzymes and acid
produced by the body to break apart the chemical bonds in food
molecules. Many of the chemicals used for digestion are produced by
accessory organs attached to the alimentary canal (Figure 17.9). These
include the salivary glands, pancreas, and liver. **Salivary glands** in the
mouth secrete saliva, which contains an enzyme that begins the chemical
digestion of starches into sugar. The tongue and teeth provide mechanical
digestion, grinding and mixing to expose more surface area of each food
particle to digestive juices for breakdown. The resulting soft mass of food
and saliva is called a *bolus*. Each organ of the digestive system works on
this food bolus to release its nutrients and energy to the body.

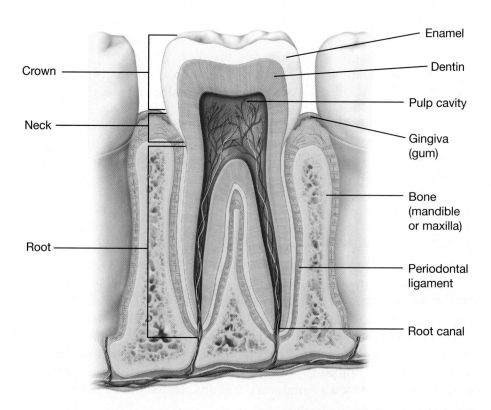

Crown

Neck

Root

Enamel

Dentin

Pulp cavity

Gingiva
(gum)

Bone
(mandible
or maxilla)

Periodontal
ligament

Root canal

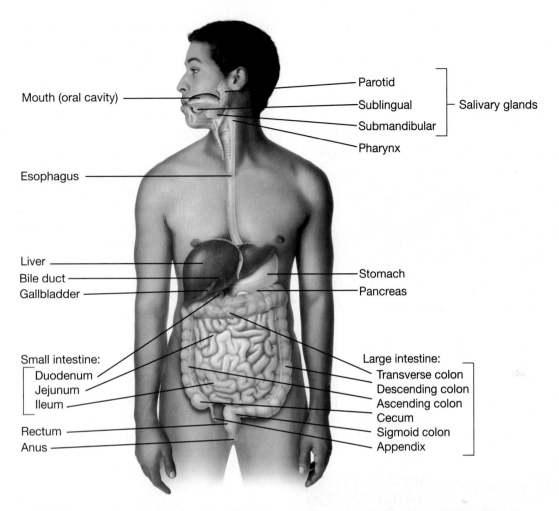

Mouth (oral cavity)

Parotid
Sublingual
Submandibular
Pharynx
Salivary glands

Esophagus

Liver
Bile duct
Gallbladder

Stomach
Pancreas

Small intestine:
  Duodenum
  Jejunum
  Ileum
Rectum
Anus

Large intestine:
  Transverse colon
  Descending colon
  Ascending colon
  Cecum
  Sigmoid colon
  Appendix

Animation

Figure 17.9   Food passes through the organs of the alimentary canal as it goes through the digestion process. How are accessory organs different from those of the alimentary canal? Can you identify which organs in this diagram are accessory organs and which are included in the alimentary canal?

The bolus is pushed from the mouth down the pharynx (FA-rinks), or *throat*, as you swallow. It is squeezed along the **esophagus** (eh-SAH-fuh-guhs) from the mouth to the stomach by involuntary waves of muscle contractions called **peristalsis**. In the muscular **stomach**, the bolus is churned together with hydrochloric acid to break down carbohydrates and proteins. The lining of the stomach produces mucus for protection against the strong acid. The food and acid mixture, called **chyme** (kIm), is held in by round sphincter muscles at the top and bottom of the stomach until it is time for the food to move on to the intestines. Heartburn is the pain you feel when acid escapes through the lower esophageal sphincter. This is a symptom of gastroesophageal [*gastr* = stomach, *esophag* = esophagus, *eal* = pertaining to] reflux disease, or *GERD*.

After several hours of digestion in the stomach, food is released into the duodenum (doo-AH-deh-nuhm). This first section of the small intestines receives digestive enzymes from the liver and pancreas. The **pancreas** produces more enzymes to digest carbohydrates, fats, and proteins. Pancreatitis sometimes occurs when the duct to the duodenum is blocked, causing the pancreas to become inflamed and damaged by its own digestive enzymes.

The pancreas also has an endocrine function. Islets of Langerhans cells within this organ make the hormones insulin and glucagon (GLOO-kuh-gahn) to help maintain proper levels of sugar in the blood. Diabetes is considered an epidemic in the United States, with nearly 26 million cases, and the number is growing. In this condition, the body stops producing or responding to insulin, causing sugar to build up in body tissues. Symptoms include excessive thirst, frequent urination, hunger shortly after eating, and infections or wounds that don't heal quickly. The exact cause of type 1 diabetes is still unknown, but it typically shows up by puberty and requires daily insulin injections. Type 2 diabetes usually develops as a result of poor dietary habits and obesity. Type 2 diabetes used to be considered an adult's disease, but it is now being diagnosed in more and more children (Figure 17.10).

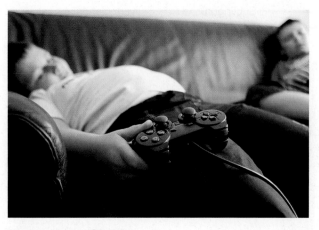

Figure 17.10   Obesity is causing a growing epidemic of type 2 diabetes in children in the United States.

The **liver** is the body's largest internal organ, weighing about three pounds. It is located in the upper right quadrant of the abdomen, above the stomach. It receives blood from the intestines, spleen, and heart. The liver breaks down and removes toxic substances, drugs, bacteria, and dead red blood cells from the body. Hemoglobin from dead red blood cells provides the pigment bilirubin, which is used by the liver to make **bile**. Bile helps mix fat with digestive enzymes so that it breaks down in the intestines.

Jaundice, a yellow color in the skin and eyes, is caused by a poorly functioning liver that allows excess bilirubin to build up in the blood. This is a common condition at birth when the liver is immature (Figure 17.11). Phototherapy uses a full-spectrum light to break down bilirubin in the skin.

Hepatitis [*hepat* = liver, *itis* = inflammation] is a common cause of liver failure. There are many types of hepatitis, each with different causes and symptoms. Hepatitis A is commonly spread through contaminated food; hepatitis B, through blood and body fluids; and hepatitis C, by contaminated needles. Childhood immunizations

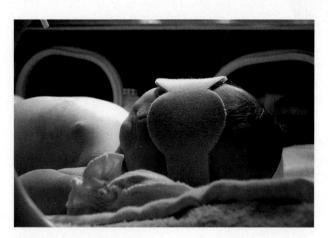

Figure 17.11   Jaundice produces a yellow color in the skin and eyes. When jaundice occurs in infants, they are treated with phototherapy.

have reduced the incidence of hepatitis A by 90 percent and hepatitis B by 80 percent. The liver is involved in so many body processes that we cannot live without it. Luckily, it is able to regenerate damaged sections.

Bile from the liver can be stored in the **gallbladder** until it is needed. Signals from the stomach trigger the release of bile from the liver and gallbladder into the duodenum. Sometimes this flow is blocked by gallstones, which are created from cholesterol and pigments in the bile. Laparoscopic [*lapar* = wall, *scop* = to view, *ic* = pertaining to] surgery uses several small cuts in the abdomen to insert a light, camera, and surgical tools to remove the stones. This technique also allows doctors to remove the gallbladder with a shorter recovery and less pain than traditional surgery, which involves larger incisions.

Absorption occurs through **villi** in the lining of the small intestines (Figure 17.12). These finger-like projections increase the inside surface area of the intestines. Nutrients are absorbed through contact with the villi. Capillaries and lacteals close to the outside surface of the intestines take in nutrients as they pass through the thin lining of the intestines. Celiac disease damages the small intestines, destroying villi and resulting in poor nutrient absorption.

The 20 to 30 feet of the small intestines are divided into three sections, each designed to absorb different nutrients. Iron is absorbed in the duodenum. The middle section of the small intestines, the jejunum (jih-JOO-nuhm), absorbs carbohydrates, proteins, fats, vitamins, and minerals. The ileum, the last section of the small intestines, absorbs remaining vitamin B$_{12}$ and bile salts. The nutrient-rich blood from the small intestines is carried through the portal vein to the liver to be detoxified.

Liquid feces that remain after nutrients are absorbed continue down the alimentary canal through the large intestine. This tube is about five feet long and separated from the small intestines by the cecum (SEE-kuhm). Water is absorbed from the feces as it moves through the different sections of the large intestine. The undigested waste travels up the ascending colon, across the transverse colon, and down the descending colon. By the time it reaches the S-shaped sigmoid colon, the feces, or *stool*,

absorption
the act of taking up a substance into a tissue, such as the movement of nutrients from the small intestines into the bloodstream

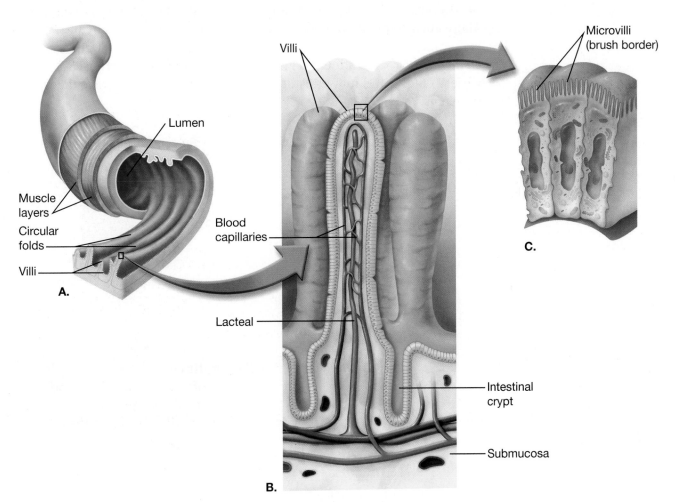

Figure 17.12   The villi in the small intestine absorb nutrients. What disease destroys the villi?

are semisolid. The muscular walls of the sigmoid colon push the stool into the **rectum** for storage.

The last step in the process of digestion, called **excretion**, occurs when feces are pushed out of the anus. If the feces have moved through the colon too quickly, diarrhea [*dia* = through, across, *rrhea* = flow, drainage] may result. When the feces spend too long in the colon, too much water is absorbed and results in constipation, with a firm stool that is difficult to expel. Piles, or *hemorrhoids*, are inflamed veins in the anal canal. They are aggravated by constipation and may cause rectal bleeding. Sometimes this blood is mistaken as a sign of colon cancer.

Colonoscopy [*colon* = large intestine, *scopy* = process of viewing] is a form of screening for colon cancer that is recommended for people 50 years of age and older. When cancer blocks the intestines, a colostomy [*col* = large intestine, *ostomy* = to create an opening] must be performed. This is a surgical procedure that brings the intestine to the surface of the abdomen. The procedure creates a stoma where a bag is attached to collect feces (Figure 17.13). Hemorrhoids, cancer, and many other digestive disorders can be avoided or improved by a healthy diet that is high in fiber and offers a variety of nutrients.

How do you describe a digestive problem to your doctor? With so many different organs involved, one of the challenges of working with the digestive system is to determine which organ is causing the problem. There are also many interactions between the digestive system and the endocrine, nervous, and circulatory systems. A gastroenterologist [*gastr* = stomach, *enter* = intestines, *ologist* = specialist in the study of] uses a wide variety of tests and may consult with other specialists to resolve digestive problems.

excretion
the removal of waste products from the body

Figure 17.13   **When part of the colon is damaged, a colostomy must be performed to allow waste to leave the body.**

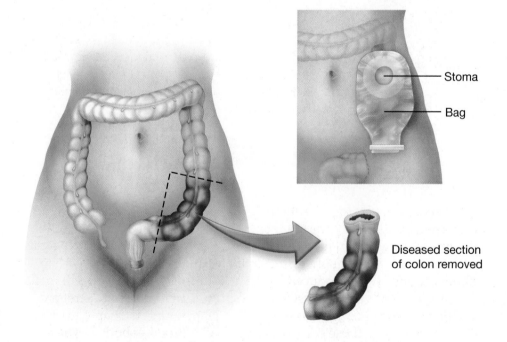

Stoma

Bag

Diseased section of colon removed

RECALL YOUR READING

1. _____, which are needed in larger amounts, include protein, _____, and fat.
2. The _____ graphic, developed by the USDA, helps balance food _____.
3. _____ and _____ digestion are used to break food down into usable molecules through four stages: _____, digestion, absorption, and _____.
4. Food is digested as it moves through the organs of the _____. The _____ organs contribute digestive juices but do not carry food.
5. Common digestive problems include GERD, _____, jaundice, _____, and _____ disease.

Complete the *Map Your Reading* graphic organizer for the section you just read.

The Excretory (Urinary) System

Waste produced by the body can provide clues about how the body is working and whether its systems are in balance. Water, vitamins, minerals, hormones, and other substances must be retained in the proper proportions for the body to work efficiently and maintain health.

The Support Services Worker: Juanita

A great deal can be learned about the body by studying its excretions. As a human resources manager, Juanita uses this information to make employment decisions at her healthcare facility. All of her employees undergo a urine test for drug screening as a condition of employment. She knows it isn't legal or ethical to test for other conditions, such as pregnancy or genetic diseases, during an employment screening. She is careful to protect the private results of these tests in her records. Juanita's role in healthcare is to ensure that patients have the best possible caregivers.

The Excretory System and Waste Removal

In their study of the excretory system, some books discuss organs such as sweat glands of the skin. The sweat glands remove excess water and mineral waste and help dissipate the heat produced during physical activity. These books might also discuss the lungs, which expel carbon monoxide and water produced by the cells. This text, however, will focus on the role of the urinary system. Further information about excretory functions of the sweat glands and lungs can be found in chapters 9 and 13, respectively, as these organs are grouped with other body systems.

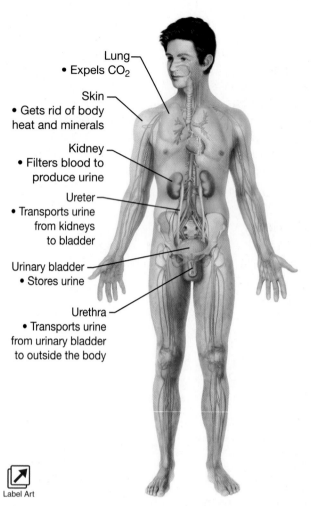

Lung
• Expels CO_2

Skin
• Gets rid of body
heat and minerals

Kidney
• Filters blood to
produce urine

Ureter
• Transports urine
from kidneys
to bladder

Urinary bladder
• Stores urine

Urethra
• Transports urine
from urinary bladder
to outside the body

Label Art

Figure 17.14 The organs of
the excretory system. What
happens if your kidneys fail?

Figure 17.15 Dialysis uses
equipment to filter waste
from the blood when the
kidneys no longer can.

Animation

Although the digestive system excretes
waste, it is not typically included as a part of
the excretory system. Digestive wastes are the
remains of food intake that are not useful in cell
metabolism. They are not the wastes produced by
cellular work. The liver is important for filtering
metabolic waste, but it is usually considered a
digestive organ.

As your body functions, the cells create waste
that builds up in the blood. If allowed to build up,
this waste becomes toxic to the body. The organs
of the excretory system are shown in Figure 17.14.
The kidneys, ureters, bladder, and urethra are
involved in filtering waste from the blood. If the
kidneys fail, the body is slowly poisoned to death.

When the kidneys no longer function properly
to filter waste and balance water, vitamins,
minerals and hormones in the blood, a dialysis
machine must be used (Figure 17.15). Dialysis
technicians monitor the patient during these
lifesaving treatments. The technicians test the
patient's blood, monitor the vital signs, and care
for the equipment used in dialysis. They may
see the same patients on a regular basis and can
observe the change in patients before and after
treatment. This is very different from laboratory
technicians who work in a lab setting, testing
labeled samples. Both careers provide valuable information and support
patient health, but in different ways.

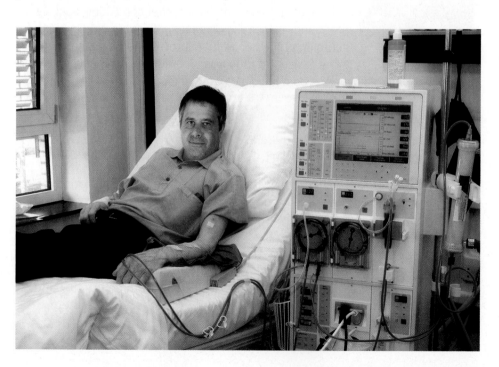

The Urinary System and Blood Filtration

Many people confuse the roles of the digestive and urinary systems. The digestive system allows the body to collect nutrients from food. Undigested food is removed as feces, but the digestive system does not form urine. Nutrients from food are filtered by the liver and delivered to the cells through the circulatory system. As cells use the nutrients, they create waste. The liver changes those waste products into urea. That waste is carried by the blood to the **kidneys**, which are located just below the liver in the lower back. The kidneys filter, concentrate, and remove waste from the blood to form urine (Figure 17.16). The urinary system does not directly filter the products of the digestive system.

About 45 gallons of blood flow through the renal [*ren* = kidney, *al* = pertaining to] arteries to the kidneys each day. Blood flow to the kidneys is essential for filtration to occur. When blood flow or blood pressure to the kidneys decreases, their ability to filter and remove waste is reduced. Heart disease, high blood pressure, and diabetes are common conditions that make the kidneys less efficient. The elderly are particularly susceptible to kidney failure because they are more likely to have one of these related conditions.

Although we can live for weeks without food, we can only live a few days without water. Dehydration also reduces blood flow to the kidneys and causes electrolyte imbalances that can result in death. Experts recommend drinking eight glasses of water per day to avoid dehydration and keep blood flowing through the kidneys.

There are three steps to urine formation in the kidneys (Figure 17.17 on the next page). **Filtration** occurs in the capillary beds that lie in the renal cortex. This dark red, blood-rich, outer portion of each kidney contains millions of glomeruli (glah-MER-yuh-lI). Each glomerulus is

filtration
the process of separating substances, such as solid from liquid, large from small, or impure from pure

Figure 17.16   The structure of the kidney. Where are the kidneys located in the body?

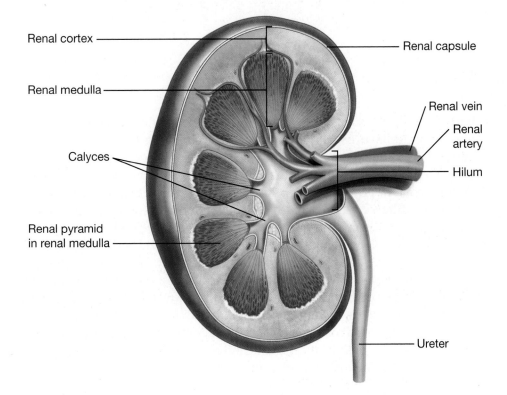

Renal cortex

Renal medulla

Calyces

Renal pyramid in renal medulla

Renal capsule

Renal vein

Renal artery

Hilum

Ureter

Figure 17.17   The steps in urine formation. Where does each step take place?

Animation

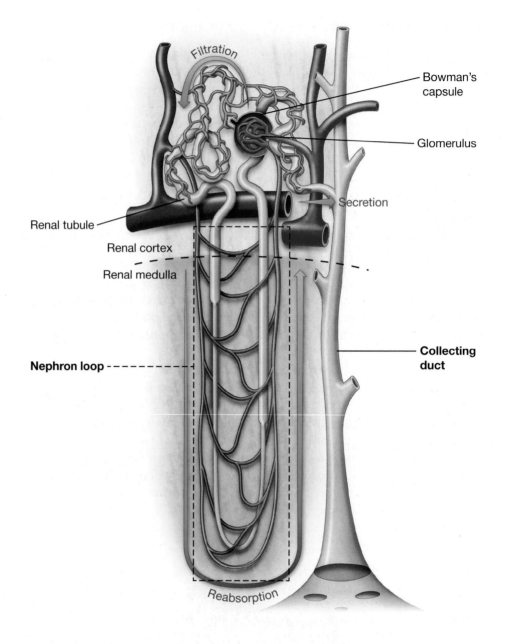

Filtration

Bowman's capsule

Glomerulus

Secretion

Renal tubule

Renal cortex

Renal medulla

Nephron loop

Collecting duct

Reabsorption

a ball of capillaries surrounded by a Bowman's capsule that collects water, sugar, salts, urea, and other waste from the blood. Blood cells and protein stay in the blood vessels unless they are damaged by disease. The waste-filled liquid flows through a collecting tubule. The glomerulus and tubules form a **nephron** [nephr = kidney]. More than a million nephrons (NEH-frans) filter the blood in each kidney. Capillaries wrap around the nephron loop of the collecting tubule, where **reabsorption** balances water, sugar, and salts. Needed substances are returned to the body.

Secretion is the last phase, in which the remaining toxins, drugs, ions, and metabolic waste are pulled back into the collection tubule to form urine. After waste products are removed, the blood is returned to the circulatory system through the renal vein to collect more toxins from the body.

The renal medulla contains pyramid-shaped groups of collection tubules. These tubules empty into ducts that merge to form calyces (KAY-luh-seez), which collect the urine. Calyces connect to form the renal pelvis at the center of the kidney. A **ureter** exits each kidney at its

reabsorption
the act of returning a substance to the part of the body from which it was previously filtered out

secretion
the release of a liquid substance from blood, cells, or tissues

hilum, a depression on the medial side of the kidney toward the center of the body. This long, thin ureter carries urine from the kidney to the bladder. Sometimes urine flow is blocked by a kidney stone. This painful collection of crystals can occur anywhere in the urinary tract. The ureter is a common site because it is a narrow passage. A procedure called *lithotripsy* [*lith* = stone, *tripsy* = to crush] uses shock waves to break apart kidney stones without surgery. The tiny pieces flow out with the urine during urination.

When urine reaches the **bladder**, it is stored there temporarily. The bladder, like the stomach and rectum, is a muscular sac. It has folds called *rugae* (ROO-gee) that allow it to expand without causing damage. Sphincter muscles keep the bladder's exit point closed until it is "time to go." When the brain tells the sphincter muscles to relax, urine flows down the **urethra** to be eliminated.

In females, this tube is only about 1½ inches long, making them more prone to urinary tract infections (UTIs) because bacteria can easily travel the short distance up to the bladder. The urethra is longer in males, meaning they are less prone to UTIs. Males are more likely to contract urethritis [*urethr* = urethra, *itis* = inflammation], which is inflammation of the urethra. In males, the urethra also serves as a passageway for the reproductive system, which puts them at risk for a variety of sexually transmitted infections (STIs) that can affect the urethra. Painful urination may be a symptom of either urethritis or an STI.

Urination is a problem for many people. *Urinary incontinence* is the inability to control when you urinate. Pregnant women may have urinary accidents because of the pressure the developing baby places on the bladder. Older women who have gone through vaginal childbirth may continue to have stress incontinence when they sneeze or laugh.

The inability to urinate completely, called *urinary retention*, is most common in men with enlarged prostates. The prostate gland surrounds the urethra like a donut. Conditions such as benign prostatic hyperplasia (BPH) and testicular cancer cause an increase in the number of cells in the prostate. This enlargement presses against the urethra and may restrict urine's ability to flow through the urethra. Sometimes, a tube called a *catheter* may be inserted through the urethra to help drain the bladder. Nocturia is the need to get up at night to urinate. Frequent urination may indicate urinary retention or diabetes. All of these urinary conditions are treatable, and symptoms should be reported to your doctor.

A healthy urinary system excretes about 10 cups of light yellow urine per day. Urine exiting the body can provide a lot of information. For instance, dark-colored urine can indicate dehydration, while cloudy urine may signal a UTI. Urine tests can determine diabetes, pregnancy, drug use, kidney disease, and a variety of other conditions in a patient (Figure 17.18).

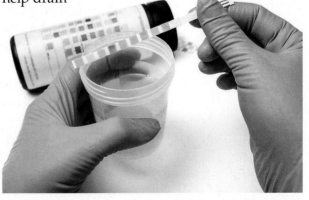

Figure 17.18   Urine testing can indicate a variety of conditions.

The Kidneys' Role in Maintaining Homeostasis

The kidneys balance the body's fluids and minerals. During the production of urine, the kidneys sense the amounts of different substances in the blood. Healthy kidneys either return or excrete different substances to maintain a proper proportion of each substance in the blood.

The kidneys influence blood pressure. When you don't have enough fluid in your body and your blood pressure drops, the kidneys produce renin. This enzyme helps raise the blood pressure in the kidneys to improve their filtering. Renin signals the adrenal cortex, an endocrine gland sitting on top of each kidney. The adrenal cortex then produces aldosterone, a hormone that tells the body to keep sodium and excrete potassium ions. As a result, an antidiuretic hormone (ADH) from the brain increases thirst. This cycle increases water retention and raises blood pressure. High blood pressure is often controlled by medications that interrupt this renin, aldosterone, and ADH production cycle.

The kidneys also influence the body's pH level. The body closely regulates its acid-base balance, keeping the blood pH between 7.35 and 7.45. Both the kidneys and the lungs affect pH by reducing the number of free hydrogen ions in the body. The lungs achieve this by expelling carbon dioxide (CO_2) and water (H_2O). The kidneys influence pH by reabsorbing bicarbonate (HCO_3) into the blood and excreting hydrogen ions in urine. Without this tight regulation on pH, serious conditions such as acidosis can result in death.

In addition, the kidneys produce and react to hormones and enzymes that control other body functions. When the kidneys sense a low number of red blood cells, they make erythropoietin (ih-rihth-roh-POY-eht-ihn) [*erythr* = red, *poietin* = to make], a hormone that tells the bone marrow to make more red blood cells. This process helps prevent conditions such as anemia. The kidneys also make *calcitriol*, a form of vitamin D_3. Calcitriol tells the intestines to absorb calcium from food and tells the kidneys to retain calcium in the blood. This process increases during breastfeeding because of the greater demand for calcium to produce milk.

The close relationship between the urinary, endocrine, and cardiovascular systems makes it difficult to change one excretory function without having an effect on other body processes. This means a patient may need to consult two or more specialists for any given condition. A patient advocate performs a wonderful support role in this type of complicated medical situation. The advocate helps the patient find his or her way through the healthcare system and can assist in understanding a doctor's diagnosis, arranging appointments, and filing insurance claims. Advocacy is a growing support services career area that brings together many different areas of knowledge.

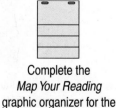

Complete the
Map Your Reading
graphic organizer for the
section you just read.

RECALL YOUR READING

1. Waste from the blood is removed by the organs of the _____ system.
2. Waste is _____ by the nephrons, certain substances are _____ into the body, and waste is _____ from the body as urine.
3. Common conditions of the _____ system include kidney stones, _____, _____, and retention.
4. Blood pressure, blood pH, _____ production, and _____ levels are influenced by the _____.

The Reproductive System

While the digestive and excretory systems maintain good health, only the reproductive system can generate new life to continue the species. The reproductive system includes all of the organs required to produce sperm, eggs, and sex hormones, as well as the organs connected to fertilization, pregnancy, and the development of new life.

Reproduction is a complex process controlled by hormones. Many jobs have emerged as a result of our ability to control reproductive options. Marriage and family counselors often find themselves helping couples through the emotions and decisions related to reproduction and sexual relationships. Genetic counselors identify testing options and discuss the risks of disease inheritance. Clinical fertility coordinators help patients experiencing infertility follow the complicated schedule of appointments and activities required for in vitro fertilization. People in these careers enjoy a stable daytime schedule, medical office environment, and growing demand for their skills.

The Male Reproductive Organs

The role of the male reproductive system is to produce and deliver sperm to the female for reproduction (Figure 17.19). Two oval **testes**, the male **gonads**, produce the **sperm**. These tadpole-shaped male **gametes** carry 23 chromosomes, half of a zygote's genetic information. Males are

gametes
reproductive cells that have half the normal number of chromosomes and unite during fertilization; sperm in males and ova in females

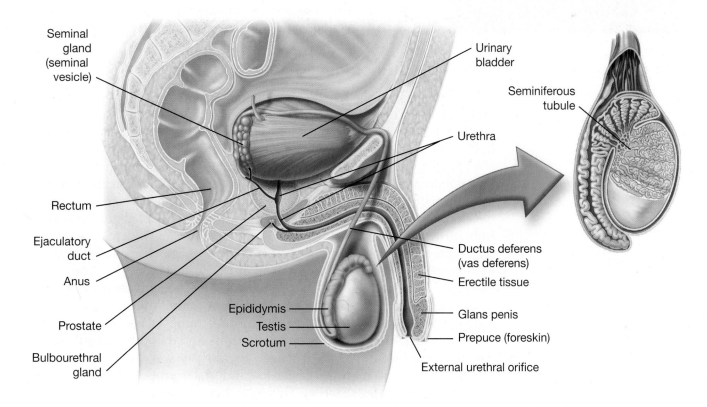

Figure 17.19   The male reproductive system. What are the male gonads and gametes?

not born with sperm, but they produce millions of them each day. Sperm are formed in long, thin seminiferous tubules of the testes.

Sperm production begins at puberty and continues into old age, although the number of sperm produced declines with age. The sperm mature in the **epididymis** at the top of each testicle and are stored until they are ready for release. The **scrotum** is a sac that holds the testes on the outside of the body. Muscles in the scrotum tighten in cold temperatures and loosen when warm to maintain a constant environment ideal for sperm production. Sperm leave the testicle through the **vas deferens**, which is sometimes called the *ductus deferens*. Connective tissue called the *spermatic cord* wraps around this tube and supports each testicle in the scrotum.

The vas deferens picks up secretions from the testes, seminal vesicles, prostate, and bulbourethral (or *Cowper's*) glands. This thick, milky white fluid called **semen** supports millions of sperm on their way to the uterus. The seminal vesicles provide nourishment for the sperm. The prostate and bulbourethral glands produce fluid to neutralize acidity in the urethra and vagina that would harm the sperm.

The **penis** is made up of vascular erectile tissue. Stimulation increases blood flow, filling the tissue to make the penis erect. The nerve impulses that cause an erection also stimulate the bulbourethral glands to secrete lubricating mucus. During sexual intercourse, about 40 million to 150 million sperm are released into the female's vagina. These small, active cells live for 48 to 72 hours. During this time, they must swim to reach the egg in the fallopian tube and break through the surface of the egg to fertilize it (Figure 17.20). After ejaculation delivers the sperm and semen, the blood in the erectile tissue dissipates, and the penis returns to its normal size. An erection is not under voluntary muscle control.

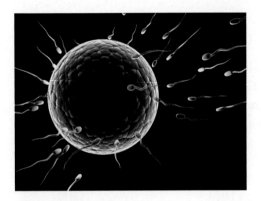

Figure 17.20   Sperm attempting to penetrate an egg.

The Female Reproductive Organs

The purpose of the female reproductive system is to house, nourish, and protect the egg and fetus during development. Females play a larger role in the continuation of the species than males because the fetus grows in the uterus for nine months.

The major organs of the female reproductive system are found in the lower abdomen (Figure 17.21). The **ovaries** are the female gonads. Ovaries store immature **ova** (eggs), the female gametes, waiting to be released for development. Females are born with their life's supply of about a million immature ova.

Beginning at puberty, around 10 to 13 years of age, one ovum matures each month. This continues into a woman's forties, when her hormone production gradually slows. The older a woman is, the greater her risk of having a child with birth defects. Her risk of complications during pregnancy, such as gestational diabetes or preeclampsia, is also greater after 40 years of age. **Menopause**, the end of fertility and monthly menstruation, usually begins around 50 years of age.

When an ovum matures, finger-like fimbriae funnel the ovum into the **fallopian tube** for fertilization. This tube then carries the ovum on to the **uterus**. This hollow, muscular organ is the shape of an upside-down pear. Each month, the uterine lining develops a thick layer, called the *endometrium*,

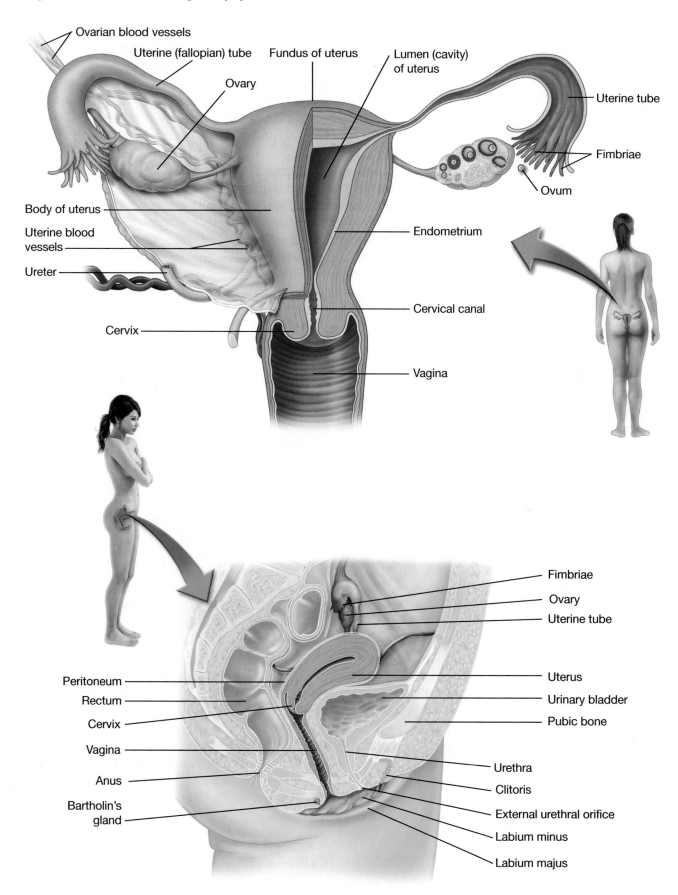

Figure 17.21   The female reproductive system. What are the female gonads and gametes?

in preparation for a developing embryo to implant. If an embryo does not attach to the endometrium, the ovum and lining of the uterus are shed, and they will redevelop during the next monthly hormone cycle.

The uterus houses and protects the growing fetus during pregnancy. The top of the uterus is called the *fundus*. The **cervix** is the narrower neck at the bottom of the uterus that connects to the vagina. Sperm and the menstrual flow are able to pass through the closed cervix between the vagina and uterus. During birth, the cervix dilates to 10 centimeters so the baby can pass down the birth canal.

From the outside, the vaginal opening is enclosed and protected. In young women, the opening of the vagina is partly covered by a thin mucous membrane called the *hymen*. In some cultures, an intact hymen is an important sign of virginity. The *labia* are folds of skin that cover the vagina, urethra, and clitoris. The clitoris is the sensitive female erectile organ. When the clitoris is stimulated, Bartholin's glands—located beside the vaginal opening—produce mucus to lubricate the vagina.

Sexually transmitted infections are the most common cause of disease within the reproductive system. Milky-colored discharge or sores on the penis or labia are a sign of possible STIs. Unfortunately, many people have no symptoms, and sores inside the vagina or urethra can't easily be seen. Condoms provide a barrier that can help reduce the spread of STIs, but abstinence is the only sure way to prevent infection.

The Genetic Uniqueness of Offspring

The male and female reproductive systems allow us to produce offspring and introduce new gene combinations into the population. Most human cells divide through **mitosis** to create two identical cells with 46 chromosomes each (Figure 17.22). Sperm and ova divide through **meiosis** (mI-OH-sihs) to make genetically unique cells. During meiosis, a cell copies all of its chromosomes, and then divides the chromosomal material between two daughter cells. Each of these daughter cells divides again to produce four daughter cells, each with a unique combination of 23 chromosomes. The ovum and sperm join during **fertilization**. The genetically unique cell that results is called a **zygote**. It has 46 chromosomes, half from each parent.

Heredity describes the process of passing on genetic characteristics from one generation to the next. Inherited characteristics are controlled by chromosomes in our genes. With paired chromosomes, there are two alleles for each characteristic. Some alleles are dominant and always express their trait. Others are recessive and may only show if both alleles are recessive. We often think of eye or hair color when discussing inheritance, but genetic disorders such as Down syndrome and hemophilia are also passed on this way. Some traits are easily traced from parents to children, while others may skip generations. A genetic counselor helps families understand the likelihood of genetic disorders being passed on to their children.

Reproductive Hormones

Both the male and female reproductive systems produce and respond to hormones that trigger puberty and the development of secondary sexual characteristics. The pituitary gland in the brain produces

mitosis
the asexual process of cellular reproduction that creates two identical copies of a cell, each with a full set of 46 chromosomes

meiosis
the sexual process of cell division that produces four new haploid cells, each with a unique combination of 23 chromosomes

heredity
the passing of traits (such as eye color, height, and some diseases) from parent or ancestor to offspring through chromosomes

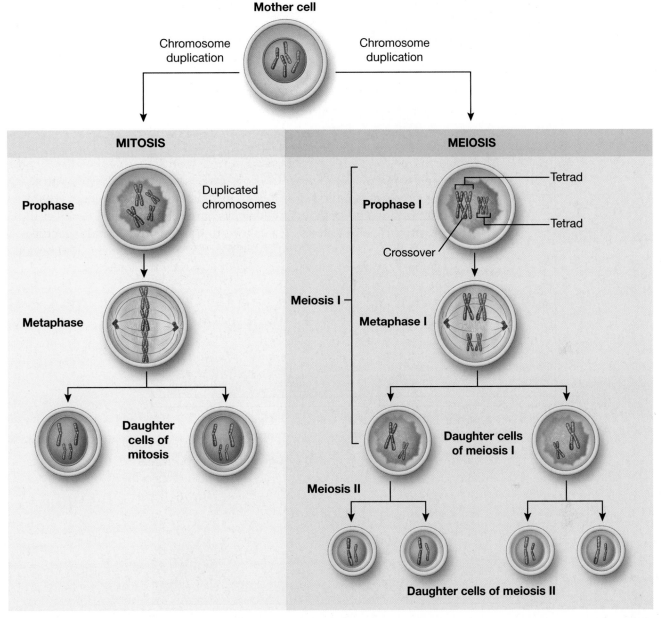

Figure 17.22   Daughter cells of mitosis have 46 chromosomes identical to the mother cell. Daughter cells of meiosis II each have a unique combination of 23 chromosomes.

Animation

luteinizing hormone (LH) and follicle-stimulating hormone (FSH). These hormones tell the male's testes to make sperm and **testosterone**. Testosterone is responsible for the development of a deep voice, facial hair, and muscle bulk at puberty. In the female, LH and FSH stimulate the ovaries to produce **estrogen** and **progesterone**, which regulate the menstrual cycle each month. Estrogen is responsible for the development of breasts, the growth of pubic hair, and an increase in body fat during puberty. Progesterone prepares the uterine lining for an egg to implant.

In females, a monthly hormone cycle matures an ovum and prepares the uterus for a possible pregnancy (Figure 17.23 on the next page). The first menstrual cycle is called *menarche*. The first day of the cycle is marked by the first day of menstruation and hormone levels are low. During menstruation, the endometrium is shed from the uterus. From

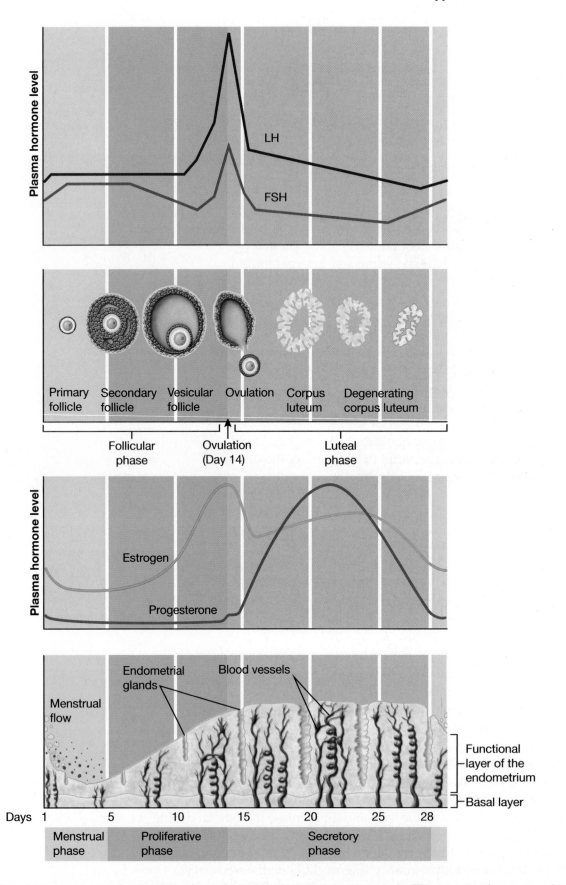

Figure 17.23   Hormonal and structural changes during the female hormone cycle. The events of one complete female cycle, lasting 28 days, are shown. The time scale, shown horizontally at the bottom, applies to all four panels of the figure.

days 6 to 12, estrogen helps to rebuild the endometrium in the uterus, while FSH tells the ovaries to mature an ovum follicle. Around day 14, LH and FSH levels increase to trigger ovulation. After the ovum is released, LH and FSH levels decrease until the next cycle. Progesterone from the ovaries continues to build the endometrium through day 28 of the cycle. If an egg is not fertilized or hormone levels are not high enough to support a pregnancy, the endometrium begins to break down and the cycle starts again. If an egg is fertilized, a different hormone process begins.

Hormones also control the processes of pregnancy. Progesterone from the ovaries and human chorionic gonadotropin (kor-ee-AH-nihk goh-nad-oh-TROH-pihn), or *hCG*, from the placenta maintain the placenta during pregnancy. Toward the end of pregnancy, relaxin and prostaglandin help soften the ligaments in the pelvis and relax and open the cervix in preparation for birth. Oxytocin starts the contractions of the uterus that will push the baby out (Figure 17.24). Endorphins trigger an emotional high at the end of labor that helps with pain management. The uterus also secretes prolactin at the end of pregnancy to stimulate milk production in the mammary glands. Increased production of all these hormones can affect a woman's emotions. After birth, the sudden drop in hormone levels may cause postpartum [*post* = after, *partum* = birth, labor] depression in some women.

Hormonal changes continue after birth. When a baby nurses, more oxytocin is released to help shrink the uterus and release milk from the breasts. Nursing maintains hormone levels and may delay the release of ova for several months after birth.

Birth control pills take advantage of the role of hormones in controlling these processes. These pills artificially regulate hormone levels to trick the body into believing it is pregnant, so no eggs are released. Unfortunately, many other side effects come with pregnancy hormones, such as fluid retention and high blood pressure. If you are pregnant or taking birth control pills, regular consultation with a doctor is important to monitor these effects.

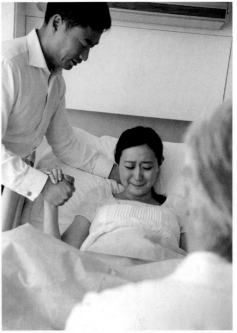

Figure 17.24   The hormone oxytocin triggers contractions that will begin labor.

Around 50 years of age, menopause begins. Estrogen levels drop, ovulation gradually ends, and women lose their reproductive abilities. Men may experience enlargement of the prostate gland and a reduction in hormone levels as they age, but they still continue to produce sperm. Hormonal changes in women during menopause cause thinning of the uterus, reduced vaginal secretions, hot flashes, night sweats, irritability, fatigue, depression, weight gain, insomnia, and forgetfulness. More hormonal changes occur around 80 years of age, causing a relaxation of ligaments, a general loss of muscle tone, and drooping of the breasts.

The Reproductive Process

During the reproductive process, a fertilized egg develops into a new baby. This process takes 10 lunar months, which is 280 days or about 9 calendar months. Much growth and development happens during this period, especially in the first few months.

Animation

Fertilization begins in one of the fallopian tubes, where the sperm and ovum meet. The resulting zygote divides quickly to produce a **morula** (MOR-yoo-luh). This solid ball of 16 cells travels down the fallopian tube to the uterus to implant. If the morula accidentally implants inside the fallopian tube, the result is an ectopic pregnancy. This is becoming more common due to the increased use of fertility treatments. An ectopic pregnancy cannot develop normally, and the woman may die from internal bleeding if it is not removed.

When the morula reaches the uterus, it attaches to the uterine lining, or *endometrium*. As it grows, the morula becomes a hollow **blastocyst** [*blast* = embryonic, *cyst* = fluid-filled sac], developing a fluid sac in its center. The inner cells of the blastocyst become the **embryo** at day seven, eventually developing into a baby. The outer cells release enzymes and hormones that help the embryo implant and form the placenta and amniotic sac. At this point, it is possible for a pregnancy test to detect hCG, but tests are most accurate about three to four weeks after conception.

The embryo is unrecognizable in this early stage of development. During the embryonic stage, blood vessels develop between the embryo and the mother's uterus, forming the **placenta**. The embryo's blood and the mother's blood must cross the placental membrane; it never meets directly. This helps prevent the spread of some illnesses between mother and fetus during pregnancy. By the fifth week, the heart begins to beat.

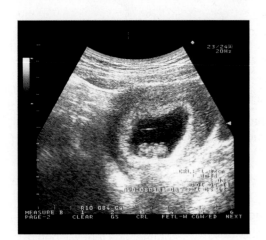

Figure 17.25   Sonogram of a fetus at three months.

By the eighth week, all of the major internal organs and external features are present. At this point, the developing baby is called a **fetus** and is more than a half-inch long (Figure 17.25). The woman has probably missed her second menstrual cycle and may be aware of her pregnancy, although it may not show for several months.

This first *trimester*, or period of three months, is a risky time for the developing fetus. During this time, when all of the body systems are forming, the woman is least aware of her pregnancy. Exposing the developing fetus to drugs, alcohol, or other harmful teratogens during this critical development period can have devastating results. Figure 17.26 shows the critical periods of development for various structures. A healthy diet that contains all the vitamins, minerals, and nutrients for growth is essential at the same time that many women report nausea or morning sickness.

At this stage, the only way to distinguish between a male and female fetus is by karyotype. This is a visual examination and pairing of the 46 chromosomes. It will show two XX chromosomes in females and an X and a Y in males. Male and female gonads develop from the same structures in the embryo. When testosterone is present, the male gonads develop into the vas deferens (ductus deferens), seminal vesicle, prostate, scrotum, and penis of a male, while the female gonads degenerate. Without testosterone, the gonads develop into the uterus, uterine (fallopian) tubes, vagina, labia, and clitoris of a female, while the male gonads degenerate. External genitalia can be seen after 8 to 12 weeks of gestation.

At 12 weeks, the fetus is about two inches long and able to make small movements. The fetal heartbeat can be detected during regular visits to the obstetrician/gynecologist (OB/GYN). During these visits, the doctor

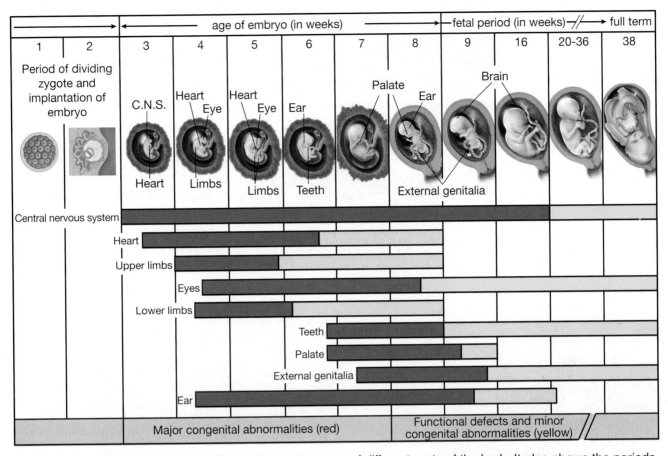

Figure 17.26 This chart shows the timing for development of different parts of the body. It also shows the periods during which major abnormalities (red) and less serious defects and abnormalities (yellow) can occur.

will take urine samples from the mother to check for signs of infection, gestational diabetes, or other conditions that may affect the pregnancy. The size of the uterus is also measured as an estimate of fetus growth. The length from the pubic bone to the fundus (the top of the uterus) will increase by about one centimeter each week.

The second trimester, from the sixteenth week until the end of the seventh month, is usually described as the easiest stage of pregnancy. Feelings of morning sickness usually go away. The mother often feels the baby kick and move in the womb. An ultrasound may be done at 20 weeks to confirm that the baby and placenta are growing properly.

The third trimester is a period of rapid growth. The fetus grows from about two pounds at 28 weeks to four pounds at 32 weeks. Half of a baby's weight is added during the last month of gestation, which explains why premature infants, or *preemies*, are so small. A preemie often remains in the neonatal intensive care unit until the full-term due date. The average baby is 20 inches long and weighs 7.5 pounds at full term. Delivery between 38 and 42 weeks is considered full-term.

Birth is a three-stage process (Figure 17.27 on the next page). It begins with the thinning and dilation of the cervix to open the birth canal. Strong contractions of the uterus stretch the cervix opening to 10 centimeters in diameter. The active phase of stage one lasts several hours and can be painful. An anesthesiologist or nurse anesthetist can help control the pain of labor with medications. A birthing coach, doula,

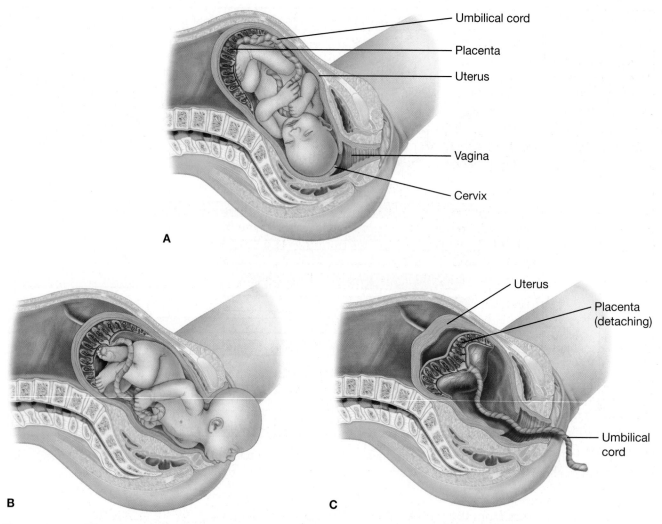

Figure 17.27   The stages of labor—dilation (A), expulsion (B), and delivery of the placenta (C). How wide is the cervix when it is fully dilated?

or midwife uses breathing, imagery, water baths, and changes in position to help the mother manage her pain.

The second stage is the birth of the baby, or *expulsion*. This happens much faster than the dilation stage. The baby should come out head first and facedown. Any other presentation can slow the delivery and may cause complications for the baby or the mother. The final stage is delivery of the placenta. The placenta, commonly called the *afterbirth*, should not detach from the uterus until after the baby is born, but it does need to come out. Some cultures have rituals related to the placenta, so it is important to discuss this with the mother before birth. They may wish to bury it, eat a portion of it, or save the blood.

After birth, hormones will begin the process of shrinking the uterus and starting the flow of breast milk to nourish the baby. Most women spend only a day in the hospital for the birth of a child. When the mother and child are released, a patient transport technician assists in safely seeing them out of the hospital. A nurse may call the new mother after she returns home. Regular checkups with the pediatrician follow the healthy development of the new baby.

Stages of Development

Human development is monitored from the time of conception through death. Recognized stages of development will occur in the physical growth of the body, mental development of the mind, emotional control of feelings, and social development through relationships with others. Being aware of the changes that normally take place during these stages of development helps parents and healthcare workers recognize problems. Knowing what to expect at different stages also helps care providers anticipate a person's needs and challenges.

Physical Development. Physical growth of the body follows two general patterns. First, development starts at the head and works its way down. Infants learn to lift their head, then to push themselves up, then to sit up, and finally to walk. Second, development radiates from the midline of the body outward. Infants learn to use the large motor muscles of their torso and arms before they can control the fine motor skills of their fingers. Parents and healthcare workers compare a child's physical growth and milestones to those of other children of the same age as a way of monitoring for problems.

Psychosocial Development. All people have the same basic needs that drive their behavior. Abraham Maslow identified five levels of needs (Figure 17.28). He recognized that our needs exist in a hierarchy, meaning that some must be met before others. After meeting basic physical needs, our attention can shift to safety and security needs. If we feel protected from harm, we can focus on developing relationships to fulfill our need for love and belonging. Once we feel accepted, we can work toward self-actualization. Different ages and cultures may meet these needs in different ways.

Our needs influence our behavior. Erik Erikson was a psychoanalyst who identified basic conflicts that must be resolved for psychosocial development to occur (Figure 17.29 on the next page). Infants must rely on others to meet their basic physical needs. They test different behaviors, such as crying and cooing, to see what works. Children want to explore and push for more independence. Parents' rules keep them safe and help them fulfill their needs. Children must learn to create their own structure and form their own supportive relationships as they gain independence from their family. Autism is an emerging developmental disorder that limits a child's ability to form relationships with others.

Healthcare workers need to remember that illness affects patients' basic needs and may affect their behaviors and reactions to others. Sudden illness or surgery can create feelings of insecurity, pain, and stress. Medications and illness can alter patients' mental states or affect their ability to interact with others or the environment. Try to anticipate

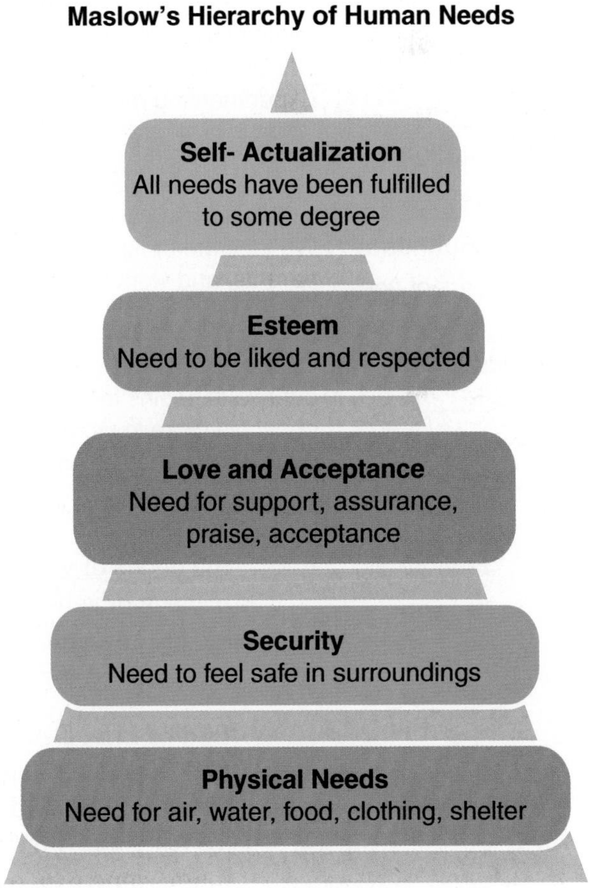

Maslow's Hierarchy of Human Needs

Self- Actualization
All needs have been fulfilled to some degree

Esteem
Need to be liked and respected

Love and Acceptance
Need for support, assurance, praise, acceptance

Security
Need to feel safe in surroundings

Physical Needs
Need for air, water, food, clothing, shelter

Figure 17.28 The five levels of need, as determined by Abraham Maslow. Why are these arranged in a hierarchy?

Figure 17.29 Erikson's Stages of Psychosocial Development

Age	Stage Description	Main Challenge
Infancy birth to 18 months	We experience rapid growth but are not yet able to control our bodies or fend for ourselves. We need to be fed, bathed, clothed, and kept safe and warm by caregivers. We have difficulty expressing our needs.	learning to trust others to meet our needs for food, care, and affection
Early childhood 18 months–3 years of age	We begin to control our bodies and assert our independence, but we need others to keep us safe by providing limits.	developing self-control and autonomy without a loss of self-esteem to build will power
Preschool 3–5 years of age	We use our growing independence to explore the world and exert control over our environment.	developing initiative and a sense of purpose without guilt
School age 6–11 years of age	We begin school and experience extended separation from our parents. We form new friendships and learn to cope with demands to perform well in school.	needing praise and reassurance in our accomplishments so we don't feel inferior to others
Adolescence 12–18 years of age	We go through a period of self-discovery, with increasing responsibilities and independence in relationships, money control, and decision-making. Our peers have more influence than our parents. Experimenting may lead to risky behaviors.	needing loyalty, acceptance, and self-identity to avoid role confusion
Early adulthood 20–40 years of age	We feel the stress of building a new career and a family apart from our parents.	needing intimacy and love versus isolation
Middle adulthood 40–65 years of age	We face the pressures of parenthood, aging parents, and work responsibilities.	being productive and caring for others so we don't become self-absorbed
Late adulthood 65 years of age and older	We look back on life as friends and family are aging, our health begins to fail, and we experience the loss of people close to us. We face shrinking financial resources and social opportunities with retirement.	accepting accomplishments and loss without despair

the needs of your patients and their families. Be sensitive to their need for privacy or self-expression. Reactions will vary, and they may be affected by age and culture. It is important to be patient and encourage them to talk about their feelings.

End of Life. Death is the final stage of life. Dr. Elisabeth Kübler-Ross identified five stages of death and dying. It was later realized that these stages could also apply to grief surrounding other times of major loss or crisis (Figure 17.30). Not all people experience these stages in the same way or at the same time, but the breakdown provides some understanding of what to expect. It can help to know that your experience is normal, although you may still need support from others to get through it. Some people may not progress through all of the stages. As a healthcare worker, being able to recognize the stages will help you understand your patients and not take it personally when they lash out.

Hospice care is available for people with six months or less to live. Hospice is a philosophy of care that supports dignity and comfort in death.

Palliative care is provided to relieve pain, but the focus is no longer on finding a cure. Some facilities are dedicated specifically to providing hospice care, but this type of care may be provided by a care team in any setting. Working with patients at the end of life can be very rewarding, but it is also stressful for caregivers. Supportive care and self-awareness are important to the well-being of families and healthcare workers. Hospice social workers, chaplains, support groups, and other grief services are available to anyone who is experiencing loss due to death, even if the loved one was not a hospice patient. Nonprofit hospices have a charitable mission of serving those in need.

Figure 17.30 The Stages of Grief	
Stage	**What It May Be Like**
Denial We refuse to believe the truth.	ignoring the facts or sad news • "There must be a mix-up." • "I feel fine. I'm sure their estimates are off."
Anger We become angry when we can no longer deny the truth.	feeling upset with doctors and others • "Why me?" • "This is your fault." • "That doctor's a quack. He didn't keep me well."
Bargaining We accept death but want more time.	trying to make deals with the doctor, family members, or God • "If I stop smoking, can you just keep me alive until my grandchild is born?" • "If I take more medications and exercise better, can you get me a few more years?"
Depression We realize that death will come soon.	extreme sadness that interferes with life activities • crying easily • poor memory and concentration • sleeping a lot; restless when awake
Acceptance We understand and accept that we are going to die.	acceptance of the loss as real and beginning to move on • making a will and getting affairs in order • ability to talk about life after you're gone • shifting concern to those who will be left behind

RECALL YOUR READING

1. Sperm are produced in the _____, mature in the _____, and are released through the _____.

2. Upon release from the _____, an ovum can be fertilized while in the _____ and implant in the _____.

3. Most human cells divide through _____, a process that results in two identical cells that each have _____ chromosomes. _____ is the process of sexual reproduction, creating four daughter cells that each have _____ chromosomes.

4. Hormones control the monthly cycle of _____, and, around 50 years of age, _____.

5. According to Maslow, human needs can be identified as _____, _____, _____, _____, and _____.

Complete the *Map Your Reading* graphic organizer for the section you just read.

SUMMARY

 Assess your understanding with chapter tests

- Surveying, previewing, and questioning your reading material will help you to make sense of and remember information.

- The body needs macronutrients (carbohydrates, proteins, fats) in larger quantities and micronutrients (vitamins and minerals) in smaller amounts.

- The process of breaking down food for use by the body includes ingestion, digestion, absorption, and excretion.

- Digestive problems, such as GERD, diabetes, jaundice, gallstones, and celiac disease, demonstrate the importance of each organ in the digestive system.

- The excretory system, which includes the urinary organs, removes waste from the body.

- The renal cortex of the kidneys contains millions of nephrons that filter waste from the blood, reabsorb substances needed by the body, and secrete the waste as urine.

- The kidneys help maintain homeostasis in the body by making and responding to a variety of hormones and enzymes. The kidneys influence blood pressure, blood pH, red blood cell production, and calcium levels.

- Male testes produce millions of sperm from puberty until death. They mature in the epididymis and are released through the vas deferens.

- Females house, nourish, and protect the ovum and fetus during development. They are born with about one million immature ova.

- Reproduction produces new gene combinations in offspring. Heredity of dominant and recessive traits is controlled by chromosomes.

- The reproductive system produces new life through a complex process controlled by hormones.

- Birth is a three-stage process. Dilation and thinning of the cervix opens the birth canal. Contractions of the uterus push the baby out. The placenta is delivered last.

- Recognized stages of development occur in the physical growth of the body, the mental development of the mind, emotional control of feelings, and social development through relationships with others.

MAXIMIZE YOUR PROFESSIONAL VOCABULARY

 Build vocabulary with e-flash cards, games, and audio glossary

Listed below are the essential, yellow-highlighted terms and the additional professional vocabulary that you encountered in this chapter. Complete the activities that follow the list to make all of these terms part of your everyday professional vocabulary.

absorption	calories	estrogen
accessory organs	cervix	excretion
alimentary canal	chyme	fallopian tubes
amino acids	digestion	fertilization
bile	embryo	fetus
bladder	epididymis	filtration
blastocyst	esophagus	gallbladder

gametes	ova	semen
gonads	ovaries	sperm
heredity	pancreas	stomach
ingestion	penis	testes
kidneys	peristalsis	testosterone
liver	placenta	ureter
meiosis	progesterone	urethra
menopause	reabsorption	uterus
mitosis	rectum	vas deferens
morula	salivary glands	villi
nephron	scrotum	zygote
nutrients	secretion	

VOCABULARY DEVELOPMENT

Matching. Match the essential terms from this chapter with the best descriptions below by writing the letter of the description next to the number of the essential term on your answer sheet.

1. absorption
2. digestion
3. excretion
4. filtration
5. gametes
6. heredity
7. ingestion
8. meiosis
9. mitosis
10. nutrients
11. reabsorption
12. secretion

a. the asexual process of cellular reproduction that creates two identical copies of a cell, each with a full set of 46 chromosomes

b. the release of a liquid substance from blood, cells, or tissues

c. the process of separating substances, such as solid from liquid, large from small, or impure from pure

d. term for the mechanical and chemical breakdown of food into nutrients that can be absorbed and used by the body

e. a sex gland that produces gametes; the testes in males and the ovaries in females

f. the act of taking up a substance into a tissue, such as the movement of nutrients from the small intestines into the bloodstream

g. the passing of traits (such as eye color, height, and some diseases) from parent or ancestor to offspring through chromosomes

h. the sexual process of cell division that produces four new haploid cells, each with a unique combination of 23 chromosomes

i. the act of returning a substance to the part of the body from which it was previously filtered out

j. reproductive cells that have half the normal number of chromosomes and unite during fertilization; sperm in males and ova in females

k. the stage of digestion in which food is taken into the body through the mouth

l. molecules such as carbohydrates, proteins, fats, vitamins, and minerals used by the body to grow and maintain body processes

m. the removal of waste products from the body

13. **Term Snap.** Make flash cards for each word part listed in the table shown here. Sit in circles of 3 to 5 students and shuffle your cards, keeping them all facing in the same direction. The first player turns over a term card to reveal the definition and places it in the center, "term side" facing up. Other players go around the circle, taking turns to discard one card at a time with the definition side facing up. When the definition matching the term card in the center of the circle is discarded, the first to notice must slap the matching card. That player takes all the cards in the middle and draws the next term card. Play continues until the time is up or players run out of cards. The player with the most term cards at the end of play is the winner.

Medical Word Parts			
Prefixes	**Root Words**		**Suffixes**
macro-	blast/o	lapar/o	-ostomy
micro-	col/o, colon/o	lith/o	-partum
post-	cyst/o	lip/o	-poietin
	enter/o	nephr/o	-rrhea
	esophag/o	ren/o	-scope
	gluc/o	urethr/o	-tripsy
	hepat/o		

14. **Diagram and Terms.** Draw or trace a diagram of the digestive or urinary system. Using the medical word parts in the table shown here, label the organs and processes associated with the system you chose.

REFLECT ON YOUR READING

15. Review your Vocabulary Sorting Organizer you created for the *Connect with Your Reading* activity. Share your "clinical diagnosis" of the new term you selected with a partner. Does your partner agree with your diagnosis? Why or why not? Ask them to add an idea of their own to it.

BUILD CORE SKILLS

16. **Reading.** Review the reading strategies at the beginning of the chapter. Then select an article related to the research and findings of Abraham Maslow, Erik Erikson, or Elisabeth Kübler-Ross. Use the strategies you learned to read and comprehend the article you found. Evaluate the source of the reading and the purpose for writing it. Skim through the headings to understand the topic and its organization. Turn the headings into questions, then take notes that include your questions and their answers. Write the notes in your own words, including any new terms you circled or underlined. Review the notes you've made and underline the key points to separate them from details.

17. **Writing.** Do some research and then write a five-paragraph essay describing an aspect of human development across the life span. The five-paragraph essay follows a common format. Introduce the topic and your three main points in the first paragraph, focus on one major point and its supporting details in each of the next three paragraphs, then summarize by restating the thesis and adding any closing thoughts in the last paragraph.

18. **Critical Thinking.** Use Figure 17.3 to analyze the carbohydrate, protein, and fat contents of various foods. Determine the top three healthiest food choices for a young adult. Use the nutritional data in the figure and what you learned about nutrients to explain your choices.

19. **Problem Solving.** For each of the following physical conditions, research the body system or systems it relates to, the signs or symptoms associated with it, and the healthcare professional or professionals the patient or client would have to consult.

    - benign prostatic hyperplasia
    - autism
    - diabetes
    - jaundice
    - Down syndrome
    - kidney failure

20. **Critical Thinking.** Name your favorite cartoon character and analyze which stage of psychosocial development he or she is in. Use one of their conflicts to support your answer.

21. **Problem Solving.** The chapter mentions several medical procedures related to body systems for maintenance and support. For each of the following procedures, write out the medical description and then write or explain it in simpler terminology. Which specific organs are involved in each of these procedures?

    - colonoscopy
    - colostomy
    - dialysis
    - catheterization
    - vaginal childbirth

22. **Math.** Demonstrate the exponential spread of sexually transmitted infections. Keep a list of every person you touch or talk to for one day. Compare your list with the lists of everyone else in your class. Highlight the names of anyone on your list who is also on someone else's list. Choose one name on the list and count how many other people had that name on their list. Then count all the other names on the lists that contain this one name. If this one person had herpes, and these interactions were sexual interactions, how many people would have been exposed?

ACTIVATE YOUR LEARNING

23. Demonstrate the importance of mechanical digestion by comparing the effect of water on a teaspoon of sugar granules versus its effect on a solid sugar cube. Place a teaspoon of sugar and a sugar cube in the bottom of separate cups and add water. Note what happens. Then stir each mixture. Which dissolves fastest—the loose sugar granules or the sugar cube? Use your observations to explain how chewing and mixing are important to digestion.

24. Simulate filtration in the kidney. Use a large pan of sand and gravel mix to represent the blood content delivered to the kidney for filtration. Use a sifter to represent the kidney's filter and a cup for the desired amount of sugar, salt, and water in the blood. Filters allow only specific sizes of material to pass through—what would the gravel in the sifter represent? Where does the overflow from the cup go? Explain how this process results in homeostasis. How do hormones play a role in this process?

THINK AND ACT LIKE A HEALTHCARE WORKER

25. Shawna believes she is pregnant. As her primary care physician, what tests would you use to determine if she is truly pregnant or not? If she is pregnant, what additional risks and tests would you discuss with her about pregnancy, prenatal, and postnatal care? What dietary information will she need to maintain a healthy weight and get the right nutrients during pregnancy?

GO TO THE SOURCE

26. Go to the MyPlate website or the USDA website. Insert your personal data (age, sex, weight, height, and physical activity level) to find a daily meal plan that fits your physical criteria. Consider the value of these sites for a preschooler, mom, or teenager. Take time to check out the sites and the information they offer. If you were a dietitian or nutrition counselor, how would you use these websites to help your clients? Report back to the class with your observations and insights.

Unit 5
Biotechnology

While studying, look for the online icon to:

- **Listen** to the audio Glossary and review e-flash cards
- **Assess** learning with quizzes and online exercises
- **Expand** knowledge with animations and activities
- **Simulate** healthcare tasks and employability skills

www.g-wlearning.com/healthsciences

Companion G-W Learning

Study on the Go
Use your mobile device to practice vocabulary and assess learning
www.m.g-wlearning.com

Mobile G-W Learning

Career Pathway

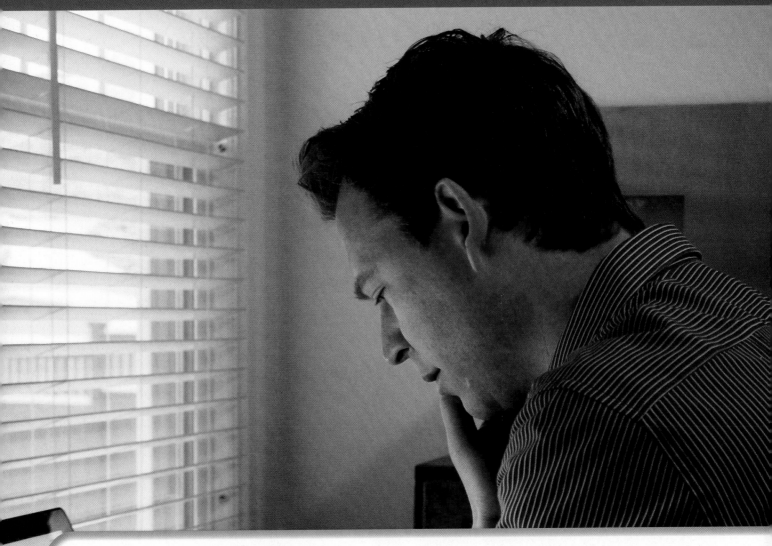

Healthcare Insider: *Brett—Sales Representative*

As a sales rep, my job is to effectively negotiate, sell, and service equipment and disposable products. This means that I make presentations, talk directly to customers, and help them when equipment and products need repairs. The products that I specifically work with are used for minimally invasive spinal procedures. It's my responsibility to foster a good relationship with my customers. I do that by providing quality service in a timely manner, handling all product complaints appropriately, training physicians and staff members on products, and assisting with product application during procedures.

Chapter 18
Career Skills in Biotechnology Research and Development

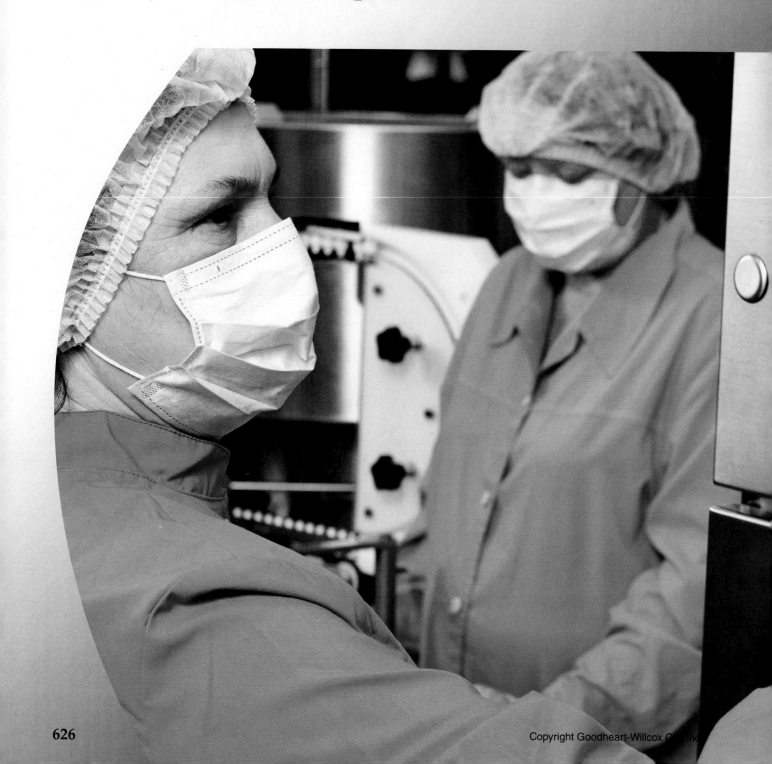

PROFESSIONAL VOCABULARY

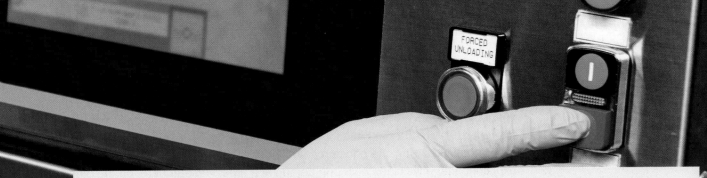
E-flash Cards

You will need to learn the essential terms listed below before you begin your reading. These terms will help you understand the main concepts of the chapter. These terms, which will be highlighted in yellow within the text, will become part of your professional vocabulary.

In addition to the essential terms, you will see bold terms throughout the chapter. The meanings of these terms are explained where the terms first appear. The bold terms, like the essential terms listed here, will also become part of your professional vocabulary and deepen your understanding of the topics presented.

assay analysis done to determine the presence and amount of a substance or to determine the potency of a drug

autoclaves chambers for sterilizing items with steam under pressure

biohazard term that describes a biological agent, infectious organism, or insecure laboratory procedure that constitutes a danger to humans or the environment

biotechnology the manipulation of living organisms to produce useful products

biotechnology research laboratories research facilities that develop new products or treatments and are located on college campuses, in hospitals, and in private biotechnology companies

business-to-business selling exchanging goods between businesses rather than between businesses and individuals

clinical laboratories facilities that examine materials taken from the human body to discover information related to diagnosis, prognosis, prevention, or treatment of disease

clinical trial an experiment performed on human beings to evaluate the comparative effectiveness of two or more treatments

electronic balances measuring instruments that display the weight of a substance digitally and are used to weigh chemicals in labs

laboratory documentation written records of observable, measurable, and reproducible findings obtained through examination, testing, research studies, and experiments

letter of resignation a written document that formally states an employee's decision to leave a job

micropipette an instrument designed for the measurement of very small volumes

personal and professional development term that describes steps taken to improve personal, educational, and career-related performance

personal leadership style an individual approach to giving directions, implementing plans, and motivating people

professional organization an association formed to unite and inform people who work in the same occupation

sales presentation a prearranged meeting in which a salesperson presents detailed information and often a demonstration of a product

CONNECT WITH YOUR READING

Make a list of five improvements made to medical care during your lifetime. These may be procedures, equipment, or treatments. Compare and discuss your list with a classmate. Did you list the same improvements or different ones?

Next, identify the types of workers involved in creating each new procedure, piece of equipment, or treatment on your list. Once again, compare your list with a classmate. Consider these workers as you read about biotechnology, research, and development careers in this chapter.

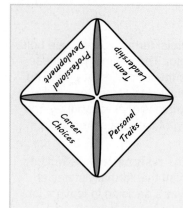

MAP YOUR READING

Create a visual summary of this chapter, just as you did in chapter 2. Begin with a square sheet of paper—an 8½-inch square works well. Fold each of the four points of the square to the center. Label each of the four resulting flaps with one of these topics: *Personal Traits*, *Career Choices*, *Team Leadership*, and *Professional Development*. When you finish reading each of these sections in the chapter, open the corresponding flap and draw a picture or symbol to illustrate what you have read. Ask yourself what each topic looks like, how you could draw it, and what graphic or symbol best represents it. Finally, for each of the four topics, write two words that explain how the topic relates to you personally in the center square of your visual summary.

Whether they are developing a new drug, building a surgical robot, marketing artificial heart valves, or maintaining sterile conditions where medicines are produced, biotechnology research and development workers fill a wide variety of work roles.

In this chapter, you will learn about job opportunities in the biotechnology research and development pathway and study the qualities of effective team leaders. You will be introduced to guidelines for laboratory safety and practice basic procedures performed by biotechnology workers. Finally, you will learn how professional development activities can improve your skills and enhance employment options.

The Biotechnology Research and Development Worker: Annika

Annika was excited about finally finishing her PhD program. After completing her undergraduate degree and six years of postgraduate research, she was ready for the next step in her career. However, that step was causing a problem.

Annika had enjoyed science in high school and had chosen that field for her college coursework. Part-time work in a research lab during her undergraduate years convinced her that research was the direction her career should take. Her postgraduate work in stem cell research was energizing, and she spent many hours perfecting her laboratory research and scientific writing skills to prepare for a career in biotechnology research.

When asked why she chose research instead of medicine, Annika always explained that physicians help one person at a time. Researchers, on the other hand, can help many people and change the delivery of healthcare with their discoveries. Her program supervisor and lab director encouraged her to pursue an academic research career. That had always been her goal, but lately she wasn't quite sure.

Annika observed the high level of commitment shown by academic research lab directors and saw how the work consumed them. She had also experienced that singular focus as her postgraduate research consumed her life. Did she really want her career to be the main focus of her life? Maybe she should consider a career working for a pharmaceutical or other biotechnology company. She could still use her research skills, but she would have more time to pursue personal goals. Either way, Annika knew she would find her career niche in the expanding field of biotechnology research and development.

Personal Traits

Do you enjoy science classes? Do you find lab experiments interesting? If so, you might find a satisfying career in **biotechnology** research and development. If you pay attention to details and take pride in performing work precisely and accurately, then you possess qualities required for successful work in a research laboratory.

Rob's friends teased him about his class binder. He had the best notes in the class and routinely made lists of tasks to complete every assignment (Figure 18.1). His teacher commented that he had the most organized binder she had ever seen. Though Rob didn't know it, he had an **aptitude**, or natural inclination, for documenting experimental data. Habits that came naturally to him are strengths of skilled lab workers.

Do you also like to figure out why things happen or come up with your own ideas to solve problems? Then you may enjoy the challenge of working as a lab scientist, developing and testing new biotechnology products. Are you persistent but also patient? Since it takes many years to develop and test new products, these qualities will keep you from becoming discouraged during the research process.

Do you enjoy working with computers? As a result of DNA sequencing, large databases of biological information are becoming common in research settings. Biotechnology research and development scientists will need computation skills for working with large data sets.

Can you be discrete about sharing information? In a competitive research environment, teamwork moves a project forward and can help increase the documentation of results. However, sharing research ideas and information inappropriately can cost a researcher years of work. If that information is leaked, someone else might publish similar research findings first.

Nora, a lab technician for a biotechnology research company, says that honesty is important for all research workers. When test results are inaccurate because of poor lab practices, or when research data is falsified so a project will look successful, real harm can be done to patients. Physicians rely on research results that are valid, legitimate, and accurate when they develop treatment regimens for their patients. **Validity** is important in scientific research because patients expect new treatments to be beneficial. In Nora's lab, a broken beaker in step seven means starting over from step one to prepare the designated formulation. That means Nora might have to stay late to finish so that the steps in the research study are not interrupted and the results are reliable.

Are you a likeable person with great listening skills? Do you like a team-oriented environment and enjoy working with people who have different types of personalities? Then you might find your career in biotechnology sales and support. While sales representatives focus on

biotechnology
the manipulation of living organisms to produce useful products

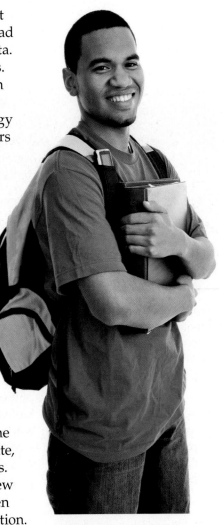

Figure 18.1   If you have organized class notes like Rob, you may have a natural aptitude for skills needed by lab workers.

building relationships with potential customers, they must also become **consultants** for any healthcare worker who uses the products they sell. This means they give professional advice or provide training seminars for those healthcare workers. Sales reps need self-motivation, determination, and resilience to be successful in selling products. They also need good time management and organizational skills to educate and support the people who use their products.

Biotechnology Research and Development Career Choices

You might choose a career in biotechnology so that you can cure diseases, feed the hungry, or improve the environment. People who work in this field discover new drugs, improve food crops, preserve the environment, and manufacture medical devices. Biotechnology is a growing industry that provides job opportunities for people who have studied the biological sciences and have good laboratory and computer science skills.

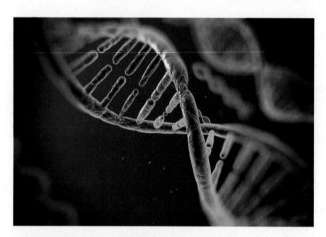

Figure 18.2 In the field of biotechnology, DNA molecules become the building blocks for research tools and diagnostic tests.

assay
analysis done to determine the presence and amount of a substance or to determine the potency of a drug

What exactly is biotechnology? This field uses advances in life sciences to create products that come from the living things we call organisms. The science of biotechnology uses the DNA molecules found in the cells of all living organisms to create new and helpful tools (Figure 18.2).

Historically, we have used the concept of biotechnology—modifying living organisms for human purposes—when we domesticate animals or cultivate plants using artificial selection or hybrid development during breeding. Modern biotechnology, however, began in the 1970s when scientists modified a DNA molecule by "recombining" DNA from two different organisms. They combined an insulin gene with a bacterium cell and multiplied it millions of times to harvest the insulin. Insulin is used to treat diabetes, and this manufactured insulin is far more plentiful and less expensive than extracting insulin from animals. Today, the science of biotechnology is used to formulate drugs; create **assays** and other biological research tools; and develop diagnostic tests used in medical research, diagnosis, and treatment.

The science of biotechnology is also used in agriculture, industry, forensics, mining, environmental cleanup, and the creation of biofuels. Yet healthcare continues to be the most active sector of biotechnology. Since the 1970s, biotechnology has been used to sequence the human genome and clone mammals. It is used to create drugs that treat diseases, vaccines that prevent diseases, and tests and devices that diagnose diseases (Figure 18.3).

Currently, researchers are working to develop gene therapies with the goal of curing genetic diseases by using modified viruses to deliver healthy DNA to cells. They are using stem cells to develop treatments for spinal cord injuries and chronic diseases such as diabetes and

Treatments	Diagnostics
drugs to treat cancer, AIDS, arthritis, asthma, heart disease, and hemophilia	home pregnancy test
antibiotics, birth control pills, vitamins, and growth hormones	tests to diagnose prostate cancer, cholera, and high cholesterol
vaccines to prevent hepatitis, meningitis, influenza, rotavirus, and chickenpox	test to determine a woman's predisposition to breast cancer
skin replacements for burn victims	screen to ensure that blood is safe and doesn't carry diseases from donors

Figure 18.3   Since the 1970s, the list of accomplishments achieved through biotechnology research and development in the area of human health has continued to grow. What are some other treatment-related and diagnostic advancements?

Parkinson's. As medicine becomes more personalized, providers will use a patient's own genomic sequence to tailor that person's medical treatment.

The field of biotechnology research and development also includes the industries that develop new products, equipment, and devices used to improve the delivery of medical care. MRI machines, CT scanners, radiation therapy machines, DNA sequencers, surgical robots, and automated specimen analyzers are all examples of the advancements made through the research and development of medical products.

Careers That Focus on Research and Development

Laboratory assistants, technicians, and scientists work in academic research labs located in hospitals, on university campuses, and in the commercial labs of biotechnology companies. Laboratory support employs entry-level workers in the lab and requires a high school diploma. These workers maintain the basic equipment used in a lab. They clean and store glassware, maintain inventory and reorder supplies, and test glassware to verify that it is sterile.

Lab assistants and technicians most commonly hold an associate's degree in biological science. Many technicians have completed or are working to complete a bachelor's degree as well. These employees work with scientists on biotechnology experiments. They follow directions using a high degree of accuracy according to **standard operating procedures (SOPs)**. These procedures spell out the exact steps used when completing any laboratory task. Workers know and follow **good laboratory practices (GLPs)**, which are regulations that describe how laboratories must operate.

Lab technicians use recombinant (ree-KAHM-bih-nuhnt) DNA techniques and basic molecular biology procedures as they perform experiments. They also analyze and graph data from the experiments.

Successful lab technicians have excellent math skills and can work carefully at repetitive tasks to maintain accuracy. Greater demand for

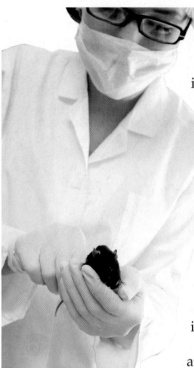

Figure 18.4 Animal caretakers provide for the daily care of laboratory animals used in biotechnology research.

clinical trial
an experiment performed on human beings to evaluate the comparative effectiveness of two or more treatments

biotechnology research is expected to increase the need for lab technicians, but there will be strong competition for available jobs. Applicants with lab experience will have the best job opportunities. Other entry-level positions focus on the plants or animals used in research. For example, animal caretakers provide for the daily care of laboratory or farm animals used in biotechnology research. In addition to feeding, cleaning, and grooming the animals, caretakers maintain records to comply with research regulations and may administer medication to the animals in their care. This entry-level job requires a high school diploma and documented experience in caring for animals. Students can gain experience by volunteering at an animal shelter, zoo, or veterinary clinic (Figure 18.4).

Animal caretakers do lots of walking, lifting, and carrying. While they love animals and receive satisfaction from working with them, seeing the effects of illness can be stressful. Forty-hour workweeks are typical, and working nights, weekends, and holidays is common in a research setting. Jobs related to caring for animals are expected to increase, with the highest number of job openings occurring in pet care services and veterinary clinics.

Laboratory technicians with a bachelor's or master's degree and at least a few years of lab experience may become research associates. In addition to supervising the work of technicians and assistants, they may be responsible for developing the SOPs for the lab. Associates often have experience in specific biotechnology laboratory techniques or specialized areas of research. They are responsible for writing reports or making presentations about their research. They may also develop new protocols for research projects. Research associates work in many areas of biotechnology, including developing new products, testing new medications, and developing processes for manufacturing new products.

Medical scientists hold a PhD and sometimes an MD. They plan and direct the studies that investigate human diseases and methods for preventing or treating those diseases. Medical scientists can form a **hypothesis** and develop the experiments needed to test that hypothesis, or *theory*. They lead the teams of research associates and lab technicians who will carry out their experiments.

When their research leads to a new treatment or medication, scientists conduct a **clinical trial** using patient volunteers in cooperation with the volunteers' physicians. Patients in a drug-related clinical trial receive either the trial drug or a **placebo** (pluh-SEE-boh), which is a harmless substance that contains no medication. Patients don't know if they are taking the drug or the placebo. Scientists analyze data from all the patients in the trial to see if the trial drug worked better than the placebo. They also determine which particular patients had the most or least desirable outcomes. Finally, scientists write up their findings and publish them in a formal lab report, case study, or research article.

Medical scientists who work at universities are also responsible for writing and submitting grant proposals to organizations such as the National Institutes of Health or the National Science Foundation to secure funding for their research. Scientists employed in the private sector focus on developing new medications or medical instruments and typically have less freedom to select their areas of research. While they don't have to write grant proposals, they do have to justify their research plans to company managers. Scientists employed by government agencies also conduct research on human diseases and health, and they may focus on exploratory research using nonhuman subjects or on overseeing clinical trials (Figure 18.5).

Careers That Focus on Manufacturing and Services

Once a product has been developed and tested, the manufacturer prepares for full-scale production. Once again, the government regulates the manufacturing process to ensure the manufacture of safe and reliable medical products. Medical manufacturers follow GLPs as well as **good manufacturing processes (GMPs)** in the production process. The use of these standards is required by law.

Medical manufacturing companies produce a wide variety of products, with pharmaceuticals and vaccines making up a large segment of the industry. In addition, **bioassays** are made for use in conducting medical research, and tests for screening or detecting genetic illnesses or chronic diseases are continually being developed and improved. For example, a colonoscopy is effective in detecting colon cancer, but many people avoid the test because of the unappealing test preparation process. Scientists are working to develop an alternate screening process that is less invasive and eliminates the colon-cleansing preparation stage.

Medical devices and equipment represent another area of medical manufacturing. Picture all of the equipment you encounter as a patient in a hospital or clinic. In addition, consider all of the equipment used in medical laboratories. This includes digital microscopes, **centrifuges** (SEHN-truh-fyooj-ehs) for separating fluids, and analyzers for DNA or blood to name just a few.

Material handlers are entry-level workers in biotechnology manufacturing. They work in warehouses, unpacking and checking incoming supplies and packing products for shipment. They may work with biological products that have a limited life span and with products that require a temperature-controlled environment. For example, some products may be packed in dry ice to maintain proper temperature during the shipping process.

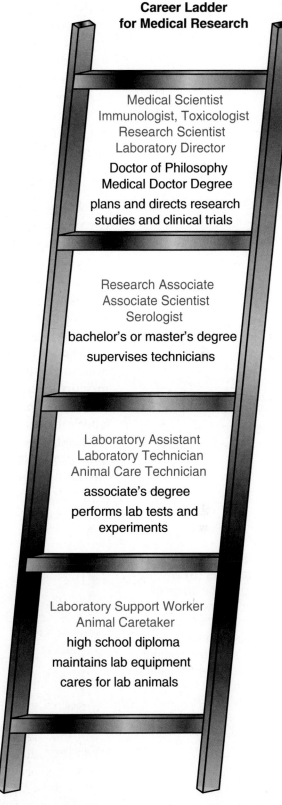

Career Ladder for Medical Research

Medical Scientist
Immunologist, Toxicologist
Research Scientist
Laboratory Director

Doctor of Philosophy
Medical Doctor Degree

plans and directs research studies and clinical trials

Research Associate
Associate Scientist
Serologist

bachelor's or master's degree

supervises technicians

Laboratory Assistant
Laboratory Technician
Animal Care Technician

associate's degree

performs lab tests and experiments

Laboratory Support Worker
Animal Caretaker

high school diploma

maintains lab equipment

cares for lab animals

Figure 18.5   The career ladder for medical research workers.

Material handlers feel comfortable lifting heavy materials and can operate conveyors, forklifts, and other equipment. Requiring only a high school diploma, this job provides an opportunity to learn about a company and its products. Employees may take advantage of company educational benefits to continue their studies and advance to other jobs within the company.

Manufacturing assistants have a high school diploma or an associate's degree. They work with **fermentors** or **bioreactors** to produce drugs or enzymes for use in the biotechnology industry (Figure 18.6). They may work in a "clean room" and wear special clothing to maintain a sterile environment. They operate equipment to fill, label, and package products. They may be exposed to disease-causing bacteria or viruses or poisonous chemicals, so their ability to follow safety procedures is critical.

Manufacturing technicians oversee the assistants' production work. Technicians typically have an associate's degree or a bachelor's degree along with work experience in biotechnology manufacturing. They frequently use automated and robotic equipment and are responsible for sterilizing equipment, setting up the machines used to fill sterile containers, and completing routine equipment maintenance.

Monitoring equipment to ensure that SOPs and GMPs are followed is an important part of the technician's job. Since medications must be produced using the exact procedures approved by the FDA, mistakes during the process cost companies time and money. Medications can't be sold if correct procedures have not been followed and documented.

Engineers have at least a bachelor's or master's degree and some have a PhD. Manufacturing process engineers design the methods and equipment used to manufacture a product. They apply scientific principles to the production of goods to make better products at the lowest possible cost.

Figure 18.6   Fermentors (A) and bioreactors (B) are used to produce drugs or enzymes for use in the biotechnology industry. Which biotechnology research and development workers use fermentors and bioreactors?

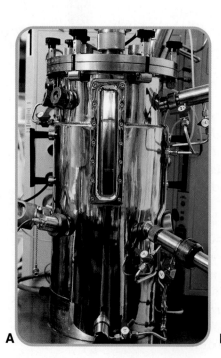

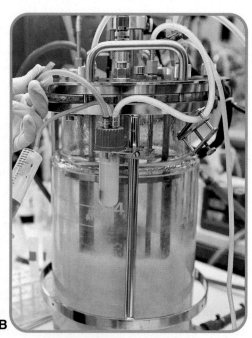

A   B

Biomedical engineers combine their knowledge of biology and engineering to design and develop products such as artificial organs, prostheses, and machines for diagnosing medical problems. These engineers can analyze the needs of patients and enjoy problem solving to design medical products. They frequently work directly with patients, therapists, physicians, and medical scientists. Because of this, they must be skilled communicators who are able to incorporate the ideas of other professionals during the design process. Rapid advances in technology are expected to create new job opportunities for biomedical engineers.

Biotechnology workers can also provide services in crime laboratories. For example, **forensic DNA analysts** work in crime labs to extract and match DNA from samples that are used as evidence to solve crimes (Figure 18.7). DNA samples from crime scenes can help identify and convict people who have committed crimes. Analysts use samples of human tissue from blood, urine, or saliva to create a DNA profile that is unique for each individual.

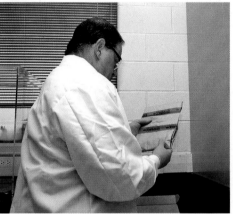

Since forensic analysts work in law enforcement, they must pass drug tests and background checks. In addition to a bachelor's or master's degree in biological sciences, analysts need to complete coursework in crime detection and investigation. Forensic analysts also need strong speaking and writing skills. Their laboratory notes are submitted as court documents, and they may be called to testify in court cases.

Careers in Sales and Technical Support

Figure 18.7   Forensic DNA analysts find information that may be used as evidence.

Sales representatives contact and meet potential customers to sell their company's products. They need a bachelor's degree in marketing or science combined with additional training in medical sales. Medical sales reps study medical terminology, anatomy, disease states, and specific product knowledge before completing exams to prove their knowledge of company policies and government regulations.

Sales reps are excellent communicators. They listen to the needs of their clients and can demonstrate a product, answer technical questions about its use, and check to make sure it is working correctly. In some cases, they train the healthcare workers who will use their products. They also use writing skills as they analyze sales data, write sales reports, and keep careful records of sales contacts. The field of sales is appealing to individuals who enjoy traveling and working with people.

Technical service representatives have strong technical and science skills, but they are also good at working with customers. They usually have a bachelor's degree in biological sciences and have often worked as lab technicians. They solve technical problems that customers encounter. Reps usually communicate by phone or e-mail, but they may go to the customer's business to install products. These reps know about product updates and receive training for all of the company's new products. They track customer complaints to identify problems with a product and report those problems to supervisory staff. They may also complete research and lab work to find solutions to technical problems.

Careers That Focus on Quality and Regulation

Health and safety specialists focus on making the workplace safe for all employees and ensuring that safety regulations are followed. As part of the emergency response team, the health and safety specialist responds to hazardous spills, fires, and accidents that occur in the workplace.

A bachelor's degree in environmental science, safety, or hazardous materials technology prepares you for this career. Health and safety specialists write safety procedures for their companies, investigate workplace accidents, and train employees regarding safety regulations and emergency procedures. These workers are also responsible for the safe storage, use, and disposal of any hazardous materials used at their company. A health and safety specialist needs strong communication skills and the ability to work with all company employees, especially during an emergency. While certification through the Institute of Hazardous Materials Management is not required, employers prefer certified job applicants.

Quality assurance specialists make sure that the manufacturing process follows required guidelines and procedures. They analyze data, write reports, and document every step in the manufacturing process. Their work shows the FDA that regulations have been followed so that a product will be approved for sale. Entry-level qualifications include a bachelor's degree in biology, engineering, or computer science and work experience in a manufacturing environment. These workers need good lab skills, attention to detail, and excellent organizational skills.

Quality control technicians perform inspections at every step in the manufacturing process. They examine raw materials used in manufacturing to make sure they meet quality requirements. Technicians also monitor the work environment to make sure that clean or sterile conditions are maintained (Figure 18.8). They test the finished product and check its packaging and labeling.

Technicians need a bachelor's degree in the biological sciences and some work experience in biotechnology lab work or manufacturing. They may specialize in biotechnology, microbiology, or chemical analysis. However, all technicians need good lab and problem-solving skills. They must continue to learn the changing regulations affecting the biotechnology industry. A working knowledge of SOPs, GLPs, and GMPs is expected. With experience, technicians can advance to analyst positions, which also require technical writing skills. Certification is voluntary and is available through the American Society for Quality.

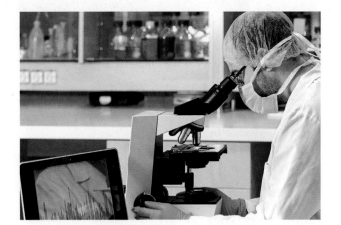

Figure 18.8   Biotechnology manufacturing follows strict regulations to produce products that are safe for human use. What is the role of a quality control technician in following these regulations?

Additional Career Opportunities

Bioinformatics scientists use their computer skills to organize the expanding overload of data created by improved DNA sequencing technologies. These workers combine biology and computer science to develop organized databases of biological information and to write

algorithms or sets of rules that computers follow to process and analyze the information. For example, they may write a program to track and analyze influenza outbreaks across the country or one that evaluates the genetic codes of thousands of individuals to develop personalized medicine. These scientists have at least a master's degree with an extensive background in life science and computer science.

Epidemiologists (ehp-ih-dee-mee-AHL-uh-jihst) study the spread of diseases. You will find them working in public health, research, and hospital settings. Epidemiologists solve medical mysteries by answering the question "What caused it?" Research epidemiologists figure out how to eliminate or control a disease, while clinical epidemiologists investigate outbreaks of infection. Epidemiologists have a master's degree in public health with an emphasis in epidemiology. Advanced epidemiologists have a PhD. Epidemiologists are meticulous, analytical, and logical and possess a strong desire to help people. Indeed, their work has the potential to save many lives.

Geneticists (juh-NEHT-ih-sihsts) are medical scientists who study genes, heredity, and the variation of organisms. However, you may like science, but would prefer not to work in a lab setting. Genetic counseling combines a focus on science with the opportunity to interact with families affected by genetic disease. **Genetic counselors** need a master's degree and must complete extensive coursework in biology, genetics, and counseling. These professionals meet with clients to gather medical information (Figure 18.9). They construct a detailed health history to inform clients about possible genetic disorders and to help them understand and manage existing disorders. They put families in touch with resources that can assist them, such as support organizations or healthcare specialists. Counselors can work in a variety of specialty areas, such as cancer counseling, prenatal counseling, or pediatrics. Most employers require certification by the American Board of Genetic Counseling, and some states require licensure.

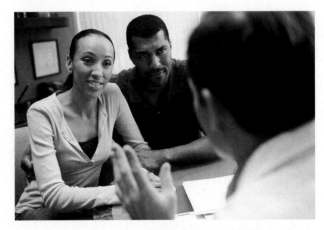

Figure 18.9   Genetic counselors may work in specialty areas such as cancer counseling, prenatal counseling, or pediatrics. How might counselors help a couple wanting to start a family?

The Biotechnology Research and Development Worker: Jesse

Jesse never expected to work in the field of health science. He is a creative individual who enjoys working with computers. During high school, he did some photo retouching. Then a class speaker from a career college got him interested in computer graphics, animation, and game design. While attending college, he learned about an internship opportunity from a friend. That internship led to a full-time job working for a foundation that conducts biomedical research.

Today Jesse is a graphic Web user interface designer. He works to promote the foundation's goal to make science accessible, exciting, and relevant for students of all ages. He does this by designing computer games that teach scientific concepts. He develops educational games so that students learn by playing, making complex medical concepts user-friendly. The results are interactive and intuitive games that don't overwhelm you with instructions. Jesse loves the flexible and collaborative work environment that gives him access to experienced medical scientists as consultants during game development. He loves his job and says, "I still pinch myself because I can't believe work is this fun!"

Complete the
Map Your Reading
graphic organizer for the
section you just read.

RECALL YOUR READING

1. Biotechnology uses _____ molecules found in all living _____ to create new tools.
2. Lab assistants and technicians must follow standard _____ procedures and good _____ practices.
3. Medical manufacturing companies' products include _____ and vaccines, but also _____ and tests for detecting genetic diseases.
4. Sales reps often _____ the healthcare workers using their products and technical _____ reps solve technical problems for customers.
5. Genetic counselors can work in various areas, including _____ counseling, _____ counseling, and _____.

Team Leadership

All people assume leadership roles at various times in their personal and work lives. When we choose to lead, we usually find a leadership task that fits our own personality. These leadership opportunities feel comfortable, and we are confident about our skills.

For example, Sally works as a medical secretary at a local healthcare clinic. When she joins the local chamber of commerce as a representative of her company, she is willing to act as the organization's secretary. She is comfortable taking notes and feels confident about her ability to produce accurate minutes of each meeting.

Emily, on the other hand, dreaded being made the team leader for a group project. Although Emily was a good leader in her classroom every day as she willingly helped other students who were struggling with the course content, she believed she could never be a successful leader. Because of Emily's quiet nature, managing a team and organizing the work of her classmates felt uncomfortable. How could she be effective at doing something she didn't like?

Leadership Styles

personal leadership style
an individual approach
to giving directions,
implementing plans, and
motivating people

Each of us has a **personal leadership style** that relies on our own preferences and attributes. Like the connection between personality and career choices, there is a connection between personality and leadership styles. Do any of the descriptions in Figure 18.10 match your leadership preferences?

John Holland Type	Characteristic	Leadership Style
Figure 18.10 Characteristics of Leadership Styles		
Realistic Doer	likes mechanical, hands-on activities	Role Model • takes action • sets an example by doing what is asked of others
Investigative Thinker	is an analytical problem solver	Pioneer • analyzes and compares other situations • develops a long-term view of the future
Social Helper	is cooperative and people-oriented	Facilitator • encourages and mentors people • builds personal relationships and cares for others
Enterprising Persuader	is a competitive leader	Innovator • tries new things and likes change • creates new work-related opportunities
Conventional Organizer	pays attention to detail	Monitor • observes and organizes the work of different people • sets clear goals and manages resources
Artistic Creator	exhibits creativity and originality	Motivator • shows passion for key issues • supports the current cause

Knowing your personal leadership style helps you assess how effective you will be at accomplishing a leadership task. Because different tasks require different styles, you may need to expand your leadership skills to accomplish your goals. In the same way that you learn the technical skills and knowledge required for your job, you can also learn the skills required for various leadership roles.

Leadership Skills

Leadership uses many familiar skills (Figure 18.11 on the next page). Developing leadership skills begins with developing all the skills that make you a good worker. When you are asked to take on or are assigned a leadership role, remember that a true leader unites people and works to achieve a positive result. Notice that the focus of a leader is not on himself or herself. Effective leaders are not trying to prove that they are better than others or show that they are in charge. Instead, they model the behavior they want to see in team members. They encourage and help team members to perform work tasks effectively.

From informal team working sessions to formal gatherings to transact the business of an organization, effective leaders are frequently called upon to conduct meetings. These leaders usually set the agenda that lists the topics to be discussed and acted upon. For the more formal meetings they may guide the meeting's progress using parliamentary procedure.

Figure 18.11 Leadership Skills

Familiar Skills for Leaders	How Leaders Put Those Skills to Use
Effective leaders practice personal health maintenance.	They set realistic goals and manage their time to effectively achieve their goals.
Effective leaders are effective workers.	They have developed excellent technical skills for the job tasks they perform.
Effective leaders use an organized system for managing the tasks of everyday work and life.	They use problem-solving techniques to make decisions when conflicts and problems arise.
Effective leaders are team players.	They use a positive attitude and assertive communication skills to improve relationships with coworkers.

Based on Robert's Rules of Order, parliamentary procedure is a set of rules that maintains order and allows all members to participate in the meeting. Leaders know how to call a meeting to order, handle a variety of motions, and address a motion to adjourn or end the meeting. In a well-run meeting, people take turns speaking, and only one idea is discussed at a time.

Members present their ideas by making a motion. Everyone is given an opportunity to discuss or debate each motion before voting to accept or reject it. Ideally both the leader and the members of the group are familiar with the several different kinds of motions. If everyone speaks clearly and uses parliamentary procedure correctly, the group's business is more likely to be accomplished in an effective, timely manner.

Effective leaders also accept the challenge of learning new leadership skills. They develop self-confidence and learn to make decisions in the face of disagreement. Team leaders make the best choice after considering all of the information, but they understand that some team members may not like the decision. Effective leaders know their personal leadership preferences, but they are willing to learn different styles of leadership that are a better fit for their current leadership task (Figure 18.12).

Figure 18.12 When to Use or Avoid a Leadership Style

Leadership Style	When to Use	When to Avoid
Role Model	when team members lack motivation and are not focused on accomplishing tasks	when team members are focused on achievement rather than on quality of work
Pioneer	when long-term change is needed	when it's important to fix current problems
Facilitator	when there are sensitive situations or when support from others is necessary	when decisions need to be made quickly
Innovator	when the group is stuck in the same routines	when there are too many new procedures already in progress
Monitor	when there is a lack of organization and expectations are unclear	when there are so many goals and procedures that it's difficult to focus on work tasks
Motivator	when the group has lost its sense of identity	when a problem needs to be solved objectively

Leadership Styles: Margo

Margo spent multiple hours planning her hospital department's budget. She analyzed previous purchases, reviewed equipment usage trends, and tried to anticipate future needs. Before committing to major purchases based on her plan, she sought the advice of her supervisor, Janelle. However, her supervisor told her to move forward with major purchases without even looking at Margo's plan. Janelle wanted to discuss a change in the color of scrubs worn on each hospital unit. Margo was dumbfounded. She couldn't believe that her boss was more interested in uniforms than in a major spending initiative.

A few weeks later, Margo attended a leadership training workshop and learned about leadership styles. Now her supervisor's actions and her own reactions began to make more sense. Margo learned that she has a pioneer style, which causes her to focus on plans for the future. Janelle has a role model style of leadership. She prefers to focus on the smaller activities that can be decided and completed now. Neither leadership style is right or wrong. However, effective leaders learn to change their preferred style to fit the current task.

Great leaders are developed rather than born. Effective leaders begin by building excellent work skills, but they are willing to step beyond their comfort zone to learn new skills for leading others' work. They understand that true leaders promote positive changes by inspiring others. Effective leaders are innovators, motivators, and facilitators rather than pessimists, opponents, or referees.

RECALL YOUR READING

1. People often choose _____ tasks that fir their personalities.
2. Knowing your _____ leadership style will help you assess your effectiveness at different tasks.
3. Great leaders are willing to _____ their leadership skills to accomplish their goals.
4. Effective leaders _____ the work behaviors they want to see in team members.
5. Sometimes leaders must learn different _____ of leadership for their current task or situation.

Complete the *Map Your Reading* graphic organizer for the section you just read.

Technical Skills for Biotechnology Research and Development Workers

Many employees in the biotechnology research and development pathway work in laboratory or manufacturing environments where it is clear that safety and accuracy are critical. Research and development workers learn and follow specific guidelines and protocols to ensure safety and validity. However, everyone involved in this pathway—from research planning to sales—needs to be concerned with the safety and effectiveness of the products they offer. For that reason, healthcare marketing professionals provide advanced training and technical support to their customers to ensure that highly specialized products are used correctly.

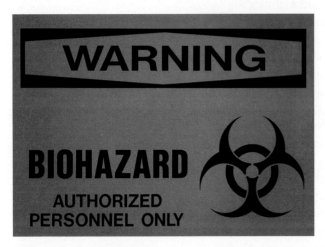

Figure 18.13   Entrances to areas containing biohazardous materials display the universal biohazard symbol. This means biological material that could pose a risk to human health may be present.

biohazard
term that describes a biological agent, infectious organism, or insecure laboratory procedure that constitutes a danger to humans or the environment

autoclaves
chambers for sterilizing items with steam under pressure

Biosafety Guidelines

All laboratory workers focus on safety measures that protect them from physical and chemical hazards created by fires, faulty electrical equipment, and toxic chemicals. However, medical laboratory workers in both clinical and research settings must also focus on safety measures that provide protection from infectious agents. The term **biohazard**, and the presence of the biohazard symbol, warns of a risk or hazard to health or the environment from infectious agents (Figure 18.13). Workers must know and use the appropriate measures to prevent exposure.

Biological agents are classified according to their level of risk. Biosafety Level One (BSL-1) agents represent the lowest level of risk, while Biosafety Level Four (BSL-4) agents pose the highest level of risk. There are four corresponding levels of biological containment to protect against biohazards. Each level of containment has guidelines for laboratory facilities to follow, including safety equipment requirements and laboratory practices and techniques.

For example, a BSL-1 lab is common in high schools and colleges that teach introductory microbiology courses. Lab coats and gloves are worn here and surfaces and equipment are decontaminated using chemical disinfectants or steam autoclaving. Autoclaving uses pressurized steam to sterilize instruments, glassware, and other materials (Figure 18.14).

A BSL-2 lab has restricted access. Workers wear gloves, lab coats, and face protection. **Autoclaves** are used for decontaminating waste materials and a biological safety cabinet is available (Figure 18.15). Positive air pressure keeps infectious materials inside the cabinet and air is drawn away from the worker into a vent or filter. BSL-3 and BSL-4 labs use separate buildings with double-door entry and directional inward airflow, as well as many special procedures and protective devices.

Laboratory Safety Protocols

Before beginning any lab procedure, healthcare workers must be trained in standard precautions as well as the use of personal protective equipment (PPE) and equipment such as a safety shower or eyewash that is used to limit exposure to biohazards. Laboratory personnel also learn work practice controls. These controls consist of safe work habits that limit the possibility of exposure, such as hand washing after removing gloves. Every laboratory develops an **exposure control plan** that explains how specimens, contaminated equipment, contaminated work surfaces, and contaminated waste materials can be handled safely. The following safety protocols apply to all lab settings:

1. Wear pants or a skirt that fully covers your legs and shoes with closed toes. Tie your hair back and away from your face. Do not wear loose clothing, dangling chains or earrings, or large rings.

2. Wash your hands before and after all lab procedures, after removing gloves, and before leaving the lab.

3. Wear a lab coat or gown, gloves, and appropriate face protection such as goggles, a face shield, or a mask when working with strong chemicals or when splashing is possible.

4. Know the location of exit doors, a fire extinguisher and fire blanket, the safety shower, and the eyewash station so you can respond to an emergency or accident.

5. If a reagent splashes your face or eyes, wash for several minutes at the eyewash station. Use the safety shower if a reagent splashes on any exposed skin or soaks through your clothing.

6. Follow exposure control plan guidelines to treat contaminated work surfaces and clean up spills immediately.

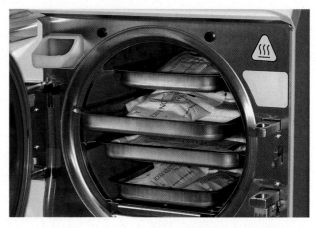

Figure 18.14   Autoclaves use pressurized steam to sterilize lab equipment. Why are autoclaves important equipment for a lab?

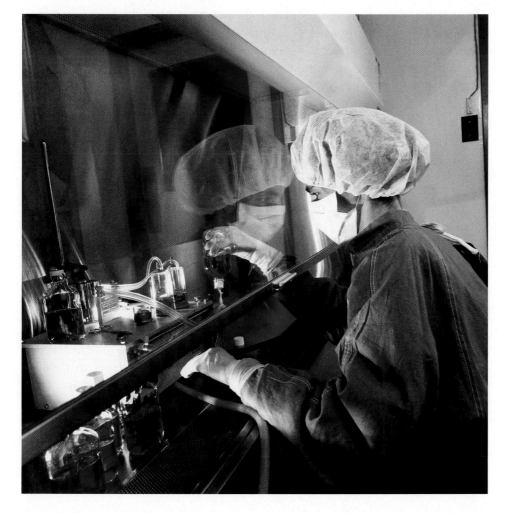

Figure 18.15   A biological safety cabinet protects lab workers by preventing infectious materials from escaping into the lab.

7. Report all accidents and exposure incidents to the lab supervisor *immediately* after using the eyewash or shower.

Lab workers also follow rules of laboratory etiquette that promote a safe and pleasant work environment. These rules include the following:

1. No eating, gum chewing, or drinking is permitted in a lab setting. Do not bring food, beverages, tobacco products, or cosmetics into the lab.

2. Clean your work area before and after lab procedures and whenever needed. Put away all supplies and equipment before leaving the lab.

3. Leave your lab coat, equipment, samples, and reagents in the lab.

4. Do not allow visitors into the lab work area unless they are properly dressed and have been instructed in patient confidentiality and safety precautions. Follow facility guidelines for visitors.

Tasks Performed by Laboratory Workers

Valid results rely on accurate measurements. Especially in biotechnology lab settings, technicians frequently measure miniscule amounts and small mistakes can cause major errors. Labs use metric units of measurement (Figure 18.16). In addition to taking correct measurements, lab workers must keep accurate records and know how to clean and sterilize equipment.

Measuring Mass. Biotechnologists measure reagents, which are chemical substances used in preparing a product or detecting a component in another substance. A common example is a reagent strip used by a lab worker to test a urine specimen. The chemical reagents in this case are attached to a plastic strip, and they react to a specific substance. The strip is inserted in the sample, and when the specific substance is present, it reacts with the chemical reagent and produces a color change. The

Figure 18.16 Metric Units Used in the Lab		
Prefix	**Symbol**	**Meaning**
kilo	k	1,000
base unit		
meter	m	1
gram	g	1
liter	L	1
centi	c	.01
milli	m	.001
micro	μ	.000001
nano	n	.000000001

color change indicates the amount of the substance that is present in the sample.

Because biotechnology reagents are often measured in small amounts or masses, lab workers use precision instruments such as **electronic balances** for lab measurements. There are several different types of balances (Figure 18.17). Tabletop balances measure amounts weighing between 1 gram (g) and 1,000 grams. Analytical balances are more precise and can measure amounts between 10 milligrams (mg) and 1,000 milligrams. A microbalance will measure even smaller amounts. Follow these steps for measuring mass using an electronic balance:

1. Turn the balance on and press the control bar. Wait for zeros to appear, showing that the scale is ready for use.

2. Use a weighing container for all substances. Place the empty weighing container on the balance pan and close the doors.

3. Tare the container by briefly pressing the control bar. The display will show zero with the container sitting on the pan. This allows the mass of your sample to be read directly. You will not need to subtract the empty weight from the filled container weight.

4. Remove the weighing container and add the substance to be weighed. Be careful not to spill chemicals on the balance.

5. Return the filled weighing container to the balance pan and close the chamber doors. Read the display to find the mass of your sample.

Measuring Volume. Volumes are measured using graduated cylinders, pipettes (smaller amounts), and **micropipettes** (very small amounts). Flasks and beakers hold substances, but they are not used for measuring volume because they are not very accurate.

Always use the smallest size cylinder or pipette possible for your specific measurement because the markings on a smaller instrument are more precise. This will ensure accuracy and minimize error. For example, when measuring 9 milliliters (mL), a 10-mL pipette is more accurate than a 25-mL pipette. Use a graduated cylinder for measuring volumes between 10 mL and 5 liters (L) (Figure 18.18 on the next page). Follow these protocols for measuring volume in a cylinder:

electronic balances
measuring instruments that show the weight of a substance digitally and are used to weigh chemicals in labs

 Expand

micropipette
an instrument designed for the measurement of very small volumes

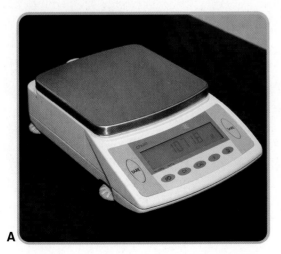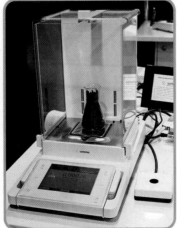

A   **B**

Figure 18.17   A tabletop balance (A) measures amounts weighing between 1 gram and 1,000 grams, while an analytical balance (B) measures amounts between 10 milligrams and 1,000 milligrams.

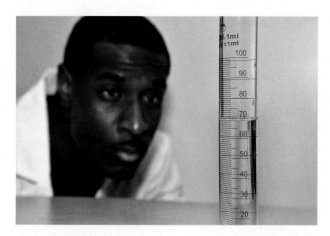

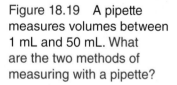

Figure 18.18   Graduated cylinders measure volumes between 10 mL and 5 L. For accuracy, always read the volume at eye level from the lowest point of the meniscus. What measurement is shown here?

1. Check to verify the total volume of the cylinder and the value of each marking on the cylinder.
2. Place the cylinder on a level surface and add the substance to be measured.
3. Locate the **meniscus** (meh-NIHS-kuhs). This is a curve at the surface caused when liquid sticks to the walls of the cylinder, but it is lower in the middle of the cylinder.
4. Read the volume measurement at eye level from the lowest point of the meniscus.

Pipettes measure volumes from 1 mL to 50 mL. They are inserted into a pipettor tool that creates suction and draws liquid into the pipette (Figure 18.19). Follow these protocols when using a pipette:

1. Insert the top of the pipette into the pipettor.
2. Insert the bottom tip of the pipette into the liquid to be measured.
3. Keep the pipette in a vertical position to avoid contaminating the pipettor.
4. Draw fluid up into the pipette and fill it slightly above the capacity desired.
5. Slowly lower the meniscus to the correct capacity line and read the measurement at eye level while holding the pipette vertically.
6. Move the pipette to the receiving container and press the button to empty the pipette.
7. Expel the pipette into the correct discard container.

In the "blowout" method of measuring, which is described in the pipette measuring protocol, the pipette is completely emptied. The pipette tool delivers a puff of air to "blow out" the liquid. Lab workers never

Figure 18.19   A pipette measures volumes between 1 mL and 50 mL. What are the two methods of measuring with a pipette?

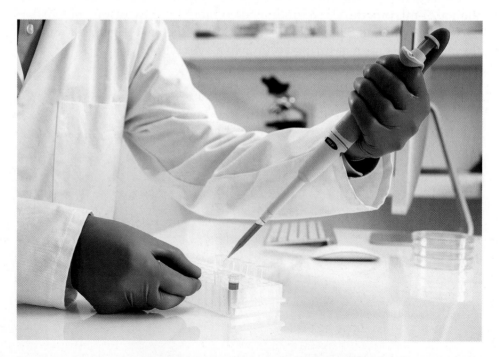

actually blow on the pipette because of the risk of contamination and illness. When using the point-to-point method for measuring, you pipette a volume between two measurement lines and do not need to "blow out" the pipette (Figure 18.20).

Micropipettes measure very small volumes in microliter (μL) amounts. Micropipettes measure volumes from 0.1 μL to 1 mL and are available in different sizes. For example, a P-1000 measures from 100 μL to 1,000 μL (1 mL), while a P-10 measures from 0.5 μL to 10 μL.

Cleaning and Sterilizing Equipment. Health science laboratories use autoclaves to **sterilize** the items used in both clinical and research facilities. Autoclaves keep these items free of microorganisms that could act as contaminants. The autoclave is typically used at both ends of a research project. At the beginning, it sterilizes glassware and lab instruments to ensure that the experiment is conducted free of biological contaminants. At the end of a project, the autoclave sterilizes the waste products from the experiment and inactivates any microorganisms that may be found within the waste disposal containers.

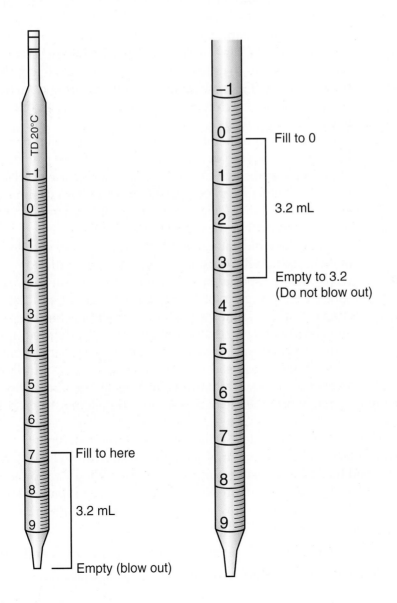

Figure 18.20   The first pipette shows how to measure volume using the "blow out" method, which completely empties the pipette. The second pipette shows how to measure volume using a "point-to-point" method. Either method will produce an accurate measurement.

An autoclave uses pressurized steam at temperatures that are high enough and for time periods that are long enough to kill most contaminants. However, autoclaves must be properly maintained to remain effective, and employees must know how to operate the autoclave correctly to prevent injury. Since manufacturers sell many types and sizes of autoclaves, employees must learn the guidelines for using their own facility's machine to sterilize the specific products used at that facility.

The goals of cleaning and sterilizing equipment remain the same whether the facility is a large hospital with employees dedicated to maintaining a central supply of ready-to-use equipment or a small dental office in which the assistant maintains equipment for the dentist and hygienist. Whether a lab runs clinical tests or research experiments, effective protocols for preventing contamination are required.

For all equipment contaminated with bloodborne pathogens or **other potentially infectious material (OPIM)**, such as other body fluids or tissues, cleaning is the first step in the contamination-prevention process. The cleaning process removes all debris, blood, body fluids, and tissue. If visible debris is not removed before equipment enters an autoclave, contaminants will bake on and stick to the items being sterilized. This compromises the sterilization process.

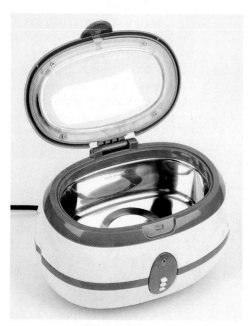

Ultrasonic cleaning is preferable to manual scrubbing and soaking because it is safer for workers. **Ultrasonic cleaners** use sound waves to create millions of water jets that gently remove debris (Figure 18.21). Ultrasonic cleaning does not sterilize equipment. Viruses and spores remain on the items even after this process.

Once the equipment is cleaned, it is ready to be sterilized. Employees wrap or package all materials before placing them in the autoclave. Several types of wraps are available, including autoclave paper, plastic or paper bags designed for autoclaving, and autoclave containers. Steam can penetrate these wraps during the autoclaving process.

Autoclave indicators are placed at the center of a group of items and on the outside of the wrap. The indicators, which include special tape or sensitive marks on bags or containers, change color during the autoclaving process. The change indicates that the package of materials has been in an autoclave. However, it does not guarantee that the equipment is sterile because it is possible for the tape to change color without being exposed for the full time or to the required level of pressure. Maintaining an autoclave's proper function and using it correctly provide the best assurance that items are properly sterilized.

Figure 18.21 Ultrasonic cleaning is preferable to manual scrubbing and soaking because it is safer for workers. How do ultrasonic cleaners work?

Many items can be autoclaved, including surgical instruments, glassware, plastic tubes, pipette tips, solutions, water, animal food and bedding, and hazardous waste materials. Take care when wrapping items in autoclave paper to ensure that all edges of the wrap are sealed (Figure 18.22). Open corners allow pathogens to enter. Follow these steps to wrap equipment for autoclaving:

1. Wash your hands and put on a gown or lab coat, a mask, and gloves.
2. Clean the items to be sterilized using an ultrasonic cleaner.

3. Select the correct type of wrap, making sure it is large enough to enclose the equipment completely. Use a single or double thickness according to your facility's policy.

4. Position the wrap diagonally with one corner pointing toward you.

5. Open hinged items so that steam can sterilize all surfaces.

6. Place the equipment and an indicator strip in the center of the wrap (A).

7. Fold the bottom corner of the wrap in toward the center and fold a small corner back, forming a tab (B and C).

8. Fold the left edge over to the center and fold the corner back (D).

9. Repeat with the right side (E).

10. Close the package by folding the remaining corner over the top of the package and tucking it in or by folding the package up from the bottom (F and G).

11. Check to see that items are wrapped securely for handling but loose enough that steam can circulate during the autoclaving process.

12. Seal the wrap with indicator tape, leaving a tape tab at one end to allow for easy opening (H).

13. Label the tape with the date, package contents, and your initials (I).

14. Remove and discard your PPE according to your facility's policy. Wash hands.

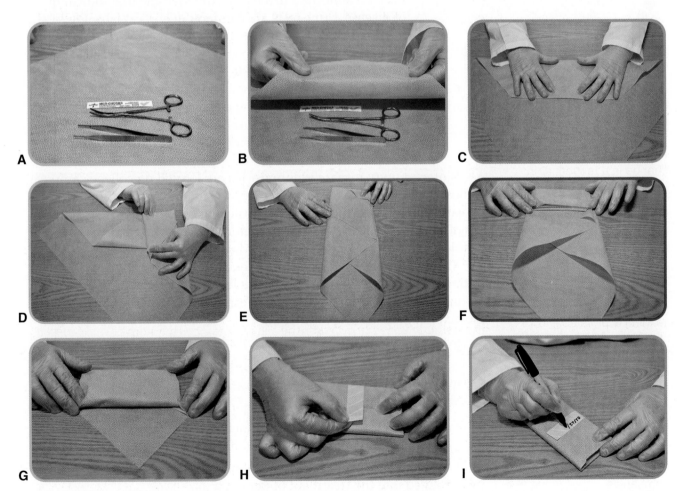

Figure 18.22   Study these images and the steps listed in the text to learn how to wrap instruments for autoclaving.

Performing Clinical and Research Laboratory Functions. Clinical laboratories are located in hospitals, physician offices, clinics, at the Department of Public Health in each state, and at the federal Centers for Disease Control and Prevention (CDC). Each lab is certified by the Centers for Medicare and Medicaid Services (CMS). The five levels of certification explain what types of tests a laboratory can perform. These range from simple tests with little risk to complex tests requiring highly trained personnel.

clinical laboratories
facilities that examine materials taken from the human body to discover information related to diagnosis, prognosis, prevention, or treatment of disease

Small clinics and physician offices perform **waived tests**. This means the CDC or the FDA has determined that the tests are so simple that there is little risk of error. Waived tests include blood glucose metering, urinalysis using reagent strips, rapid strep test, and urine specimen pregnancy tests, to name a few.

The development of small, simple-to-use analyzers has increased the use of **point-of-care testing**, which allows tests to be performed in nursing homes, emergency rooms, intensive care units, and surgery suites. Portable analyzers can measure hemoglobin, glucose, and cholesterol. Most point-of-care tests are also waived tests.

Urinalysis (yer-ih-NAL-uh-sihs) is the examination of urine to observe its physical, chemical, and microscopic properties. This is categorized as a waived clinical test. Because abnormal urine tests are often the first indication of disease, urine tests are common in clinical labs. Physical testing includes observing and recording color, odor, transparency, and specific gravity. Next, chemical testing checks pH, protein, glucose, ketones, bilirubin, and blood. Reagent strips are used for chemical testing (Figure 18.23). Finally, microscopic testing examines the formed elements in urine. A centrifuge spins out the solid particles, which are examined under a microscope to check for the presence of blood cells, bacteria, and other elements.

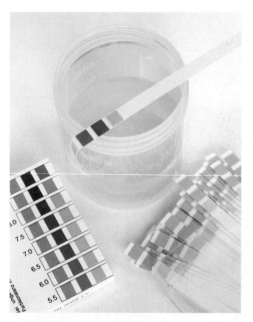

Figure 18.23   The color change in a reagent strip indicates the amount of a substance that is present in the sample, such as the amount of glucose present in a urine sample.

Expand

Biotechnology research laboratories are located on college campuses, in hospitals, and in private biotechnology companies that complete research to develop products and treatments. The FDA oversees the majority of biomedical research laboratory projects, regulating the development of human drugs and medical devices.

Medical biotechnology labs use monoclonal (mah-noh-KLOH-nuhl) antibody technology, bioprocess technologies, and genetic engineering technologies. The following are a few examples of medical uses of biotechnology in testing for diseases:

biotechnology research laboratories
facilities where research is done to develop new products or treatments, which are located on college campuses, in hospitals, and in private biotechnology companies

- tests to confirm the diagnosis of disease, such as the rapid test to detect strep throat

- tests for carrier status of inherited disorders, such as cystic fibrosis or sickle-cell anemia

- methods for prenatal testing, such as chorionic villus sampling or blood tests to screen for diseases and disorders like Down syndrome

The following examples of medical uses of biotechnology are incorporated into the treatment of patients:

- Enzyme replacement therapy produces enzymes that are given like medicine. They function in place of the patient's own enzymes, which are deficient as the result of a genetic disorder. For example, pancreatic enzymes are given to people with cystic fibrosis to help them absorb fat and proteins. They replace missing enzymes caused by blocked pancreatic ducts.

- Gene therapy uses genes as medicine. The new gene takes over for a nonfunctioning gene or increases or regulates the activity of a faulty gene. For example, a treatment called *Glybera* compensates for lipoprotein lipase (LI-pays) deficiency (LPLD), which can cause severe pancreatitis.

- Stem cell therapy involves developing stem cells into specific tissue to replace or supplement tissue in a patient with a health problem or genetic condition. For example, bone marrow transplants replace faulty cells with healthy donor cells. Researchers are working to develop stem cells that grow skin or produce insulin.

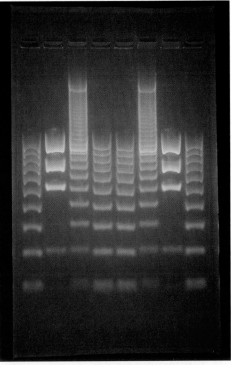

Unless you have an identical twin, your DNA is different from that of every other person in the world. That fact enables DNA fingerprinting, which is another laboratory function (Figure 18.24). Also known as *DNA typing* or *DNA profiling*, this test uses DNA to show whether two subjects are related or to identify humans, other animals, or plants. In forensic science, the DNA fingerprint can eliminate a suspect, prove that a convicted criminal is innocent of a crime, and show that a suspect was present at a crime scene. In addition to forensic applications, DNA fingerprinting can identify impurities in food products, identify human remains, determine the relatedness of family members, and identify organisms that cause disease.

Creating a DNA fingerprint uses several different biotechnology lab techniques, including restriction enzyme digestion of the DNA, gel electrophoresis (eh-lehk-troh-fuh-REE-sihs), and Southern blotting.

Figure 18.24 In DNA fingerprinting, probes with radioactive labeling attach to complementary DNA segments of the same length and "mark" the segments to make them visible. An X-ray image of the membrane shows where the probes attached to the DNA fragments. The barcode-like result shown here is the DNA fingerprint.

Expand

Completing Laboratory Documentation. The Food and Drug Administration's handbook says that if it isn't written down, it wasn't done. That is the guideline for all **laboratory documentation**. Lab information systems (LIS) use specialized software to track the testing of samples and record test results in a clinical laboratory. As the systems become more sophisticated, their functions expand to include patient check-in, order entry, specimen processing, result entry, and patient demographics. The LIS stores this information in its database for future reference. Once a provider has reviewed lab results, patients receive a letter and can often access the results more quickly using a secure Web portal and a personal password. When patients review a lab report, they see reference values to compare with their own test results. Results that are out of the normal or reference range signal that further investigation is needed.

laboratory documentation
written records of observable, measurable, and reproducible findings obtained through examination, testing, research studies, and experiments

Expand

In a biotechnology lab, the information management system processes reports and records data for large batches of samples. The information system must follow good manufacturing procedures and meet FDA reporting requirements. Documentation has several purposes, including

- recording what an individual has done and observed;

- establishing ownership for patent purposes;

- establishing criteria for production processes or product evaluation;

- tracing the manufacture of a specific product;

- proving that a procedure was done correctly; and

- developing or evaluating standard operating procedures.

Documentation is an essential skill for all biotechnology workers. While the details of documentation may vary from lab to lab, the importance of accurate documentation can't be overlooked. Excellent lab work is worthless without proper documentation. Laboratory notebooks are used to determine patent rights, product quality, and liability as well as to verify accuracy. Biotechnologists treat their notebooks as if they might be used in a court of law at any time. In fact, you can be questioned about your notebook in court.

Lab notes record not only procedures and observations, but also the equipment and materials used. Notes should indicate that these items were used in the correct manner. Information must be legible and complete so that companies cannot be fined or held liable for damages in a product lawsuit and so that rights are established for valuable **patents**, or *licenses*.

Much like the documentation in patient medical records, lab documentation is permanent rather than erasable. Information may be corrected but not removed from the record. Documentation must be clear, concise, and complete. It contains any details about the research that may influence results. Researchers must be able to answer questions about the methods and processes used in their research (Figure 18.25).

Figure 18.25   Excellent lab work is worthless without proper documentation. What are two specific purposes of documentation?

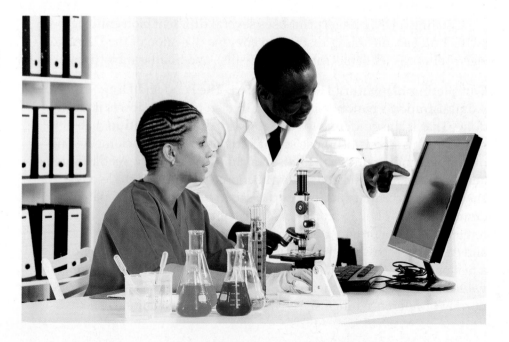

Sales and Technical Support Skills

The process of healthcare marketing includes research, planning, promoting, selling, and distributing goods and services to meet the needs of healthcare facilities and individual consumers. Because healthcare requires many specialized products that use advanced technologies, training and technical support is often part of a company's marketing plan.

Sales representatives for medical companies focus on **business-to-business selling**. This means the customer may be a large organization with multiple facilities. However, the process of selling still includes gathering information about the customer and advising the customer about which products would best suit the organization's needs.

After making contact with a potential customer, you need to focus on the **sales presentation**. For a presentation to be effective, you must first identify the customer's needs. Does the facility need to save time, provide better results for its patients, or simplify a procedure? Listening is your most important communication skill during this part of the sales process. It's a good idea to spend time "selling" the appointment for a sales presentation by learning the customer's needs and then telling the customer what he or she will receive from your presentation. For your customers, knowing that you intend to meet their needs is more important than knowing what product you intend to show.

A sales presentation gives you the opportunity to demonstrate your skills and abilities (Figure 18.26). Solid planning and preparation is essential. A physician who sees that the sales rep doesn't know the product very well will not want that rep consulting with him in the operating room. The life and health of patients rely on a physician's knowledge and skill. He can't put patients at risk because of a poorly prepared sales rep. The sales presentation must also be well organized. Healthcare workers are busy people who can't afford to waste time.

You must tailor your presentation to a specific customer. In today's market, the physician may be your first customer, but the purchasing agent or a product approval committee may also need to agree to a purchase. While product quality and performance might be the doctor's priority, equipment cost and its maintenance will be the purchasing agent's focus. Tailor your presentation to meet the needs of both customers.

Finally, knowing your presentation backward and forward lets you concentrate on the customer. Observe the customer during your presentation to pick up subtle clues. Does she look confused? Then take a moment to clarify. Does she have a question? Stop your presentation and take time to answer it. This keeps the customer's attention on the presentation. If you lose her attention, you won't make a sale.

Be prepared for **customer objections**. These are concerns, doubts, or other reasons the customer gives for not making a purchase. Anticipate objections and role-play your responses as you prepare your sales presentation (Figure 18.27 on the next page).

business-to-business selling
exchanging goods between businesses rather than between businesses and individuals

sales presentation
a prearranged meeting in which a salesperson presents detailed information and often a demonstration of a product

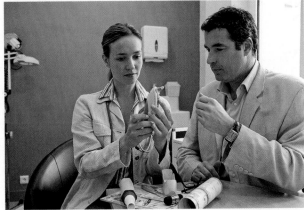

Figure 18.26   A sales presentation gives sales reps the opportunity to demonstrate their skills and abilities. What is the simple format of a sales presentation?

Expand

Figure 18.27 How to Handle Customer Objections	
Objection	**Response**
Price: "I can get the product cheaper from someone else."	Break your prices into smaller parts to show the unique services you will provide that others may not provide.
Fear of change: "It's easier to keep doing things the way we always have."	Explain what competitors are doing and show how change can make a positive improvement.
Trust: "How do I know you can really do what you say you can do?"	Provide solid information, including testimonials and references. Always be honest and consistent in your responses.
Personal obligations: "I promised to buy from my friend or relative."	Don't fight the customer's connection, but look for ways to provide services in the second phase of a project. This will keep your foot in the door for a future sale.
Authority: "My partner/boss/spouse needs to approve this."	Become a part of the decision by meeting with those who have decision-making authority. Assist your customer in answering questions about the product.
Timing: "I'm too busy right now. Call back in a few months."	Show the customer how easy it will be to work with you and how much your products will benefit them.

Expand

A sales presentation follows a simple format. Begin by introducing yourself and your company. Next, tell the customer how your product fits his needs. Use visual aids to clarify details. Compare your product with others that are available and discuss the recommended purchase proposal for your customer. Explain cost, invoicing, and your company's process for delivering the product. Take time to answer all of the customer's questions. Close your presentation with a thank you and get the customer's positive agreement to buy. If he is not prepared to purchase, invite him to contact you with further questions or to discuss a purchase quote.

When a potential customer voices an objection, listen carefully. Maintain eye contact and let the customer talk. Acknowledge the customer's objection by responding with, "I understand your point," or "Yes, other customers had similar questions." These comments don't mean that you agree with the customer, but they show that you care about the customer's concerns. When you disagree with customers or tell them they're wrong, they become defensive. That rarely leads to a sale.

Frequently, customers' questions are disguised as objections. Once you figure out the basic cause of the objection, you can respond to the concerns and questions that are preventing them from committing to a purchase. For example, a customer objecting to the design of the product really wants to know how difficult it will be to adapt to a new product design. Respond to this concern by explaining the experiences of other customers. "Yes. Other customers had that same concern about the new design, but they found that they adapted quickly and easily to the change."

Successful sales reps use many techniques for communicating with customers and presenting products, but their most important skill is following through on commitments made to customers. Something as simple as making a phone call when you promised to or remembering to check a price and call the customer back builds a trusting relationship. Although this requires a high level of personal organization and commitment, it results in long-term success in sales.

RECALL YOUR READING

1. The term _____ warns that workers are at risk for exposure to _____ agents.
2. In a lab, _____ balances are used for measurements between 1 and 1,000 grams, and _____ balances and _____ are used to measure smaller amounts of substances.
3. _____ are used to sterilize lab equipment and keep them free of _____ that cause contamination.
4. Urinalysis, a type of _____ test, is used to observe the physical, chemical, and microscopic properties of _____.
5. When preparing a sales _____, focus on the customer's needs.

Complete the *Map Your Reading* graphic organizer for the section you just read.

Employability Skills for Healthcare Workers

Healthcare is always changing and healthcare workers adapt to workplace changes by pursuing personal and professional development activities. As they move forward on their chosen career paths, successful healthcare employees exhibit positive behaviors and follow professional guidelines when changing jobs.

Continuing Personal and Professional Development

Darius is studying the hospital's new protocols for environmental safety. Briana is taking a training class to operate the lab's new analyzer. Nan is completing training in the protection of human subjects for her clinical research position. Addison hired a personal trainer to help her improve her fitness level so she can handle the long hours of standing that her surgical technologist position requires (Figure 18.28).

These are all healthcare workers. While their jobs may be very different, they have one thing in common. They are lifelong learners. All of them have already completed the education and training needed for their healthcare position. Yet they continue to learn new skills to enhance their personal and professional development.

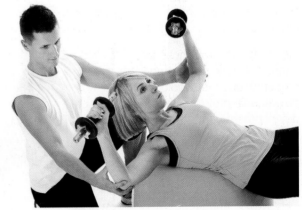

Figure 18.28   Lifelong learners continue to learn new skills to enhance their personal and professional development. How might physical fitness help you in your professional life?

personal and professional development
term that describes steps taken to improve personal, educational, and career-related performance

Personal and professional development includes activities that enhance your knowledge and skills, improve your employment opportunities, and lead you to accomplish your goals. Seeking advanced degrees, attending conferences and workshops, participating in training sessions to learn specific skills, and completing independent reading and study are all part of personal and professional development (Figure 18.29).

Healthcare workers are frequently required to obtain additional training to renew or maintain licensure or certification for the jobs they perform. For example, Janice just renewed her CPR certification, which is a requirement of her nursing assistant position at an assisted living facility. Professional development may lead to new job opportunities or job advancement. For example, Logan works as a medical assistant but continues to attend college to achieve his long-term career goal of becoming a physician assistant.

Rapid advances in medical care and continuing changes in technology make professional development necessary for long-term success in healthcare careers. It keeps your knowledge current and helps you perform your job effectively. Learn to view your professional development as an opportunity to expand your knowledge and skills rather than a burden.

There are several ways to enhance your personal and professional development. If you choose to further your education, your healthcare employer may support you by reimbursing the costs of your continuing education and training. For example, Janice is taking a medication training class so she can deliver medications to residents. You might also request additional responsibilities at your current job. Addison is a preceptor who works with future surgical technologists to guide their clinical training in the hospital setting. Finally, you can join a professional organization.

Membership in a **professional organization** supports your career development in several ways. First, professional organizations may offer certification and provide continuing education related to your specific career field. For example, the American Health Information Management

professional organization
an association formed to unite and inform people who work in the same occupation

Figure 18.29   Your hospital might offer workshops and presentations that would be valuable professional development opportunities.

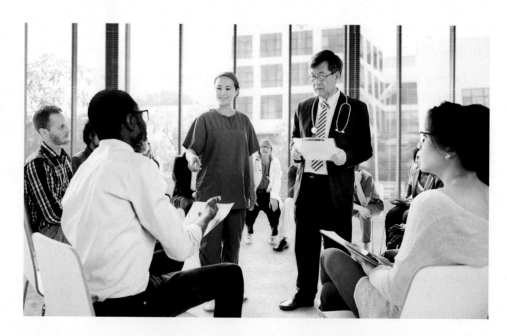

Association (AHIMA) issues credentials in health information management (HIM), coding, and healthcare privacy and security such as the Registered Health Information Technician (RHIT) certification. The association also promotes lifelong learning for HIM professionals by providing web-based training, specialty advancement institutes, workshops, and seminars.

Continuing education credits offered by professional organizations allow you to renew your certification or advance your career knowledge. A continuing education unit (CEU) typically represents one hour of instruction or other learning activity. CEUs can be granted for completing assignments or passing tests, as well as for class or workshop attendance. Your certifying agency decides which CEUs count toward your license or certificate, so always check their requirements before taking a class or attending a workshop.

Second, membership in a professional organization provides a networking opportunity for learning about job openings, staying updated on changes in your work environment, and providing information and encouragement to newer members of the profession. For example, AHIMA maintains an online networking tool that its members can use to share, problem solve, and stay informed on the latest trends in all HIM-related topics.

Third, organizations **advocate** for, or *promote*, your profession. They may publish journals and write public relations materials to inform consumers and government officials about the profession. Their members may serve on committees to establish best practices for your profession. Currently, AHIMA is working toward improving the benefits of information technology in healthcare by focusing on privacy and security, the electronic record, the national health information infrastructure, and system interoperability.

Finally, professional organizations offer you an opportunity to develop your leadership skills (Figure 18.30). Volunteer to serve on a

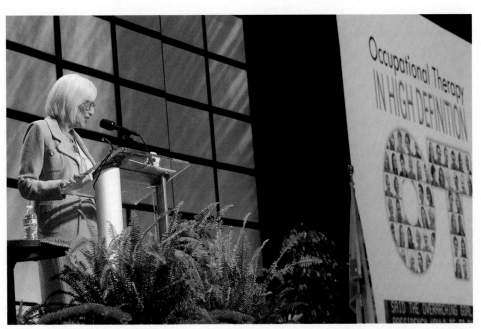

Figure 18.30 Rising to a leadership position in a national organization can be a very rewarding experience. Here, the president of the American Occupational Therapy Association (AOTA) presides over an AOTA meeting.

committee or become an officer of your organization. Your participation will broaden your knowledge and understanding of issues affecting your profession beyond your everyday work environment. At the same time, you will improve your teamwork capabilities and strengthen your organization and management skills, which may lead to future job advancement.

Healthcare professionals can choose from a wide variety of professional organizations. Some are large and well known, such as the American Medical Association or the American Nurses Association. Many others are smaller and more specific, such as the Opticians Association of America or the Association of Surgical Technologists. Some organizations focus on serving special populations, such as Doctors without Borders or Healing the Children. The National Library of Medicine offers an extensive list of organizations on its Medline Plus website. Search this list to locate health organizations and information about career fields that interest you.

Changing Jobs

Changing jobs is common, but you should try to leave your job in the right way. People change jobs for a variety of reasons, including improving pay or working conditions, moving to a new city, seeking new challenges and responsibilities, dealing with company layoffs, or seeking further education.

When you are considering a job change, think carefully about your options and weigh the pros and cons of leaving your current job for another position. Resist the urge to leave your current place of employment immediately. Complete the search for a new job before leaving your current one. Save enough money to cover your expenses until you receive a paycheck from a new job.

The Biotechnology Research and Development Worker: Sophia

Sophia worked at her first job during her junior and senior years of high school. Working part-time in a pharmacy was an excellent learning experience that fit right in with her plan to become a pharmaceutical sales representative. Now she was heading off to college in another city and needed to make a job change. She was able to leave her current job with the understanding that she could work during school breaks when she returned home. The pharmacy would be looking for workers to fill in for regular employees who were taking vacation breaks. In addition, her current supervisor recommended her to the supervisor at a pharmacy located in her college town. Eventually, she was able to work at that location as well. It was a win-win situation for Sophia.

Sometimes changes at work are out of our control. When problems arise, try to see the situation from the employer's view and avoid making decisions when you are upset.

For example, Jac was a hard-working employee at a medical equipment manufacturing company. Earning a regular paycheck was important because he had a large payment due each month for his new truck. When the number of orders for products decreased, his hours were cut. Jac was angry. "How can they do this to me?" he thought. "I need the money!" He stormed into his supervisor's office to complain. After learning that she couldn't give him more hours, he was still so angry that he quit his job. As a result, Jac has no income and no employer reference for seeking a new position (Figure 18.31).

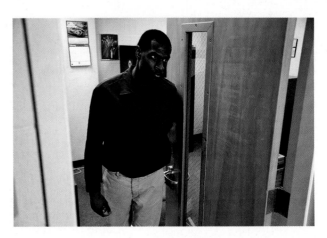

Figure 18.31   Always leave a job under the best possible circumstances. What could Jac have done differently in his situation?

Always leave a job under the best possible circumstances. Be sure to tell your employer before you tell your coworkers. Give at least two weeks' notice before leaving so your employer can find your replacement. If it's helpful and appropriate, offer to train your replacement. Give notice to your employer in person but also provide a **letter of resignation**. Your letter can be brief, but it should always be positive (Figure 18.32 on the next page). Include the following elements in the letter:

- the date of your last day of work

- the reason you are leaving, stated positively

- a thank you for the opportunity to work at the facility

- a description of how the job has been a benefit to you

letter of resignation
a written document that formally states an employee's decision to leave a job

Keep a sample letter of resignation in your career portfolio to remind you of these elements when you prepare to leave a job.

Work just as hard in your last two weeks as you always have. Let your employer remember you as a good worker. Remain positive with your coworkers. You may work with these people again in a different job. Resist any temptation to complain about your current job or brag about your new one. Instead, thank your coworkers for their help and support before you leave.

Maintaining Your Career Portfolio

Your career portfolio should currently include an introductory essay; your résumé; a personal data page; a list of career contacts; a sample application form and cover letter; copies of your current licenses and certificates; a sample letter of resignation; documentation of continuing education, awards, achievements, and service-learning activities; letters of recommendation; and copies of career assessments.

As you work in healthcare, keep your portfolio current. Add information about your employers and supervisors. Update your address and enter all of your continuing education information. Keeping all of your work records in one location greatly simplifies the process of applying for a new job or renewing your license or certification. When

Figure 18.32   Provide a letter of resignation in addition to talking with your employer in person. What elements should a letter of resignation include?

Build Portfolio

Sam Sanchez
4035 Starlight Ct.
Star Prairie, TX 74260

August 5, 2015

Shondra Lorenz
Pharmacy Manager
Star Prairie Pharmacy

Dear Shondra:

While I am happy to be heading to college, I am sorry that I will need to leave my job as a technician here at Star Prairie Pharmacy. My last day of work will be August 20.

This job has taught me so much about daily pharmacy operations. I feel well prepared for my college-level pharmacy courses because I was able to learn so much about the classifications of medications as well as their functions.

Thank you so much for being a caring boss and a great mentor. Completing an apprenticeship at Star Prairie was a fantastic learning experience.

Sincerely,

Sam Sanchez

Sam Sanchez

you apply for a scholarship or for a reimbursement of course costs, you will have all the information in one place.

HOSA Connections

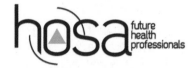

You can continue to receive the benefits of HOSA membership beyond high school by joining the postsecondary/collegiate division. You will be able to continue participating in competitive, service, and leadership events throughout your college years. When you finish your healthcare training, consider supporting and mentoring future healthcare workers as an alumni or professional member (Figure 18.33). HOSA allows you to continue your personal and professional development as you enhance the delivery of healthcare by assisting in the preparation of qualified healthcare workers.

In the meantime, consider serving on a committee, leading a service project, or becoming a HOSA officer. Just like other professional organizations, HOSA offers excellent opportunities for developing your leadership skills. In addition, competitive events will strengthen your biotechnology, research, and development skills (Figure 18.34). You can read about these events in the competitive events section of the HOSA website.

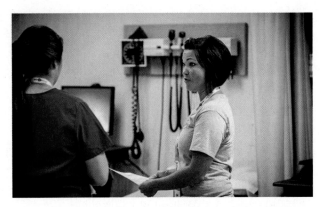

Figure 18.33   Mentor future healthcare workers as an alumni or professional member of HOSA.

Figure 18.34 HOSA Events	
Event Name	**Event Description**
Medical Law and Ethics	written test
Biomedical Laboratory Science	written test and skills demonstration
Epidemiology	written test and case study responses
Forensic Medicine	written test and case study analysis
HOSA Bowl	written test and oral question responses
Biomedical Debate	written test and oral debate
Medical Innovation	analyze or create a medical innovation

RECALL YOUR READING

1. Through _____ and _____ development, you can enhance your knowledge and skills, improve your _____ opportunities, and accomplish your goals.
2. A(n) _____ such as AHIMA can support your career development in many ways.
3. Professional organizations offer _____ credits that help you renew your certification.
4. When leaving a job, always give _____ weeks' notice and provide a letter of _____.

Complete the
Map Your Reading
graphic organizer for the
section you just read.

SUMMARY

Assess your understanding with chapter tests

- Biotechnology uses advances in the life sciences to create products that come from living things.

- The biotechnology industry employs people who have studied the biological sciences and possess good laboratory practices and computer science skills.

- Medical scientists plan and direct research studies. They oversee the work of lab technicians and research associates.

- Medical manufacturing companies produce a wide variety of products, including pharmaceuticals, vaccines, research assays, screening tests, medical devices and equipment, and provide crime investigation laboratory services.

- Biomedical engineers combine their knowledge of biology and engineering to design and develop products such as artificial organs, prostheses, and machines that diagnose medical problems.

- Medical sales representatives often serve as product consultants for the healthcare professionals who purchase their products, while technical service reps solve technical problems encountered by customers.

- Quality assurance workers promote compliance with industry regulations such as standard operating procedures, good laboratory practices, and good manufacturing practices.

- All people assume leadership roles at various times in their personal and work lives.

- Each person has a preferred leadership style that relies on personal preferences and attributes.

- Different leadership tasks require different leadership styles.

- Biotechnology laboratories are classified according to their level of risk from exposure to infectious agents.

- Lab workers measure mass using electronic balances and volume using graduated cylinders, pipettes, or micropipettes.

- To prevent contamination, lab workers use ultrasonic cleaners and autoclaves to clean and sterilize laboratory equipment.

- Clinical laboratories are certified by the Centers for Medicare and Medicaid Services to perform varying levels of tests.

- Documentation is an essential skill for all biotechnology workers because excellent lab work is worthless without proper documentation.

- Sales representatives for medical companies focus on business-to-business selling.

- Personal and professional development activities enhance your knowledge and skills, improve your employment opportunities, or lead you to accomplish your goals.

- Continuing education is a requirement for renewing many healthcare licenses and certifications.

- Professional organizations offer continuing education, professional networking, and leadership development opportunities.

- Maintaining your career portfolio simplifies the process of applying for a new job or renewing your license or certification.

MAXIMIZE YOUR PROFESSIONAL VOCABULARY

 Build vocabulary with e-flash cards, games, and audio glossary

Listed below are the essential, yellow-highlighted terms and the additional professional vocabulary that you encountered in this chapter. Complete the activities that follow the list to make all of these terms part of your everyday professional vocabulary.

advocate	autoclaves	biomedical engineer
algorithms	bioassay	bioreactor
aptitude	biohazard	biotechnology
assay	bioinformatics scientists	biotechnology research laboratories

business-to-business selling

centrifuge

clinical laboratories

clinical trial

consultant

customer objections

electronic balances

epidemiologists

exposure control plan

fermentor

forensic DNA analyst

genetic counselors

geneticists

good laboratory practices (GLPs)

good manufacturing practices (GMPs)

hypothesis

laboratory documentation

letter of resignation

meniscus

micropipette

other potentially infectious material (OPIM)

patents

personal and professional development

personal leadership style

placebo

point-of-care testing

professional organization

sales presentation

standard operating procedures (SOPs)

sterilize

ultrasonic cleaners

urinalysis

validity

waived tests

VOCABULARY DEVELOPMENT

Matching. Match the essential terms from this chapter with the best descriptions below by writing the letter of the description next to the number of the essential term on your answer sheet.

1. assays
2. autoclaves
3. biohazard
4. biotechnology
5. biotechnology research laboratories
6. business-to-business selling
7. clinical laboratories
8. clinical trial
9. electronic balances
10. laboratory documentation
11. letter of resignation
12. micropipette
13. personal and professional development
14. personal leadership style
15. professional organization
16. sales presentation

a. chambers for sterilizing items with steam under pressure

b. an association formed to unite and inform people who work in the same occupation

c. an instrument designed for the measurement of very small volumes

d. an experiment performed on human beings to evaluate the comparative effectiveness of two or more treatments

e. term that describes a biological agent, infectious organism, or insecure laboratory procedure that constitutes a danger to humans or the environment

f. facilities where research is done to develop new products or treatments, which are located on college campuses, in hospitals, and in private biotechnology companies

g. analysis done to determine the presence and amount of a substance or to determine the potency of a drug

h. a prearranged meeting in which a salesperson presents detailed information and often a demonstration of a product

i. facilities that examine materials taken from the human body to discover information related to diagnosis, prognosis, prevention, or treatment of disease

j. an individual approach to giving directions, implementing plans, and motivating people

k. written records of observable, measurable, and reproducible findings obtained through examination, testing, research studies, and experiments

l. the manipulation of living organisms to produce useful products

m. exchanging goods between businesses rather than between businesses and individuals

n. measuring instruments that show the weight of a substance digitally and are used to weigh chemicals in labs

o. term that describes steps taken to improve personal, educational, and career-related performance

p. a written document that formally states an employee's decision to leave a job

17. **Write It, Define It.** Select one or more of the professional vocabulary terms from the chapter. Write the terms you chose on slips of paper. Put the slips of paper in a basket or bowl with all of your classmates' terms. Pass the bowl or basket around the class, each student selecting a term at random. When you select a term, define it and explain how it connects it to biotechnology research and development in the field of healthcare. Keep passing the bowl or basket of words around until they have all been taken.

18. **Career Story.** Write a short story describing the development of a new and beneficial healthcare product or medication, from the research stage to the use of the new product. In your description, highlight the biotechnology research and development workers who play a role in the story and include professional vocabulary terms where appropriate.

REFLECT ON YOUR READING

19. Look at the biotechnology workers you listed in the *Connect with Your Reading* activity. Organize them under these headings: *Research and Development Careers*, *Manufacturing and Services Careers*, *Quality and Regulation Careers*, and *Additional Career Opportunities*. Were any of your headings empty? Complete your chart by adding at least two career opportunities for each section of the chart.

BUILD CORE SKILLS

20. **Critical Thinking.** Review the personal traits sections in this chapter as well as in chapters 2, 6, 10, and 14. Analyze your own personal traits and describe which healthcare career pathways most closely match your own personal traits.

21. **Reading.** Research a healthcare-related biotechnology company located in your community or state. What product or products does the company produce? Are the products still in the development and testing stage or are they available for purchase? How have the company's products improved healthcare?

22. **Critical Thinking.** Research one of these topics: SOPs, GLPs, or GMPs. Use the Internet to learn the definition, purposes, settings, and examples that describe your topic. Form a group of three students whose combined research includes all of the topics. Prepare a 3-section T-chart using *SOP*, *GLP*, and *GMP* as your horizontal headings and *definition*, *purposes*, *settings*, and *examples* as your vertical headings. Record your information. Analyze your information to identify similarities and differences. Post your T-chart and compare the results of all the research groups.

23. **Writing.** Write a 2-paragraph explanation that compares and contrasts clinical and research labs.

24. **Problem Solving.** For each of the following urine descriptions, identify the part of a urinalysis (physical, chemical, or microscopic testing) that would identify the abnormal sign.
    - high bacteria count
    - strong smell
    - high pH level
    - presence of ketones
    - presence of red blood cells
    - cloudy liquid
    - high protein level
    - presence of bilirubin and blood
    - medium to dark color
    - high glucose level

25. **Problem Solving.** Review DNA fingerprinting as explained in the chapter and use the Internet to create a list of situations in which DNA fingerprinting techniques would be useful. Explain how DNA fingerprinting would be helpful in those situations.

26. **Speaking and Listening.** Develop and deliver a sales presentation for the fictional product you previously created for your career story. Include responses to at least three common objections you might face.

ACTIVATE YOUR LEARNING

27. Watch a demonstration or video of cleaning and sterilizing lab equipment. Assemble the necessary supplies and practice wrapping equipment for autoclaving.

28. Review lab protocols and the procedures for measuring mass and volume as described

in the chapter. Assemble the necessary supplies and practice measuring the mass and volume of substances provided by your instructor.

29. Search for biohazard symbols in the school setting. What biohazards exist? Where are they located? What precautions are used to prevent exposure?

THINK AND ACT LIKE A HEALTHCARE WORKER

30. Read the following situations. Determine which leadership style would be most helpful to accomplish each task or activity. Justify your answer, especially if more than one style could be applied to the situation. Refer to Figure 18.12 if needed.

- Ronnie has a caring and compassionate personality. Feeling concerned about coworkers who seem less than happy or enthusiastic when interacting with patients, Ronnie has made it a personal goal of his to reach out to coworkers in a friendly way. Ronnie realizes that happy and satisfied workers result in healthier outcomes for patients.

- The clinic needs more space and a new addition is being proposed. The board of directors has asked Martina to spearhead the project and share potential plans.

- Ashley works in a local nursing home. One of her coworkers is having difficulty relating to fellow employees and several residents. Ashley has offered to work with this person to make the work environment more positive for everyone.

GO TO THE SOURCE

31. Locate three professional organizations related to a healthcare career of your choice. Research their websites to identify two professional development opportunities offered by each organization.

32. Use the Internet to search for information on prosthetics. In addition to limbs and braces, what other products have been developed to replace or support body parts?

33. Demonstrate your ability to effectively participate in meetings, both as a leader and a member of a group. Divide into small groups, each group discussing actions the group can take to learn more about topics discussed in this chapter. Each member is to take a turn as the leader. After your group has developed a plan of action for acquiring more information, discuss the group's effectiveness for conducting the meeting. How could the group's business have been conducted more effectively?

34. Use the Internet to learn more about careers in biotechnology research and development. Select two careers of interest to you and complete a career profile page for each one. Use at least one site that ends in .gov and one site that ends in .org. Record the following information for each career:

- name of career
- tasks involved in this career
- personal traits and abilities needed
- educational requirements
- type of credential needed and how it is obtained
- work conditions
- wages and benefits
- job outlook for the future
- the websites you accessed

How do the two careers compare? Why might you prefer one to the other?

DEVELOP YOUR HEALTH SCIENCE CAREER PORTFOLIO

35. Write a sample letter of resignation using Figure 18.32 as a guide.

36. Organize your career portfolio. Include all the items listed in the text.

37. Review the leadership styles described in Figure 18.10. Identify your preferred leadership style. Select a HOSA leadership opportunity of interest to you. How will this experience demonstrate the skills, characteristics, and responsibilities of a leader?

38. Review all of the HOSA competitive events and select two. Explain how your participation in these events will help you achieve your personal and professional development goals.

Chapter 19
Fundamental Skills in Biotechnology Research and Development

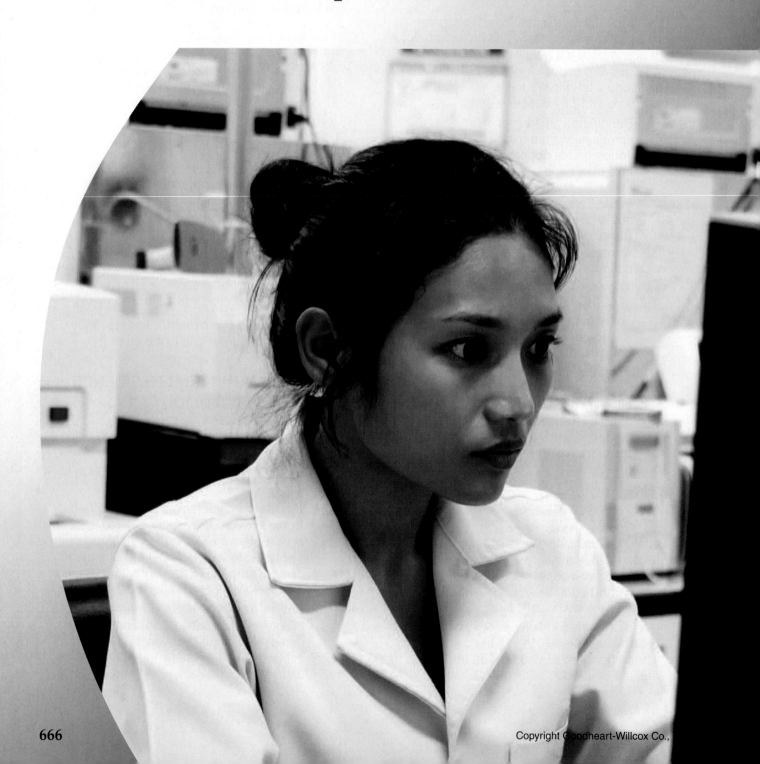

PROFESSIONAL VOCABULARY

 E-flash Cards

You will need to learn the essential terms listed below before you begin your reading. These terms will help you understand the main concepts of the chapter. These terms, which will be highlighted in yellow within the text, will become part of your professional vocabulary.

In addition to the essential terms, you will see bold terms throughout the chapter. The meanings of these terms are explained where the terms first appear. The bold terms, like the essential terms listed here, will also become part of your professional vocabulary and deepen your understanding of the topics presented.

absolute risk ratio of the number of people who have a medical event to those who could have the event because of a medical condition

bias a systematic error that produces a research finding that deviates from a valid finding

bioinformatics a scientific discipline that combines the tools and techniques of mathematics, computer science, and biology to understand the biological significance of data

number needed to treat (NNT) the number of patients who must be treated to prevent the occurrence of the condition under examination

personal health record (PHR) a file that contains information about your own health that you store electronically for easy reference

primary source a document that describes research in which the authors directly participated

relative risk ratio of the chance of a disease developing among people who are exposed to a specific factor compared with those who are not exposed

risk assessments methods used to calculate and describe a person's chance of becoming ill or dying of a specified condition

scientific communication a type of technical communication used by scientists and nonscientists to provide information and promote understanding

secondary source a document that summarizes the results of several studies

statistical data numerical information gathered through research that is used to draw conclusions about research findings

tertiary source a document compiled from primary and secondary sources that gives an overview of a specific topic

CONNECT WITH YOUR READING

Eat too many carrots during pregnancy and your baby will be born with rabbit ears. Feed your infant too many carrots and the child's skin will turn orange. Take this product and build muscle overnight. For the best muscle-building results, rest each muscle group at least 24 hours between workouts.

Some false health claims are easy to spot, but others that appear to be false may actually be true. We know that research changes healthcare knowledge, which leads to changes in healthcare practices. Your great-grandmother was likely advised to drink a little wine during pregnancy for its relaxing effects. However, research has shown that alcohol has negative effects on fetal development. That advice would never be given today.

Recall a time when you were confused or fooled by a healthcare news report or product claim. Describe the situation and explain how you learned the truth. Did you try the product or follow the recommendations in the news report? What happened as a result?

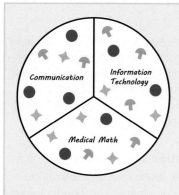

MAP YOUR READING

Create a visual summary by drawing a large circle on a blank sheet of paper. Divide the circle into three pizza slices. Label one slice *Communication*, another *Information Technology*, and the last one *Medical Math*. As you finish reading each section of the chapter, place these following "toppings" on your pizza:

- Draw "pepperoni" circles containing the main ideas, or the "meat" of the information.
- Draw "mushroom" shapes containing bits of information that are new or interesting for you and kept you from "vegging out" as you read.
- Draw "mystery" toppings (you create the shapes) that contain questions you still have about your reading.

As you learned in chapter 18, workers in the biotechnology research and development pathway often work in labs, where they have to compile and record data. That data may then be communicated to a variety of people and groups. Scientific communication can be used in those situations. This chapter describes the goals of scientific communication, a specific type of technical communication that provides information about medical research.

In this chapter, you will learn techniques for reading scientific papers and practice scientific writing to produce documents that are objective, precise, and clear. As you consider the benefits of a personal health record, you will learn how to locate reliable sources of health information. The field of bioinformatics will be introduced, as well as basic methods for analyzing research results, interpreting statistical data, and assessing health risks.

Scientific Communication

scientific communication
a type of technical communication used by scientists and nonscientists to provide information and promote understanding

Scientific communication is a specific subset of technical communication. Scientific communication can be a simple explanation of a medical condition in language that a child can understand, or it can be a complex report detailing innovative research to be shared with fellow researchers involved in similar studies. Scientific communication appears in documentaries, news articles, professional journals, health-related websites, popular magazines, and government and university publications and presentations.

Because it is technical, scientific communication's primary goal is to inform. Accuracy and validity are important components of scientific communication. Validity is achieved when a conclusion can be verified or proved to be true. Students studying health sciences need to learn how to read and evaluate scientific articles and how to write reports that are clear and objective.

Scientific Communication: Dr. Workman

Dr. Workman was putting in some long hours in front of his computer. The deadline for a major grant proposal was approaching quickly, and he needed to finalize all sections of the document before submitting his team's proposal. The research team had been meeting frequently to outline the content for each section and collate the data to support their research request. They spent many hours discussing and developing measurable goals in the hope that the foundation would grant the funds needed to continue their research project.

Now it was up to Dr. Workman to make sense of all that information and present it in a logical and convincing way. How could he make the review team at the foundation see the value of his team's research and the urgency for focusing on this new study? Dr. Workman is a scientist by training, but he's also a writer. He uses scientific communication skills both to fund his research and to document the results of that research.

Understanding is also a common goal of scientific communication. When the public or average citizens are your audience, you must communicate information in ways that help readers understand scientific concepts. Medical writers usually have strong backgrounds in science. They can read and interpret scientific research documents. They can also focus on their purpose and tailor material to their audience to produce documents that readers can understand.

Scientific Reading

Scientific research papers communicate research results and ideas between scientists. Medical professionals read scientific literature to stay informed about healthcare advances and potential changes in diagnosis and treatment. However, all people read or learn about scientific topics through media sources. Should you take calcium supplements? Will they strengthen your bones or damage your blood vessels? Is childhood obesity truly an epidemic? What does this mean for the future health of our adult population and how will it affect healthcare delivery? Since we use what we read to make decisions about our own healthcare, we must know how to select valid sources of information.

Primary, Secondary, and Tertiary Sources. Health science information can be primary, secondary, or tertiary (Figure 19.1 on the next page). **Primary sources** are original research. Scientists complete research in the laboratory, then write it up and publish it in formal lab reports, case studies, or research articles. You will find primary research documents in health science journals. Primary sources contain detailed descriptions of experiments as well as references to experiments completed by other

primary source
a document that describes research in which the authors directly participated

Figure 19.1 Sources of Healthcare Information		
Primary Sources (original research)	**Secondary Sources** (analysis of research by others)	**Tertiary Sources** (topic overview)
Examples: • lab report • case study • research article	Examples: • healthcare journal article • newspaper article • science news website	Examples: • almanac • manual • encyclopedia

researchers. These sources tell you the latest findings about a topic, but they can be difficult to read unless you are an expert in the specific subject area of the research. This is because primary sources are targeted toward people in the writer's field, who understand the common terminology.

secondary source a document that summarizes the results of several studies

Secondary sources talk about the original research of others. They summarize, analyze, and interpret information found in primary source documents. For example, you might read about research results in an article in the *Journal of the American Medical Association*, the health section of the *New York Times*, or on the Science Daily website. These articles will provide some facts and a summary of the research. They are written in language that is easier to understand but do not contain detailed descriptions of the experiments that are part of the primary source. However, the articles do provide citations so you can locate and read the primary source for more details.

tertiary source a document compiled from primary and secondary sources that gives an overview of a specific topic

Tertiary sources provide an overview of a topic. They sort and compile information from both primary and secondary sources. Almanacs, diagnostic and treatment manuals, dictionaries, and encyclopedias are tertiary sources.

Reading Scientific Papers. You've just read a news article about sleep deprivation, which included the surprising statistic that 70 percent of adolescents are sleep deprived. Since you need to pick a topic for a science paper, you decide to do some research on this topic. You search for the work of the scientist who is quoted in the article and find a presentation she gave to a professional association. You read the PowerPoint slides from the presentation, which are a primary source for information.

Next, you go to the Centers for Disease Control and Prevention (CDC) website, which is listed as a source in the article. You read results from a survey about adolescent lifestyles and find information about sleep habits. Finally, you log in to your school's media site and enter a database containing health science journal articles.

Your search locates a full text article about the sleep habits of adolescents. It was recently published in a professional health science journal. This article looks great—until you start reading. Unlike the previous sources, this one is written for other professionals in the field of health science. While you can read most of the words, you're not certain you understand what they're saying. Since you want to pursue a career in health sciences, you decide to take on the challenge of deciphering the content of this research article. Where do you begin?

First, determine which type of scientific paper you are reading. **Review articles** give an overview of a specific topic. They summarize the data and conclusions from several different studies. These articles provide a good starting point because they contain more background information about what has been happening in the field.

Primary research articles provide the original data and conclusions of researchers who conducted experiments. You will learn how the researchers organized their experiments and see charts of the resulting data. Primary research articles contain the following sections:

- **Abstract.** This is a summary of the paper. It highlights the research question, key results of experiments, and the researcher's conclusions. Abstracts are often available online at no cost. Reading the abstract helps you decide if the article presents the information you want to study.

- **Introduction.** The introduction provides background information about the research topic and identifies the specific questions addressed by the research. The footnote marker numbers found in the introduction link to resources listed in the references section. Use these to locate additional articles for your research. If you have difficulty understanding the introduction, the rest of the paper will frustrate you as well. In this situation, try reading other resources such as a textbook to learn more about the topic, or enlist the help of a mentor to guide your reading.

- **Materials and methods.** This section tells you exactly how the experiments were performed. Understanding the methods helps you determine the validity of the researcher's conclusions.

- **Results.** This section shows data from the experiments. Spend time looking at the figures, graphs, tables, and other visuals to understand the research findings. As you gain experience in reading scientific papers, you can begin to draw your own conclusions about different aspects of the research, including its accuracy, validity, and usefulness.

- **Discussion.** In this section, researchers give you their opinions about the results of their experiments and compare those results to previous findings or talk about a new direction for research. This provides a way for scientists to exchange ideas. Remember, you are reading opinions rather than facts in this section.

- **References.** This is a list of all the other papers referred to in the article. It contains enough information for you to locate a source in a library or online.

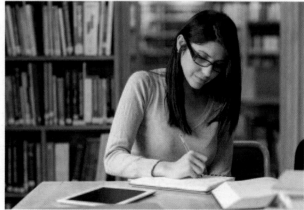

Figure 19.2   Read scientific material slowly and reread when you need to improve your understanding of specific sections. How can you determine the value of what you have read?

Reading a scientific article goes slowly. You must look up unfamiliar vocabulary and reread sections to gain understanding (Figure 19.2). Once you have conquered the content of the article, you can begin to analyze the value of the research. The best studies are clinical trials with control groups and several years of data. This type of research can show cause and effect. In some research studies, participants are surveyed and the results of those surveys are analyzed to find connections or associations between behaviors. Other studies examine and compare information found in de-identified patient records.

Different studies can find the same behavior both beneficial and detrimental. For example, one study found an increased risk of breast cancer for women who drink even small amounts of alcohol. However, another study cited the cardiovascular benefits of moderate alcohol consumption. As a result, healthcare decisions become complex because there is no single best course of action.

Healthcare professionals use **evidence-based practices** to guide diagnosis and treatment for a patient. This means they implement methods of diagnosis and treatment based on the best available current research, their clinical expertise, and the patient's needs and preferences. When there is conflicting research, the patient must ultimately make a choice. Healthcare providers who continue to learn the latest research findings can offer the best range of options to their patients.

Scientific Writing

While the majority of a scientist's time might be spent in a laboratory with other scientists, a research scientist also has to write reports for administrators and explain ideas to supervisors. Writing skills allow scientists to share their knowledge, secure research funding, and improve their employment options. In addition to research papers, scientific writing can include **proposals** and **recommendation reports**.

Proposals, as their name indicates, propose or suggest something. Sales proposals attempt to sell a product or service. Research proposals seek approval for a research study. Grant proposals ask for funding for a project, and planning proposals try to persuade the audience to take a certain action.

When HOSA members wanted to conduct a service project promoting healthy exercise for elementary school students, they needed money. This money would go toward buses to get to the elementary school, pedometers and other supplies to complete the activities with the students, and the bus chaperone required by their school district. Their advisor suggested that they write a service-learning grant. They spent the next four weeks refining their ideas and completing the grant proposal (Figure 19.3). Two months after submitting their proposal, they received an award letter and $2,000 to fund their project.

Proposals can be brief and informal. A request to order thermometers from a different supplier is written to the head of your department and may be just one or two pages. On the other hand, a research grant proposal to conduct a specific project for several years may be hundreds of pages.

The requirements of your audience determine the detail and formality of your writing, yet all proposals have two things in common. They describe a problem and suggest a solution. Successful proposals persuade the audience to invest in their solution.

Recommendation reports also consider problems and solutions. They provide a written answer that shows how to meet a need in the workplace. Because there can be more than one solution to a problem, a recommendation report helps readers make a choice by identifying

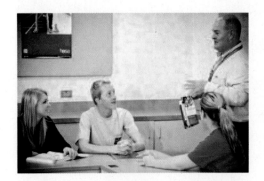

Figure 19.3 Successful proposals, such as grant requests, persuade your target audience to invest in your solution. What two elements do all proposals have in common?

the best solution. These reports can recommend which equipment to purchase or the best location for a new hospital.

Scientific Communication: Addison

Addison is a surgical technologist. She also serves on a healthcare team researching the installation of an MRI scanner in the surgical suite of the hospital where she works.

First, the team met to discuss and list the difficulties of doing surgical procedures without the guidance of ready images. Next, they visited other surgical suites with imaging equipment and interviewed healthcare workers at each site to learn the benefits and possible drawbacks of surgical suite imaging. Finally, they obtained cost estimates for the purchase and installation of new imaging equipment. Now they are ready to write a recommendation report that does the following:

- defines the problem

- explains and compares the possible solutions along with the criteria used to evaluate the solutions

- makes a recommendation by choosing the best solution after considering all factors, including costs, patient outcomes, and effects on healthcare workers

---

Scientific writing presents data or ideas with enough detail to let the reader judge the validity of the conclusions by using the facts in the document. To achieve this goal, scientific writing must be objective, precise, and clear.

Objective writing draws a conclusion from the facts. It makes no assumptions. Do not use your intuition or emotions to form conclusions.

Correct: "The data shows that…"

Incorrect: "We believe that…"

Objective writing can use the active voice, but it avoids beginning a sentence with *I* or *we*. This keeps the focus on the data and procedures instead of the researcher.

Correct: "Blood pressure measurements indicate…"

Incorrect: "We think the blood pressure measurements mean that…"

Precise writing uses concrete rather than figurative language. Be as specific as possible to avoid confusion.

Correct: "Inflate the cuff to 140 mmHg."

Incorrect: "Inflate the cuff until it feels tight like a tourniquet."

Precise writing requires quantitative descriptions that can be measured rather than qualitative descriptions that list characteristics.

Correct: "Blood pressure measurements increased by 20 mmHg at each reading."

Incorrect: "Blood pressure measurements showed a steady increase."

Clear writing uses simple language to explain ideas that may be complex.

Correct: "The text uses effective strategies to explain hypertension."

Incorrect: "Utilization of efficacious strategies to elucidate hypertensive symptoms is a hallmark of the text."

Clear writing also avoids wordiness.

Correct: "Discomfort with the procedure may elevate blood pressure readings."

Incorrect: "It is interesting to note the fact that discomfort with the procedure may elevate blood pressure readings."

These guidelines are important to follow when writing scientific reports. Chaunte is reviewing data from patient records to select patients who could benefit from wellness programs. She looks for changes in average blood pressure readings over a period of several years. She selects 10 patients and records average blood pressure readings for each patient at 20, 40, and 60 years of age. She assembles her data and writes a report (Figure 19.4).

Figure 19.4   Chaunte's first draft report.

Patient #	Avg. BP at age 20	Avg. BP at age 40	Avg. BP at age 60
1	110/75	120/80	135/85
2	118/72	128/78	148/92
3	98/68	108/72	115/72
4	140/88	145/95	155/98
5	115/70	120/74	145/95
6	135/85	150/105	120/80
7	130/80	125/75	130/80
8	110/72	130/78	120/75
9	128/78	135/84	148/95
10	113/67	125/75	150/100

Title: Hypertension Data Review

Introduction: Our goal is to help patients make lifestyle changes that reduce hypertension. The purpose of this study is to review patient data so we can select patients who will benefit from learning how to reduce hypertension.

Method: I selected 10 patients and reviewed their average blood pressure readings at ages 20, 40, and 60. I entered the data into a table (see table above).

Results: The blood pressure readings of most patients increased with age. One patient had hypertension and three patients had prehypertensive readings at age 20. Two patients had hypertension and four patients were prehypertensive by age 40. At age 60, five patients had hypertension and two patients had readings indicating prehypertension.

Conclusions: It looks like age really increases your blood pressure. We could really help the patients!

After reviewing the guidelines for scientific writing, Chaunte makes several changes to her report to make her writing more objective, precise, and clear (Figure 19.5).

Title: Hypertension Data Review

Introduction: SunView Medical wants to help patients make lifestyle changes that reduce hypertension. The purpose of this study is to review patient data to select patients who will benefit from learning how to reduce hypertension.

Chaunte removed the words our, we, and I from her report because scientific writing focuses on data rather than the researcher.

Method: Ten patient records were selected. Average blood pressure readings at ages 20, 40, and 60 were entered into the following table.

Patient #	Avg. BP at age 20	Avg. BP at age 40	Avg. BP at age 60
1	110/75	120/80	135/85
2	118/72	128/78	148/92
3	98/68	108/72	115/72
4	140/88	145/95	155/98
5	115/70	120/74	145/95
6	135/85	150/105	120/80
7	130/80	125/75	130/80
8	110/72	130/78	120/75
9	128/78	135/84	148/95
10	113/67	125/75	150/100

Chaunte moved this table to the "method" section of her report to show the quantitative data she collected.

Results: Between ages 20 and 60, eight patients had increased blood pressure readings, one remained the same, and one had decreased readings. One patient had hypertension and three patients had prehypertensive readings at age 20. Two patients had hypertension and four patients were prehypertensive by age 40. At age 60, five patients had hypertension and two patients had readings indicating prehypertension.

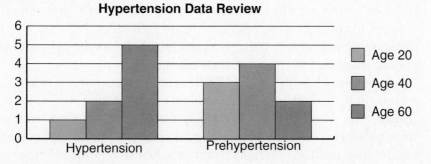

Chaunte replaced the word most with an exact number because scientific writing uses concrete language and quantitative descriptions. She drew a bar graph to make the results easier to visualize.

Conclusion: Data shows that 40 percent of 20-year-old patients could benefit from learning about lifestyle changes to reduce blood pressure. It is anticipated that improving lifestyle choices of the youngest patients will provide long-term health benefits by eventually reducing the incidence of prehypertension and hypertension at all ages.

Chaunte rewrote her conclusion to include specific data because scientific writing draws conclusions from data rather than intuition or emotion.

Figure 19.5   After reading the guidelines for scientific writing, Chaunte makes some changes to her report. Can you suggest ways to make Chaunte's conclusion even clearer?

Explaining complex scientific results in objective language takes time, thought, and practice. Remember, you are not trying to impress your audience with your own intelligence. You are trying to expand their scientific knowledge by drawing valid conclusions supported by facts learned through research.

Complete the
Map Your Reading
graphic organizer for the
section you just read.

RECALL YOUR READING

1. Accuracy and validity are components of _____, which is used to provide _____ and promote _____.
2. While a scientific topic is summarized by an overview in _____ and _____ sources, the original research is explained in _____ sources.
3. Proposals might seek to sell _____ and services, gain approval for a(n) _____, ask for _____, or persuade a(n) _____ to take a specific action.
4. When drafting a scientific paper, your writing must be _____, _____, and _____.

Information Technology

Today, individuals can use technology to manage their personal health records. Communicating health information electronically is fast and convenient, but patients and healthcare workers now share the responsibility for guarding their private information.

Electronic Health Records: Personal Health Records

Technology is changing the way we manage our personal health. Health information technology (HIT) is not just for healthcare providers. Patients can use it to learn more about their personal health status and share information with their healthcare providers. HIT allows patients to access health information more quickly and directly through online sources, to communicate with healthcare providers electronically, and to take actions to improve their personal health. It has the power to make the patient a key part of the healthcare team.

personal health record (PHR)
a file that contains information about your own health that you keep on a computer for easy reference

A **personal health record (PHR)** is similar to an electronic health record (EHR), but the patient controls the information that goes into it (Figure 19.6). The PHR helps you keep track of information from your doctor visits because it creates a digital storage center for important health information such as emergency contacts, health history, allergies and medications, lab test results, and immunization dates. Because you can import medical record information from different providers, the PHR can offer a more complete record of your health history.

The PHR can also reflect your personal health goals. Patients can use smartphone apps to track personal health indicators such as food intake, exercise, or blood pressure readings. The PHR can provide additional information about healthcare outside the doctor's office by recording habits such as over-the-counter medication use or sleep patterns. In some cases, the PHR can link to the healthcare provider's EHR to share information electronically with a provider.

The HIPAA Privacy, Security, and Breach Notification Rules cover PHR systems that are offered by a healthcare provider or health insurance plan. Other companies that offer PHR systems must comply with the Federal Trade Commission's Health Breach Notification Rule. This means they will notify you if your protected information is released to or used by unauthorized third parties. However, when you post your own information online—on a message board about a health condition, for example—it is not protected by HIPAA. Never post any private information online.

Secure your own computer files and use passwords for your e-mail system. This will ensure that your personal information has some protection if your computer is lost or stolen. Medical identity thieves try to steal personal and health insurance information to access medical treatments and get prescription drugs. Always verify your recipient's identity before sharing any personal or medical information. When discarding paper copies, be sure to shred health insurance forms, copies of prescriptions, and physician's statements.

Biotechnology Research and Development Applications

Advances in information technology have rapidly increased the amount of healthcare data and information that is generated. This means that everyone must review online information carefully to find trustworthy sources. In the field of bioinformatics, methods for storing, accessing, and using research data to advance healthcare have been developed.

Reliable Sources for Health Information. When scientific information was printed on paper, you could easily see who wrote it and when. Today, we use electronic resources to access most of this information. Anyone can publish information on the Internet. How can you sort out which information comes from a reliable source?

Look at the site address for basic clues. Addresses that end in .gov are most likely reliable government websites. They will offer statistics and objective reports. Site addresses ending in .edu are typically educational institutions. However, be aware that these sites may be a student posting personal opinions rather than a university research publication. Remember that sites ending in .com are commercial sites whose main purpose is to sell a product. While some .org sites contain excellent information, proceed with caution if they contain links to sites that sell products. These are general guidelines that provide a good way to begin narrowing your search.

When you research health information, always remember that health fraud scams abound on the Internet (Figure 19.7 on the next page). Read all medical claims with skepticism. Be on the lookout for these common online scams:

With a PHR you can...

...have an informed discussion with your healthcare provider.

...provide information to new caregivers.

...access your health information while traveling or when your medical office is closed.

...track your progress toward a personal health goal.

... review physician instructions, medications, and insurance claims.

...track appointments, vaccinations, and other healthcare services.

Figure 19.6 The advantages of a personal health record (PHR).

Figure 19.7   Remember that anyone can post information on the Internet. Do you think these headlines are scams? Explain how you arrived at this answer.

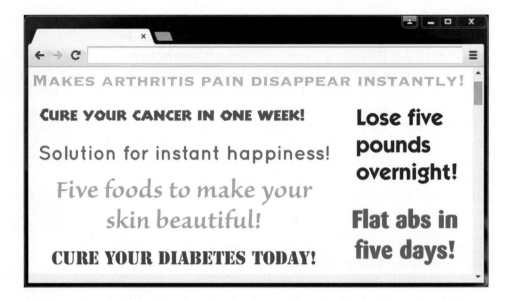

- **Miracle cures.** If the claim seems miraculous, don't believe it. Remember, it isn't true just because you see it in print. Be suspicious of "breakthroughs," "secret ingredients," and sites that use lots of technical jargon to make the product sound impressive.

- **Celebrity endorsements.** Famous people, and especially medical experts, sell products. However, the "celebrities" may be look-alike imposters.

- **Trial periods.** If the product is good, why do you have to buy it now? The words "act now" and "limited quantity" are red flags. In addition, when you do order, the sales agreement may be manipulated so you can't change your mind about future deliveries and end up owing additional money.

- **Blogs.** Personal health stories help others facing similar challenges, but be aware that "fake blogs" exist as marketing tools to get you to buy a product. Again, be skeptical of a blog that talks about a secret ingredient, a breakthrough, or the "only product that works."

- **Phony testimonials.** When you see product endorsements that are written by customers, look to see if they are all written on the same or similar dates. If you can't add your own comments, then the creators of the website posted those endorsements.

- **Missing contact information.** Check for the company name, address, and phone number before ordering. If you can't find it on the website, don't order. You won't be able to resolve any problems with the product or the amount you are charged.

- **Seal of approval.** When you purchase supplements, look for the Unites States Pharmacopeia (far-muh-koh-PEE-uh) seal. This means that the product has been tested and verified for quality. You can trust the product label regarding the purity and potency of a supplement. Without the USP seal, you truly have no idea what's in that bottle!

How can you know whether online health information is reliable? The National Library of Medicine offers solid guidelines to follow when evaluating health information you find on the Internet.

1. Find out who is responsible for the content.

   • Click on the "About Us" tab at the bottom of the homepage. Is the site administered by the federal government, a nonprofit or educational institution, a professional organization, a health system, a commercial organization, or an individual?

   • Look for a listing of professionals who reviewed the content of the website rather than an individual who established the website after being diagnosed with an illness.

   • Valid websites have a way to contact the organization. Is there an e-mail or a street address?

2. Check for funding sources.

   • Does the site use advertisements? If so, are they clearly labeled as ads, or do they look like health information with a link that leads to an online store?

   • Is the site sponsored by a nonprofit organization and funded by donations? Is it an educational institution or government site funded by tax revenue, or does the information favor the sponsor of the site?

3. Evaluate the quality of the information.

   • Look for a description of the process for selecting and approving information, often called the *editorial, selection*, or *review policy*. Is the material reviewed before posting? Do the reviewers have expertise in the site's subject?

   • Look for the author of the information and the original source for the data and research. "Written by James Smith, MD," or "Copyright 2012, American Diabetes Association" are good examples.

   • Look for dates on documents to show that information is current rather than outdated. Click on site links. If they are broken, the site may not be up-to-date.

4. Investigate privacy policies.

   • Does the site have a privacy policy, and does it tell you what information the site collects?

   • Does the site ask for your personal information, and does it tell you how that information will be used?

   • Are you comfortable with how your information will be used? Remember, health information should be confidential.

Take the time to evaluate your sources. Your knowledge and understanding of a healthcare topic will only be as good as the sources of information you use to learn about it.

Data Management. Handling data is a major task in biotechnology research and development. For example, mapping the human genome has created enormous amounts of data at increasingly faster speeds. The **Human Genome Project** completed the first DNA sequence over a period of 10 years at a cost of $3 billion. Just a few years ago, wealthy individuals were paying $300,000 for their personal DNA sequence. Today, DNA

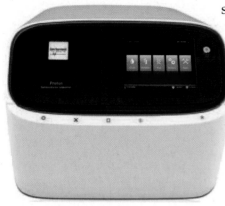

Figure 19.8 DNA sequencers are becoming smaller and faster. A tabletop machine like this can complete a genome sequence in one day.

sequencing technology uses semiconductor chips that "read chemistry" and digitize the information (Figure 19.8). Using this technology, an individual DNA sequence can be completed in one day and costs about $1,000.

By comparing DNA maps, healthcare professionals hope to target treatments to fit the specific needs of each individual. Scientists have already identified specific genes that increase risks for developing breast cancer, colon cancer, and Alzheimer's disease. Currently, researchers are studying the uses of genomic sequencing in pediatrics, cancer care, and clinical medicine. They anticipate that targeted therapies will provide more effective treatments at reduced costs.

In the meantime, the field of genomics is caught in an avalanche of data. The ability to determine DNA sequences is starting to outrun the ability of researchers to store, transmit, and especially analyze the data. The cost of analyzing a genome is greater than the cost of sequencing the genome. As a result, the field of bioinformatics is expected to expand rapidly.

Computer skills are important for managing healthcare data. From the entry-level assistant to the lead researcher, biotechnology research workers use computers to record and analyze data.

Data Management: Nina

Nina is a clinical administrative assistant at a company that conducts medical research studies. She is responsible for supply inventory for inpatient clinical studies. Since her facility had no organized system for maintaining inventory, she decided to develop a spreadsheet for ordering routine supplies. Spreadsheets store data in a grid of horizontal rows and vertical columns. Nina lists all of the supplies along with container sizes and ordering information in her spreadsheet. Each week, she quickly checks the items and lists the amount needed for reorder. She sends the form to her company's central supply location by e-mail.

Nina's simple form speeds up the ordering process and keeps her from forgetting items. The company recognized that her spreadsheet worked well, so now they use it at all of their clinical sites across the United States. Nina knows how to use her computer to manage the data and information required for her job.

bioinformatics
a scientific discipline that combines the tools and techniques of mathematics, computer science, and biology to understand the biological significance of data

Bioinformatics combines biology, computer science, and information technology into a single field of study. Genome sequencing is creating massive databases of biological information. The field of bioinformatics develops tools that allow easy access to this information and make it possible to manage the large amounts of genomic data. In addition, new mathematical formulas are being developed to analyze and extract information from large sets of data, such as locating a specific gene in a sequence.

Biology is becoming not only a lab-based science, but also an information science. Using a process called *database mining*, bioinformaticists can analyze and compare vast amounts of data to find patterns. For example, you could compare the outcomes for patients treated with different drug **regimens** (REH-juh-mihns), or *plans*, for treating the same disease and determine which treatments work the best.

The challenges of storing information include the additional challenges of securing and guarding that information. While researchers can benefit from sharing the results of their studies, information can be damaging in the hands of the wrong people. Recently, scientists altered a deadly flu virus to make it more contagious and assess the risk of a pandemic. They temporarily stopped their research because of fears that terrorists could use the virus. Researchers across the globe who were sharing their studies of the virus also voluntarily stopped publishing their detailed research. It was determined that the information could potentially be used to create a biological weapon.

Many research studies employ information technology specialists to develop data protection protocols. These protocols spell out the steps taken to prevent the theft or loss of important research data. They include methods for protecting access to data, the computer system itself, and the integrity of electronic data. Protecting the integrity of data involves recording the original date and time for all files, using encryption and electronic signatures to track changes made to files, routinely creating backup files, and ensuring that data that is no longer needed is properly destroyed.

Technology is also creating **biorepositories** (bI-oh-rih-PAH-zih-tor-ees), which act as libraries of biological information. When patients grant permission for the collection and storage of leftover blood or tissue samples, robots extract the DNA from each sample and match it with the patient's de-identified electronic health record. All of the information is stored in a secure environment and may be accessed for medical research. This creates a large library of specimens from diverse populations and can significantly shorten research study times. A study may not have to recruit individual participants because the information it needs is in the biorepository. Using the biorepository, researchers might improve diagnostic procedures, enhance treatment therapies, or increase the ability to prevent disease.

RECALL YOUR READING

1. A(n) _____ is different from an electronic health record because the _____ controls the information that goes into it.

2. Health insurance plans and healthcare providers that offer PHR systems must comply with HIPAA Privacy, _____, and _____ Notification Rules.

3. When doing health science _____ online, you should narrow your search to site addresses that end in _____, _____, and _____.

4. Data _____ is a major task for biotechnology _____ and _____ organizations.

5. The field of _____ develops tools that allow easy access to information and help manage large amounts of _____ data.

Complete the *Map Your Reading* graphic organizer for the section you just read.

Medical Math

Data in research studies must be analyzed and interpreted through mathematical procedures. Healthcare workers carefully analyze research studies to determine whether any form of bias has influenced the results. They learn how to interpret statistical data and understand the risks involved with a given course of treatment.

Analyzing Research Results

bias
a systematic error that produces a research finding that deviates from a valid finding

High quality research studies strive to produce valid results, but research free of bias is nearly impossible to conduct. **Bias** is anything that produces a systematic yet unexpected change in the results of a study. While researchers want to know the true relationship between their prediction and the outcome of their research, they struggle to separate the subjects of the study from other factors that influence them (Figure 19.9). As you analyze the results of a research study, consider whether bias may affect the data and your conclusions.

There are multiple sources of bias that researchers try to avoid as they design research studies. The following are examples of types of bias:

- **Selection bias.** If you run a survey online, only individuals with Internet access can participate. If you select fewer participants, intentionally or unintentionally, your results can be biased because your participants may not represent all the people who are affected.

- **Attrition bias.** Consider the effect of people who drop out of a study. If participants who are not losing weight drop out, then a weight-loss study will appear successful because the only results reported will be for the people who lost weight.

- **Measurement bias.** If your equipment is faulty, your survey participants forget to include information, or your participants cannot read or understand your questions, then your results will not be valid.

- **Researcher bias.** If you or another researcher have a strong belief and try to prove that belief, the research methods may include "leading" questions that influence participants' responses.

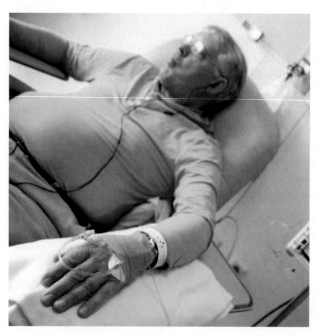

Figure 19.9   Patients who participate in clinical trials are vital to medical research. What factors do researchers consider to avoid bias in their research results?

- **Publication bias.** Successful results are published more often than studies that show a treatment to be ineffective or even detrimental. As a result, a treatment may be judged safe and effective because that is the only information available to healthcare providers.

When you read about a new medical research finding, the National Institutes of Health (NIH) recommends that you consider several questions as you analyze the results of the research study:

- Was the study conducted with people in everyday situations rather than with animals or in a lab setting? Better yet, were the people similar to you in age, gender, ethnicity, health concerns, and lifestyle? If so, then the study results are more likely to apply to you.

- Was the research a randomized, controlled clinical trial that involved thousands of people? These studies provide the best information about whether a treatment or lifestyle change is effective.

- Where was the research conducted? Large hospitals and medical schools have the resources to lead complex experiments and can employ scientists who may have more experience with a research topic.

- Do the reports agree with previous studies? Unexpected results must be verified in multiple studies before they are considered valid.

- Are the results presented in numbers that are easy to understand? Are the results statistically significant? This means the results are probably not due to chance, but they still might not be important to your own health decisions.

- What are the side effects? Side effects can sometimes be as negative as the condition being treated. The treatment may even cause another health condition to get worse.

- Who paid for the study? Does the funder have a financial interest in the outcome of the research? A nonprofit foundation may fund research because it believes the topic is important, but a company may fund research to develop a product for sale.

- Where did you find the results? News articles alert you to new research results, but further study of the research and discussions with your physician are needed to determine whether the study results will affect your healthcare decisions (Figure 19.10).

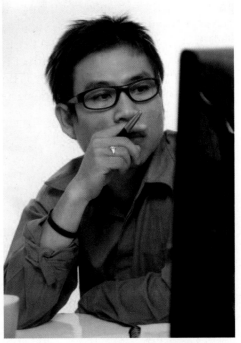

Figure 19.10 Many researchers utilize online databases to find scientific news articles and journals.

While new research results are exciting, always remember that progress in medical research takes many years. The results of a single study must be considered along with the results of similar studies conducted in different locations and over a significant period of time before they can be accepted as general medical practice.

Interpreting Statistical Data

"One in Ten Chance," "40% Improvement," "Very Low Risk," or simply "It Worked for Me!" All of these headlines grab our attention for the purpose of improving our healthcare knowledge or selling us a product. How do you know which claims are true or even what the statistics actually mean?

Health news reports affect how we feel about a product or treatment and influence our healthcare decisions. Therefore, it's important to understand **statistical data** and healthcare **risk assessments** so we can draw valid conclusions about healthcare information (Figure 19.11 on the next page).

Interpreting statistical data begins with understanding percentages. For example, you can convert a proportion into a percentage. If a person has a 1 in 1,000 chance of having an allergic reaction to a medication, this is a 0.1% chance.

statistical data
numerical information gathered through research that is used to draw conclusions about research findings

risk assessments
methods used to calculate and describe a person's chance of becoming ill or dying of a specified condition

Figure 19.11   Understanding healthcare data begins with understanding percentages and types of risk assessment, as shown by these examples.

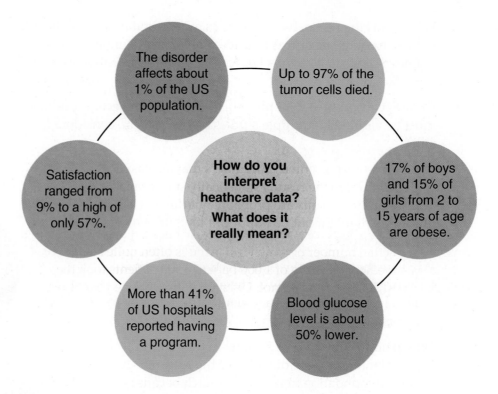

Example: $1 \text{ in } 1{,}000 = \dfrac{1}{1{,}000} = 1 \div 1{,}000 = 0.001$

$0.001 \times 100 \text{ (to convert to percentage)} = 0.1\%$

Conversely, or working from the opposite data format, you can convert a percentage into a proportion. For example, a person has a 10 percent chance of having an allergic reaction to a medication. This is a 10 in 100 chance because percentage is the rate or proportion per 100. If 1,000 people take this drug, how many people do you expect to experience an allergic reaction? Set up a proportion equation to solve this problem:

$$\dfrac{10}{100} = \dfrac{x}{1{,}000}$$

1. Cross multiply to get $100x = 10{,}000$
2. Divide each side by the number in front of x.

    $100x \div 100 = 1x$

    $10{,}000 \div 100 = 100$

3. $x = 100$

You would expect 100 people to experience an allergic reaction.

Risk is the chance that something bad will happen, such as getting a disease or being involved in an accident. However, risk is never 100 percent predictable. We can assess the level of a risk and use that information to make healthcare decisions, but we can never be certain about the outcome.

Mathematicians use the laws of **probability** to assess risk. For example, if you flip a coin using the same motion 1,000 times, how many times do you predict it will land on heads? Because there are two sides to a coin, you would expect heads to appear about half of the time. That does not mean, however, that you will have exactly 500 flips showing heads.

Because there is a 50-50 chance for each coin toss, the results could show heads 200 times, 800 times, or any number of times between 1 and 1,000. Since there are so many possible outcomes, such as 450-550, 512-488, 900-100, and so on, the probability of getting exactly 500 each of both heads and tails is low. Outcomes that are further and further from a 50-50 split become more and more unlikely. Probability tells you how likely or unlikely the chances are that something will or won't occur, but it can never tell you that something *definitely* will or won't occur.

Understanding Risk Assessments. When a magazine reports that a medication causes a 50 percent increase in heart attacks, it sounds alarming. However, the actual number of patients affected is often quite small. For example, in a medication study of 1,000 patients, 500 patients took the medication, and 500 patients did not. Over the course of one year, three patients who took the medication had heart attacks. In the group not taking the medication, two patients had heart attacks. This increase of 1 patient, from 2 to 3, is the 50 percent increase reported by the magazine.

The example above involves comparing risk. Researchers use **relative risk** to compare the risks in two groups of people, or the same group of people over time. Relative risk can be expressed as a ratio, such as the following ratio for heart attack risk in the medication example:

$$RR = \frac{\text{risk to people taking the medication (3)}}{\text{risk to people not taking the medication (2)}} = \frac{3}{2} = 1.5$$

Another way of expressing this ratio is 3:2.

When the relative risk is greater than one (as it is above at 1.5), there is an increase in risk; when it's less than one, there is a reduction in risk. A ratio of exactly 1.0 would mean that there was no increase or decrease—the groups had the same risk.

So how did the magazine arrive at a 50 percent increase? The percentage increase describes the increase in heart attacks for the people taking the medication ($3 - 2 = 1$) divided by the number of heart attacks among the people who did not take the medication (2).

$$\text{Percentage of increased risk} = \frac{1}{2} = .50 \times 100 \text{ (to convert to percentage)} = 50\%$$

Absolute risk, which describes the incidence of a condition in a population, provides a clearer understanding of the difference in risk for the population as a whole. Suppose, for example, that the normal incidence of heart attack in a specific population is 2 heart attacks in 1,000 people. Among people who take the medication, a 50 percent increase is one more person, or 3 heart attacks in 1,000 people. Stated in this way, the additional risk does not seem so alarming.

Absolute risk is the percentage of people affected. As a percentage, the absolute risk of having a heart attack for people who do not take the medication is 2 heart attacks in 1,000 people.

$$AR = \frac{2}{1,000} = .002 \text{ or } 0.2\%$$

relative risk
ratio of the chance of a disease developing among people who are exposed to a specific factor compared with those who are not exposed

absolute risk
ratio of the number of people who have a medical event to those who could have the event because of a medical condition

For the people who took the medication, the risk is 3 heart attacks in 1,000 people.

$$AR = \frac{3}{1,000} = .003 \text{ or } 0.3\%$$

The increased risk is the difference between the two groups.

0.3% − 0.2% = 0.1% increased risk

Understanding health risks means learning to live with uncertainty. By reading the data in Figure 19.12, you can see that smoking increases your risk of dying from lung cancer. However, the risk of lung cancer for nonsmokers is very low, but it is not zero. Some people, who have never smoked, die of lung cancer. Conversely, women with BRCA breast cancer genes have a high risk of developing that disease. But there are also women with those genes who never develop breast cancer.

While you may not have the statistical skills to calculate risk levels, considering the following questions will help you interpret health risk data:

- What is the risk outcome? If the data refers to dying from a disease, then it does not tell you about your risk of having symptoms or developing the disease. Having regular screenings for a disease does not prevent the disease. At best, screening detects a disease in its early stages when it is easier to treat effectively. However, it is also important to remember that screening tests are not 100 percent effective. False negative and false positive results do occur.

- What is the length of time? Data covering a period of 10 years is more meaningful than lifetime risk data. Risk changes over time, often increasing with age. A period of 10 years is long enough for you to make lifestyle and treatment changes to reduce your risk.

- How big is the risk? Look for data expressed in absolute terms, such as "1 out of 1,000 female nonsmokers 45 years of age die of lung disease within 10 years." Comparisons can also be helpful. For example, "A 50-year-old woman who smokes is about 10 times more likely to die from lung cancer than from an accident."

Figure 19.12 Risk of Death from Lung Cancer Among Smoking Women and Nonsmoking Women															
Age	20	25	30	35	40	45	50	55	60	65	70	75	80	85	90
Smoking Women (number of deaths in 1,000 women in next 10 years)	less than 1	less than 1	1	2	4	10	21	36	65	85	124	137	136	103	64
Nonsmoking Women (number of deaths in 1,000 women in next 10 years)	less than 1	less than 1	less than 1	less than 1	less than 1	1	2	3	5	7	10	11	11	8	5

Emotion and Risk Assessment. Emotion plays a role in our healthcare decisions, and it may cloud our judgment about health risks (Figure 19.13). For instance, a recent study looked at a group of women affected by breast cancer who chose to have a double mastectomy to prevent getting cancer in the unaffected breast. Emotion played a role in their decision with varying consequences.

First, consider that risk means living with uncertainty. While removing a healthy breast reduces the risk of developing breast cancer, it does not eliminate the risk. Some breast tissue remains after a mastectomy, and it is still possible to develop cancer in this tissue.

Next, consider the size of the risk. About 30 percent of the women who chose a double mastectomy had a higher risk of **recurrence** (return of the cancer). This was caused by a family history of ovarian cancer, two or more close relatives with breast cancer, or the presence of the BRCA breast cancer genes.

However, the other 70 percent of women who chose a double mastectomy had a very low risk of recurrence of breast cancer—about five or six percent over the next 20 years. A larger percentage of women had a lower risk of recurrence. This means that these women chose a major surgery and risked its complications even though they had a 95 percent chance of the breast cancer never returning.

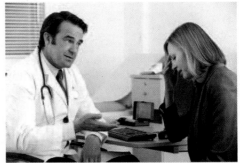

Figure 19.13   Emotions such as fear and anxiety can affect how we evaluate health risks.

When asked about their decision, 90 percent of the women said they were afraid that the cancer would return. They used emotion rather than data to make the decision. If they had considered the question objectively, they probably would not have chosen the surgery. After all, their risk of getting breast cancer a second time was very low to begin with, and removing a healthy breast does not reduce the risk of recurrence in the tissue left from the cancerous breast that was removed.

When emotion clouds our ability to make healthcare decisions, we should consider stepping back and taking some time to look at the risks and benefits. Healthcare professionals suggest that patients think about what they would recommend if they were helping another person make this decision. This technique may help patients weigh benefits and risks more objectively and less emotionally.

Comparing Harms and Benefits. Medical treatments can have **harms** as well as **benefits.** Reducing your risk of illness or death from a disease is a clear benefit. However, inconvenient or even life-threatening risks are also associated with medications and surgical procedures. The value of any treatment is determined by comparing its benefits and risks. Knowing the absolute risk numbers and expressing risks through a **number needed to treat (NNT)** makes your choices clearer.

For example, imagine you are offered a medication that will reduce your risk of experiencing a heart attack. However, you're told that the medication will also increase your risk of developing colon cancer. You read the research and learn that there was a clinical trial involving 200 patients. One hundred patients received the medication, and 100 received a placebo, which is a fake medicine that does not contain any of the medication to prevent heart attacks. People involved in the study did not know whether they were receiving the medication or the placebo. Three heart attacks occurred in the treated group and six in the placebo group.

number needed to treat (NNT)
the number of patients who must be treated to prevent the occurrence of the condition under examination

There were three cases of colon cancer in the treated group and one in the placebo group. The following shows what your evaluation of the benefits and harms of the medication might look like:

Benefits: Using relative risk, you can accurately say that the new drug *reduces* heart attack risk by 50 percent or cuts the risk of heart attack in half:

$$RR = \frac{\text{risk to people taking the medication (3)}}{\text{risk to people not taking the medication (6)}}$$

or $3 \div 6 = 0.50 \times 100$ (to convert to percentage) $= 50\%$

Using absolute risk, the heart attack risk is *reduced* by three percent. The change in absolute risk is the difference between the two groups:

$$\begin{matrix}\text{percentage of heart attacks} \\ \text{in the placebo group}\end{matrix} - \begin{matrix}\text{percentage of heart attacks} \\ \text{in the treated group}\end{matrix}$$

(6 of 100) or 6% – (3 of 100) or 3% = 3%

Harms: Using relative risk, you can accurately say that the risk of developing colon cancer *increased* by 200 percent:

$$RR = \begin{matrix}\text{number of people} \\ \text{developing colon} \\ \text{cancer in the} \\ \text{treated group}\end{matrix} - \begin{matrix}\text{number of people} \\ \text{developing colon} \\ \text{cancer in the} \\ \text{placebo group}\end{matrix} \div \begin{matrix}\text{number of people} \\ \text{developing colon} \\ \text{cancer without} \\ \text{treatment}\end{matrix}$$

$3 - 1 = 2 \div 1 = 2 \times 100$ (to convert to percentage) $= 200\%$

Using absolute risk, you can accurately say the risk of developing colon cancer *increased* by two percent:

$$AR = \begin{matrix}\text{percentage of people developing} \\ \text{cancer in the treated group}\end{matrix} - \begin{matrix}\text{percentage of people developing} \\ \text{cancer in the placebo group}\end{matrix}$$

(3 of 100) or 3% – (1 of 100) or 1% = (2 of 100) or 2%

Note that relative risk makes the benefits or harms look larger and absolute risk makes them look smaller. Understanding how a percentage increase or decrease affects actual numbers is beneficial and, for a true comparison, the benefits and the harms should be expressed in the same terms—relative risk or absolute risk When studies report an increase or decrease of a given percentage, it is generally compared to the original number. Notice how percentage increases or decreases affect the final quantity (Figure 19.14).

Knowing the number needed to treat (NNT) to produce a benefit or the **number needed to harm (NNH)** helps you evaluate risk data. You calculate these numbers by dividing 100 by the absolute reduction or increase in percentage points in risk.

$$\text{NNT or NNH} = \frac{100}{\begin{matrix}\text{absolute reduction or increase} \\ \text{in percentage points of risk}\end{matrix}}$$

Benefit: $NNT = \dfrac{100}{3} = 33.3$

This means that 33 people must be treated with the medication to prevent one heart attack.

Harm: $NNH = \dfrac{100}{2} = 50$

		Figure 19.14 Understanding Percentage Increase and Decrease		
Initial Quantity	**Percentage Increase/Decrease**	**Final Amount Compared to Initial Amount**	**Calculation**	**Final Quantity**
100	10% increase	110%	100% of initial + 10% of increase = 110% of initial	1.10 of the original
100	100% increase	200%	100% of initial + 100% of increase = 200% of initial	double the original
100	500% increase	600%	100% of initial + 500% of increase = 600% of initial	6 times the original
100	40% decrease	60%	100% of initial − 40% of decrease = 60% of initial	0.60 of the original

This means that for every 50 people treated with the medication, you could expect to see one additional case of colon cancer. Therefore, 1 in every 33 people taking this medication will be spared a heart attack, but 1 in every 50 people will get colon cancer.

As you encounter news reports about healthcare research, look for **quantitative data** that can be measured rather than stories about the experiences of people. While personal stories make the material more interesting, they don't help you evaluate research data objectively. The clearest data shows absolute risk in numbers and provides a time frame such as "This medication reduced the risk of heart attack from 6 in 100 to 3 in 100 over 10 years."

Base rates, such as "reduced from 20% to 10% or 0.0002% to 0.0001%," help you see the significance of a change that is given in percentages. Both of these examples show a 50% reduction, but 20% to 10% is a far more significant change.

Media formats that are designed to sell a product typically list its benefits in large print and harms in fine print or quickly read audio. Be aware that many news articles, which have limited space, will omit the **study limitations**. When you read about a 200% reduction in the symptoms of a disorder that affects you personally, remember to read the details. Yes, a 200% reduction is great, but if the study only looked at a small number of people over a short period of time, the chances that the treatment will work for you are far less likely.

RECALL YOUR READING

1. When you analyze research results, consider whether _____ affects your data or _____.
2. Studies in different locations with similar findings and those done over a(n) _____ period of time must be considered before data becomes part of _____ practice.
3. _____ tells you the chance that something is likely or unlikely to occur, but it cannot tell you that something _____ will or won't occur.
4. _____ risk makes benefits or harms of a treatment look smaller, whereas _____ risk makes them look larger.
5. In news reports, _____ stories are not as helpful as _____ data.

Complete the *Map Your Reading* graphic organizer for the section you just read.

SUMMARY

Assess your understanding with chapter tests

- Researchers use scientific communication to fund their research and document the results of research.

- Scientific communication is accurate and valid, informs the reader, and promotes the understanding of scientific concepts.

- Primary sources document original research, while secondary and tertiary sources summarize research and provide overviews of scientific topics.

- Healthcare professionals use research findings to improve diagnoses and treatments for their patients.

- Scientific writing is objective, precise, and clear and includes research papers, proposals, and recommendation reports.

- Patients use personal health records to learn more about their own health status, share information with healthcare providers, and track progress toward personal health goals.

- PHR systems offered by healthcare providers or health insurance plans comply with HIPAA Privacy, Security, and Breach Notification Rules.

- Website addresses that end in .gov, .edu, and .org are a good place to begin narrowing your health science research online.

- Always evaluate health information sources. Your knowledge and understanding of a healthcare topic will only be as good as the information sources you use to learn about it.

- Managing data is a growing task for those in the biotechnology research and development field.

- Bioinformatics combines the fields of biology, computer science, and information technology to develop tools for accessing, analyzing, and securing healthcare data.

- Research bias produces changes in research study results and can affect the study's data and conclusions.

- Progress in medical research takes many years. Each study is considered along with similar studies in different locations and over a significant period of time before findings become part of general medical practice.

- Understanding statistical data and healthcare risk assessments helps you draw valid conclusions about healthcare information.

- Probability tells you the chances that something will or won't occur, but probability can never tell you that something definitely will or won't occur.

- When emotion clouds our ability to make healthcare decisions, we should consider stepping back and looking at the risks and benefits.

- Relative risk makes the benefits or harms of a medication or treatment look larger, and absolute risk makes them look smaller.

- As you encounter news reports about healthcare research, look for quantitative data that can be measured rather than stories about the experiences of people.

MAXIMIZE YOUR PROFESSIONAL VOCABULARY

Build vocabulary with e-flash cards, games, and audio glossary

Listed below are the essential, yellow-highlighted terms and the additional professional vocabulary that you encountered in this chapter. Complete the activities that follow the list to make all of these terms part of your everyday professional vocabulary.

absolute risk	bioinformatics	harms
base rates	biorepositories	Human Genome Project
benefits	clear writing	number needed to harm (NNH)
bias	evidence-based practices	number needed to treat (NNT)

objective writing	quantitative data	risk assessments
personal health record (PHR)	recommendation reports	scientific communication
precise writing	recurrence	secondary source
primary research articles	regimens	statistical data
primary source	relative risk	study limitations
probability	review articles	tertiary source
proposals		

VOCABULARY DEVELOPMENT

Matching. Match the essential terms from this chapter with the best descriptions below by writing the letter of the description next to the number of the essential term on your answer sheet.

1. absolute risk
2. bias
3. bioinformatics
4. number needed to treat (NNT)
5. personal health record (PHR)
6. primary source
7. relative risk
8. risk assessments
9. scientific communication
10. secondary source
11. statistical data
12. tertiary source

a. a scientific discipline that combines the tools and techniques of mathematics, computer science, and biology to understand the biological significance of data

b. a file that contains information about your own health that you keep on a computer for easy reference

c. a document compiled from primary and secondary sources that gives an overview of a specific topic

d. a type of technical communication used by scientists and nonscientists to provide information and promote understanding

e. ratio of the chance of a disease developing among people who are exposed to a specific factor compared with those who are not exposed

f. the number of patients who must be treated to prevent the occurrence of the condition under examination

g. a systematic error that produces a research finding that deviates from a valid finding

h. numerical information gathered through research that is used to draw conclusions about research findings

i. a document that summarizes the results of several studies

j. methods used to calculate and describe a person's chance of becoming ill or dying of a specified condition

k. ratio of the number of people who have a medical event to those who could have the event because of a medical condition

l. a document that describes research in which the authors directly participated

13. **Tag Team Vocabulary.** Review the professional vocabulary list at the end of this chapter. Select any word from the list and give a brief definition and explanation of how that word connects to biotechnology research and development. The connections must be thoughtful to show an understanding of the terms. Each student will make a connection for a different term until there are no more terms left. If someone gets a response incorrect or can't make a connection, other students can offer their own connections.

14. **Fold and Review.** Fold a blank piece of lined paper in half vertically. Select 25 professional vocabulary terms and list them in a column on the front side of the folded page. As you read each term, provide an example of it. If you can't give an example, review the meaning of

the term and write an example on the inside of the folded page. Continue to study until you can provide examples for all of the terms.

REFLECT ON YOUR READING

15. Refer to the thoughts you recorded for the *Connect with Your Reading* activity. Use the Internet to find a health-related news article. Read the article and write a one-paragraph summary. Next, analyze the article more closely. Evaluate the source. Is it primary, secondary, or tertiary? Is it a reliable source? Review data supplied in the article. Is it quantitative or qualitative? Does the data show harms, benefits, and study limitations? How have these strategies helped you avoid the confusion you recorded in the *Connect* activity?

BUILD CORE SKILLS

16. **Reading.** Locate at least five different sources of information about a specific health-related topic. List the titles of these sources and label them as *primary*, *secondary*, or *tertiary*.

17. **Problem Solving.** Identify which section of a primary research article would contain each of the following statements. If needed, review the information on primary research articles in the chapter. Do not use *abstract*, the summary of the article, as a choice.

    - The published data suggests a low rate (3/9,000) of malignancy in United States white female population.
    - Systematic literature review was used as the data source.
    - Only studies reporting on the United States population were included.
    - Further research is needed to include prevalence in additional ethnic populations.
    - The prevalence in the United States white population ranged from 4.7% to 8.2%.
    - To estimate the risk of malignant transformation in the white population.

18. **Reading.** Select a healthcare topic and list a few questions you have about the topic. Locate three research papers written about it. Read the abstract for each paper and explain which paper best fits your topic.

19. **Writing.** Complete a simple science experiment from Science Kids or another website. Write a lab report documenting your findings. Use the principles of good scientific writing as described in this chapter.

20. **Critical Thinking.** Review the lab report you wrote for the experiment you completed in the previous activity. Analyze your research. Do you detect any bias in your methods?

21. **Writing.** Print a paragraph from a primary source document and underline unfamiliar vocabulary terms. Rewrite the paragraph using more familiar terms. Make the paragraph easier to read but retain the document's original meaning.

22. **Problem Solving.** Explain the differences between an electronic health record and a personal health record. List elements that may be found in a PHR. Find out if your healthcare provider has a PHR program you can use.

23. **Critical Thinking.** Using the Internet, find the most outrageous and unbelievable medical claim possible. Share your findings with the class. Discuss why people would believe these claims and even spend money on the products.

24. **Critical Thinking.** Locate an article about bioinformatics or biorepositories. Briefly describe how you believe these concepts will influence healthcare.

25. **Math.** Review the following data. Convert all proportions to percentages and percentages to proportions.

    a. 3 chances out of 50 that a stroke will occur

    b. 15% risk of an allergic reaction among 500 people

    c. 4 occurrences of cancer in 3,000 cases

    d. 7.6% chance that the medication will not be effective in a group of 600 people

26. **Math.** Review the following research results and reorder them from clearest and most useful to least useful for understanding benefit or harm.

    a. Men and women who consumed 15% less fat in their diet were less likely to die of heart attacks in comparison to those who consumed more.

    b. Eight out of ten people who have cancer are below the dietary requirements for daily intake of vitamin D.

c. Elderly people who exercised for at least 30 minutes at least three times a week over the course of five years were 15 times less likely to be diagnosed with depression.

d. Women who are carriers of the arthritis gene were found to have reduced joint range of motion compared to non-carrier women.

e. Eating at least 1 cup of blueberries per week can reduce a woman's risk of heart attack by 25%.

27. **Math.** Based on the results of the following clinical trial, calculate RR, AR, NNT, and NNH for the targeted disease, and RR and AR for kidney stones.

There were 300 participants in a clinical trial performed by a pharmaceutical company testing a preventive medication. The medicine being tested was given to 150 participants and the other 150 were given a placebo. Five people developed the disease in the treated group and 15 people in the placebo group developed the disease. However, 10 people in the group receiving medication developed kidney stones. In the group taking the placebo, three people developed kidney stones.

28. **Critical Thinking.** Which of the following statements represent the objective, clear, and precise style of writing required for scientific communication? Be prepared to explain your responses.

- It is believed that chronic dry eye disease causes dryness and itchy eyes.
- It is possible that doing housework has the same benefits for the heart as aerobic exercise.
- According to data results from the National Institutes of Health, losing 5% of one's body weight can cut one's risk of heart problems and related health problems, such as diabetes, 25% or more.
- Adults with low levels of vitamin D are two times more likely to suffer from heart disease.
- Lower bone density can occur in people who don't like milk.
- People believe that the UV light used to harden gel nail polish poses a cancer risk.

- Pneumonia occurs more often in people with COPD.
- After the first year of quitting smoking, the risk of heart disease drops by 50%.

ACTIVATE YOUR LEARNING

29. Identify two potential field trip opportunities for your health science class or HOSA organization. Both trips are valuable, but you can only be sponsored for one field trip. Using information on recommendation reports and proposals in this chapter, work with a small team of classmates to write a recommendation report identifying one trip as the better option. Include a description of the two field trips, the research your team completed, a cost comparison, your recommendation, and the reasons for your choice. List your names and the date of your report as well as a list of sources you used. Edit each other's writing to make sure it is objective, clear, and precise.

THINK AND ACT LIKE A HEALTHCARE WORKER

30. Shukare works in the neonatal unit of a large hospital. Recently, there have been several cases of early viral respiratory infections in premature newborns. Shukare wants to learn more about the causes of these infections and the long-term effects on her patients. Create some suggestions for Shukare. Explain how to locate reliable information on the Internet and how to evaluate whether information you are reading is valid.

GO TO THE SOURCE

31. The actor Howie Mandel recently revealed that he has a health condition called *atrial fibrillation*. Search the Internet to find the website for *NIH Medline Plus*, the magazine. Locate the article that features Howie Mandel describing his diagnosis. Using your guidelines for Shukare in the previous question, evaluate this source of healthcare information. Explain your findings.

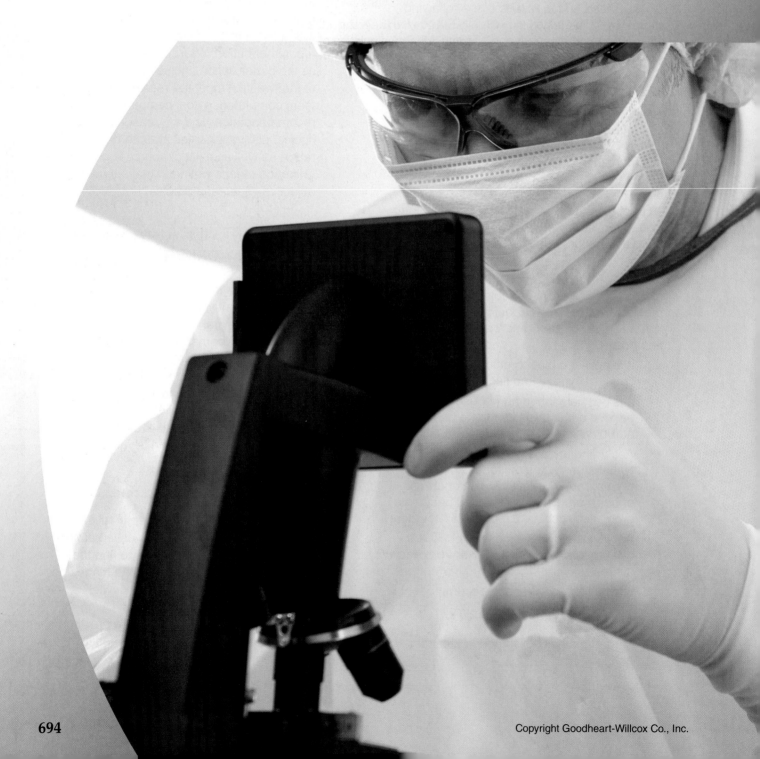

Chapter 20
Professional Knowledge in Biotechnology Research and Development

PROFESSIONAL VOCABULARY

E-flash
Cards

You will need to learn the essential terms listed below before you begin your reading. These terms will help you understand the main concepts of the chapter. These terms, which will be highlighted in yellow within the text, will become part of your professional vocabulary.

In addition to these essential terms, you will see bold terms throughout the chapter. The meanings of these terms are explained where the terms first appear. The bold terms, like the essential terms listed here, will become part of your professional vocabulary and deepen your understanding of the topics presented.

bioethics   the study of ethical practices in medical research and the use of advanced technology to treat patients

Common Rule   a set of regulations adopted in common by a number of federal agencies to ensure the safety of testing on human subjects

gene   term for a combination of DNA found on the 46 chromosomes inside each human cell that determine the unique genetic makeup of an individual and carry the code for building human cells, tissues, and organs

genetic discrimination   the use of genetic information by employers and insurance companies to deny employment or insurance coverage or to treat individuals differently because of a genetic condition

genetic engineering   the deliberate manipulation of genetic materials to eliminate harmful traits or to ensure the presence of desirable traits

genetic test   the examination of a person's cells to analyze his or her genes and identify possible genetic disorders

incident report   a form used to record the details of an unusual event, such as an accident or injury

personalized medicine   term for medical treatments that are tailored to a person's genetic makeup and individual needs

recombinant DNA   genetically engineered DNA that usually includes segments from two or more different genetic sources

reproductive cloning   the creation of exact genetic duplicates

select agent   a highly dangerous and strictly controlled substance that can potentially be used to develop biological or chemical weapons

stem cell   a cell that can duplicate itself many times and has the ability to develop into many different types of cells

CONNECT WITH YOUR READING

Are healthcare workers who have direct contact with patients more important than other healthcare workers?

Kimberley goes to work every day believing this is the day her research could make a difference. She works in a lab that is trying to develop a new way to fight antibiotic-resistant bacteria. Some bacteria have become strong enough that they cannot be killed by the usual antibiotic treatment or even the strongest drugs. These bacteria are causing serious problems for people around the world.

Kimberley is one of many workers in her company doing research at the cellular level to find a solution to this problem. Her approach is to look for a virus that will eat the specific bacterium she is investigating. Finding one won't be the end of the work, of course. She'll also have to make sure that the virus itself won't cause any harm. Then her team will have to determine if this treatment will have any side effects on patients. Finally, they'll have to see if they can mass-produce the virus. But all of that is down the road. Today, Kimberley has to run more tests on the virus with which she's currently working. After she puts on her scrubs, gloves, and goggles and walks into the lab, she thinks to herself, *Who knows? Maybe today is the day we have a breakthrough.*

Kimberley is one of hundreds of thousands of workers in biotechnology research and development. If you've ever taken a medication to treat an illness, you can thank these workers for helping you get better. They have no direct contact with patients, but they are an important part of the healthcare system. How would healthcare be different without biotechnology research and development workers?

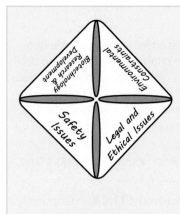

MAP YOUR READING

Can you identify the important role of biotechnology research and development workers in healthcare? Create a visual summary to record your ideas. Begin with a square sheet of paper—an 8½-inch square works well. Fold each of the four points of the square to the center. Label each of the four resulting flaps with one of these topics: *Biotechnology Research and Development*, *Environmental Constraints*, *Legal and Ethical Issues*, and *Safety Issues*. When you finish reading each of these sections in the chapter, open the corresponding flap and draw a picture or symbol to illustrate Kimberley's role in this situation. Ask yourself how biotechnology research and development workers impact the healthcare system, legal and ethical issues, and safety. Finally, write three or four keywords below each drawing that help highlight these important topics.

Biotechnology research and development workers perform lab research to create new equipment and treatments for healthcare. In the process of this research, workers may find themselves in ethical dilemmas. They also have to be aware of the safety measures required for their research. Difficult decisions must be made to balance what is possible with what is appropriate in biotechnology research and development.

In this chapter, you will be introduced to the advances made possible by this pathway, as well as the issues those advances create. These issues include forces outside the healthcare industry that affect biotechnology, the legal and ethical debates that surround various projects, and the constant need for attention to safety for both researchers and subjects.

Systems Theory in Medical Research

Approximately 1.4 million people in the United States currently work in biotechnology. The main focus of biotechnology in healthcare has been to improve human health and increase life span. More than 250 biotechnology healthcare products have been approved by the Food and Drug Administration (FDA) since 1996, including vaccines and synthetic insulin, which were the first to enter the market.

Biotechnology, the manipulation of living cells or organisms to solve problems and create useful products, is drawing attention from many people outside of the healthcare industry. While the study of genetics is more than a century old, recent advances have enhanced our understanding of inherited characteristics and diseases. In 2011, the knowledge gained from the Human Genome Project was applied in reverse, building chemical base pairs into the first synthetic cell that could replicate on its own. While we have solved the puzzle of the human genome, we still don't fully understand the role of each **gene** and all of the variables that affect genes. This will be the focus of research and debate, both within and outside of the medical community, for many years to come.

Genomic research has created ethical, social, and legal issues for society. People need to be educated about these issues so they can deal with the challenges in a responsible way. Ethical, legal, financial, and social implications of this research lead to environmental constraints that

gene
term for a combination of DNA found on the 46 chromosomes inside each human cell that determine the unique genetic makeup of an individual and carry the code for building human cells, tissues, and organs

affect biotechnology research and development. From political influence and legal restrictions to public opinion and funding, there are many outside influences on the current use of and future developments in biotechnology research in the medical field.

The Politics of Medical Research

Medical research has undergone major changes in the past few decades. Since the cloning of Dolly the sheep, the possibilities of what biotechnology *can* do has created fear about what scientists *will* do, if allowed. The power to clone humans and manipulate genetics could be misused or abused. Past history and Hollywood movies have planted images of a "superior race," "designer babies," and cyborgs in our minds. There are also moral objections to tampering with natural selection or the creation of life. Public and political debates around these topics have the ability to affect research, legislation, and funding.

Government regulation, public opinion, and funding all have an impact on the rate of advancement in biotechnology (Figure 20.1). When research is funded by government grants, the process of decision making is slowed by political structures. There is also the potential for bias based on political agendas. For many years, political leaders have attempted to influence biotechnology research and development to please their voters or fit the views of others in their political party. For example, the most recent Bush administration restricted stem cell research, embryo research, and human cloning.

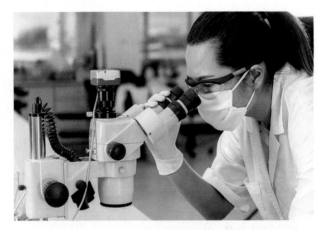

Figure 20.1   **Although lab workers may feel isolated while performing their research, many outside factors can influence their work.**

Government Regulations

Various public policies regulate contentious issues in biotechnology research and development. In addition to President Bush's position against biotechnology research methods in the first decade of the new millennium, strict guidelines have been imposed for product development and human testing. These regulations affect the development, availability, and safety of medications, products, and procedures in the healthcare industry.

Regulation of Human Testing. Beginning with the United Nations' Universal Declaration of Human Rights in 1948, the United States has joined many other countries in signing agreements that govern medical research involving human subjects. This research is required when companies develop potential treatments for an illness like influenza or a medical condition such as obesity. Researchers can only determine the effectiveness and safety of a treatment by testing it on human subjects. Human testing is also needed to determine the nature and severity of any side effects of a treatment. However, the rights of a test subject must come before the interests of the research group.

Since the United Nations declaration, the federal government has tried to ensure the safety and dignity of human subjects during testing.

Common Rule
a set of regulations adopted in common by a number of federal agencies to ensure the safety of testing on human subjects

One way they have done this is by issuing a set of regulations called the **Common Rule**. The name is based on the fact that a number of federal agencies have adopted the same regulations. The regulations apply to all research projects funded by the federal government and, more broadly, to all research that a federal agency has the authority to regulate.

One key protection provided by the Common Rule is that human trials must be reviewed and approved by an ethics panel before the testing can begin. This is to ensure that adequate measures to protect the physical safety, dignity, and privacy of the subjects are in place. In addition, everyone who participates in medical tests must receive information on the nature of the treatment, any risks or discomfort that may be involved, and any available alternatives to the treatment. Voluntary informed consent is required from each participant before testing can begin.

Product Approval. The FDA regulates the production and sale of drugs, vaccines, and other medical products based on effectiveness and safety. While it does not test drugs or medical devices itself, the FDA requires that companies put new treatments through a rigorous approval process before they can be sold. The process of testing and approval for a new drug follows these general steps:

1. Based on laboratory studies or tests using animal subjects, a company decides that a substance could be effective as a treatment (Figure 20.2). The company submits evidence from the studies and an application to the FDA requesting approval to test the substance on human subjects.

2. FDA scientists review the initial application and either order that further testing be put on hold or allow it to continue.

3. If the FDA does not put a hold on tests, the company can begin clinical trials. These are controlled experimental studies in which the medicine being developed is given to a group of people who have the disease or condition the drug is meant to treat. In addition to determining effectiveness, these trials also aim to identify any potential side effects of taking the drug. Clinical trials typically involve three phases, each with increasing numbers of participants. This can take many years to complete. In the final phase, the new drug is tested against any existing treatments for the targeted disease or condition to ensure that it is at least as effective as current medications.

4. If the drug is effective, the company applies to the FDA for its approval, submitting all the data from clinical trials as well as other information that proves the drug's safety and effectiveness.

5. FDA scientists from various disciplines review the clinical trial information and, if they judge the drug to be both effective and safe, recommend its approval.

The government regulates some of the more advanced biotechnical research as well. Federal rules require that any experiment giving altered genes to human subjects receive approval from the National Institutes of Health (NIH) before it can proceed.

The process is rigorous and time-consuming, but it has benefits. In the 1950s, German researchers developed the drug *thalidomide* as a sleeping pill. It was also found to help treat morning sickness in pregnant women. Thalidomide was sold over the counter in Germany and was available by prescription in the United Kingdom. Only after its release did researchers and the rest of the medical community learn that the drug also caused severe birth defects. While several thousand children in Europe were born with these defects, the impact on the United States was limited to those involved in clinical trials. The FDA refused to approve thalidomide for sale in this country because of a lack of research data demonstrating its safety and effectiveness.

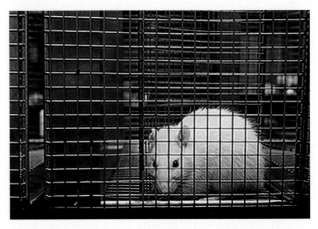

Figure 20.2 Medications are often tested on animals before they are tested on humans. What is the purpose of animal testing?

The US drug approval process worked effectively in the case of thalidomide. It is not foolproof, however. Drugs and medical devices are still sometimes approved for use and later found to cause problems. In an effort to combat these problems, the Kefauver-Harris Amendments of 1962 were passed. These required that drugs be proven both safe and effective for their intended use before they are marketed.

The National Drug Experience Reporting System began collecting data on the adverse, or *negative*, effects of drugs in 1971. The FDA Adverse Event Reporting System (FAERS) is mandatory for drug and biologics manufacturers and distributors. MedWatch also collects voluntary reports of adverse effects from consumers and health professionals.

Because these systems weren't standardized and didn't include complete information, the FDA implemented the Sentinel Initiative in 2008. This system uses electronic healthcare data to actively monitor the safety and effectiveness of drugs and medical devices after they become available to the public. Those that are not safe—or individual lots or production runs that are unsafe for some reason—can be *recalled*, or withdrawn from the market. The FDA cannot order this action, but it does encourage manufacturers to recall products voluntarily. In addition, the FDA publicizes the information when it judges the safety issue to be a major threat to public health.

Public information often pushes the recall process forward. In 1997, the diet drugs used in the combination known as *Fen-phen* were pulled from pharmacy shelves when reports suggested that as many as a third of those using the combination suffered from heart valve complications. The two drugs were approved as safe and effective individually, but the combination enhanced their negative side effects and made them unsafe. In 2010, the manufacturer of infant liquid forms of Tylenol, Motrin, Zyrtec, and Benadryl issued a voluntary recall of 43 products after the FDA cited them for manufacturing problems.

Product Regulation. The FDA also regulates the marketing, labeling, and sale of medical products. Doctors write more than 2.2 billion prescriptions per year in the United States. Physicians are often involved in clinical trials or receive sample medications from drug companies that are marketing or testing new products (Figure 20.3 on the next page). These companies spend an average of $12,000 per doctor per year on marketing, including grant funding, conference attendance, and other gifts. When

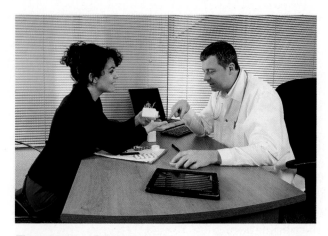

Figure 20.3   Doctors receiving free samples from pharmaceutical companies or being paid by those companies to push certain drugs can cause a conflict of interest.

a doctor may benefit from recommending a particular medication or procedure, this creates a conflict of interest that can put patients' health at risk.

There has been increasing concern that gifts from pharmaceutical companies may inappropriately influence physicians' medication recommendations. The cost of medications has risen faster than all other areas of medical expenditures in federal healthcare programs over the last 15 years. Professional organizations of physicians and drug companies have not been effective in preventing these practices through ethical guidelines. The skyrocketing costs led to fraud investigations and polices issued through the Office of the Inspector General. Government regulation has increased in an attempt to reduce inappropriate influences on doctors by pharmaceutical companies.

Prescription drug labeling is also regulated by the FDA. Package labels and inserts must contain a summary of the safe and effective uses approved for the drug, its dosing instructions, and warnings of any known risks or contraindications. The main purpose of labeling is to give doctors the information they need to prescribe drugs appropriately. This information must be based on data from human clinical trials. The label cannot contain false or misleading promotional information.

Off-label prescribing is the practice of a doctor using a medication in a way that is not specified in the product information. There may be evidence that an off-label drug use is safe and beneficial, but it has not been through rigorous testing. Some drugs are prescribed to take advantage of known side effects, such as drowsiness. They may also be prescribed for an age group that is not listed in the drugs' information. Because prescribing is regulated by the medical industry and not the FDA, off-label prescribing is not illegal, but it may be risky.

There is an increased incidence of negative side effects and dangerous outcomes from off-label prescribing. For example, there is a higher risk of suicide in children who are given psychiatric medications to treat attention deficit disorders. A more rigorous testing process would avoid these risks, but that would also slow the introduction of much-needed new medications. Would you consider taking a drug that was prescribed off-label if there were no other medications available?

Funding Biotechnology Research

Funding affects which biotechnology research projects are completed. Some areas of research are easily paid for by profits from the product that is produced. When an area of research won't produce a product that can be patented or sold, it must be backed by financial support or it will not be completed.

Federal grant money from organizations such as the National Science Foundation and NIH is a common source of funding for biotechnology research and development. Several billion dollars are spent each year on researching cancer, HIV, heart disease, and mental disorders. Funding priorities shift with political agendas and social events, covering broad areas such as health, space, energy, defense, and general scientific understanding.

Some of these topics may sound like they are far removed from biotechnology or healthcare. However, advances in one industry, such as space science, can produce technology that advances the study of another area, such as healthcare. Tools that we use every day in our homes and hospitals, such as the infrared thermometer and water purification systems, were developed through space science research.

Tax credits and cooperative research agreements are another way the government encourages companies to invest in research that will benefit society. Using public dollars for this research can be justified by the benefits provided to society or the public good. Research can focus on health problems that affect large segments of the population, such as cancer or heart disease. The growth of biomedical research also provides a training ground for the next generation of scientists who will continue building on these scientific gains. This gives the United States a competitive edge over global competition in biotechnology.

Funding from private foundations and organizations has also grown in the United States, particularly in the area of pharmaceutical research. A company may choose to invest in research to develop a drug or technology that will be profitable for that company to sell. These are typically products marketed to large numbers of people, such as new treatments for arthritis or high blood pressure. The development of new drugs is risky, costly, and time-consuming (Figure 20.4). It is estimated that the cost to produce a new drug approved by the FDA is between $500 million and $2 billion. Without incentives, private companies are less willing to invest in research to develop treatments for rare diseases. These "orphan drugs," which are used by a very small number of people, would not be profitable.

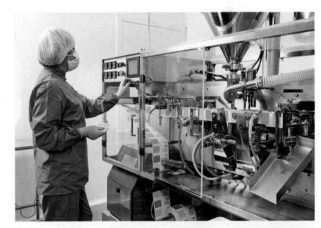

Figure 20.4   The lengthy development and approval process for new drugs can be expensive. How does this relate to funding for biotechnology research?

Some companies would like to patent their genetic research as a way to protect their financial investment. Biological patents that prevent someone else from making or selling the same biological product or gene sequence are being debated in courts around the world. A patent on a naturally occurring breast cancer gene was allowed in Australian courts in 2013 but was not granted in US courts because isolating the gene was not considered inventive or creating something new. If the process is changed in some way to make it more useful, then it might qualify for a 20-year patent in the United States.

Recombinant DNA, synthesized sequencing of DNA, stem cell production lines, and lines of genetically modified organisms (GMOs) for research have all been granted US patents. Specialized techniques for diagnostic testing have also been patented. Each patent carries the potential for huge profits because anyone wanting to conduct research using the patented product or technique must pay the patent holder for the right to do so. Once a patent expires, competitors can develop **generic drugs** or comparable products. Generics are chemically identical to brand-name products and meet the same standards for quality and performance, but they are usually less expensive. Thus, the patent holder has an incentive to charge high prices for the product while it has patent protection. This allows the patent holder to recover research and development costs.

Issues in Biotechnology

Advances in biotechnology also affect the healthcare system regarding throughput. This is done through changes in the methods and outcomes of patient care.

Personalized Medicine. The ability to tailor medications to a person's individual genetic makeup promises better outcomes for patients. However, this **personalized medicine** is not necessarily easy to implement or guaranteed to succeed. Skeptics say that it will cost too much and take too long to collect and process DNA samples from an individual and tailor the treatment to his or her genetic markers. The smaller the number of consumers, the fewer people there are to share the cost of developing the treatment. The expected high cost of new treatments also raises questions about equal access to healthcare (Figure 20.5).

personalized medicine
term for medical treatments that are tailored to a person's genetic makeup and individual needs

Pharmacogenomics is concerned with an individual's response to medications. The drug and dosage can be adjusted for each person to gain the most benefit with the smallest amount of unwanted side effects. We already calculate dosages according to the height, weight, and age of a patient. We can test bacteria to know which antibiotics work best to treat specific types of infection. It is also possible to monitor patient response to and metabolism of a drug and adjust the dosage to his or her individual needs and usage.

The popularity of personal electronics and smartphones has led to the development of many new health-tracking devices that are affecting personalized medicine. There are phone apps that can check your heart rate, monitor your activity level, and track your food intake. This increased involvement with their health can motivate patients to improve their lifestyle and help them communicate more accurately with healthcare workers and practitioners.

Personal monitoring devices, such as an echocardiogram for the heart or real-time blood sugar monitor, are also available as attachments to smartphones. These items can bring lab testing right into the doctor's office, where it can be discussed and acted on without the patient having to come back for another appointment. Patients may even wear the device at home and send the data electronically to their doctors in real time. This means the doctor can monitor patients at home and contact them or send them to the hospital before a small change becomes life threatening.

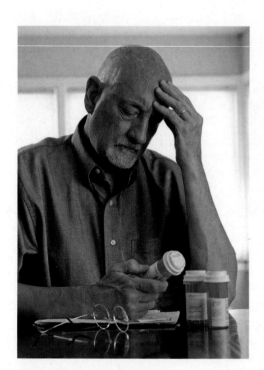

Figure 20.5   The high cost of certain medications can mean that some people do not have access to the healthcare they require.

Nanotechnology. The needs of researchers and physicians have resulted in creative new nanotechnology products that can benefit the field of medicine. This branch of technology uses very small devices to manipulate structures within the body that are smaller than the width of a human hair.

A nano-sized particle can be used to encourage new bone growth after injury or osteoporosis. Nanoparticles provide "stealth technology" by coating chemotherapy medications so these drugs can deliver their treatment before being destroyed by the immune system. Nanosponges can be used to absorb and remove toxins from the blood. Nanosensors injected under the skin can measure the levels of various chemicals in the blood. Many nanotechnology products are awaiting FDA approval and more ideas, such as nanorobots, are in the planning stages. What would you design a nanoparticle or nanorobot to do?

The potential hazards of nanoparticles are unknown. Very small particles interact differently with cells than larger particles that can't fit through a cell membrane. It is possible that nanoparticles may result in toxicity at lower levels. Because of their small size, harmful nanoparticles may be infused into the body without the victim being aware of it. The possibilities for bioterrorism are endless.

Fighting Bacterial Resistance. As you read in chapter 12, the increased use of antibiotics has led to the growing problem of drug-resistant bacteria. These are strains of a treatable bacterium that have developed the ability to resist normal antibiotic treatment. Some strains have even developed resistance to multiple drugs or to the most powerful antibiotics used for a particular infection. For instance, vancomycin is the most potent antibiotic used against the most severe cases of intestinal infections, such as *Enterococcus* bacterium. This drug is no longer effective in more than 20 percent of patients with those infections (Figure 20.6).

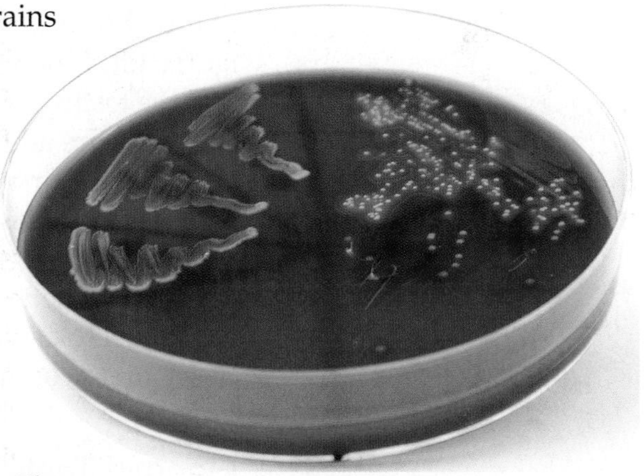

Biotechnology may offer solutions to the problem of bacterial resistance. Researchers are pursuing several different approaches, including the following:

Figure 20.6   *Enterococcus* is just one type of bacterium that has become drug-resistant. What other drug-resistant bacteria have you heard about in the news?

- **Bacterial interference.** In this method, an individual is injected with non-infecting bacteria. These beneficial bacteria attach to the walls of body cells, preventing the infecting bacteria from doing so. As a result, the infecting bacteria cannot find sources of food. They may also be attacked by the body's immune system.

- **Bacteria-killing viruses.** This approach is actually a return to a technique commonly used from the 1920s through the 1940s, before the widespread use of antibiotics. It relies on injecting an infected individual with *bacteriophages*, which are viruses that kill bacteria. The traditional technique can be improved if the genetic material of the bacteriophage can be changed to target specific bacteria.

- **Manipulation of bacterial genes.** Some approaches rely on altering the genetic makeup of bacteria to make them more vulnerable. One possibility is to change a bacterium's genetic makeup to provoke the body's immune system to attack it. Another is to find ways of stopping the bacterium's ability to reproduce itself.

Complete the
Map Your Reading
graphic organizer for the
section you just read.

RECALL YOUR READING

1. Outside influences in biotechnology include _____ influence and _____ restrictions.
2. The _____ regulates drugs, vaccines, and other medical products based on _____ and _____.
3. While much of the funding for research comes from government sources, funding from _____ foundations and organizations has grown, especially in _____ research.
4. The tailoring of medications to individuals based on their _____ makeup is called _____ medicine.
5. _____ uses very small devices to _____ structures within the body.

Legal and Ethical Issues in Biotechnology

In the last few decades, the huge advances scientists have made through biotechnology research and development and the possibilities of future discoveries have raised many ethical issues. These issues focus on the kinds of research being done, the application of research results, and the testing of potential treatments based on research. These serious questions are addressed within the field of **bioethics**.

Since the first in vitro fertilization (IVF) resulting in a "test tube baby" in 1978, the idea of tampering with the creation of life has been controversial (Figure 20.7). More recently, debates have centered on issues related to genetics and cloning. A fuller understanding of human genetics has made it possible to manipulate genes and create new cells. These possibilities continue to raise new legal and ethical concerns.

bioethics
the study of ethical practices in medical research and the use of advanced technology to treat patients

Genetic Testing

Better understanding of the human genome has added to the existing body of knowledge about the genetic causes of certain diseases and conditions. Researchers have identified several thousand **genetic disorders**—diseases or conditions that result from damaged, incorrectly located, or abnormal genes. Researchers believe that as many as 1 in 10 adults have some kind of genetic defect. Genetic disorders are thought to cause half of all miscarriages and nearly a third of all infant mortality cases.

Several serious diseases and conditions can be identified through **genetic tests**. These tests are done by taking a small number of cells from a person's body to analyze his or her genetic makeup. Fetal genetic testing can be used to identify a few dozen diseases or disorders, including cystic fibrosis, Tay-Sachs disease, and sickle-cell anemia. Adults can be tested for hundreds of different conditions. Tests can determine whether someone is genetically at risk for developing some cancers or Alzheimer's disease. Adults can also be tested to determine if they carry a genetic disorder that can be passed on to their children.

genetic test
the examination of a person's cells to analyze his or her genes and identify possible genetic disorders

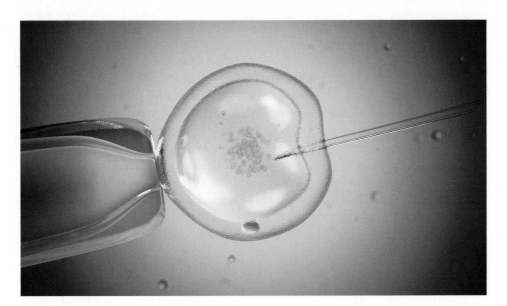

Figure 20.7   The first in vitro fertilization, which was done in 1978, was just the beginning of ethical concerns related to biotechnology.

These tests can provide people with important information. Knowledge that you may pass on a genetic disorder can be useful when making decisions about whether or not to have children. Adults with a genetic tendency for Alzheimer's disease or other conditions can try to alter their lifestyle to reduce the likelihood that they will develop the disease. In some cases, they can begin treatment that reduces their risk of developing the disease or condition.

Genetic testing also raises concerns about how people use the results. Who should have access to genetic testing? Who should have access to the results? How should this information be used? If expectant parents learn that their unborn child has a genetic disorder or isn't the desired gender, should they be able to terminate the pregnancy based on that information? Can a child be forced to undergo genetic testing or have his or her genetic material used for the benefit of a sibling? If an employer pays for the insurance that covers genetic testing, should he or she have access to those test results? Should society or the courts be concerned that intolerance of differences may grow as a result of access to genetic testing?

Genetic Discrimination

Genetic discrimination is the use of genetic information to treat individuals with certain genetic conditions differently. As genetic testing has become more common, people have reported many cases of such treatment. Some workers lost their jobs even though there had never been any complaints about their job performance. Others were denied health insurance because they had a genetic disorder, sometimes before they even showed symptoms of the disease.

These situations led to a public demand for protection. Some states enacted laws to prevent genetic discrimination. The effort was boosted in 2008, when Congress passed the Genetic Information Nondiscrimination Act (GINA). That law banned health insurers from making decisions regarding enrollment, extent of coverage, or premium amounts based on genetic information. It also banned employers with more than

genetic discrimination
the use of genetic information by employers and insurance companies to deny employment or insurance coverage or to treat individuals differently because of a genetic condition

15 employees from basing decisions regarding hiring, firing, promotion, pay, or job tasks on genetic information. GINA also prohibits employers from requiring genetic testing as a condition of employment and from requesting the results of genetic tests taken by employees.

People's legal rights regarding insurance were aided further by passage of the Affordable Care Act (ACA) in 2009. By requiring insurers to issue insurance to all applicants, the ACA guarantees health insurance for people with a genetic condition. This includes people identified through genetic testing to have a predisposition, or *likelihood*, to develop a genetic condition. The ACA also prevents health insurers from increasing premiums paid by those individuals.

Genetic Engineering

genetic engineering
the deliberate manipulation of genetic materials to eliminate harmful traits or to ensure the presence of desirable traits

recombinant DNA
genetically engineered DNA that usually includes segments from two or more different genetic sources

Increased knowledge of human genetics has also led to ethical concerns about **genetic engineering**. This term refers to rearranging genetic materials with the goal of removing harmful traits or inserting desirable ones. This is usually done using **recombinant DNA**. Technicians duplicate and extract DNA from one or more desired genes, then recombine and insert it into a cell whose original DNA has been removed. The cell then follows the instructions of the new DNA.

Genetic engineering is widely used in agriculture to produce strains of crops such as corn, tomatoes, and soybeans that are more resistant to disease or insects (Figure 20.8). In healthcare, the major controversy over genetic engineering concerns modifying human genes. For instance, researchers have tried to introduce human genetic material into pigs so that the modified animals can be used to provide organs such as hearts and kidneys that are in short supply for human transplants. Athletes have used gene doping to increase the amount of hormones and protein that their cells make. Three-parent IVF procedures take the DNA from a mother and father, and then implant them into a healthy cell from a surrogate. This procedure is still experimental in the United States, but it may allow us to treat life-threatening illnesses, such as muscular dystrophy, in the womb while the body is still developing.

Not everyone is in favor of genetic modifications. Modern science often conflicts with traditional values. Some people object on the grounds that combining human and animal genes is immoral. Others worry that the introduction of animal genes into the human population could lead to the spread of animal diseases with devastating results. With the health problems shown in clones, researchers worry that children born through three-parent IVF will not have normal or healthy life spans. Others worry about the ethics of using human trials to determine the safety and effectiveness of therapies.

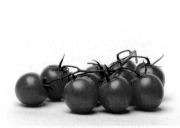

Figure 20.8   Genetic engineering has already been used in the world of agriculture. What are the main concerns of those who are opposed to genetically modified organisms, or *GMOs*?

Another set of questions revolving around genetic engineering focuses on the possibility of creating individual or large numbers of "superhumans" who have physical abilities or intelligence beyond that of most people. Will couples be able to order "designer babies" with the qualities they most desire in offspring by calling on scientists to manipulate the genes in a fetus? Some groups have raised serious objections to such activities.

There is also concern about the possibility of governments using genetic engineering in ways that harm specific populations. **Eugenics**, or the attempt to promote desirable genetic characteristics, arose in the late 19th century and gained considerable influence in the early 20th century. Eugenicists typically aimed to promote the reproduction of their own ethnic group or race and suppress others. In the United States, the eugenics movement led several states to pass laws in the early 1900s that mandated sterilization of the mentally ill. As a result, several thousand people were sterilized. These laws became models for Nazi Germany, which sterilized 300,000 to 400,000 people who were classified as mentally ill. The possibility of some future government using genetic engineering to promote racist ideology worries many people.

Reproductive Cloning

Cloning creates identical cells and is a common tool for creating the material used in biotechnical testing. **Reproductive cloning** creates exact genetic copies of a human or an animal. This process typically involves transferring the nucleus of a somatic cell into an oocyte (egg cell, or *ova*) whose nucleus has been removed. Reproductive cloning became news in 1997, when Scottish scientists announced that they had produced a cloned sheep, which they named Dolly (Figure 20.9). This marked the first time an animal as complex as a mammal had been cloned from adult cells.

reproductive cloning
the creation of exact genetic duplicates

The announcement about Dolly prompted questions about whether human cloning was possible or ethical. These questions have become more critical considering the high failure rate and shortened life span of cloned animals. In cloning experiments conducted since Dolly's birth, only about one or two out of a hundred attempts are successful. In addition, nearly a third of the animals that are born suffer from rare but serious conditions. Many do not live very long.

The possibility of putting a human life at such risk is considered immoral by many people. Both the American Medical Association and the American Association for the Advancement of Science have urged a ban on human cloning. Congress has debated such legislation but has not yet passed a federal law controlling this practice. Regulation of cloning has been left to individual states, and the laws differ in terms of what types of cloning are allowed and for what purposes. Public opinion is solidly against human reproductive cloning.

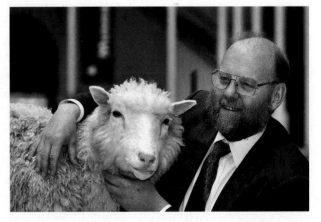

Figure 20.9   Dolly the sheep is widely known as the first successful attempt at cloning a mammal.

Stem Cell Research

One promising area of biotechnology is the use of stem cells as the basis for medical treatments (Figure 20.10 on the next page). **Stem cells** can duplicate themselves many times and develop into many different types of cells. All of the organs and tissues in your body develop from

stem cell
a cell that can duplicate itself many times and has the ability to develop into many different types of cells

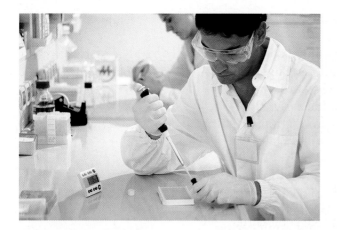

Figure 20.10 Stem cell research is done in the hopes of developing new, more effective medical treatments. What specific types of treatment could stem cells be used for?

stem cells. Stem cells also reproduce themselves to repair tissues that have been damaged. Healthy stem cells may be used to generate new tissues, such as skin, for transplant. They may restore tissues, as in bone marrow transplants. Scientists hope to use these cells' capabilities to develop cellular-level treatments for a variety of diseases and conditions, such as diabetes, heart disease, or degenerative nerve conditions. This kind of treatment is called **regenerative therapy**.

Scientists distinguish between stem cells taken from embryos (the early stages of development after a human egg has been fertilized) and those taken from adults. Embryonic stem cells have great potential for use in regenerative therapy because of their ability to reproduce so many times and because they are *unspecialized*. This means they can develop into many different kinds of cells and tissues, from blood to skin to heart cells. Because of this ability, embryonic stem cells are called **pluripotent**, meaning they have the potential to take many forms.

Adult stem cells generally make cells of the same type as the tissue from which they come. For example, blood stem cells develop into red blood cells, various types of white blood cells, or other immune system cells. In 2007, however, scientists developed *induced pluripotent stem cells* (iPSCs). These are adult stem cells that have been altered so they have the flexibility of embryonic stem cells.

The use of embryonic stem cells for research generated considerable ethical debate beginning in 1998, when the identification of human embryonic stem cells was first announced. These cells are obtained from the blastocyst stage on the fourteenth day of an embryo's development. The process destroys the embryo before it has developed a nervous system or is ready to implant in the uterus. Those who believe that life begins at the moment of conception view this procedure as murder. Many people also object to the creation of embryos specifically for the purpose of harvesting stem cells. Others warn that there is also a potential for abuse of women's rights in the harvesting of large numbers of egg cells to be fertilized for this use.

One stem cell line commonly used for medical research was obtained unknowingly from the cancerous cervix of Henrietta Lacks in 1951. Researchers discovered that her cells could be kept alive and wanted to study them further. The cells, cultured as the *HeLa* cell line, have been used around the world for medical and biological research, including the development of the first polio vaccine and the first successful cloning of a human cell. However, permission to harvest or use the cells was never obtained. In 1990, the courts ruled that discarded cells and tissues are not a person's property and can be used for commercial purposes. Legal cases such as this point to the need for balancing commercial, academic, and ethical interests when patenting new cell lines.

In 1994, President Bill Clinton ordered that no federal money could be used for research on embryos created specifically for that purpose. This did not ban privately funded stem cell research or the use of embryos left over from in vitro fertilization, abortion, or other procedures. In 2001,

President George W. Bush issued a partial ban on federal funding of stem cell research using new embryonic stem cell lines. This limited the number of cell lines available for research. This ban was lifted in 2009 by President Barack Obama. The FDA still has the power to regulate cloning for research.

Research using adult stem cells and iPSCs is less controversial. It is also less certain that these stem cells can produce as many therapies, or therapies that are as potent, as those based on embryonic stem cells. Adult stem cells are also more difficult to obtain, and a method for reproducing masses of them—which would be needed to use them in therapy—has not yet been developed.

In one respect, however, adult stem cells may be more promising than embryonic stem cells. An adult's immune system may be less likely to reject stem cells taken from that person's body, modified to produce a desired treatment, and then placed back in the body. However, this has not been proven. As with much stem cell research, huge amounts of work still need to be done before effective treatments are developed.

Equity and Diversity in Medical Research

Before the 1980s, medical research that made it to human testing was primarily conducted on white males in their mid-thirties. It was assumed that medications and treatments that worked for them would work for other populations as well. That assumption is no longer accepted.

One reason for this change was pressure placed on the industry and the government by advocacy groups and health activists. These groups complained that the health of women and members of racial and ethnic minorities was being ignored (Figure 20.11). The need to change was supported by the fact that, as researchers finally included these groups in studies, findings among populations actually differed. Results from studying white males in their mid-thirties could not be assumed to apply to women, African-Americans, Hispanics, Asian Americans, Native Americans, children, or the elderly.

Many drugs achieve different levels in the blood and different levels of effectiveness depending on factors such as body mass, which reproductive hormones are present, the ratio of muscle to body fat, and which other disease processes or medications are present. Women tend to weigh less than men, have a higher percentage of body fat, and process medicines differently. Clinical trial volunteers often don't represent the whole population. Researchers even discovered that men and women reported different symptoms for the same disease or condition. Only personalized medicine will truly adjust medication dosages to each individual's needs, but campaigns such as "I'm In" have attempted to raise awareness among minority populations about the importance of diverse participation in clinical research.

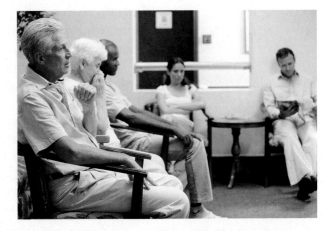

Figure 20.11   In recent years, clinical trials and studies have used more diverse subjects. What type of subject was used before the 1980s? What is the reason for the change?

Test Reliability and Validity

Questions still remain about the reliability and validity of biotechnology research. Several studies have shown that when private companies conduct clinical trials, the results are more likely to be positive than when nonprofit groups do the research. When biotechnology firms are responsible for testing and reporting to the FDA on the effectiveness of their own products, this creates a conflict of interest.

Test protocols describe how a test is done so that the results can be replicated. The design of the test must measure what it says it is measuring and interpret the information correctly to produce valid results. A test that can be repeated and produce the same results is reliable. A genetic test or medication trial that can be demonstrated to produce the same results on many different occasions means that the test results can be trusted.

An alarming number of physicians and researchers have been charged with fraud and misconduct in conducting and reporting biotechnology research and development results. Reports from the Government Accounting Office on these matters include participants being given unapproved medications, reports being falsified for tests that were not conducted, and failure to report serious adverse reactions. Research results may be falsified to gain more funding, to gain tenure within a research team, or for a variety of other reasons.

The Office of Research Integrity (ORI) at the US Public Health Service (PHS) has a legal duty to investigate research misconduct. Since 1992, at least 90 findings of research misconduct have been reported. The incidents have involved falsified data, false background information, and plagiarism.

Researchers use scientific journals to study medical research and build on their knowledge base. Researchers may repeat a study to show reliability. They may change a factor to test a similar theory. Each addition of research results helps to build a knowledge base that leads to further innovation. When the knowledge base is flawed and studies are based on invalid test results, more invalid science is produced.

Complete the *Map Your Reading* graphic organizer for the section you just read.

RECALL YOUR READING

1. Unfair treatment of individuals based on their genetic makeup, called _____, has been banned by the _____ Information _____ Act.

2. Genetic _____ has been used to modify agricultural crops, but concerns still exist about its use on humans.

3. _____ stem cells generally have greater potential than adult stem cells because they are _____.

4. Clinical trials have become more diverse in recent years because _____ and _____ work differently on different populations.

5. It is important for test results to be both _____ and _____ because diagnoses, treatments, and future research are based on these results.

Health and Safety Issues in the Research Environment

As you read earlier, government regulations aim to ensure that the research methods and products developed through biotechnology are safe and effective. The federal government has also established various rules to protect the safety of the research workplace, shipment of biological materials, and disposal of waste products.

Lab Safety

The Office of Biotechnology Activities (OBA) of the NIH has several duties regarding the study of DNA and genetic manipulation. Among them is the responsibility to ensure that such research is conducted safely (Figure 20.12). The OBA oversees a complex set of regulations that describe specific rules for handling cells and genetic material based on their belonging to one of four risk groups. Each risk group is determined by its potential harm to humans and can be described as the following:

- agents not related to any disease in healthy adult humans
- agents linked to rare human diseases for which there are treatments
- agents that cause severe or fatal diseases for which there are treatments
- agents that cause severe or fatal diseases for which there are no treatments

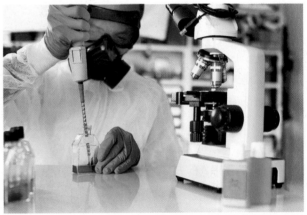

In addition, any institution conducting recombinant DNA research is required to have a special committee to oversee that work and ensure its safety. Another requirement states that lab workers must be trained in safety procedures and the use of safety equipment. Any lab worker handling blood must follow the Occupational Safety and Health Administration's (OSHA) bloodborne pathogen standards. These were discussed in chapter 12. Labs that work with plants and animals must have special safety precautions for the care and handling of them.

Facilities should also have an exposure control plan. This plan spells out the steps to be taken in a situation that poses a hazard to workers or the public at large, such as a major chemical spill.

As an extra precaution, some institutions follow medical surveillance procedures. These apply to anyone who works with hazardous substances. The procedures include taking baseline measures of workers' health statuses through blood tests and tissue samples. This is to allow for later identification of any changes, should infection or exposure to hazardous materials be suspected.

Basic Precautions. Certain precautions are common sense. Lab workers should walk and never run in a lab area. Walking prevents accidental

Figure 20.12   Research that deals with DNA and genes is subject to very strict rules and regulations, mostly for the sake of safety. What are the four risk groups for genetic material?

falls or collisions. Following established traffic patterns also prevents accidents. Workers should always walk on the right side of the hallway and use the door on the right-hand side when there is a set of double doors. Above all, lab workers need to be alert and careful. They should move through the lab and hallways with their head up and eyes focused on what's around them. They should hold anything they carry securely. Finally, lab workers need to take their setting and its potential hazards seriously. Horseplay and practical jokes have no place in a lab setting.

Personal Protective Equipment (PPE). As with medical laboratories, people working in biotechnology labs have to wear personal protective equipment (PPE). Basic PPE includes a laboratory coat or scrubs, gloves, and goggles (Figure 20.13). If the experiment increases the risk of sprays or splashes of infectious material, lab workers need to wear goggles with side shields or a face mask. If there is a danger of inhaling substances that could be harmful, researchers should wear a respirator that will filter the air they breathe. They should also change gloves often, especially when there is a possibility of contamination. Workers using acids or other hazardous materials may need to wear a rubber apron as well.

In some situations, such as labs developing nanotechnology and research that involves animals, the lab environment must be protected from contamination by the workers. In these situations, PPE is worn to prevent contamination of the sterile field.

An even greater concern is the risk of bringing hazardous substances from the lab setting out into public areas. Biotechnology research labs that work with highly infectious organisms, such as Ebola and anthrax, must use the proper protections to prevent contamination or unintended transfer of these organisms. PPE and safety procedures are established by OSHA to provide these proper protections.

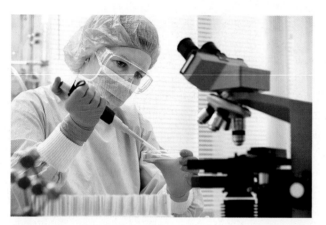

Figure 20.13   Basic PPE includes a laboratory coat or scrubs, gloves, and goggles. Why is PPE important in a laboratory setting?

Lab workers must always put on PPE before beginning work. Street clothes are not acceptable in a biotechnology lab. When they are ready to leave the lab, researchers should remove PPE, dispose of it properly, and wash their hands. They should never touch a mucous membrane, such as inside the mouth, or insert or remove contact lenses while in the lab. Mucous membranes are a portal of entry for infectious materials. Lab workers must also avoid bringing food, drink, or cosmetics into the lab or using them there. The same standard precautions and transmission-based precautions used for patient care apply to the organisms and tissue samples in a research lab.

Safety Equipment. The OBA guidelines establish procedures for ensuring that the material being worked on is contained, whether that is bacteria, or cells or DNA from plants, animals, or humans. Researchers must follow one of four safety levels, depending on the risk group of the material with which they are working. Those safety levels may include specific laboratory installations, the use of certain kinds of equipment, and strict adherence to certain procedures.

Some types of lab work can be done with chemical fume hoods, which protect the worker from hazards but protect neither the material being worked with nor the environment from contamination. Other experiments must take place in **biological safety cabinets (BSCs)**, which filter and control airflow to prevent chemical and biological material from being released into the air (Figure 20.14). Even more complex equipment and safety procedures are required during recombinant DNA research.

Regulations also try to ensure that the equipment being used is functioning properly. BSCs have to be inspected and certified at least annually and at certain other times as well. For instance, they must be inspected any time they are moved or any time a risk assessment suggests a potential problem. BSCs have alarms that sound when contamination occurs. At that point, workers should immediately stop using the equipment and take steps to address the situation.

Cleanliness Procedures. Work areas in a biotechnology lab must be kept neat and clean. This prevents contamination of the materials being studied and used, which could ruin the experiment. It also prevents contamination of the worker and others by those materials, which can introduce hazards.

When working, lab technicians are urged to keep clean and dirty materials and equipment strictly separated. In this case, *dirty* means potentially hazardous or contaminated. One way to achieve this separation is to have a pan ready in which to put used items. Workers should follow the principle of "clean to dirty," which means starting in a clean area with clean materials and equipment and only moving toward dirty surfaces, never bringing contaminants back into the clean area. Of course, workers then need to change equipment or gloves before going back to clean materials.

Specific disinfectants need to be used on specific microorganisms to ensure that surfaces and equipment are properly cleaned. For instance, a 4- to 8-percent solution of formaldehyde is useful for cleaning vegetative bacteria and lipo viruses but not bacterial spores. For spores, a lab worker could use formaldehyde gas.

Working with Sharps and Chemicals. As with medical offices, biotechnology labs have to follow proper procedures for using and disposing of sharps, such as needles, scalpels, and other tools that can puncture or cut. Chapter 12 includes a more detailed discussion of sharps use and disposal. Some labs urge workers to use plastic rather than glass equipment to reduce the potential for broken glass.

It is important to use the correct solutions when working with chemicals. Lab workers should read the label three times: when gathering materials, before using them, and after using them (Figure 20.15). Never use solutions stored in unlabeled bottles. Don't mix solutions from different containers

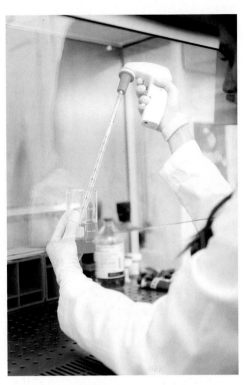

Figure 20.14   Some experiments require the use of a biological safety cabinet. What does the safety cabinet do?

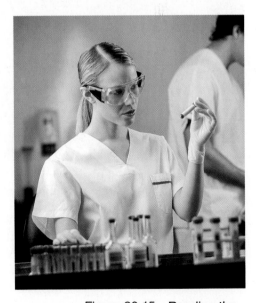

Figure 20.15   Reading the label on a chemical you are using ensures that you are choosing the correct substance. When should you read a chemical's label?

unless directed to do so by a supervisor. If an error is made, report it immediately so it can be corrected.

Some chemicals and biohazardous materials require special treatment. Any hazardous materials in the lab must have a materials safety data sheet (MSDS), as discussed in chapter 12. That sheet specifies the potential hazards and required safety precautions for the substance.

Responding to Lab Emergencies. If chemicals, hazardous materials, blood, or body fluids come in contact with a worker's skin, eyes, or a mucous membrane, the area must be flushed with water. Eyewash stations provide a stream of water to rinse the eye. The worker should never rub the affected eye because this can lead to serious complications. Some labs recommend washing the eye for as long as 15 minutes, depending on what substance entered it.

Simulate
EHR

incident report
a form used to record the details of an unusual event, such as an accident or injury

Any accident, cut, spill, malfunctioning equipment, or other problem must be reported to a supervisor. That person will ensure that an **incident report** is filled out. Careful records of all accidents must be maintained in case problems arise. After an incident, the follow-up will include an evaluation of why it happened and how to avoid similar incidents in the future. Spills or accidents that result in exposure or potential for exposure must be reported to the OBA within 30 days of the event.

If you experience a needlestick or exposure to a hazardous material in the lab, you may be asked to undergo a blood test to determine if the exposure caused any disease. If a glass container breaks, you should never pick it up with your hands. Using tongs, forceps, or a dustpan and brush is much safer.

When a spill occurs, you should notify any workers nearby so they will be alert to the possible danger. If the spill is large enough and outside a containment cabinet, all personnel should leave the room in which it occurred before the cleaning crew begins the cleanup. If the contamination is airborne, you may have to wait for a certain period of time before reentering the room and cleaning it. If the spill is small enough for you to clean up yourself, do so, then disinfect anything that requires it and dispose of or clean the contaminated material (Figure 20.16).

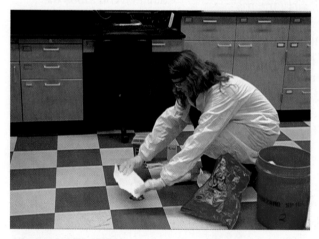

Figure 20.16   Spills in the lab must be handled and reported properly. What should you do if a spill occurs in the lab?

Bioterrorism

In the 1800s and 1900s, several governments worked to develop chemical and biological weapons. Some chemical weapons were used in World War I by both sides and in World War II by Germany (Figure 20.17). Many of these weapons were stockpiled for later use. In 1972, countries around the world agreed to ban biological weapons. Twenty years later, a United Nations conference resulted in an international agreement to ban chemical weapons. Dozens of countries have agreed to both bans.

Despite such agreements, these deadly weapons remain a threat. The possibility that terrorist groups might employ such weapons remains a serious security concern. While no attacks resulting in massive deaths have occurred, a Japanese religious sect called *AUM Shinrikyo* did release nerve gas in the Tokyo subway in 1995. That attack killed 13 people and injured thousands. Government intelligence agencies believe that other terrorist groups have sought and may still be seeking the ability to develop and deliver such weapons.

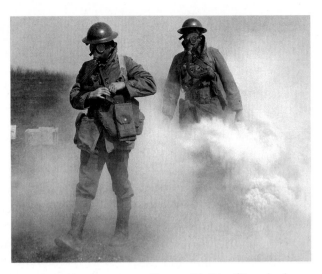

Figure 20.17   Chemical warfare was frequently used in World War I and World War II.

Security concerns were heightened in the United States when, in the weeks after the September 11, 2001 terrorist attacks on New York City and Washington, D.C., an anthrax attack killed five people. These attacks delivered anthrax spores through the mail in an envelope. The spores were released into the air when the envelope was opened, and the victims inhaled spores into their lungs.

The federal government has identified some 30 substances as **select agents**, which are highly dangerous because they can be used to develop biological or chemical weapons. These agents include the Ebola and Marburg viruses, which cause deadly diseases; *Botulinim* toxins, which are also potentially fatal; ricin, which can make a highly deadly gas; and *Yersinia pestis*, the bacterium that causes what was known in the Middle Ages as the *Black Plague*. These materials are strictly regulated by the federal government, and any lab working with them must register first and receive approval. By carefully controlling the use of these substances, the government hopes to limit the possibility of accidental release or a deliberate terrorist attack.

select agent
a highly dangerous and strictly controlled substance that can potentially be used to develop biological or chemical weapons

RECALL YOUR READING

1. The Office of _____ describes specific rules for labs engaging in the study of _____ and _____ manipulation.

2. Certain experiments require the use of a _____, which controls airflow to prevent the release of biological or chemical material.

3. If an accident occurs in the lab, a detailed written document called a(n) _____ must be completed.

4. Substances known as _____ can be used to develop biological or chemical weapons.

Complete the *Map Your Reading* graphic organizer for the section you just read.

SUMMARY

 Assess your understanding
with chapter tests

- Biotechnology refers to the manipulation of cells or chemical or structural components of cells to develop new products or new medical treatments.

- The federal government has strict rules on research involving human subjects, which include the review of plans for such research and informed consent from study participants.

- The Food and Drug Administration ensures the safety and effectiveness of medicines and medical devices by reviewing test results submitted by manufacturers and approving the products for sale and use.

- Funding of biotechnology research may come from government grants, private grants, tax credits, or the profitable sale of biotechnology products.

- Some scientists think advances in biotechnology promise personalized medicine, but skeptics think that this will be difficult to achieve and may result in costly products.

- Genetic testing can identify the presence of or predisposition toward genetic disorders that may cause illness or health conditions.

- Genetic discrimination is the unfair treatment of individuals based on their genetic makeup, such as firing or not hiring individuals with genetic disorders and insurance companies denying coverage to such individuals.

- Genetic engineering raises concerns about potential use by parents to select only certain characteristics in offspring or by governments to discriminate against minority groups.

- Stem cell research may provide ways to repair tissue or replace dead or missing tissue with new cells grown from stem cells.

- Medicines and procedures need to be tested on different ethnicities, genders, ages, and body sizes, each of which may experience different results and side effects.

- Test results need to be confirmed with further testing to be sure they are reliable and valid.

- The Office of Biotechnology Activities of the National Institutes of Health oversees the safety of research involving DNA and genetic manipulation. Research organizations must strictly follow NIH rules during research in these areas.

- Lab safety includes basic precautions, the wearing of personal protective equipment, the use of specialized safety equipment, cleanliness procedures, and working carefully with sharps and chemicals.

- The federal government tries to prevent bioterrorism by carefully controlling access to and use of select agents.

MAXIMIZE YOUR PROFESSIONAL VOCABULARY

 Build vocabulary with
e-flash cards, games,
and audio glossary

Listed below are the essential, yellow-highlighted terms and the additional professional vocabulary that you encountered in this chapter. Complete the activities that follow the list to make all of these terms part of your everyday professional vocabulary.

bioethics	genetic disorder	pluripotent
biological safety cabinet (BSC)	genetic engineering	recombinant DNA
Common Rule	genetic test	regenerative therapy
eugenics	incident report	reproductive cloning
gene	off-label	select agent
generic drug	personalized medicine	stem cell
genetic discrimination		

VOCABULARY DEVELOPMENT

Matching. Match the essential terms from this chapter with the best descriptions below by writing the letter of the description next to the number of the essential term on your answer sheet.

1. bioethics
2. Common Rule
3. gene
4. genetic discrimination
5. genetic engineering
6. genetic test
7. incident report
8. personalized medicine
9. recombinant DNA
10. reproductive cloning
11. select agent
12. stem cell

a. term for medical treatments that are tailored to a person's genetic makeup and individual needs

b. a highly dangerous and strictly controlled substance that can potentially be used to develop biological or chemical weapons

c. the examination of a person's cells to analyze his or her genes and identify possible genetic disorders

d. the creation of exact genetic duplicates

e. the use of genetic information by employers and insurance companies to deny employment or insurance coverage or treat individuals differently because of a genetic condition

f. term for a combination of DNA found on the 46 chromosomes inside each human cell that determine the unique genetic makeup of an individual and carry the code for building human cells, tissues, and organs

g. a set of regulations adopted in common by a number of federal agencies to ensure the safety of testing on human subjects

h. the study of ethical practices in medical research and the use of advanced technology to treat patients

i. a cell that can duplicate itself many times and has the ability to develop into many different types of cells

j. a form used to record the details of an unusual event, such as an accident or injury

k. the deliberate manipulation of genetic materials to eliminate harmful traits or to ensure the presence of desirable traits

l. genetically engineered DNA that usually includes segments from two or more different genetic sources

13. **Find Your Match.** Your teacher will write this chapter's professional vocabulary terms on note cards and their definitions on separate cards. As you enter the classroom, you will select a term or definition from the shuffled note cards. When you find the person with your term's definition, you should sit down with that person. At the beginning of class, each student with a term will present his or her matching definition.

14. **Least Familiar Vocabulary.** Select five of this chapter's professional vocabulary terms that are least familiar to you. In your own words, write a statement of explanation for each term that does not use the term itself. Have

a partner guess the professional vocabulary terms you are describing and add any important details that help them remember the terms.

REFLECT ON YOUR READING

15. Review the story about Kimberley at the beginning of the chapter. Using your notes taken in the *Connect with Your Reading* activity, identify the role Kimberley and her coworkers play in healthcare. What issues are raised by the field of biotechnology? Try to use your new professional vocabulary as you support your points.

BUILD CORE SKILLS

16. **Reading.** Find an article about genetic testing or genetic engineering. Read the article and answer the following questions:

    - What is the purpose of this procedure?

    - What are the potential challenges and benefits?

    - What ethical issues are associated with the procedure?

    - What new or unexpected findings did you encounter as you read the article?

17. **Speaking and Listening.** Share your findings from the article you read for the previous activity. Give a one- to two-minute oral report to the class. Plan ahead so that you are able to pronounce any difficult terms. Be prepared to answer questions about your presentation. Listen to and ask at least one question during the presentations of your classmates.

18. **Critical Thinking.** Consider the ethical issues associated with biotechnology that were mentioned in this chapter. Which do you think is the most serious? Why? What do you think are the core ethical questions involved with that particular issue?

19. **Math.** Go to the FDA's Adverse Events Reporting System (FAERS) website. View the chart of reports received and entered by year. What are three statements you can make about this data set?

20. **Critical Thinking.** Using the chart viewed in the previous question, make a prediction about the number of reports that will be made in the upcoming year. Suggest one change that might be made in healthcare or society to influence this trend. Explain your reasoning.

21. **Problem Solving.** What are some of the problems associated with drug-resistant bacteria? Briefly describe the three approaches that biotechnology offers as solutions to these problems. If you worked in a biotechnology lab, which approach would you be most interested in researching? Why?

22. **Math.** Use the Internet to research trends in nanotechnology and the financial impact of these developments. Prepare a chart or graph showing the financial impact of nanotechnology on the field of healthcare. Share your findings with the class.

23. **Speaking and Listening.** Research the topic of human cloning on the Health Research Funding website. Read the information with an open mind. Then, based on your findings, decide whether you are for or against cloning. Prepare a three- to four-minute persuasive speech supporting your position.

24. **Critical Thinking.** How are stem cells used in healthcare? Based on your understanding of stem cells, what other potential uses might they have?

25. **Writing.** Imagine that you are Henrietta Lacks. Write a letter to medical researchers regarding your feelings about the use of your stem cells.

26. **Speaking and Listening.** Explain the reasoning behind focusing early medical research and human testing primarily on white males in their mid-thirties. Discuss this concept with classmates in terms of pros and cons, results, assumptions, demographics, and implications for medications and treatments. What suggestions or support for additional testing with other populations can you identify?

27. **Critical Thinking.** What duties and responsibilities does the Office of Biotechnology Activities (OBA) have with regard to lab safety? Identify the four risk groups for genetic material stated in the chapter. Research at least two examples that fit into each of the four categories. What role does the Occupational Safety and Health Administration (OSHA) have in the monitoring of safety in the workplace? What kinds of situations are specific to OSHA? Share your findings with classmates.

28. **Writing.** Work with a group to create a series of lab safety posters that cover the six lab safety topics presented in this chapter. As a second option your group could create its own incident report for clearly recognizing and relating problems, such as accidents, spills, cuts, and technology malfunctions.

29. **Critical Thinking.** What are three safety rules that biotechnology labs and medical laboratories have in common? What are

three safety rules unique to biotechnology labs?

30. **Problem Solving.** Research a recent health safety event that put a healthcare worker in danger. Describe the circumstances of the event. What were the immediate and long-term dangers for the healthcare worker's health or safety? What steps were taken to protect the worker? What additional steps might have been taken? What was the outcome? How might it have been different if proper precautions were or were not taken?

31. **Problem Solving.** Why are incident reports so critical in lab or research settings? What types of incidents need to be reported? What actions need to be taken by supervisors or lab workers when these incidents occur?

32. **Reading.** Use the Internet to find a sample incident report. Find another sample at your school or workplace. Compare both samples with the guidelines for an incident report presented in the chapter. Is there anything missing in the one from your school or workplace? Which items are new or surprising to you? Why are incident reports crucial for employers, employees, and supervisors? Why is it important to report accurate and complete details on incident reports?

33. **Reading.** Locate an MSDS sheet on a cleaning product from the SDS binder at your school or workplace. What are the potential hazards associated with the substance? What safety precautions are required? What other information was useful to read about on this cleaning product?

34. **Problem Solving.** In a world where bioterrorism is a real threat, what actions have been taken regarding select agents? Identify at least four select agents other than those mentioned in the chapter. Explain why each of these agents is dangerous. What is the history or additional information behind each of these select agents?

35. **Math.** Go to the website for the Department of Health and Human Services' National Practitioner Data Bank. Under "Resources," use the Data Analysis Tool to look at medical malpractice rates. Build a table that shows data for medical doctors in all states, in the most recent year available, and in the malpractice payment range of $1,000,000–$1,999,999. Refer to your table to answer the following questions: How many payments were made by physicians in your state in this year? Which state made the most payments? least? Change the table to show statistics for all types of practitioners in just your state. Which type of practitioner has made the most payments? What other practitioners also made payments in your state?

ACTIVATE YOUR LEARNING

36. Suppose you work in a biotechnology research lab. Use your classroom as a hypothetical lab setting. Label certain items in the classroom as important items you might find in a laboratory. Demonstrate a basic safety procedure that all people in the lab should follow.

THINK AND ACT LIKE A HEALTHCARE WORKER

37. Imagine that you are a genetic counselor. How will you explain genetic testing to individuals who come to your company to have a test performed? Write a script and act out the scene with a classmate.

38. Suppose you have recently been hired by a biotechnology company. What minimum guidelines should be established for potential hazards to workers at this company? What do workers need to know to be protected on the job?

GO TO THE SOURCE

39. Visit the Food and Drug Administration's MedWatch Safety Information website. Select one of the safety alerts on the "Safety Information" tab. Read the report. Briefly summarize the problem and any recommendations offered.

40. Visit the CDC website. Find the page that discusses the "10 Critical Topic Areas" related to nanotechnology and workplace safety. Research one of these critical topics and report your findings to the class.

Chapter 21
Academic Knowledge: Body Systems for Regulation and Communication

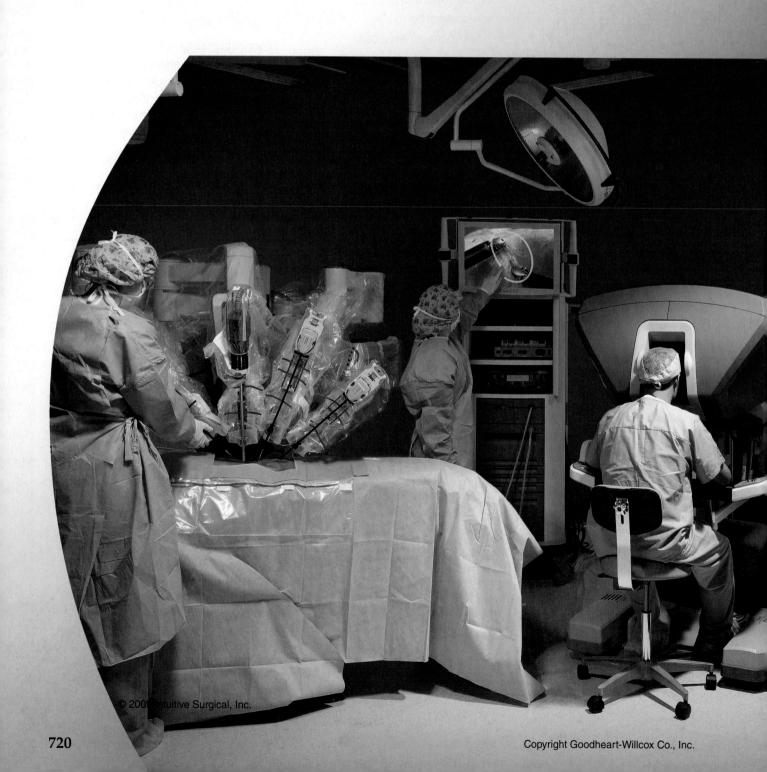

© 2009 Intuitive Surgical, Inc.

PROFESSIONAL VOCABULARY

 E-flash Cards

You will need to learn the essential terms listed below before you begin your reading. These terms will help you understand the main concepts of the chapter. These terms, which will be highlighted in yellow within the text, will become part of your professional vocabulary.

In addition to these essential terms, you will see bold terms throughout the chapter. The meanings of these terms are explained where the terms first appear. The bold terms, like the essential terms listed here, will become part of your professional vocabulary and deepen your understanding of the topics presented.

central nervous system (CNS) the brain and spinal cord

cerebrum the largest part of the brain, which is formed by the four lobes of the cerebral cortex

homeostasis a state of balance between interdependent elements

hormone a chemical used to send messages from an endocrine gland to a target organ

myelin a fatty layer that protects the axons of some nerves

negative feedback system mechanism that reduces a body function in response to a stimulus, such as a hormone

neuron a nerve cell

neurotransmitter a chemical used to carry a signal from an axon to a receptor cell to pass along a message

peripheral nervous system (PNS) term for the sensory and motor nerves that go out to the body's extremities

primary motor cortex an area of the frontal lobe that directs muscle movement through efferent neurons to muscles in the body

primary sensory cortex an area of the parietal lobe dedicated to gathering and interpreting information regarding the five senses of the body from afferent neurons

receptor a nerve cell that receives stimuli

CONNECT WITH YOUR READING

New Terms	Terms I've Heard Of	Terms I Know Well

How was the term used? What is the topic? What does the context tell you?	Opposites or non-examples of the term (what it isn't); don't use *not* or *un-*
(Term and Definition)	
Other words that relate to this term (shared word part, similar meaning)	Draw a picture to represent this term or use the word in a *meaningful* sentence.

There are many new terms to learn when you study the body systems. Some terms will require more effort to remember than others. Using the steps listed here, create a study aid to help you organize and remember these important terms. Be prepared to share your work with classmates and to learn from theirs.

1. Create a Vocabulary Sorting Organizer.

   a. Fold a piece of paper lengthwise to create three columns.

   b. Unfold the paper and label the three columns as *New Terms, Terms I've Heard Of,* and *Terms I Know Well.*

   c. Sort the terms in the Professional Vocabulary list into the columns you have created.

2. On the back of your organizer, write one of the new terms in the center of the page along with the definition given in the chapter.

3. Divide the page into four sections, and complete a "clinical diagnosis" of the new term.

   a. In one section of the page, explain how the word was used in the text. What topic is it related to? What does the context tell you about the meaning of the term?

   b. In the next section, list three or more related words that have a similar meaning or share a word part with this term.

   c. In the third section, use the word in a meaningful sentence or draw a picture of the concept described by the term.

   d. In the last section, explain the opposite of this term, or what it isn't. Avoid using the word *not* or the prefix *un-*.

Systems for
Regulation and Communication
hearing   touch   hormones
vision   smell   taste
speech/words
body language/actions

NERVOUS SYSTEM

SPECIAL SENSES

ENDOCRINE SYSTEM

MAP YOUR READING

Make a tablet organizer with two sheets of paper using the example shown here. Stack the sheets, keeping the side edges even, but move the top sheet of paper up so that its bottom edge is ½ inch to 1 inch above the bottom edge of the sheet below it. Holding both sheets of paper, fold them down so the top edge of the top sheet is ½ to 1 inch above the bottom edge of the top sheet. Crease both layers and staple at the top folded edge. Write *Systems for Regulation and Communication* on the outside flap, and list ways that body systems communicate with each other and with the outside environment to control body functions. Label the edges of the flaps below it with the headings *Nervous System*, *Special Senses*, and *Endocrine System*. As you read, add visual cues, definitions of new terms, and notes on the main functions and careers and diseases related to each system.

The educational experience can be overwhelming. You may feel like you can't possibly finish all of the reading and assignments given to you by teachers. Luckily, there are study skills you can use and steps you can follow that will help you handle your workload efficiently.

This chapter will show you how to use time management, good study habits, and test preparation methods to manage your education. You can use these skills as you read the rest of the chapter, which describes the roles of the nervous system, special senses, and endocrine system.

Study Skills for Health Science Students: Active Learning

Continual education is a part of any healthcare career. Acting like a learner, someone who is always ready and willing to learn more, will help you succeed in your ongoing training. Skills that will support you include time management, good study habits, self-advocacy, and test preparation skills. All of these skills can be developed through practice.

Time Management

From the moment you wake up until the moment you go back to sleep, you are making choices about what to do with your time. Good time management helps you move toward your goals. You can use time management to guide your schoolwork at school and at home.

Select the most appropriate classes for your needs and schedule classes for the time of day when you are mentally at your best. Use a notebook or calendar to keep track of homework assignments and plan time to complete them. Break down larger assignments, such as research papers, into specific tasks and set deadlines so you will be done on time. If you use an electronic calendar, you can set an alarm to remind you of an approaching deadline or test date.

Outside of school, set aside a block of time each day to study. Give yourself enough time for sleep so you are mentally alert. This may require difficult decisions about what to give up, such as time in front of the television or texting friends. To track your time-wasting activities, try keeping a diary of your time use for a week. Make sure your time is spent working toward your goals.

Good Study Habits

Sitting in class doesn't make you a good learner. It's what you do before, during, and after class that's important. Come to class ready to learn. If possible, read the textbook before class and take notes, leaving extra space so you can add to them. As you listen and participate in class, ask the questions you've written in your notes. Add information to the notes, paying special attention to what the teacher writes on the board or spends the most time on in class.

Create a specific time in your daily schedule to do homework, study, and review your notes. Find a quiet place to work where your brain can focus without distraction. If you have trouble staying focused, find a study partner who is also committed to doing well in school. Reviewing information out loud together will use more areas of your brain than just reading and writing. You will know that you have learned a piece of information when you can explain it to someone else in your own words.

Self-Advocacy

You will need to advocate for yourself as a learner. If you have special needs, let your teachers know how they can help you (Figure 21.1). If you don't understand something, try to determine when you became confused and what needs clarification. Choose an appropriate time and place to speak with your teacher. Ask about options for review sessions or retaking a test that did not go well. Take responsibility for your learning and look for ways to resolve problems.

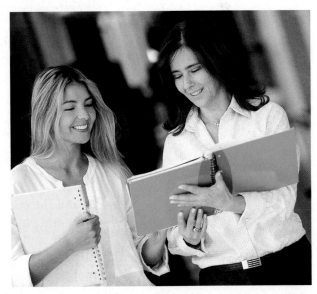

Figure 21.1   Self-advocacy often means asking for help. If you are falling behind, ask your teacher about tutor options.

Test Preparation

A focus on test taking can change the way you study and improve your test scores. When you get a test back, keep a log of the errors you've made. In addition to relearning the concepts you missed, look for problems with your test-taking skills. Common errors to watch for include the following:

- misreading the question

- focusing on the wrong information in the question

- failing to study the correct information

Practice your test-taking skills. Study your incorrect answers to find your most common errors. Ask your teacher for practice tests, or use your notes to create them. On multiple choice tests, examine the distracters used in the answer options so you understand the level of knowledge required to avoid errors.

When you take a test, begin by previewing the test to decide how much time to spend on each section. Make notes in the margin about formulas or information you will need to use. Start with the easiest or most familiar questions. Try to answer the question in your head before looking at multiple choice options. Read the entire question and all answer options before marking your answer. Use the process of elimination to narrow your options. Use all of the test time your teacher allows, rechecking difficult questions after you have completed the test.

If you've chosen the right career path, you should enjoy the content of most of your classes. That doesn't mean they will all be easy, but the effort you put into them will be worthwhile. Use your time management, study, self-advocacy, and test-taking skills to help you through the challenging times.

Complete the
Map Your Reading
graphic organizer for the
section you just read.

RECALL YOUR READING

1. To effectively manage your time, select _____ appropriate for your needs, use a calendar to keep track of _____, and get enough _____ to be mentally alert.

2. When adding to your notes, pay attention to what the _____ writes on the board and spends the most _____ on.

3. Self-advocacy means taking _____ for your learning and finding ways to resolve _____.

4. When your teacher returns a test, keep track of the _____ you made so you can avoid them next time.

Body Systems for Regulation and Communication

The body has two main systems of communication—the nervous system and the endocrine system. The nervous system gathers information through the five senses, processes and stores that information, and responds to it. The nervous system also provides centralized control for rapid and coordinated responses. It gathers information through the sensory system and carries messages back to the body through electrochemical impulses. The endocrine system uses chemical messengers to control body systems. The response of the endocrine system is generally slower and longer acting than the nervous system. Both systems work together to regulate body functions and maintain balance, or **homeostasis**, within the body.

homeostasis
a state of balance between interdependent elements

The Nervous System

The nervous system serves as the body's main control system. It connects and directs all of the other body systems. Neurosurgery, which deals with structures of the nervous system, is one of the most specialized areas of medicine. Neurosurgeons benefit from advances such as microsurgery and functional brain imaging. Microsurgery makes it possible to repair small nerves and blood vessels. Functional magnetic resonance imaging (fMRI) can show which areas of the brain are active in different situations, as well as the anatomy of brain growth and tumors (Figure 21.2). Biotechnology and genetic engineering promise new advances for repairing vertebrae and regrowing spinal nerves.

The Neuron

Nerve cells, called **neurons** [*neuro* = nerve], connect the structures of the nervous system. These cells grow and multiply in the brain as an infant develops. This development begins in the third week of embryonic growth and continues into early adulthood. Different types of neurons have similar structures (Figure 21.3).

Although their structures are similar, different types of neurons have different purposes. Sensory neurons gather information from the body. Motor neurons stimulate muscles to respond to information. Interneurons form connections between other neurons in the brain and spinal cord. Movement, thinking, and memory use these connections. Neurons can reach lengths of several feet as they grow toward their target.

Think of your body as a model for a neuron. Your chest would represent the **cell body**, where the nucleus is found. Your limbs are like **dendrites** [*dendr* = branching] that branch off the cell body to bring in information from other cells. One arm is like the **axon** that takes information from the cell body out to the muscles. The fingers are like **terminal branches** at the end of the axon that connect to other cells. Nerve cells reach out to new areas to **innervate** them, or provide them with a nerve connection to the brain. The brain contains its greatest number of neurons in childhood. Connections that are not used are reabsorbed.

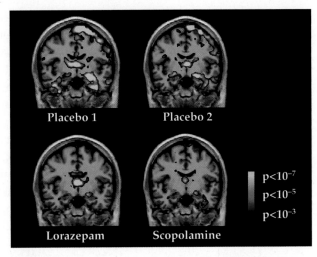

Placebo 1   Placebo 2

$p<10^{-7}$
$p<10^{-5}$
$p<10^{-3}$

Lorazepam   Scopolamine

Figure 21.2   Functional magnetic resonance imaging (fMRI) shows activity in the brain under different conditions. What might fMRI technology be used to diagnose?

neuron
a nerve cell

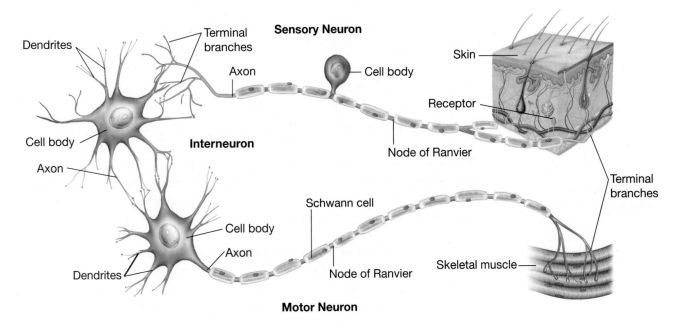

Figure 21.3   Different types of neurons may have similar structures, but they have different purposes. What are the purposes of sensory neurons, motor neurons, and interneurons?

Label Art

Development of motor neuron control in infants moves from the center of the body out to the limbs. Large muscle groups are connected first, followed by small muscles for fine motor control. Each muscle needs to be connected to the brain by an axon so it can receive the signal to contract. Neurons communicate by creating electrochemical signals that travel along the axon. The signal is passed to connecting axons through a synapse. A **synapse** is a tiny gap between an axon and a receptor cell. When a pulse of electricity reaches the synapse, it releases a **neurotransmitter**. This chemical carries the signal across the synapse and triggers a chemical response in the receptor cell. This electrochemical activity can be measured by an electroencephalogram (EEG) [*electro* = electric, *en* = within, *cephal* = head, *gram* = record]. The absence of brainwaves on an EEG is sometimes used as a legal definition of brain death.

Remember that your body can be a model of a neuron, with your chest representing the cell body and your heart as its nucleus. Your arms and legs would be dendrites and axon branches. In this model, the electrical signal sent by a neuron would travel from your limbs to your chest, across your arm, and finally to your fingers. At this point, in the terminal branches, the electrical signal would trigger a chemical signal to be transmitted across the gap to the next cell. This is how the brain sends signals to the body.

Cell bodies and dendrites lying on the surface of the brain form *gray matter*. Its dark color comes from the dark nuclei in the cell bodies. Axons have a waxy coating that gives them a light color. They form *white matter* in the brain. This waxy sheath, called **myelin**, protects axons from "cross-connections" that slow or interrupt signals in the brain. Think of the myelin sheath as a sleeve covering the axon of your arm. Schwann cells along the myelin sheath produce the myelin.

Defects in the myelin sheath can cause diseases such as schizophrenia and multiple sclerosis (MS). Schizophrenia is a breakdown of thought processes, while MS often appears as muscle weakness. In these cases, the nerves are not able to communicate properly with each other because the electrical signal is lost along the unmyelinated pathway.

The Central Nervous System

The nervous system can be divided into two main parts: the **central nervous system (CNS)** and the **peripheral nervous system (PNS)**, as shown in Figure 21.4. The CNS includes the spinal cord and brain. The PNS, discussed in detail later in this chapter, includes the sensory and motor nerves that carry communication between the CNS and the body. All parts of the nervous system work together to communicate sensations and control the body's responses.

The brain is considered the control center of the nervous system. The brain, spinal cord, and nerves are formed from the ectoderm in embryonic development. The ectoderm curls to form a neural tube (Figure 21.5). The top of the tube swells and folds forward to become the **forebrain**. The middle section folds in on itself to become the **hindbrain**. The forebrain grows large enough to cover the **midbrain** beneath it. As the brain grows and pushes for room, more wrinkles are formed until it looks like a large walnut without its shell.

neurotransmitter
a chemical used to carry a signal from an axon to a receptor cell to pass along a message

myelin
a fatty layer that protects the axons of some nerves

central nervous system (CNS)
the brain and spinal cord

peripheral nervous system (PNS)
term for the sensory and motor nerves that go out to the body's extremities

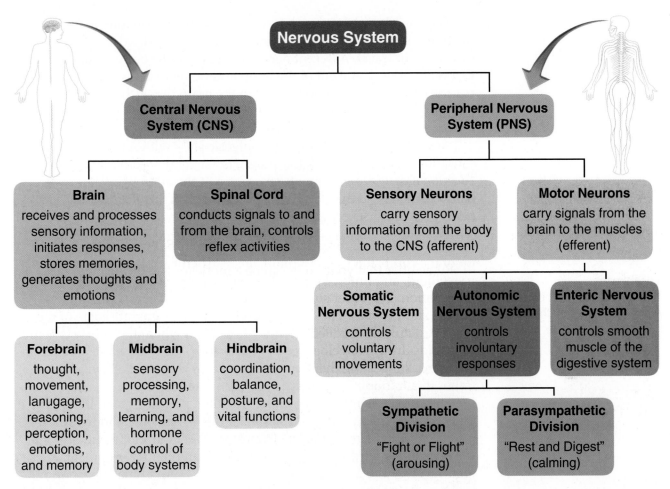

Figure 21.4   The nervous system can be divided into the central nervous system and the peripheral nervous system, each of which has its own components and purposes.

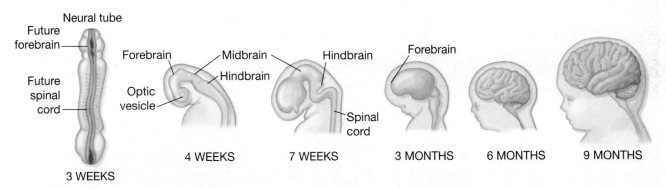

Figure 21.5   As an embryo, the brain starts off as a neural tube, which then curls and folds to form the forebrain, midbrain, and hindbrain.

The brain can be divided into two halves called the *cerebral hemispheres* [*hemi* = half]. The left hemisphere controls the right side of the body and vice versa. They are connected at the center by a large bundle of nerves called the *corpus callosum*. Each hemisphere is made up of several distinct sections, each with a different function.

The spinal cord acts as a highway, carrying information to and from the brain. Like a highway, the spinal cord is clearly divided into two directions of travel. **Afferent** nerves travel from the body up to the brain. **Efferent** nerves come out of the brain and travel to the body. Afferent neurons carry sensory information to the brain. After this information is processed, efferent neurons carry the appropriate motor response from the brain back to the body along peripheral nerves.

Anesthesiologists administer analgesic [*an* = without, *algesia* = feeling, sensation] drugs that block these signals. General anesthesia includes additional drugs to block motor response. If the afferent signals are blocked, then we don't experience pain. Can you think of other ways to block pain or muscle responses?

The Forebrain. The forebrain is the largest part of the brain. It is made up of the **cerebrum** [*cerebr* = brain, *um* = structure], basal ganglia [*gangli* = swelling], and limbic system. The cerebrum sorts and classifies information. The outer surface, called the **cerebral cortex**, has many bumps and grooves. The deepest grooves, which separate some of the brain structures, are called *fissures*. These form when the embryo's neural tube folds during development. Fissures form the same basic patterns in all brains, suggesting that the folding pattern is controlled by genetics rather than randomly created.

The surface bumps of the brain are called *gyri* (JI-rI), and the small folds between them are called *sulci* (SUHL-kI). They form individually unique patterns during the last trimester of fetal development. This suggests that environment plays a large role in their development. These folds increase the total surface area that can fit into a small space. More surface area on the cerebral cortex means more gray matter is available to process information.

The fissures, sulci, and gyri serve as landmarks for identifying major structures of the brain (Figure 21.6). The longitudinal fissure divides the cerebrum into the left and right hemispheres. Each hemisphere is divided into four lobes. The central sulcus divides the frontal and parietal lobes.

cerebrum

the largest part of the brain, which is formed by the four lobes of the cerebral cortex

Figure 21.6   The fissures, sulci, and gyri found on the brain help identify major structures.

Label Art

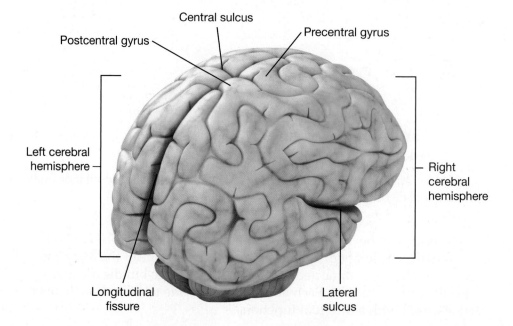

The parieto-occipital sulcus separates the parietal and occipital lobes. The lateral fissure separates the temporal lobe. Each lobe has a different function.

The **frontal lobes**, located at the forehead, are responsible for voluntary muscle control, thinking, memory, language, judgment, creativity, and personality. They are separated from the parietal lobes by the central sulcus. The precentral gyrus is a narrow strip along this groove that contains the **primary motor cortex**. It sends planned motor responses through efferent neurons from the frontal lobes to the muscles of the body.

Different parts of the primary motor cortex control muscles in different areas of the body. More neurons are needed to direct fine motor control, so more space on the motor cortex is devoted to the connections for the fingers, eyes, lips, and tongue than to those for the torso or legs. The motor homunculus is an exaggerated drawing that emphasizes this point (Figure 21.7). Broca's area, which aids in speech production, is also located in the frontal lobe.

The **parietal lobes** lie behind the frontal lobes, on the back of the central sulcus. The somatosensory [*somat* = body] cortex, or **primary sensory cortex**, located on the postcentral gyrus, brings in information from the senses. Wernicke's area, which is located in these lobes, helps people understand written and spoken language. Similar to the primary

primary motor cortex
an area of the frontal lobe that directs muscle movement through efferent neurons to muscles in the body

primary sensory cortex
an area of the parietal lobe dedicated to gathering and interpreting information regarding the five senses of the body from afferent neurons

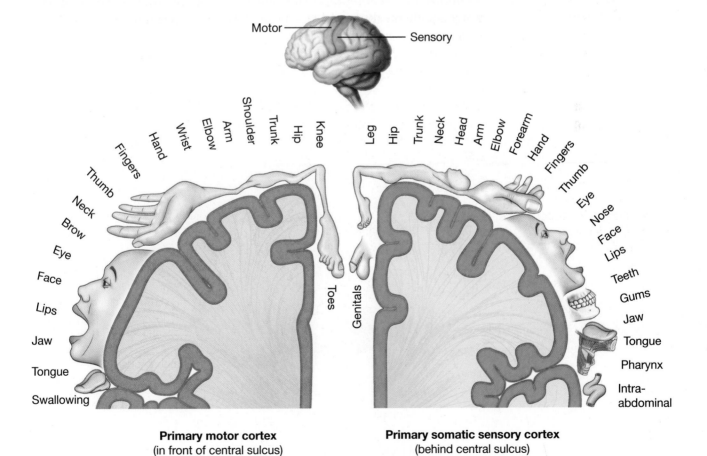

Primary motor cortex
(in front of central sulcus)

Primary somatic sensory cortex
(behind central sulcus)

Figure 21.7   The motor homunculus demonstrates how areas of the body that require fine motor control take up more space in the brain. Areas that are mainly gross motor control take up less space.

motor cortex, different amounts of space on the primary sensory cortex are devoted to different areas of the body. The space dedicated to each body area is based on the number of sensory nerves connected to it. Damage to the parietal lobes can result in problems with sensation, perception, and spatial coordination.

The **occipital lobes** are the smallest of the four pairs of lobes. They sit in the back of the skull behind the parietal lobes and under the occipital bone. They control sight, visual-spatial processes, memory, and storage. The primary visual cortex is located in this area. Damage to the occipital lobe can cause hallucinations, distorted vision, and problems with reading and writing.

The **temporal lobes** lie on the outer side of the other lobes, near the ears. They are separated from the parietal lobe by the lateral fissure. These lobes control hearing, balance, emotions, speech planning, and memory associations. The primary auditory cortex, which processes sound, is located in the temporal lobes. The temporal lobes are the last area of the brain to finish developing, so the frontal lobes help process emotions until temporal lobe development is completed around 20 years of age. This helps explain why children react physically to strong emotions.

The cingulate gyrus, basal ganglia, and limbic system connect the cerebral cortex to the subcortical brain (Figure 21.8). Basal ganglia, also called *basal nuclei*, are areas of gray matter that relay information between the midbrain and cerebral cortex. The basal ganglia are involved in motor control, body position, and the sense of direction and distance.

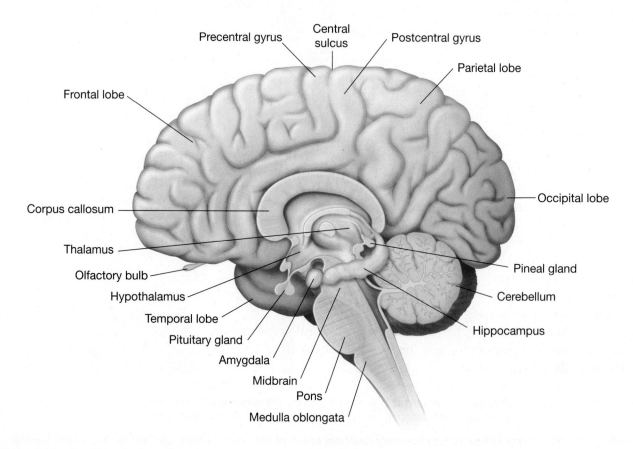

Figure 21.8 A midsagittal section shows many of the brain's structures.

The limbic system is affected by drug use. Drugs can block or trigger the transmission of neuron impulses in the synapse between two neurons. This is a good thing when you have a headache and take aspirin to relieve the pain, but it's not so good when drugs or alcohol prevent you from responding effectively to a stimulus, such as a traffic light changing to red.

The limbic system includes the amygdala (uh-MIHG-duh-luh) and hippocampus, which lie next to the thalamus. The amygdala is an almond-shaped structure located near the temporal lobe. It is involved in strong emotions such as fear, anxiety, defensiveness, sexual arousal, and aggression. These emotions are normally kept under control by a balance of neurotransmitters in the brain. In obsessive-compulsive disorder (OCD), these controls do not work, and the amygdala takes over with obsessive thinking and compulsive rituals. Completion of OCD behaviors feels rewarding and perpetuates the cycle of behavior.

The hippocampus is an arched group of nerve cells connecting the thalamus and the amygdala and ending near the temporal lobe. It is also related to emotions, as well as navigation and spatial memory. Stress releases a hormone that slows the function of the hippocampus and activates the amygdala. This explains why we can't remember things under stress.

Sensory information is initially stored in the hippocampus just long enough to be recognized. If we pay attention longer by repeating the information and making connections, that information may be transferred to long-term memory. The hippocampus is also the first area of the brain affected by mental illnesses such as post-traumatic stress disorder (PTSD), Alzheimer's disease, and depression (Figure 21.9). What common symptoms of these diseases can you connect to malfunctions of the hippocampus?

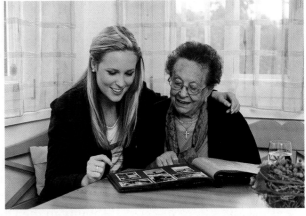

Figure 21.9   The hippocampus, which is related to memory function, is affected in those who have Alzheimer's disease. What are some things you can do to help improve your memory?

The Midbrain. The midbrain includes the thalamus, hypothalamus, pituitary gland (also called the *hypophysis*), and pineal gland (also called the *epiphysis*). Most sensory information comes through the **thalamus**. This area acts as a relay station for sorting, interpreting, and directing sensory signals to the appropriate area of the cerebral cortex. It also plays a role in attentiveness.

The thalamus controls the hormones for the sympathetic nervous system's fight-or-flight response to stressful situations. When you get excited, the sympathetic system reacts by increasing your respiration and heart rate, raising your blood pressure, and sending hormone messengers to prepare your body to respond. A panic attack is an exaggerated example of this response mechanism. After the stressful situation has passed, the parasympathetic system reverses this physical response so that your body returns to normal.

The **hypothalamus**, located just below the thalamus and behind the frontal lobe, is the brain's center for emotions and instincts. It controls pleasure, pain, sleep, hunger, and thirst. The hypothalamus stimulates the pituitary gland, located below it, to release hormones that control growth, body temperature, water balance, and sleep cycles.

The pineal gland lies near the center of the brain. It controls sleep cycles and the biological clock. It secretes melatonin to make you feel sleepy when it's dark. In the winter, when they have less exposure to natural light, people may develop seasonal affective disorder (SAD). This causes depression, sleepiness, and weight gain. Full-spectrum light therapy helps reduce symptoms of SAD. Have you experienced this difference in energy levels with winter doldrums or spring fever?

The Hindbrain. The hindbrain includes the cerebellum and the brainstem. The **cerebellum**, located below the occipital lobe, is the second-largest area of the brain. It coordinates incoming and outgoing messages to produce smooth skeletal movements. Without it, your actions would appear hesitant and clumsy. The cerebellum contributes to planning movements, motor memory, and error recognition. It looks like neatly folded layers, so you might think of it as the secretary of the brain that neatly organizes and smoothes your daily functions. Tremors, decreased muscle tone, and an inability to control movements may indicate a problem with the cerebellum.

The **brainstem** is known as the *vital functions center* of the brain. It controls the smooth muscles of the heart and lungs that are essential for breathing, heart rate, blood pressure, and sleep cycles. It also controls digestion and some reflexes like swallowing and vomiting. The brainstem has three parts: the midbrain, pons, and medulla oblongata (meh-DOO-luh ah-blawn-GAH-tuh). The sympathetic and parasympathetic nervous systems connect here. The medulla oblongata becomes the spinal cord when it exits the skull. The brainstem is generally not involved in mental disorders, but injury to it can cause seizures, coma, or death.

The Role of the Brain in Mental Health. Emotional, psychological, and social well-being combine to form **mental health**. As we have seen, many mental disorders are linked to organs of the nervous system. Mental disorders interfere with everyday living and are the leading cause of disability in the United States. According to the National Institute of Mental Health, one in five American adults is affected by a mental health disorder each year. Nearly half of those are cases of depression.

Depression is usually described as a long-lasting and overwhelming feeling of sadness. Figure 21.10 provides a helpful mnemonic for

Figure 21.10 Symptoms of Depression

Symptom	Description
Sleep changes	may sleep a lot more or experience insomnia
Overwhelming feelings	sadness, guilt, or hopelessness that lasts for several weeks
Memory problems	difficulty remembering details, concentrating, or making decisions
Behavioral changes	may stop doing activities that used to be enjoyable
Eating changes	may eat excessively or lose appetite and stop eating
Restlessness	inability to stick with one task for a long period of time; irritable

identifying depression symptoms. There are several different forms of depression, such as postpartum depression, seasonal affective disorder, and bipolar disorder. These are caused by a combination of genetic, biological, environmental, and psychological factors.

Brain-imaging techniques show that the brains of people with depression function differently and look different from the brains of other people. Some areas of the brain may be smaller in people with depression or other mental disorders. The connections between the areas of the brain, and how often the areas of the brain communicate, may also be different.

Maladaptive behaviors are some of the nonproductive ways that people deal with emotional challenges. These patterns of thinking and behavior can help reduce anxiety in the short term, but they are considered maladaptive if they are not a productive or long-term solution. Examples include the rituals of a person with OCD, the self-injury of a person with depression, or the social and emotional withdrawal by a person with anxiety disorders. Maladaptive behaviors can be harmful to ourselves and others and may be inappropriate in society. They do not help us solve our problems or adapt to life's demands.

Different mental disorders respond to different types of treatment. Some people benefit from psychotherapy, or *talk therapy* (Figure 21.11). Others may respond better to medication. Electroconvulsive therapy (ECT) has been shown to help interrupt signals in an overactive brain. Being physically active can trigger the brain's natural secretion of neurotransmitters, which is helpful for some people.

Keep in mind that mental disorders are real illnesses. You can't be talked out of having poor mental health, but emotional support can help you manage the symptoms. If you or a friend are feeling depressed or having unhealthy thoughts, you should seek help. Don't wait too long to ask your doctor or a mental health counselor for an evaluation or treatment. When treating your mental illness, remember to set realistic goals and be patient.

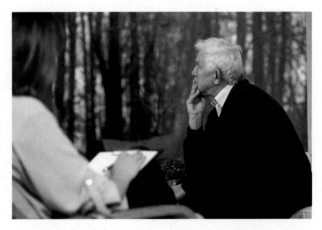

Figure 21.11   Talk therapy is often used to treat mental illnesses such as depression.

Antidepressants work differently for different people because of the complex causes of mood disorders. Research shows that mood-regulating drugs can help reduce the symptoms of these disorders for many people by balancing neurotransmitters in the brain. These drugs are most effective over a long period of time because they also help stimulate neuron growth that connects the emotion centers of the brain. There is a risk, especially with children and young adults, that antidepressant medication can increase thoughts of suicide, so its use should be monitored closely.

Protecting the Central Nervous System. The brain and spinal cord are protected by bone, cerebrospinal fluid, a blood-brain barrier, and three layers of meninges. The **meninges** (meh-NIHN-jeez) are tough layers of tissue covering the brain and spinal cord (Figure 21.12 on the next page). The three layers include the dura mater (the outer layer), arachnoid mater (the middle layer), and pia mater (the layer closest to the brain and spinal cord).

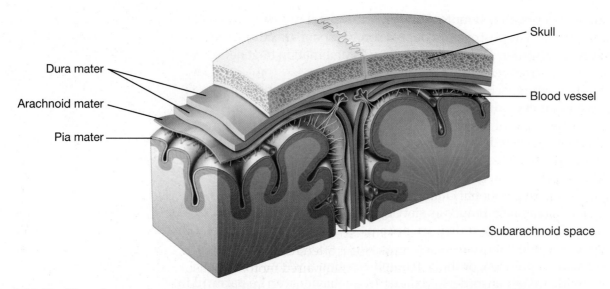

Figure 21.12   Three layers of meninges cover the brain and spinal cord to provide protection. What are the symptoms of meningitis, an inflammation of these meninges?

Like the skin, the meninges keep viruses and bacteria out of the brain. Bacterial meningitis is a serious inflammation of the meninges. It is spread through respiratory secretions during close contact. This illness affects about 1,000 people each year. Symptoms include headaches, fever, neck stiffness, and nausea. These symptoms may be mistaken for a mild flu, but meningitis can cause convulsions, brain damage, or death in as little as a few hours. The meningococcal vaccine is recommended for teenagers with a booster given before college.

The blood-brain barrier sounds like a lining that covers the brain, but it actually exists in the blood vessels of the CNS. Capillaries in the CNS have smaller gaps between their cells than in other parts of the body. These blood vessels are very selective. They do not allow large molecules, highly charged molecules, or fat-soluble molecules to pass through the barrier.

This barrier protects the CNS from common bacterial infections, the influence of outside hormones or neurotransmitters, and other foreign substances that could cause harm. Active transport is required to move glucose across the barrier. Unfortunately, this barrier also makes it difficult to deliver antibiotics or other helpful drugs to the brain. Research is underway to develop new techniques for delivering materials such as medications and contrast dyes to the brain.

Bones also protect the brain and spinal cord. The skull shields the brain, and vertebrae surround the spinal cord. These bones protect against the force of a blow to the head or back, but they don't offer cushioning. A concussion is bleeding and swelling on the surface of the brain. This can happen when the head whips back and forth quickly, bouncing the brain against the inside of the skull.

If infants are shaken, their soft brain may be damaged even more easily than an adult's. Their neck bones also have less support from muscle and may allow the spinal cord to stretch enough to cause damage. This results in a condition known as *shaken baby syndrome.*

Spinal injuries emphasize the importance of vertebrae for protecting the spinal cord. When vertebrae are fractured or dislocated, the spinal cord may be bruised or damaged. Spina bifida (spI-nuh BIH-fih-duh) is a birth defect caused when some vertebrae do not fully form around the spinal cord (Figure 21.13). This leaves the spinal cord exposed to injury. The result of these injuries is weakness or **paralysis** [*para* = beyond, *lysis* = destruction] below the point of the injury. This limits the ability to move certain parts of the body. There may also be complications from infection or swelling in the spinal cord. The risk of having a child with spina bifida can be reduced by taking folic acid supplements before becoming pregnant. Breakfast cereals are often fortified with folic acid to prevent this birth defect.

Quadriplegia (kwa-druh-PLEE-jee-uh) [*quad* = four, *plegia* = weakness] is paralysis or weakness in all four limbs, most often resulting from damage to the cervical vertebrae. Paraplegia is impaired motor or sensory function of the legs. It is usually caused by damage to the thoracic, lumbar, or sacral regions of the spine.

Cerebrospinal fluid (CSF) "floats" the brain inside the skull and cushions it to protect against concussions. Additional CSF also fills the ventricles inside the brain, the central canal of the spinal cord, and the subarachnoid space between the meninges of the spinal cord. The fluid provides glucose and other nutrients for the brain and spinal cord. A spinal tap, or *lumbar puncture*, uses a needle to draw CSF out of the spinal column for testing. A medical technologist examines the fluid for red and white blood cells, cultures it for bacteria, and measures the levels of protein and other substances that don't belong. These tests will reveal hemorrhaging, infections, syphilis, and cancers affecting the brain or spinal cord.

The Peripheral Nervous System

The PNS uses neurons to connect the CNS to the rest of the body. The beginning of this chapter discussed the main concepts of neurons and neurotransmitters. The next body system section will focus on the special

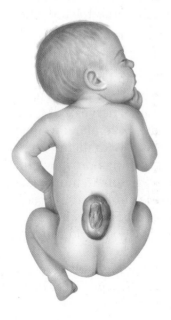
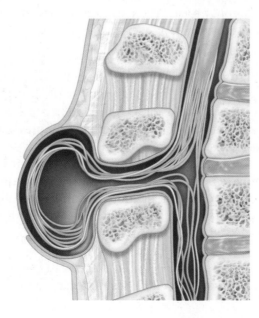

Figure 21.13   The condition known as *spina bifida* can lead to spinal cord inury. In which limbs would you expect this child to experience weakness and paralysis?

senses. This section focuses on nerve pathways and message relays. As shown in Figure 21.4, the PNS can be further divided into the somatic [*soma* = body], autonomic [*auto* = self], and enteric [*enter* = intestine] nervous systems.

All divisions of the PNS can produce involuntary responses. The enteric nervous system controls the smooth muscles of the digestive system. Enteric responses are all involuntary. We don't think about moving food through our digestive system or changing the speed at which it moves. Similarly, we don't think about our heart rate or blood pressure, which are autonomic responses. The autonomic nervous system (ANS) provides involuntary control over smooth muscles of the circulatory and endocrine system. This includes the body's "fight-or-flight" response of the sympathetic nerves as well as the opposite "rest-and-digest" response of the parasympathetic nerves. However, it is important to note that some autonomic responses can be consciously controlled, such as breathing.

The somatic nervous system provides voluntary control of skeletal muscles. You can remember that motor neurons are efferent because it takes *effort* to move your muscles. Sensory neurons are afferent, and you will feel the pain *after* working your muscles. Somatic responses are usually voluntary, but an involuntary response can also be produced. **Reflexes** are involuntary responses of the nervous system (Figure 21.14). They are predictable and will produce the same response each time. What reflex responses are familiar to you?

The purpose of a reflex is to maintain homeostasis in the body and protect the body from harm. A reflex uses a shortcut to produce a faster response in the body. When a sensory neuron gathers information from the body, it typically sends it up the spinal cord to the brain for processing. The information is sorted and a response is returned via a motor neuron, through the spinal cord, to the body. In an emergency situation, a reflex arc will connect the sensory message directly to a motor neuron in the spinal cord rather than going up to the brain. The brain may not process the pain sensation of an injury until after the body has already reacted.

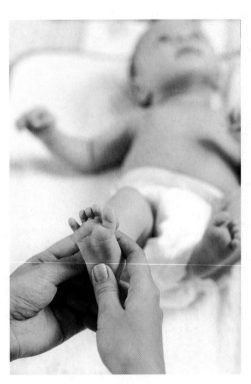

Figure 21.14 If you stroke the bottom of an infant's foot, the toes will fan outward. This is an example of a reflex.

Cranial and Spinal Nerves. There are 12 pairs of **cranial nerves** (Figure 21.15). They provide connections from the brain to the head and neck. Most of these pathways contain motor neurons, but some contain sensory neurons or a combination of both. The cranial nerves exit the skull through *foramina*, which are holes in the bone. Several nerves may use the same foramina, and blood vessels may travel with them.

Nerves are generally named for their location or function, much like muscles. The cranial nerves are also numbered with Roman numerals. If you view the underside of the brain, the nerves are numbered in order, beginning with the olfactory nerve as cranial nerve I. Figure 21.16 on page 738 provides information about the names, locations, and functions of the cranial nerves.

Similar to the cranial nerves, 31 pairs of **spinal nerve** roots connect the spinal cord to the rest of the body (Figure 21.17 on page 739). They are

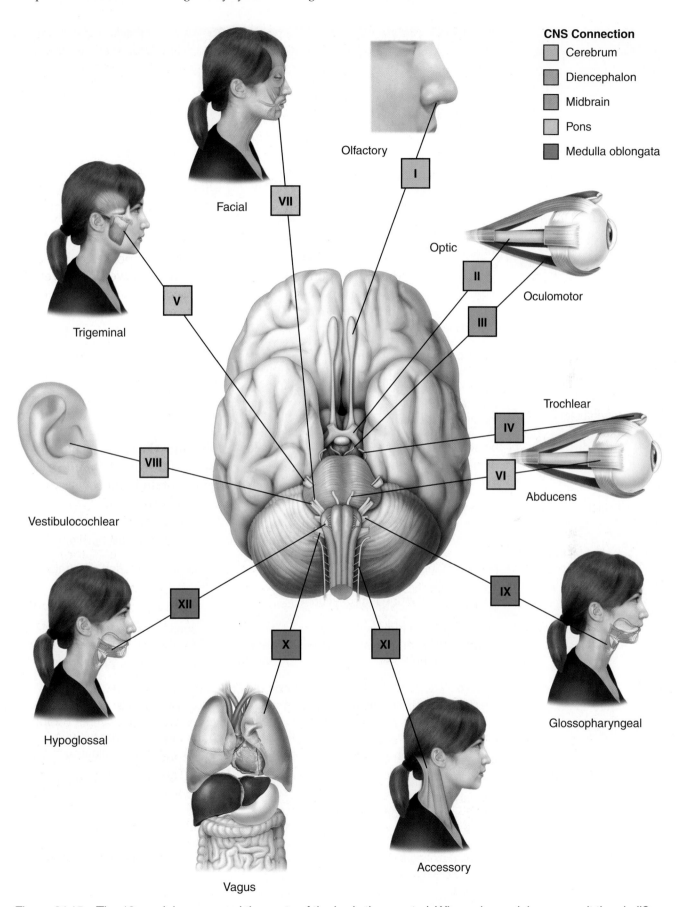

Figure 21.15   The 12 cranial nerves and the parts of the body they control. Where do cranial nerves exit the skull?

Figure 21.16 Name, Location, and Function of the Cranial Nerves

Nerve name	Location	Motor or Sensory	Function
I—Olfactory	below the frontal lobe, exiting through the ethmoid bone into the nasal cavity	sensory	sense of smell
II—Optic	below the frontal lobe, exiting through the sphenoid bone into the eye socket	sensory	visual signals
III—Oculomotor	below the frontal lobe, exiting through the sphenoid bone into the eye socket	motor	muscle innervation to move and focus the eyes
IV—Trochlear	below the frontal lobe, exiting through the sphenoid bone into the eye socket	motor	muscle innervation to move the eyes up, down, and inward
V—Trigeminal: V1—ophthalmic V2—maxillary V3—mandibular	in the pons, exiting in three locations: sphenoid bone into the eye socket, sphenoid wing behind the maxilla, sphenoid wing behind the zygomatic arch	both sensory and motor	muscle innervation for chewing; sensory innervation of the face
VI—Abducens	below the frontal lobe, exiting through the sphenoid bone into the eye socket	motor	muscle innervation to move the eyes outward (abduction)
VII—Facial	brainstem, between the pons and medulla, exiting through the auditory canal of the temporal bone	both sensory and motor	sense of taste; muscle innervation of the face, salivary glands, and tear ducts
VIII—Vestibulocochlear (Acoustic)	brainstem, between the pons and medulla, exiting through the auditory canal of the temporal bone	sensory	sense of hearing and balance
IX—Glossopharyngeal	medulla, exiting through the jugular foramen between the temporal and occipital bones	both sensory and motor	sense of taste from the back of the tongue; muscle innervation of salivary glands and tonsils; swallowing
X—Vagus	medulla, exiting through the jugular foramen between the temporal and occipital bones	both sensory and motor	some sense of taste from epiglottis; muscle innervation of larynx and pharynx for speech and swallowing
XI—Accessory (Spinal Accessory)	cranial and spinal roots, exiting through the jugular foramen between the temporal and occipital bones	motor	muscle innervation of neck
XII—Hypoglossal	medulla, exiting below the tongue through the hypoglossal canal to the neck	motor	muscle innervation of tongue

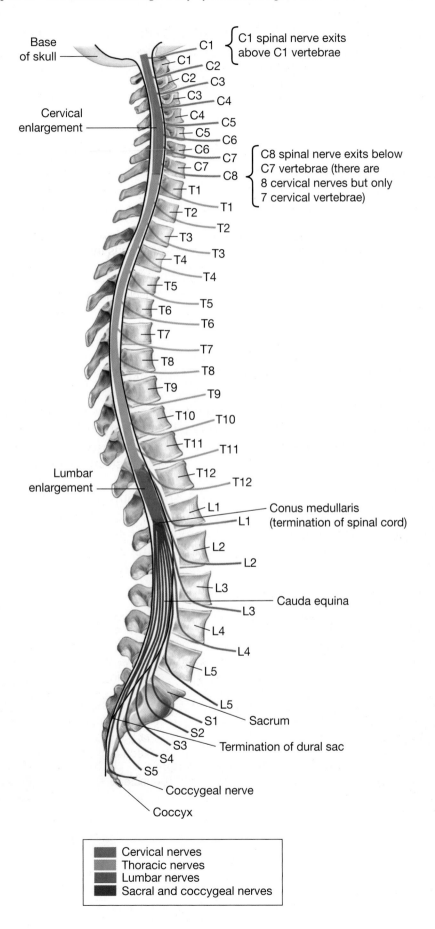

Base of skull

Cervical enlargement

Lumbar enlargement

C1 — C1 spinal nerve exits above C1 vertebrae

C1
C2
C2
C3
C3
C4
C4
C5
C5
C6
C6
C7
C7
C8 — C8 spinal nerve exits below C7 vertebrae (there are 8 cervical nerves but only 7 cervical vertebrae)

T1
T1
T2
T2
T3
T3
T4
T4
T5
T5
T6
T6
T7
T7
T8
T8
T9
T9
T10
T10
T11
T11
T12
T12

L1
L1 — Conus medullaris (termination of spinal cord)
L2
L2
L3
L3 — Cauda equina
L4
L4
L5
L5

S1 — Sacrum
S2
S3 — Termination of dural sac
S4
S5
Coccygeal nerve
Coccyx

Cervical nerves
Thoracic nerves
Lumbar nerves
Sacral and coccygeal nerves

Figure 21.17   The 31 spinal nerves that connect the spinal cord to the rest of the body. How are spinal nerves named?

named with a letter and number according to the vertebrae where they exit. For example, the nerve exiting above the first cervical vertebra is C1, C2 exits the spinal canal between the first and second cervical vertebrae, and so on. The sacrum is fused as one bone, but its nerves exit through holes in the bone. There are eight pairs of cervical nerves (C1–C8), twelve pairs of thoracic nerves (T1–T12), five pairs of lumbar nerves (L1–L5), five pairs of sacral nerves (S1–S5), and one coccygeal nerve. The spinal cord and its meninges extend down to a swelling at the second lumbar vertebra. Beyond that, the nerves separate into the cauda equina (kaw-duh ee-KWI-nuh) [*caud* = tail, *equin* = horse], which is Latin for *horse's tail*. Beyond L2, the nerves are not gathered together in the spinal cord.

Nerve Pathways and Message Relays. Spinal nerves help direct messages entering and leaving the spinal cord (Figure 21.18). The ANS requires two neurons to make the connection from the brain to the body. The connection between the two neurons forms a **ganglion**, or *swelling*. Chains of these ganglia run down both sides of the spinal cord. The preganglionic [*pre* = before, *ganglion* = swelling, *ic* = pertaining to] neuron starts in the brain, runs down the spinal cord, and ends at the sympathetic ganglion. The postganglionic [*post* = after, *ganglion* = swelling, *ic* = pertaining to] neuron runs from the ganglion out to the target organ. All ANS neurons are part of a network connected by ganglia.

Spinal nerves act as on-ramps and off-ramps to the spinal cord's highway of information. They are a collection of many separate axons gathered together. Their messages pass through a **plexus**, or *braid*, of interwoven spinal nerve roots that are similar to highway interchanges. The cervical, lumbar, and sacral nerve plexuses continue to divide into trunks, divisions, and cords (Figure 21.19). These pathways become smaller as they spread out to their separate body regions, like neighborhood streets branching off local highways. Then neurons separate from the nerve tract to connect nerves to body parts in that region, like neighborhood streets taking traffic directly to and from individual houses.

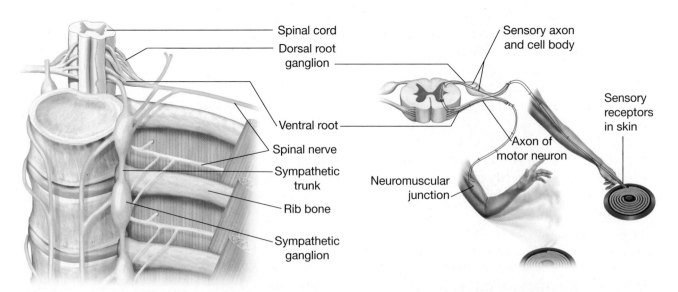

Figure 21.18 A sensory receptor is stimulated by a hot surface, sending an afferent signal to a sensory axon in the spinal cord. The signal is then transferred by an interneuron directly to a motor neuron, stimulating quick removal of the hand from the hot surface. These neurons are connected at a ganglion.

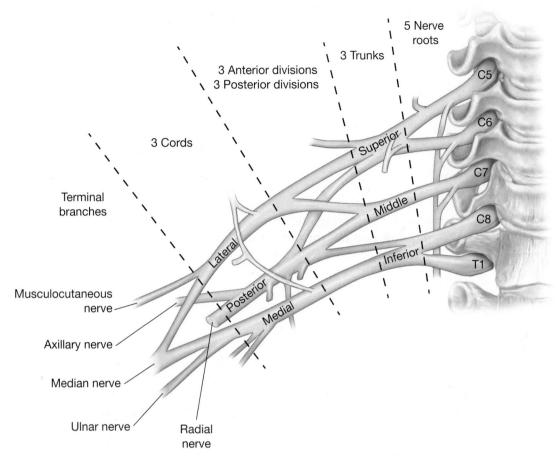

5 Nerve roots
3 Trunks
3 Anterior divisions
3 Posterior divisions
3 Cords
Terminal branches
C5
C6
C7
C8
T1
Superior
Middle
Inferior
Lateral
Posterior
Medial
Musculocutaneous nerve
Axillary nerve
Median nerve
Ulnar nerve
Radial nerve

Figure 21.19   Spinal nerve plexuses begin as roots and then branch out into trunks, divisions, and cords.

The brachial plexus provides an example of how nerve trunks divide into anterior and posterior divisions. Anterior nerves generally innervate flexor muscles, while posterior nerves innervate extensors. In the shoulders, the cervical [*cervic* = neck] plexus and brachial [*brachi* = arm] plexus are formed by cervical and thoracic [*thorac* = chest] nerve roots. Down the front of the arm, anterior divisions form the musculocutaneous, median, and ulnar nerves that flex the upper arm, wrist, and finger muscles. Down the back of the arm, posterior divisions form the axillary and radial nerves that innervate the upper arm, forearm, wrist, and finger extensor muscles.

The thoracic spinal nerves are connected directly to the muscles of the ribs, back, and abdomen. These nerves do not travel through plexuses. Their roots branch directly off the spinal cord to their target organs. These nerves are important to muscles that support breathing and balance.

Major nerves travel along the same pathways as major blood vessels (Figure 21.20 on the next page). Nerves require a constant supply of oxygen and glucose to transmit their nerve impulses. The lumbar and sacral plexuses serve the pelvis, legs, and feet. The lumbar plexus branches into the femoral nerve. The femoral nerve, artery, and vein run together in a sheath through the inguinal, or *groin*, region. The saphenous nerve and artery branch off from the femoral nerve and artery, traveling together down the inner side of the knee to the ankle and foot. The sacral

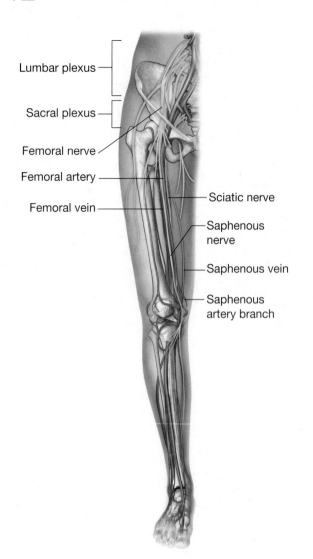

Lumbar plexus

Sacral plexus

Femoral nerve

Femoral artery

Femoral vein

Sciatic nerve

Saphenous nerve

Saphenous vein

Saphenous artery branch

Figure 21.20   Major nerves require a constant supply of oxygen and glucose to transmit their impulses, so they travel along the same pathways as major blood vessels.

Complete the *Map Your Reading* graphic organizer for the section you just read.

plexus branches into the sciatic nerve through the buttocks and down the legs. Most of us have experienced numb legs from sitting too long in a position that cuts off the blood supply to this nerve.

The fact that blood provides glucose for nerve impulses helps explain why diabetic patients have increased nerve pain and numbness. Their high blood sugar level increases the potential for those nerves to send impulses, even when there is no true pain demanding a response. This is one cause of peripheral neuropathy [*neuro* = nerve, *pathy* = disease], or nerve damage.

The nervous system serves all of the other body systems. It gathers and directs sensory and motor information that connects the functions of the other systems. The systems theory model in chapter 4 explained that no system operates in isolation. The body systems are another example of this interconnectedness. A change in one system impacts the others.

Healthcare professionals need to be aware of connections between the body systems. With the trend toward specialization, medical professionals need to connect with specialists in other fields to solve many medical challenges. If a patient has very low blood pressure, there may be a connection to cardiovascular, kidney, or lung function. The patient may be dehydrated or taking a medication that lowers blood pressure as a side effect. Making a change to one system, such as the heart, and its medications may affect other body systems. General practitioners have a broad view of all body systems. New medical careers, such as hospitalists, are also focused on coordinating care among a variety of different specialists.

RECALL YOUR READING

1. The nervous system is connected by _____, whose parts include the cell body, a(n) _____, _____ branches and _____, and a myelin sheath.

2. Each _____ of the brain is made up of lobes, including the frontal, _____, temporal, and _____ lobes, each with a different _____.

3. The parts of the _____ include the thalamus, _____, pituitary gland, and _____.

4. Sometimes people manage their _____ challenges in nonproductive ways by exhibiting _____ behaviors.

5. Nerves travel along the same pathways as major _____ and form an interweaving _____ as they leave the spinal cord.

The Special Senses

The special senses are part of the nervous system, but they are sometimes studied separately as the sensory system. There are five senses: touch, taste, smell, vision, and hearing. Each special sense has many afferent, or *sensory*, **receptors**. These specialized neurons respond to different types of stimuli and gather different types of information.

receptor
a nerve cell that receives stimuli

Touch

There are many types of sensory receptors in the skin. These neurons can detect light touch, firm pressure, pain, vibration, temperature, and position. Each receptor is responsible for a specific area of skin. Some areas, such as the fingertips and lips, are more sensitive. They have more receptors per square inch of skin than other areas, such as the thigh.

Different areas of the skin have different types of receptors (Figure 21.21). For instance, hairy skin has nerve fibers wrapped around the hair follicles to sense when hairs move. *Ruffini endings* detect pressure in the dermis, while *Pacinian* (puh-SIH-nee-uhn) *corpuscles* sense deep pressure and vibration in the hypodermis of both hairy and non-hairy skin. *Merkel disks* sense continuous touch and *Meissner corpuscles* feel light touch in non-hairy skin. *Krause corpuscles* sense cold, pressure, and low vibrations in mucous membranes. Free nerve endings in the epidermis detect pain, touch, and temperature in many different skin types. Without a variety of receptors, we would not be able to distinguish between touch,

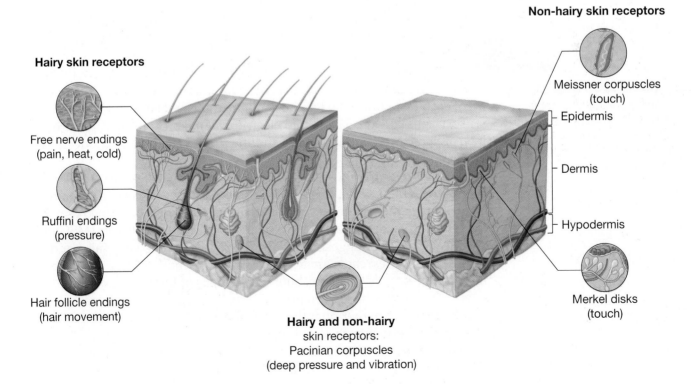

Hairy skin receptors

Free nerve endings (pain, heat, cold)

Ruffini endings (pressure)

Hair follicle endings (hair movement)

Non-hairy skin receptors

Meissner corpuscles (touch)

Epidermis

Dermis

Hypodermis

Merkel disks (touch)

Hairy and non-hairy skin receptors: Pacinian corpuscles (deep pressure and vibration)

Figure 21.21 Hairy and non-hairy skin have some different types of skin receptors. Choose one type of skin receptor shown here and explain what it senses.

Animation

vibration, and pain. It would be difficult to carry out everyday tasks, such as typing or picking up an object.

Information from skin receptors is carried to the spinal cord and up to the brain for interpretation. The sensory information is sorted in the thalamus, then passed on to the postcentral gyrus in the parietal lobe. This is the location of the primary sensory cortex, where the sense of touch is interpreted. The lips, face, fingers, and feet are the most sensitive parts of the body. These areas have the most cell bodies in the postcentral gyrus (see the sensory homunculus in Figure 21.7).

The sense of touch can be reduced by infection, disease, or damage to the neurons or spinal cord. Touch, pain, and temperature sensations also decrease in old age because the number of receptors per square inch declines.

Taste

Gustation [*gust* = taste, *ation* = action of], the sense of taste, is a combination of several different sensory inputs. Both flavor and smell molecules activate taste receptors in the tongue and mouth (Figure 21.22).

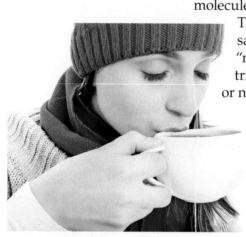

These receptors can identify many different combinations of sweet, salty, sour, bitter, and savory flavors. Moisture, temperature, and "mouth feel" are also important to taste perception. These inputs trigger memories and emotions. Taste can be enjoyable, unpleasant, or nostalgic.

As you bite into food, escaping molecules activate odor receptors in the nose. Smell enhances taste, and food memories help trigger saliva production. Saliva is important because food molecules must dissolve in fluid to access the taste sensory cells. Saliva and food molecules flow across the tongue and down the throat. **Papillae** (puh-PIH-lee) [*papill* = nipple-like] on the sides, tip, and back of the tongue become coated with saliva (Figure 21.23). A groove, or *moat*, around each papilla brings food molecules in the saliva to microvilli at the

Figure 21.22   Flavor and smell both activate taste receptors, so smell is important in perceiving taste.

tip of each **taste bud**. The tongue contains thousands of taste buds. These sensory cells convert flavors into electrical signals. Their messages are interpreted by the limbic system, and the frontal cerebral cortex decides on a response.

Current research shows that there are five basic tastes: sweet, salty, sour, bitter, and umami. Umami is the newest flavor discovery. Its name is taken from the Japanese word for *delicious*. Umami is described as a rich and savory flavor found in meat and *monosodium glutamate* (MSG). Its chemical structure suggests that it is a combination of sweet, salty, and sour flavors. Researchers are also investigating whether there is a taste receptor for fat. Old theories about which areas of the tongue are able to sense which tastes have been proven wrong. Although specific receptors may be found in higher quantities in some areas, each taste bud may contain a variety of taste receptors.

The sense of taste may be affected by damage to taste cells. Extreme heat, which might come from eating food that is too hot, can damage taste buds. Drugs, such as cancer treatments, may also destroy taste cells. Although new taste buds develop every 7 to 10 days, we gradually produce fewer taste buds. We have about 10,000 at birth and only about

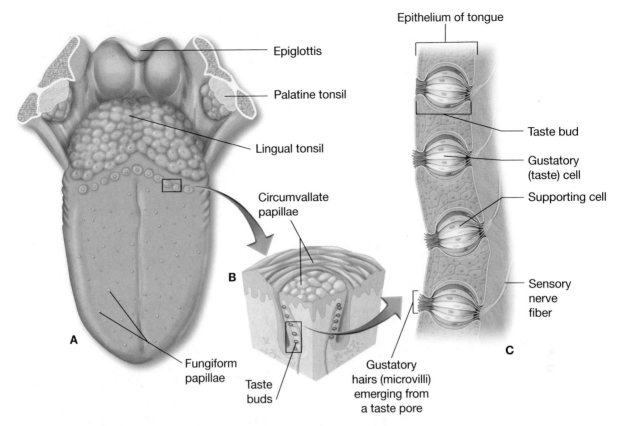

Figure 21.23   The taste sensory organs include papillae and taste buds.

4,000 as adults. In old age, a reduced sense of taste may lead to a lack of appetite or a desire for more seasoning in food.

Anything that affects molecules' ability to reach their receptors will affect your ability to smell or taste. Smoking, a dry mouth, or thick mucus caused by a cold can all reduce the sense of taste and smell. The business of creating new taste enhancers and ingredient substitutes for sugar, salt, and fat continues to be an area for research.

Smell

Olfaction [*olfact* = smell, *ion* = action of] is the sense of smell. It is a chemical sensory system that works in a similar way to taste, but it is much more sensitive (Figure 21.24 on the next page). We have about two dozen different kinds of olfactory receptors. Most odors are a combination of chemicals, so thousands of unique smells are possible.

When you inhale, scent molecules travel to the back of your nasal passage. Once there, the molecules dissolve into a small area of mucus covering the olfactory receptor cells. The sense of smell enhances taste, and some scent molecules may pass down the pharynx to taste receptors in the back of the mouth. A cold may cause thick mucus to block access to the receptor cells. This can reduce both taste and smell.

When scent chemicals trigger chemoreceptors in the olfactory cilia, the messages are passed to the brain. The chemoreceptors' axons pass through small holes in the skull to the **olfactory bulb**. Scent messages begin the sorting process with hundreds of glomeruli in the olfactory

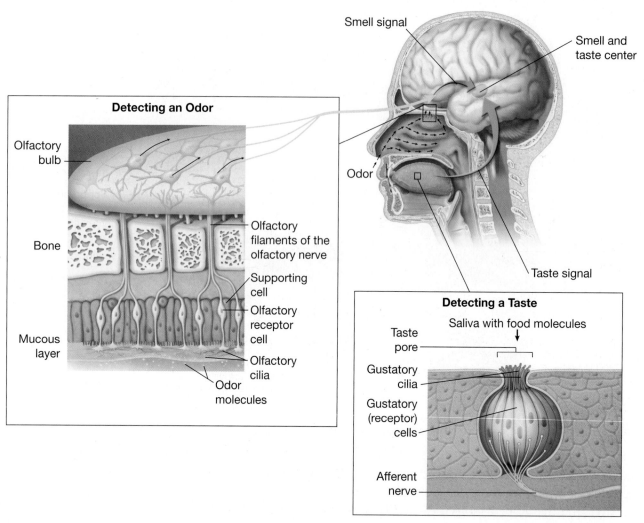

Figure 21.24 The sensory organs for smell and taste are similar, which means that detecting an odor can be connected to detecting a taste.

bulb. Neurons link the olfactory tract to the limbic system. This explains the strong connection between odors, memories, emotions, and compulsive behaviors such as overeating.

Hearing

The ear is an instrument for detecting sound waves. Sounds are actually waves of molecular vibrations picked up by the ear and converted to electrical impulses that are sent to the brain.

The ear can be divided into three sections: the outer ear, inner ear, and middle ear (Figure 21.25). The outer ear includes the pinna and ear canal. The pinna is the flap of cartilage on the side of the head that we recognize as an ear. It funnels sound waves into the auditory canal. The **tympanic membrane**, or *eardrum*, divides the outer and middle ear. This thin membrane changes sound waves into vibrations.

The **ossicles** [*oss* = bone, *icle* = tiny] are bones that transfer vibrations from the middle ear to the inner ear. The largest ossicle, the *malleus*, sits against the tympanic membrane. Its vibrations move the other ossicles, the *incus* and *stapes* (STAY-pehz). The stapes, in turn, pushes against the

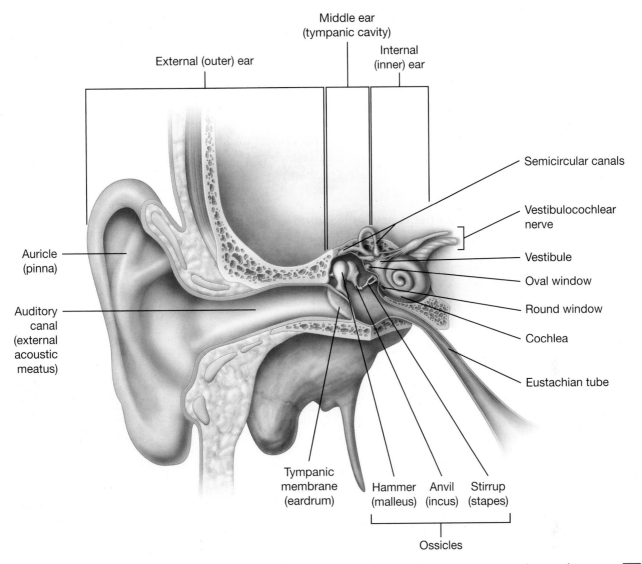

Figure 21.25   The structures of the outer ear, middle ear, and inner ear. Where is the tympanic membrane, or *eardrum*, located?

Label Art

oval window of the vestibule. This is the entrance to the two fluid-filled chambers of the inner ear. These chambers are the **cochlea**, used for hearing, and the vestibular canals, used for maintaining balance. Inside the snail-shaped cochlea, the *organ of Corti* holds tiny hair receptor cells. These nerve receptors are moved by the fluid waves created as the stapes vibrates. Different receptor cells wave in response to different pitches of sound. The receptor movement and location are transmitted by the cochlear nerve to the temporal lobe of the brain so the sounds can be identified, remembered, or responded to.

Balance and position are also sensed in the inner ear. The **vestibular canals** sense movement of fluid. This gives you information about the position of your head. You can detect movements up and down, side-to-side, and tilting. Vertigo is a problem with balance that may also include dizziness and nausea.

An audiogram is a graph that shows the results of a hearing test. It shows the frequency, or *pitch*, in hertz (Hz) and the volume in decibels (dB) measured for each ear. We can hear sounds ranging from a volume of about 20 to 20,000 Hz and a pitch of about –10 to 150 dB before experiencing pain. Normal speech ranges from about 50 to 500 Hz and 45 to 65 dB. The speech banana in Figure 21.26 shows where speech sounds fall on an audiogram. Notice that consonants are generally higher pitched and more softly spoken than most vowels. Hearing loss within the speech banana can affect a child's ability to learn language or an adult's ability to understand what others are saying. Speech therapists help patients produce clear speech and understand receptive speech. This growing career area requires a master's degree due to the many complexities of speech and hearing problems.

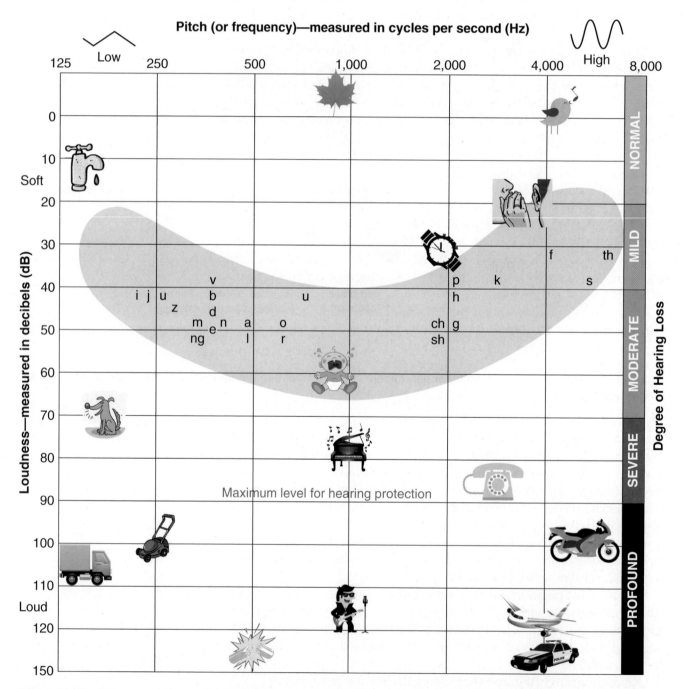

Figure 21.26   The speech banana in this illustrated audiogram shows the range of hearing required to detect speech sounds.

An audiologist may perform a variety of tests for measuring hearing. The method of testing often depends on the ability of the patient to participate. For example, auditory brainstem response (ABR) involves attaching electrodes to the head to pick up brainwaves in response to hearing. An otoacoustic emission (OAE) test measures the inner ear's echo responses to sound. Behavioral observation audiometry looks for behavioral changes in response to sound. People being tested may be asked to raise their hand when they hear a tone (Figure 12.27).

Hearing should be checked at birth because approximately 3 in 1,000 newborns have hearing loss. This limits their ability to collect and process information and communicate with the world around them. Late diagnosis may result in permanent effects on speech, language, and social development.

Some types of hearing loss may be inherited. Both dominant and recessive genes have been identified as causes of hearing impairment. Surprisingly, in 9 out of 10 children born with an inherited impairment, either one parent or both parents have no impairment. Inherited hearing loss is only responsible for 20 percent of all cases of hearing loss. A loss of hearing that results from infection or injury will not be passed on.

Some mild to moderate hearing loss, called *presbycusis* (prehz-bih-KYOO-sihs), is a normal part of the aging process. This condition is distinctly different from other types of hearing loss. It particularly relates to sounds in the higher frequencies. The audiogram shows a gradual drop in the highest frequencies. Older people find it particularly hard to understand high-pitched voices in women and children. They also may not hear softer speech sounds such as *v*, *p*, and *s*. Background noise can often interfere with their hearing. An inability to hear can be frustrating and embarrassing, affecting family, work, and social life.

Noise-induced hearing loss (NIHL) occurs when sensory hair cells in the cochlea are damaged by loud sounds that last too long. High-frequency sounds cause the most damage. The harmful effects of exposure also add up over time, so regular exposure increases your risk

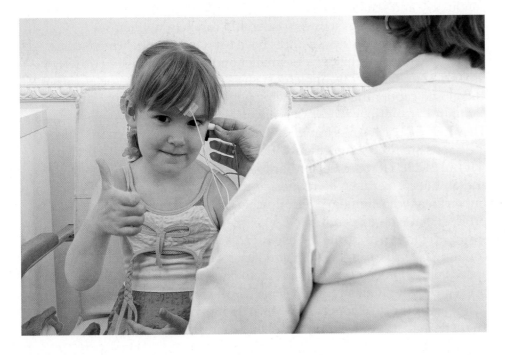

Figure 21.27   In a hearing test, participants are asked to signal when they hear a tone.

for hearing loss. You know you may have NIHL when you have to raise your voice to be understood by someone near you, when noise hurts your ears, or when you develop a ringing sound or temporary reduction in hearing after being exposed to loud noise.

Workers who are exposed to noise at 85 dB or higher for extended periods of time are required to wear hearing protection, such as earplugs or earmuffs (Figure 21.28). It's important to note that portable music devices play at much higher levels than 85 dB. Parents and children are encouraged to develop healthy hearing habits to prevent NIHL. For example, turn down the sound on TVs and portable devices. Block loud noises with earplugs or earmuffs, or move farther away from the noise.

Hearing loss is ranked as mild, moderate, severe, or profound. There are also three specific types of hearing loss. Conductive hearing loss occurs when a sound wave is not carried through from the outer ear to the eardrum and into the cochlea. On an audiogram, conductive hearing loss results in a loss of sensitivity across the entire range of frequencies and may affect only one ear. This may be due to a buildup of earwax against the eardrum, a hole in the eardrum, fluid in the middle ear, or the ear bones having a limited ability to vibrate. If the cause is treated, hearing may be restored.

Sensorineural hearing loss may be caused by exposure to loud noises, drug use, or illnesses that damage the cilia. It may also be hereditary. This includes NIHL. On an audiogram, NIHL creates a characteristic dip in the high-pitched sounds around 4 kHz. Sensorineural damage is usually permanent but may be treated with cochlear implants for people who have profound hearing loss. These electronic devices can provide some sound information to support hearing, but the information is different from what others hear. Mixed hearing loss occurs when a person has both conductive and sensorineural hearing loss.

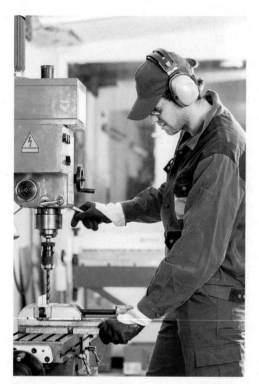

Figure 21.28 Workers in environments with loud, persistent noises must wear protective earplugs or earmuffs.

Hearing aids make sounds louder and can help to filter out background noise. Many advances have been made in hearing aid technology to make the devices smaller and more sensitive to different types of sound. Other technology such as computers, teletype (TTY), and closed captioning can also help people with a hearing impairment communicate with or follow the conversations of hearing people. They may also use American Sign Language (ASL), a system in which the hands are used to represent letters, numbers, words, and phrases (Figure 21.29). This can be similar to speaking a foreign language, and an interpreter may be requested to help a patient with a hearing impairment who signs to communicate with a hearing healthcare professional who does not.

Hearing is an important sense for a variety of purposes. It helps us communicate, learn, and understand each other, and it is important to speech development. It helps alert us to danger and lets us locate a person or scene. Living with a reduced sense of hearing requires adaptation. Members of the deaf community have their own cultural norms, rules of etiquette, and a positive attitude toward being deaf.

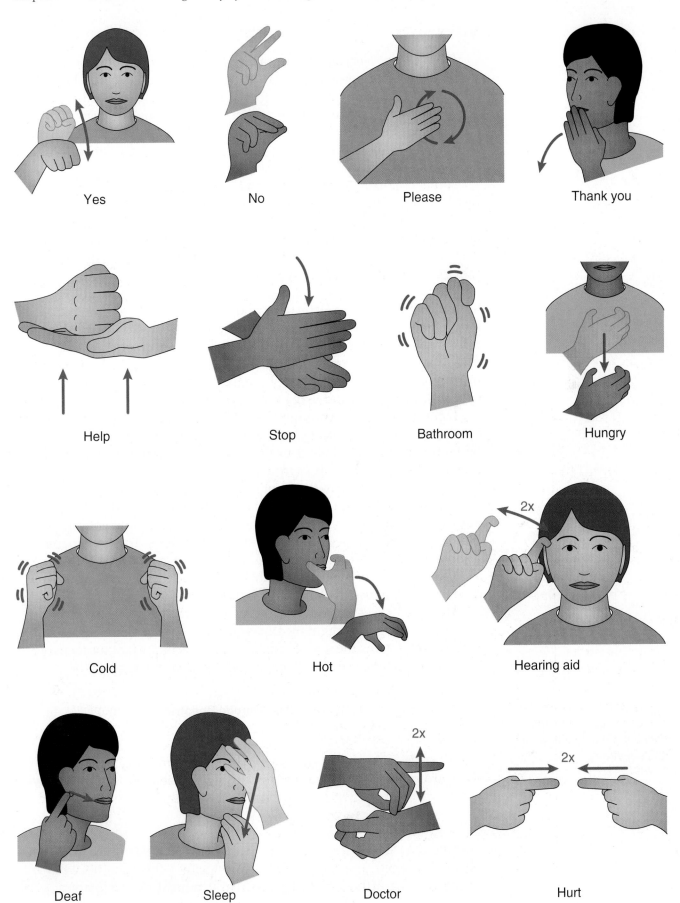

Yes   No   Please   Thank you

Help   Stop   Bathroom   Hungry

Cold   Hot   Hearing aid

Deaf   Sleep   Doctor   Hurt

Figure 21.29   These are some important signs in American Sign Language that might be used in a healthcare setting.

Vision

Our eyes are *photosensitive*, meaning they can detect light within the visible spectrum (Figure 21.30). That light passes through several layers of the eye to reach the photoreceptors. Aging, eye disease, and hereditary conditions can all cause a loss of vision. Ophthalmologists [*ophthalm* = eye, *ologist* = specialist] define legal blindness as vision that is less than 20/200. What a person with this diagnosis sees from 20 feet away can be seen by a person with normal vision from 200 feet away.

A diet that includes vitamin A and omega-3 fatty acids is important for eye health. The eyes are also physically protected by the structures around them. The eyelids lubricate and shade the eyeballs. Touching the eyelashes triggers a reflex to close the eye. Tear glands produce a fluid to help cleanse the eye. Excess tears drain away to the nasal cavity through the nasolacrimal duct. That's why your nose runs when you cry.

The white of the eye, or **sclera**, covers the eyeball (Figure 21.31). Six extraocular muscles [*extra* = beyond, *ocul* = eye, *ar* = pertaining to] attach to the sclera to turn the eyes toward the object you want to see. Strabismus, or *crossed eyes*, occurs when the muscles do not keep the eyes focused on the same point. Microsurgery, performed with surgical microscopes and microscopic tools, makes it possible to surgically correct eye muscle problems and many other eye conditions.

Light enters the eye through the transparent **cornea** at the front of the eye. Next, light passes through the **aqueous humor** [*aqu* = water, *ous* = pertaining to, having]. This clear fluid in the front of the eye maintains pressure and nourishes the cornea and lens. Glaucoma is a condition in which high pressure in the front of the eye can cause blindness. The light must pass through the **pupil** to reach the lens. A circular band of muscles called the *iris* contracts to limit the amount of light entering the eye. Tiny ciliary muscles control the shape of the **lens**. This transparent, flexible structure focuses light at the back of the eye. The lens becomes less flexible and more yellowed with age. A cloudy lens, caused by age or cataracts, will reduce the amount of light entering the eye.

The lens focuses light on photoreceptors at the back of the eye to perceive an image. The light must pass through the **vitreous humor**, a fluid that maintains the eye's shape. Eye shape is important for focusing light that enters the eye. A misshapen eye focuses an image on the

Figure 21.30   The eyes are photosensitive, meaning they can detect light within this spectrum.

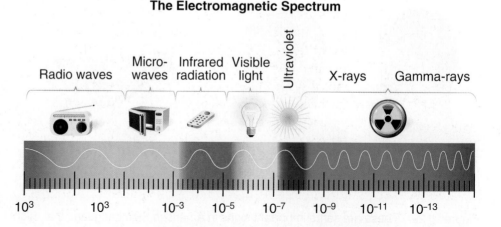

The Electromagnetic Spectrum

Radio waves   Micro-waves   Infrared radiation   Visible light   Ultraviolet   X-rays   Gamma-rays

10^3 10^3 10^{-3} 10^{-5} 10^{-7} 10^{-9} 10^{-11} 10^{-13}

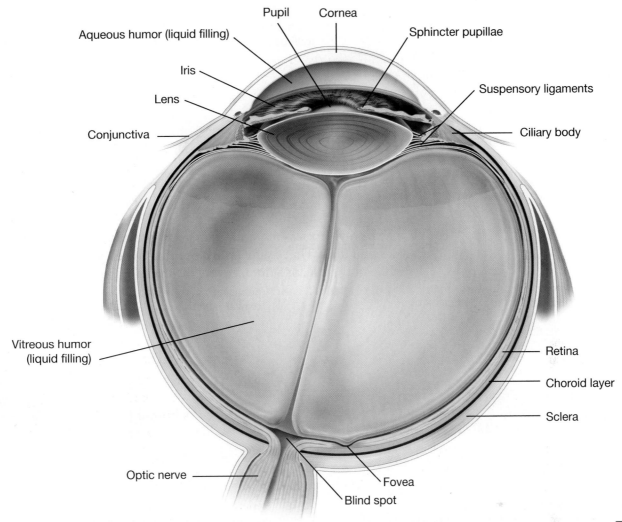

Figure 21.31   The structures of the eye. Which structure limits the amount of light that enters the eye?

Label Art

wrong area of the eye, resulting in blurry vision (Figure 21.32 on the next page). Myopia [*my* = muscle, *opia* = condition of the eye], known as *nearsightedness*, results from an eyeball that is too curved or too long. If the eye is too flat or too short, hyperopia [*hyper* = more than normal, *opia* = condition of the eye], or *farsightedness*, occurs. An astigmatism [*a* = without, *stigmat* = mark or place, *ism* = condition] results when an eye is irregular in shape. Glasses, contact lenses, or refractive surgery can correct vision by changing the focal point.

The **choroid**, located at the back of the eye, is a membrane that supplies blood to the eye and controls the light reflected to the retina. "Red eye" occurs in photos when the flash of a camera reflects off the blood-filled retina at the back of the eye. Melanin is a pigment in the choroid that gives the iris its color and absorbs excess light reflection. The less melanin, the lighter the eye color, and the more sensitive the person will be to light. The absence of melanin, in the case of albinism, causes low vision in bright light and abnormal development of the retina.

Two types of photoreceptors—rods and cones—in the retina interpret light as a visual image. Rods are the most sensitive to light. They are

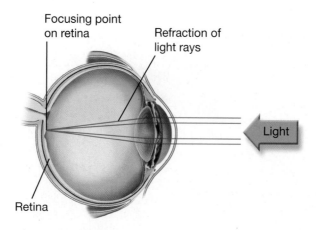

Focusing point
on retina

Refraction of
light rays

Light

Retina

A   Normal vision:
light rays focus on the retina

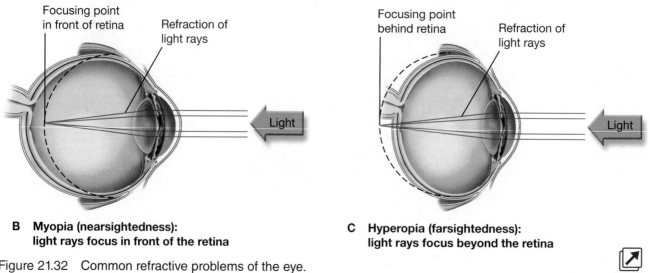

Focusing point
in front of retina

Refraction of
light rays

Light

B   Myopia (nearsightedness):
light rays focus in front of the retina

Focusing point
behind retina

Refraction of
light rays

Light

C   Hyperopia (farsightedness):
light rays focus beyond the retina

Figure 21.32   Common refractive problems of the eye.

Animation

concentrated in an area called the *macula* at the back of the retina. They can pick up images in dim light but do not provide fine detail. A loss of rod function results in night blindness. Macular degeneration, in which the macula is damaged, can make the center of your field of vision look blurry, dark, or distorted. It is the leading cause of blindness in older adults.

Cones are the photoreceptors that interpret color and take in small details. Cones are most concentrated in the fovea at the center of the macula. Red, green, and blue cone receptors each respond to a different range of light wavelengths. Problems with color vision are usually hereditary. The genes for red and green cones are both on the X chromosome, so red-green color blindness affects about 8 percent of males but only 0.5 percent of females.

Each eye gathers information from its own visual field. More than a million axons carry visual information from the eyes to the brain. The blind spot, where the optic nerve leaves the eye, has no room for photoreceptors. The axons join at the optic chiasma. Stem cell research has generated new photoreceptors for the eye, so new cures for blindness may be on the horizon.

RECALL YOUR READING

1. The variety of _____ in the skin allows us to distinguish between pain, _____, and vibration.
2. The five basic tastes, which are detected by _____ on the tongue, are sweet, salty, _____, bitter, and _____.
3. The _____ bulb sorts messages from _____ in the olfactory cilia.
4. Hearing is the result of the ears changing _____ into _____, which are converted into _____ that are sent to the brain.
5. Light enters the eye at the _____ and passes through the _____ and _____ before reaching the lens.

Complete the *Map Your Reading* graphic organizer for the section you just read.

The Endocrine System

The endocrine [*endo* = inside or within, *crine* = to secrete] system is an important control mechanism for the body (Figure 21.33). It works closely with the nervous system to stimulate, regulate, and coordinate activities to maintain homeostasis. Maintaining this stable system allows the body to function most efficiently. While the nervous system tends to produce a rapid, short-lived response with electrical stimuli, the endocrine system works much more slowly and over a longer period of time.

The Use of Hormones for Communication

Endocrine glands produce and secrete **hormones**, which are chemical messengers for the body. They regulate growth and metabolism, maintain fluid and chemical balances, and control sexual processes. The endocrine glands are located in many different areas around the body. Figure 21.34 on the next page lists some of the hormones and effects produced by endocrine glands. Hormones communicate their messages to different organs than those in which they are produced.

Endocrine glands don't have ducts, so hormones are secreted directly into the bloodstream. Each hormone is designed to cause a response in a specific target organ. The hormone must travel through the circulatory system from where it is produced to the target organ. When it reaches the target organ, the hormone locks onto cell receptors, then sends its chemical instructions into the cell (Figure 21.35 on page 757). This takes much longer than the direct nerve stimulus action of the nervous system.

Blood screening can measure the amount of a hormone or other substance controlled by the endocrine system that is present in the body. Because blood is filtered by the urinary system, urine tests can also be used to assess hormone levels. Reagent strips change color to indicate

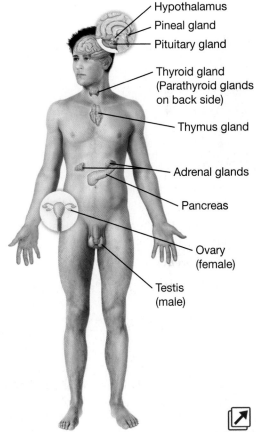

Hypothalamus
Pineal gland
Pituitary gland
Thyroid gland
(Parathyroid glands on back side)
Thymus gland
Adrenal glands
Pancreas
Ovary (female)
Testis (male)

Label Art

Figure 21.33   The major organs and glands of the endocrine system.

hormone
a chemical used to send messages from an endocrine gland to a target organ

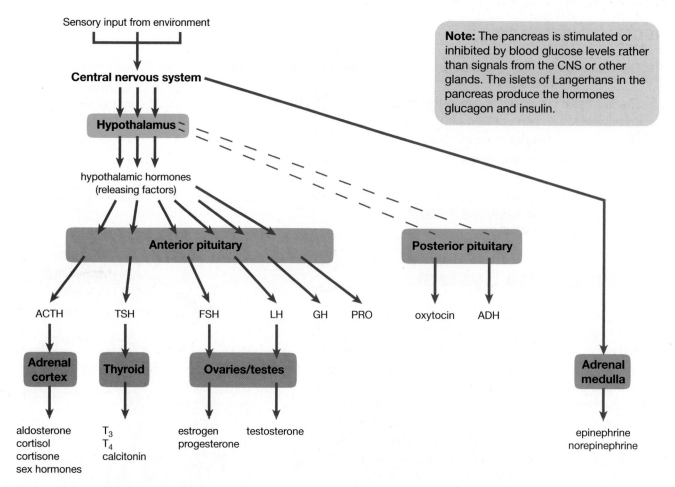

Figure 21.34   Hormones are sent to organs other than the ones in which they originated. Where are hormones from the anterior pituitary sent?

the amount of a hormone or other body substance in the urine (see Figure 18.23).

Under- or overproduction of hormones can cause physical problems. Because the endocrine system is slow acting, symptoms of an endocrine disorder may take years to develop or become noticeable. Acromegaly (ak-roh-MEHG-uh-lee) [*acr* = extremities, *megaly* = enlargement] is a condition characterized by an oversecretion of growth hormone, usually caused by a tumor of the pituitary gland. This most commonly results in enlarged bones in the hands, feet, and face. The condition may go undiagnosed in adults because they are not screened for growth changes as regularly as children are.

Sometimes, people take additional hormones that are not produced by their own body. For instance, women in menopause may use hormone replacement therapy to counteract their decreasing estrogen level. Anabolic steroid abuse is a growing problem among athletes and teens. It is illegal to use these synthetic testosterone hormones without a prescription. They can cause unpleasant physical changes, such as shrunken testicles, development of breast tissue, acne, body hair growth, and baldness. In addition, they can have serious health consequences, such as weight gain, blood clots, high blood pressure, liver damage, and even cancer.

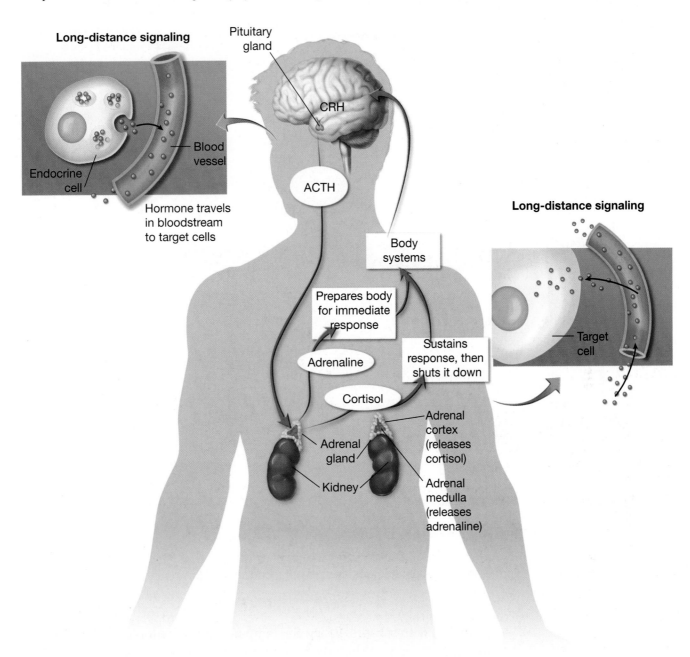

Long-distance signaling

Pituitary gland

CRH

ACTH

Blood vessel

Endocrine cell

Hormone travels in bloodstream to target cells

Body systems

Prepares body for immediate response

Adrenaline

Sustains response, then shuts it down

Cortisol

Long-distance signaling

Target cell

Adrenal gland

Kidney

Adrenal cortex (releases cortisol)

Adrenal medulla (releases adrenaline)

Figure 21.35   Hormones travel through the circulatory system to reach their target organ.

Hormones work to maintain homeostasis. Blood chemistry, nerve stimulation, or hormones from other glands tell an endocrine gland to release its hormone when the system is out of balance. Many hormones occur in antagonistic pairs that work in opposition to each other, such as insulin and glucagon. They may also operate on a **negative feedback system**. This system reverses a condition that is above the normal range to restore homeostasis.

When a body activity is out of balance, a hormone is released to encourage the activity to change (Figure 21.36 on the next page). When the activity level is high enough, hormone production ends or another hormone is triggered to decrease the activity. This is similar to the action of a home heating system. Suppose the thermostat is set at 70°F and is

negative feedback system
mechanism that reduces a body function in response to a stimulus, such as a hormone

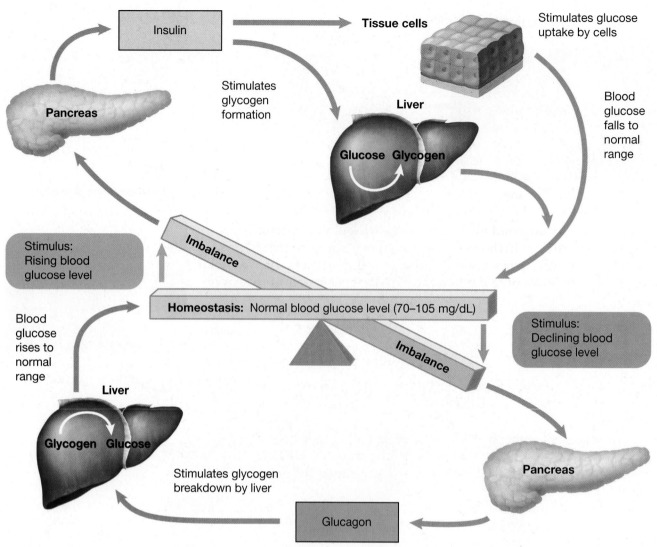

Figure 21.36   Hormones help the body maintain homeostasis, or balanced levels. How does insulin contribute to this process?

Animation

equipped with sensors. When the temperature drops too far below 70°F, the heat comes on. When the temperature rises to a point at or above 70°F, the heat shuts off. Endocrine glands act in a similar way to keep body systems in balance.

Connection to the Nervous System

The nervous system and endocrine system are linked by the hypothalamus gland. The hypothalamus is located beneath the thalamus in the center of the brain. It encourages or discourages the activity of the pituitary gland.

The **pituitary gland** is called the *master gland* because it releases hormones that affect the operation of many other glands in the body. This small gland is attached to the brain by a short stalk just below the hypothalamus. The pituitary gland has two parts, an anterior lobe and a posterior lobe. Hormones produced in the anterior lobe control activities of the thyroid, adrenal, and reproductive glands. The posterior lobe does not produce its own hormones, but it does store hormones produced by the hypothalamus and releases them when stimulated by nerve impulses.

Functions of Endocrine Glands

There are many different glands in the endocrine system. The **thyroid gland** is the largest endocrine gland in the body. It is made up of two lobes that sit like a bowtie on either side of the larynx. This gland controls energy, metabolism, and calcium levels in the blood. It requires iodine to produce its hormone. To get enough iodine in our diets, we use iodized table salt. When the body struggles to make thyroid hormone, a swelling around the neck called a *goiter* may develop.

Four tiny **parathyroid glands** sit on the back of the thyroid. They help balance calcium in the blood by secreting a hormone that triggers the release of calcium from bones. Calcium is important in many cellular activities. Low levels of calcium in the blood trigger spontaneous nerve impulses and muscle contractions.

The **adrenal glands** are located just above the kidneys and have two parts that function separately. The adrenal cortex on the outer surface produces a small amount of sex hormones. This becomes important when a woman reaches menopause and stops producing sex hormones from the ovaries. The inner part of the adrenal gland, the adrenal medulla, makes two important hormones, epinephrine (ehp-ih-NEHF-rihn) and norepinephrine.

The release of epinephrine, or *adrenaline*, and norepinephrine is triggered by the sympathetic nervous system when we are stressed, producing the "fight-or-flight" response (Figure 21.37). The body prepares itself by increasing the heart and respiration rates, making glucose available for energy, increasing muscle contractions, and slowing other body processes. People have been known to perform superhuman feats of strength in response to stress, such as lifting a car off a person being crushed. After the stress has passed, the parasympathetic nervous system

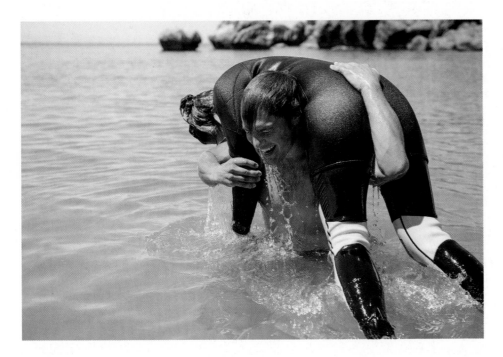

Figure 21.37   The release of adrenaline in stressful or emergency situations can allow people to perform amazing feats, such as rescuing a drowning person.

returns the body to its "rest-and-digest" mode. What regulation system is this an example of?

The pancreas secretes hormones that are important during digestion. This endocrine and digestive organ sits under the stomach. It secretes digestive enzymes into the duodenum and hormones into the bloodstream. Clusters of cells on the pancreas, called **islets of Langerhans**, make the hormones insulin and glucagon. Insulin is produced when blood sugar levels are high. This hormone helps move sugar into the cells for use and lowers the body's blood sugar level. Glucagon responds to low blood sugar by helping the liver convert glycogen back to glucose. This raises the blood sugar level.

Diabetes mellitus is a chronic illness caused by decreased sensitivity to or secretion of insulin. Type 1 diabetes, or *juvenile diabetes*, begins in childhood and usually requires regular insulin injections. Type 2 diabetes, or *adult-onset diabetes*, generally begins later and is more common in people who are overweight. Symptoms of excessive thirst, frequent urination, fatigue, and slow healing may go undiagnosed for many years. Type 2 diabetes has become an epidemic and is even occurring in children due to obesity (Figure 21.38). It can often be controlled through diet and exercise. The buildup of sugar in the tissues caused by diabetes can slowly damage the blood vessels, kidneys, and nerves. It also slows healing and leads to nerve disorders such as neuropathy and detachment of the retina.

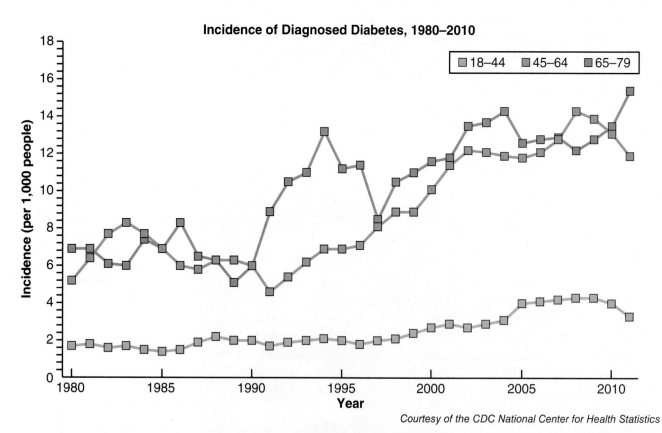

Courtesy of the CDC National Center for Health Statistics

Figure 21.38   The incidence of diabetes diagnosis, grouped by age. Which age group had the most diagnosed cases of diabetes after 2010?

Several other glands also serve both the endocrine system and another body system. The thymus is a collection of lymph tissue that lies in the center of the chest. It produces thymosin, which plays an important role in the immune system's production and development of T-cell lymphocytes. The kidneys produce erythropoietin when blood oxygen is low. This hormone tells the bone marrow to make more red blood cells. Cells in the mucous lining of the stomach and intestines also have endocrine functions. They produce hormones that influence digestive secretions and the movement of substances through the intestines.

The reproductive system uses hormones to regulate the development of sexual characteristics, the production of gametes, and the reproductive cycle. In women, the ovaries produce estrogen and progesterone that prepare the uterus for pregnancy, regulate menstruation, and develop secondary sexual characteristics such as breast tissue and body fat. During pregnancy, the placenta is a temporary endocrine gland that produces progesterone and human chorionic gonadotropin (hCG). These hormones maintain the pregnancy and tell the breasts when to release milk.

In men, the testes produce testosterone, which is responsible for the development and maintenance of male sexual characteristics. Testosterone supports the development of the testes, increased growth of bones and muscles, enlargement of the larynx, growth of body hair, and increased male sex drive.

There are inherited differences in sensitivity to hormone production. For example, hirsutism is a condition characterized by excessive facial and body hair in women caused by an inherited oversensitivity to testosterone. Endocrinologists specialize in diagnosing and treating hormone imbalances. Pharmacogenetics [*pharmac* = drugs, *gen* = production] focuses on predicting and improving individual metabolic responses to new treatments.

As the body ages, a decrease in hormones may affect sleep patterns, bone density, digestion, urinary function, and regulation of other body activities. Hormones are broken down more slowly in older people than in younger people. With age, the body also becomes less able to handle stress.

RECALL YOUR READING

1. _____ help regulate _____ and metabolism, maintain _____ and _____ balance, and control _____ processes.

2. Under- or overproduction of hormones can cause physical problems, such as _____, which is caused by oversecretion of growth hormone.

3. The _____ system reverses a condition that has exceeded the normal range for homeostasis.

4. The _____ gland has two parts—a(n) _____ lobe and a(n) _____ lobe.

5. The release of _____ and _____ results in a "fight-or-flight" response.

Complete the *Map Your Reading* graphic organizer for the section you just read.

SUMMARY

↗ Assess your understanding with chapter tests

- Time management, good study habits, self-advocacy, and test preparation skills can help you reach your goals when studying challenging material.

- The nervous system and the endocrine system are the body's two main pathways for communication and maintaining homeostasis.

- The central nervous system includes the brain and spinal cord. The peripheral nervous system includes the nerves that extend out to the rest of the body.

- Neurons connect the nervous system. Their basic structures include a cell body, an axon, terminal branches and dendrites, and a myelin sheath.

- Sensory, or *afferent*, neurons gather information from the body. Motor, or *efferent*, neurons signal a response.

- The forebrain includes the frontal, parietal, temporal, and occipital lobes of each hemisphere. The midbrain includes the thalamus, hypothalamus, and pineal gland.

- The hindbrain includes the cerebellum and brainstem.

- The CNS is protected by the meninges, the blood-brain barrier, bones, and cerebrospinal fluid. Despite these protections, birth defects, diseases, and injuries can cause paralysis.

- Nerves are named for their location and function. There are 12 pairs of cranial nerves and 31 pairs of spinal nerves.

- The senses use special sensory receptors to gather information. Pain, pressure, vibration, stretch, and temperature are all sensed by different receptors in the skin.

- A change in the senses can impact a person's ability to communicate and gather information from their environment.

- Hormones each have a different function in regulating body growth, development, and many system functions. They operate in antagonistic pairs on a negative feedback system to keep the body in homeostasis.

MAXIMIZE YOUR PROFESSIONAL VOCABULARY

↗ Build vocabulary with e-flash cards, games, and audio glossary

Listed below are the essential, yellow-highlighted terms and the additional professional vocabulary that you encountered in this chapter. Complete the activities that follow the list to make all of these terms part of your everyday professional vocabulary.

adrenal glands	dendrites	midbrain
afferent	efferent	myelin
aqueous humor	forebrain	negative feedback system
axon	frontal lobes	neuron
brainstem	ganglion	neurotransmitter
cell body	hindbrain	occipital lobes
central nervous system (CNS)	homeostasis	olfactory bulb
cerebellum	hormone	ossicles
cerebral cortex	hypothalamus	papillae
cerebrum	innervate	paralysis
choroid	islets of Langerhans	parathyroid glands
cochlea	lens	parietal lobes
cornea	meninges	peripheral nervous system (PNS)
cranial nerves	mental health	

pituitary gland	reflex	terminal branches
plexus	sclera	thalamus
primary motor cortex	spinal nerves	thyroid gland
primary sensory cortex	synapse	tympanic membrane
pupil	taste bud	vestibular canals
receptor	temporal lobes	vitreous humor

VOCABULARY DEVELOPMENT

Matching. Match the essential terms from this chapter with the best descriptions below by writing the letter of the description next to the number of the essential term on your answer sheet.

1. central nervous system (CNS)
2. cerebrum
3. homeostasis
4. hormone
5. myelin
6. negative feedback system
7. neuron
8. neurotransmitter
9. peripheral nervous system (PNS)
10. primary motor cortex
11. primary sensory cortex
12. receptor

a. a fatty layer that protects the axons of some nerves
b. the largest part of the brain, which is formed by the four lobes of the cerebral cortex
c. term for the sensory and motor nerves that go out to the body's extremities
d. a nerve cell that receives stimuli
e. an area of the parietal lobe dedicated to gathering and interpreting information regarding the five senses of the body from afferent neurons
f. the part of the nervous system that is made up of the brain and spinal cord
g. a nerve cell
h. a chemical used to carry a signal from an axon to a receptor cell to pass along a message
i. an area of the frontal lobe that directs muscle movement through efferent neurons to muscles in the body
j. a chemical used to send messages from an endocrine gland to a target organ
k. mechanism that reduces a body function in response to a stimulus, such as a hormone
l. a state of balance between interdependent elements

13. **Term Connections.** Make term cards for the word parts in the table shown on the next page. Play *Term Connections* using the following directions:

- Shuffle together two sets of term cards for every three players joining the game. Pass out seven cards to each player and place the remainder in the center as a "draw pile." Turn over the first card from the draw pile and place it term-side up to begin playing.
- The player to the left of the dealer goes first. Each player will attempt to get rid of his or her cards by discarding a term card that matches or coordinates with the card that is showing on the discard pile.
- A discard may "coordinate" with your term card if it has the same meaning, relates

to the same part of the body, or rhymes with it. Stretch your brain to come up with creative connections!

- If the card is challenged by the entire group, then it must be placed back in the player's hand and a penalty card must be drawn.
- If a player is unable to find a coordinating card in his or her hand, the player must also draw a card.
- If play goes all the way around the group without anyone being able to play, then a new card may be turned over from the draw pile and play continues.
- The winner is the first player to get rid of his or her cards, or the player with the fewest cards left at the end of play time.

Medical Word Parts			
Prefixes	**Root Words**		**Suffixes**
en-	acr/o	ocul/o	-algesia
extra-	aqu/a	olfact/o	-ar
hemi-	brachi/o	ophthalm/o	-crine
para-	cephal/o	papill/o	-icle
	cerebr/o	pharmac/o	-ism
	cervic/o	scler/o	-megaly
	dendr/o	som/a	-opia
	gangli/o	somat/o	-pathy
	gust/o	stigmat/o	-plegia
	neur/o		

REFLECT ON YOUR READING

14. Review the Vocabulary Sorting Organizer you created for the *Connect with Your Reading* activity. Select five terms from the "New Terms" column. Create a multiple choice question for each term and write them on a note card, using the text to create distracting options for the answers. They should be close to correct but have important differences from the correct answer. The distracters may also lead the test taker to confuse one term with another similar or related term. Write the correct answer on the back of the card. Give the note cards to your teacher for a class review activity.

BUILD CORE SKILLS

15. **Reading.** Reread the sections in this chapter that compare the endocrine and nervous systems. How are they alike? How are they different? Find an example from the chapter for each system that supports your answers.

16. **Critical Thinking.** Using your knowledge of brain structures, answer the following questions. What is the value of wearing quality helmets for sports like football, snowboarding, or bicycling? From a medical perspective, what types of brain injuries could be avoided by using a helmet?

17. **Critical Thinking.** Which type of sensory deficit or loss would have the largest impact on your social life and acceptance by others? Why? Explain your response.

18. **Writing.** Do research to identify biological and chemical processes that maintain homeostasis. Write a three to five paragraph paper describing your examples.

19. **Problem Solving.** In the endocrine system, what is the role of the thyroid gland? What are the potential effects of a thyroid hormone imbalance? When the body is out of balance, what is a common cause and how can you help the body return to homeostasis?

20. **Math.** Healthcare workers need to be able to read and interpret information presented in graphs and charts. What information can you gather from Figure 21.38? What conclusions can you draw? What questions come to mind when you read this information?

21. **Math.** Use the Internet to investigate when items such as video games, the World Wide Web, and smartphones became popular. Plot these dates on a graph. Compare

the graph you've created to Figure 21.38. Then discuss how these and other historic events may have affected the occurrence of diabetes.

ACTIVATE YOUR LEARNING

22. Experience a simulation that shows how the senses or muscle control can be compromised with age or illness. Work in pairs, switching roles so that each person is able to perform the tasks. Record and share your results with the class. Which activities best simulated the feeling of having a disability? How did that make you feel?

   - Vision—Put petroleum jelly on sunglasses to simulate the loss of transparency and ability to focus the lens due to aging or disease. Then perform simple tasks like reading or tying a shoe while wearing the sunglasses.

   - Speech—Chew two pieces of bubble gum while reading a selection from a book out loud to simulate the potential effects of a stroke on muscles required for speech.

   - Hearing—Walk through a hallway with cotton balls or earplugs in your ears to block the transmission of sound waves. Then walk through the same hallway without anything in your ears and pay close attention to any sounds you missed the first time. To increase your focus on hearing, try this blindfolded with a partner silently guiding you.

   - Touch—Perform simple tasks such as writing your name, using a cell phone, or buttoning a shirt with your non-dominant hand to simulate retraining of the brain that is needed following a stroke. You can also complete these activities after wrapping your finger joints with aluminum foil and then covering them with the gloves to simulate arthritis.

   - Taste—Suck on a peppermint or wintergreen candy, or chew a fresh piece of mint gum for two to three minutes. Spit the candy or gum out, then put on a blindfold and have your partner offer you water flavored with small amounts of spices or drink mixes. Were you able to distinguish the flavors offered?

   - Pain—Tape a few kernels of unpopped popcorn to the bottom of your sock at the toes, ball, or heel of the foot. Try walking to simulate the effects of bunions, corns, or arthritis.

   - Mobility—Place a clean, unsharpened pencil in your mouth with the eraser hanging out. Use the eraser to turn the pages of a magazine and type your name on a keyboard without the use of your hands.

THINK AND ACT LIKE A HEALTHCARE WORKER

23. Richard is an audiologist who works with older adults to check their hearing capabilities. Use the speech banana in Figure 21.26 to help him determine which words from the following list use sounds that his patients will be likely to lose first:

   - wish
   - hello
   - coffee
   - animal
   - catch
   - today

GO TO THE SOURCE

24. Review Figure 21.10. Visit the National Institute of Mental Health website and the Mayo Clinic website. Use the information there to answer the following questions.

   - What are additional facts about depression not covered in the textbook?

   - Select one of the forms of depression. What are signs and symptoms of this particular depression? What are some potential causes? Who is most at risk? How is it diagnosed? What treatments are recommended?

   - How could you best support someone experiencing depression?

Photo Credits

Figure 10.30 Body Scientific International, LLC; Figure 10.31A Paul Stringer/Shutterstock.com; Figure 10.31B Roman Sotola/Shutterstock.com; Figure 10.31C Courtesy of Ennovation CO; Figure 10.32 Life in View/Science Source; Erin Highwaystarz-Photography/iStock/Thinkstock; Figure 10.33A 360b/Shutterstock.com; Figure 10.33B 360b/Shutterstock.com; Figure 10.34A Wavebreakmedia Ltd/Wavebreak Media/Thinkstock; Figure 10.34B wavebreakmedia/Shutterstock.com; Figure 10.35A RetroClipArt/Shutterstock.com; Figure 10.35B Dn Br/Shutterstock.com; Figure 10.35C hvezdap4/Shutterstock.com; Figure 10.36A Courtesy of the American Red Cross; Figure 10.36B Courtesy of the American Red Cross; Figure 10.37 Monkey Business Images/Shutterstock.com; Figure 10.38 iofoto/Shutterstock.com; Figure 10.39 bevangoldswain/iStock.Thinkstock; Figure 10.40 Firma V/Shutterstock.com; Figure 10.41 Monkey Business Images/Shutterstock.com; Stacy Wards Forest Media, LLC. **Chapter 11:** Figure 11.0 Rocketclips, Inc./Shutterstock.com; Trinity kurhan/Shutterstock.com; Figure 11.1A Geo Martinez/Shutterstock.com; Figure 11.1B wavebreakmedia/Shutterstock.com; Figure 11.1C Darren Baker/Shutterstock.com; Figure 11.1D Copyright © CMSP / Custom Medical Stock Photo — All rights reserved. Figure 11.4 ybonce/Shutterstock.com; Figure 11.5 monkeybusinessimages/iStock/Thinkstock; Figure 11.8A Kzenon/Shutterstock.com; Figure 11.8B © Daryl Visscher/arabianEye/Corbis; Figure 11.8C Olga Rosi/Shutterstock.com; Figure 11.11 Rocketclips, Inc./Shutterstock.com; Figure 11.13 artemisphoto/Shutterstock.com; Celia Stock-Asso/Shutterstock.com; Figure 11.14 ChameleonsEye/Shutterstock.com; Figure 11.17 Wavebreakmedia Ltd/Lightwavemedia/Thinkstock; Figure 11.20 ©Ortho Clinical Diagnostics Inc. 2009, VITROS 3600 Immunodiagnostics System is a trademark of Ortho Clinical Diagnostics Inc.; Figure 11.21 © Karen Kasmauski/Science Faction/Corbis; Figure 11.23 monkeybusinessimages/iStock/Thinkstock; Figure 11.26 Incombile/Shutterstock.com. **Chapter 12:** Figure 12.0 science photo/Shutterstock.com; Figure 12.1 Lisa F. Young/Shutterstock.com; Figure 12.2 Tyler Olson/Shutterstock.com; Figure 12.3 hightowernrw/Shutterstock.com; Figure 12.4 Tyler Olson/Shutterstock.com; Figure 12.5 Ingram Publishing/Thinkstock; Figure 12.6 cobalt88/Shutterstock.com; Figure 12.7 Huntstock/Thinkstock; Figure 12.8 Bork/Shutterstock.com; Figure 12.9 Chaikom/Shutterstock.com; Figure 12.12 PrinceOfLove/Shutterstock.com; Figure 12.14 Elena Elisseeva/Shutterstock.com; Figure 12.15 sfam_photo/Shutterstock.com; Figure 12.16 Dmitry Kalinovsky/Shutterstock.com. **Chapter 13:** Figure 13.0 Mike Watson Images/moodboard/Thinkstock; Figure 13.1 wavebreakmedia/Shutterstock.com; Figure 13.2 CandyBox Images/Shutterstock.com; Figure 13.3 Body Scientific International, LLC; Figure 13.5 Body Scientific International, LLC; Figure 13.6 Body Scientific International, LLC; Figure 13.7 Body Scientific International, LLC; Figure 13.8 Body Scientific International, LLC; Figure 13.9 Body Scientific International, LLC; Figure 13.10 Monkey Business Images/Shutterstock.com; Figure 13.11 Monkey Business Images/Shutterstock.com; Figure 13.12A iStackphotons/iStock/Thinkstock; Figure 13.12B Peeradach Rattanakoses/Shutterstock.com; Figure 13.12C Andre Nantel/Shutterstock.com; Figure 13.12D micro_photo/iStock/Thinkstock; Figure 13.12E MichaelTaylor3d/Shutterstock.com; Figure 13.12F defun/iStock/Thinkstock; Figure 13.13 Laurent/Science Source; Figure 13.14 Body Scientific International, LLC; Figure 13.15 Body Scientific International, LLC; Figure 13.16 Gila Photography/Shutterstock.com; Figure 13.17 Photographee.eu/Shutterstock.com; Figure 13.18 Dr. H.C. Robinson / Science Source; Figure 13.19 Body Scientific International, LLC; Figure 13.20 Body Scientific International, LLC; Figure 13.21 Body Scientific International, LLC; Figure 13.22 Stockbyte/Stockbyte/Thinkstock; Figure 13.23 Body Scientific International, LLC; Figure 13.24 Body Scientific International, LLC; Figure 13.25 Lisa F. Young/Shutterstock.com. **Unit 4 Opener** Courtesy of Lauren Elm, Director of Public and Community Relations, Shriners Hospitals for Children—Twin Cities. **Chapter 14:** Figure 14.0 Courtesy of Beth Israel Deaconess Medical Center; Gloria spwidoff/Shutterstock.com; Figure 14.1 mangostock/Shutterstock.com; Figure 14.3 wavebreakmedia/Shutterstock.com; Figure 14.5 Andrey_Popov/Shutterstock.com; Figure 14.6 Dmitry Kalinovsky/Shutterstock.com; Figure 14.7 Guy Shapira/Shutterstock.com; Figure 14.9 Robert Kneschke/Shutterstock.com; Figure 14.11 Iakov Filimonov/Shutterstock.com; Figure 14.12 Robert Kneschke/Shutterstock.com; Figure 14.13 Monkey Business Images/Shutterstock.com; Figure 14.15 Andresr/Shutterstock.com; Figure 14.18 Wisconsin Department of Health; Figure 14.19 Monkey Business Images/Shutterstock.com; Figure 14.20 Wards Forest Media, LLC.; Figure 14.21A Africa Studio/Shutterstock.com; Figure 14.21C val lawless/Shutterstock.com; Figure 14.21E Wards Forest Media, LLC.; Figure 14.21F Mario7/Shutterstock.com; Allie USDA, Photo by Stephen Ausmus; Figure 14.27 Alexander Raths/Shutterstock.com; Figure 14.29 Wards Forest Media, LLC.; Figure 14.30 Wards Forest Media, LLC.; Figure 14.35 bikeriderlondon/Shutterstock.com; Figure 14.36 DenisNata/Shutterstock.com; Marco Syda Productions/Shutterstock.com; Figure 14.40 TFoxFoto/Shutterstock.com; Jean Edyta Pawlowska/Shutterstock.com; Jake Sabphoto/Shutterstock.com; Figure 14.42 Fer Gregory/Shutterstock.com; Figure 14.43 Aaron Amat/Shutterstock.com. **Chapter 15:** Figure 15.0 Wavebreakmedia Ltd/ Wavebreak Media/Thinkstock; Figure 15.1 Creatas/Creatas/Thinkstock; Salina Blend Images/Shutterstock.com; Figure 15.2 Ammentorp Photography/Shutterstock.com; Figure 15.3 *Dietary Guidelines for Americans*, 2010, Tischenko Irina/Shutterstock.com, Brian Chase/Shutterstock.com; Figure 15.5 *Dietary Guidelines for Americans*, 2010; Figure 15.6 ©iStock.com/KatarzynaBialasiewicz; Figure 15.9 Blend Images/Shutterstock.com; Beth ©iStock.com/monkeybusinessimages; Figure 15.10 © Bernd Wüstneck/dpa/Corbis; Figure 15.11 RFID reader; Courtesy of Bradford Systems; Figure 15.12 Goodheart-Willcox, Inc.; Figure 15.13 SuperTracker example; Courtesy of the USDA; Gerry PathDoc/Shutterstock.com; Figure 15.14 Wards Forest Media, LLC.; Figure 15.15 Courtesy of the USDA; Figure 15.18 Photographs taken by Susan Blahnik; Figure 15.19 © Medline Industries, Inc., 2013; Figure 15.20A Rob Byron/Shutterstock.com; Figure 15.20B Rob Byron/Shutterstock.com; Figure 15.20C MARGRIT HIRSCH/Shutterstock.com; Figure 15.22 Maxx-Studio/Shutterstock.com. **Chapter 16:** Figure 16.0 Alexander Raths/Shutterstock.com; Figure 16.1 Monkey Business Images/Shutterstock.com; Figure 16.2 Lopolo/Shutterstock.com; Figure 16.3 Tyler Olson/Shutterstock.com; Figure 16.4 Monkey Business Images/Shutterstock.com; Figure 16.5 Copyright © ASL Services, Inc. and www.ASLServices.com, 2010–2014; Figure 16.6 Goodheart-Willcox, Inc.; Figure 16.7 Goodheart-Willcox, Inc.; Figure 16.8 Africa Studio/Shutterstock.com; Figure 16.9 wavebreakmedia/Shutterstock.com; Figure 16.10 Monkey Business Images/Shutterstock.com; Figure 16.11 Jupiterimages /Stockbyte/Thinkstock; Figure 16.13 David Buffington /Blend Images/Thinkstock; Figure 16.14 Monkey Business Images/Shutterstock.com; Figure 16.15 Wards Forest Media, LLC.; Figure 16.16 ©iStock.com/monkeybusinessimages; Figure 16.17 Goodheart-Willcox, Inc.; Figure 16.18 Goodheart-Willcox, Inc.; Figure 16.19 Thomas M Perkins/Shutterstock.com, Valeev/Shutterstock.com; Figure 16.20 Apples Eyes Studio/Shutterstock.com; Figure 16.21 Edwin Verin/Shutterstock.com; Figure 16.22 upixa/Shutterstock.com; Figure 16.23 ©iStock.com/Fotosmurf03; Figure 16.24 arnet117/Shutterstock.com. **Chapter 17:** Figure 17.0 ©iStock/monkeybusinessimages; Figure 17.1 wavebreakmedia/Shutterstock.com; Figure 17.2 Monkey Business Images/Shutterstock.com; Tyler wavebreakmedia/Shutterstock.com; Figure 17.4 Sandra Caldwell/Shutterstock.com; Figure 17.7 stockshoppe/Shutterstock.com; Figure 17.8 Body Scientific International, LLC; Figure 17.9 Body Scientific International, LLC; Figure 17.10 bikeriderlondon/Shutterstock.com; Figure 17.11 Cindy Minear/Shutterstock.com; Figure 17.12 Body Scientific International, LLC; Figure 17.13 Body Scientific International, LLC; Juanita Monkey Business Images/Shutterstock.com; Figure 17.14 Body Scientific International, LLC; Figure 17.15 gopixa/Shutterstock.com; Figure 17.16 Body Scientific International, LLC; Figure 17.17 Body Scientific International, LLC; Figure 17.18 Alexander Raths/Shutterstock.com; Figure 17.19 Body Scientific International, LLC; Figure 17.20 Nejron Photo/Shutterstock.com; Figure 17.21 Body Scientific International, LLC; Figure 17.22 Body Scientific International, LLC; Figure 17.23 Body Scientific International, LLC; Figure 17.24 XiXinXing/Shutterstock.com; Figure 17.25 sittipong/Shutterstock.com; Figure 17.26 Body Scientific International, LLC; Figure 17.27 Body Scientific International, LLC. **Unit 5 Opener** Photo by Leah Garczynski. **Chapter 18:** Figure 18.0 Dmitry Kalinovsky/Shutterstock.com; Annika Milkovasa/Shutterstock.com; Figure 18.1 Flashon Studio/Shutterstock.com; Figure 18.2 vitstudio/Shutterstock.com; Figure 18.4 anyaivanova/Shutterstock.com; Figure 18.6A Hank Morgan/Science Source; Figure 18.6B borzywoj/Shutterstock.com; Figure 18.7 ©iStock.com/Supersport; Figure 18.8 Belushi/Shutterstock.com; Figure 18.9 Monkey Business Images/Shutterstock.com; Jesse wavebreakmedia/Shutterstock.com; Margo Cheryl Savan/Shutterstock.com; Figure 18.13 David W. Leindecker/Shutterstock.com; Figure 18.14 Robert A. Levy/Shutterstock.com; Figure 18.15 R. Maisonneuve/Science Source; Figure 18.17A Ron Kloberdanz/Shutterstock.com; Figure 18.17B Dikiiy/Shutterstock.com; Figure 18.18 Wards Forest Media, LLC.; Figure 18.19 18percentgrey/Shutterstock.com; Figure 18.20 Goodheart-Willcox, Inc.; Figure 18.21 anaken2012/Shutterstock.com; Figure 18.22 Wards Forest Media, LLC.; Figure 18.23 Christina Richards/Shutterstock.com; Figure 18.24 Jarrod Erbe/Shutterstock.com; Figure 18.25 michaeljung/Shutterstock.com; Figure 18.26 Image Point Fr/Shutterstock.com; Figure 18.28 Kamil Macniak/Shutterstock.com; Figure 18.29 ©iStock.com/Rawpixel; Figure 18.30 AOTA President Florence Clark, PhD, OTR, FAOTA, presiding over a meeting of the American Occupational Therapy Association in 2013. Copyright American Occupational Therapy Association. Used with permission.; Sophia Tyler Olson/Shutterstock.com; Figure 18.31 Wards Forest Media, LLC.; HOSA logo appears courtesy of HOSA-Future Health Professionals; Figure 18.33 Courtesy of HOSA-Future Health Professionals. **Chapter 19:** Figure 19.0 Milkovasa/Shutterstock.com; Dr. Workman l i g h t p o e t/Shutterstock.com; Figure 19.2 wavebreakmedia/Shutterstock.com; Figure 19.3 Courtesy of HOSA-Future Health Professionals; Addison wavebreakmedia/Shutterstock.com; Figure 19.4 Goodheart-Willcox, Inc.; Figure 19.5 Goodheart-Willcox, Inc.; Figure 19.8 Copyright © 2013 Life Technologies Corporation. Used under permission.; Nina Matthew Ennis/Shutterstock.com; Figure 19.9 ©iStock.com/nebari; Figure 19.10 william casey/Shutterstock.com; Figure 19.13 Monkey Business Images/Shutterstock.com. **Chapter 20:** Figure 20.0 Sebastian Gauert/Shutterstock.com; Figure 20.1 Bullstar/Shutterstock.com; Figure 20.2 ©iStock/lculig; Figure 20.3 sylv1rob1/Shutterstock.com; Figure 20.4 Dmitry Kalinovsky/Shutterstock.com; Figure 20.5 Burlingham/Shutterstock.com; Figure 20.6 Zaharia Bogdan Rares/Shutterstock.com; Figure 20.7 Sebastian Kaulitzki/Shutterstock.com; Figure 20.8 JIMPhotography/Shutterstock.com; Figure 20.9 Gusto/Science Source; Figure 20.10 stefanolunardi/Shutterstock.com; Figure 20.11 ©iStock/monkeybusinessimages; Figure 20.12 science photo/Shutterstock.com; Figure 20.13 Alexander Raths/Shutterstock.com; Figure 20.14 Minerva Studio/Shutterstock.com; Figure 20.15 Tyler Olson/Shutterstock.com; Figure 20.16 Courtesy of Iowa State University Environmental Health and Safety; Figure 20.17 Everett Historical/Shutterstock.com. **Chapter 21:** Figure 21.0 ©2008 Intuitive Surgical, Inc.; Figure 21.1 Andresr/Shutterstock.com; Figure 21.2 Sperling, R., D. Greve, A. Dale, R. Killiany, J. Holmes, H. Rosas, A. Cocchiarella, P. Firth, B. Rosen, S. Lake, N. Lange, C. Routledge, and M. Albert. "Functional MRI Detection of Pharmacologically Induced Memory Impairment." Proceedings of the National Academy of Sciences 99.1 (2002): 455-60. Web. Copyright 2002 National Academy of Sciences, U.S.A.; Figure 21.3 Body Scientific International, LLC; Figure 21.4 Alila Medical Media/Shutterstock.com; Figure 21.5 Body Scientific International, LLC; Figure 21.6 Body Scientific International, LLC; Figure 21.7 Body Scientific International, LLC; Figure 21.8 Body Scientific International, LLC; Figure 21.9 Lisa S./Shutterstock.com; Figure 21.11 Photographee.eu/Shutterstock.com; Figure 21.12 Body Scientific International, LLC; Figure 21.13 Body Scientific International, LLC; Figure 21.14 Dmytro Vietrov/Shutterstock.com; Figure 21.15 Body Scientific International, LLC; Figure 21.17 Body Scientific International, LLC; Figure 21.18 Body Scientific International, LLC; Figure 21.19 Body Scientific International, LLC; Figure 21.20 Body Scientific International, LLC; Figure 21.21 Body Scientific International, LLC; Figure 21.22 Mendelex/Shutterstock.com; Figure 21.23 Body Scientific International, LLC; Figure 21.24 Body Scientific International, LLC; Figure 21.25 Body Scientific International, LLC; Figure 21.26 lineartestpilot/Shutterstock.com; Igor Zakowski/Shutterstock.com, Pixotico/Shutterstock.com; Schwarzhana/Shutterstock.com, OmniArt/Shutterstock.com, xanirakx/Shutterstock.com, Pretty Vectors/Shutterstock.com, RetroClipArt/Shutterstock.com, Macrovector/Shutterstock.com, bioraven/Shutterstock.com, Dooder/Shutterstock.com, art marta/Shutterstock.com, lavitrei/Shutterstock.com, kotss/Shutterstock.com, Johnny-ka/Shutterstock.com, Mario Boutin/Shutterstock.com; Figure 21.27 Capifrutta/Shutterstock.com; Figure 21.28 Kzenon/Shutterstock.com; Figure 21.29 Goodheart-Willcox, Inc.; Figure 21.30 Designua/Shutterstock.com; Figure 21.31 Body Scientific International, LLC; Figure 21.32 Body Scientific International, LLC; Figure 21.33 Body Scientific International, LLC; Figure 21.34 Body Scientific International, LLC; Figure 21.35 Body Scientific International, LLC; Figure 21.36 Body Scientific International, LLC; Figure 21.37 Roy Pedersen/Shutterstock.com; Figure 21.38 Goodheart-Willcox, Inc.

Glossary

24-hour clock   a method of telling time that assigns a number to each hour of the day; also known as *military time*

8 and 80 system   a system that allows an employee to work more than five 8-hour days in one week and fewer days in the following week without receiving overtime

A

abdominal quadrant   one of the four regions used to divide the abdomen into sections

abdominal region   one of nine equal areas of the abdomen that are named and used as reference points when discussing the body

abdominopelvic cavity   the part of the ventral cavity that lies below the diaphragm muscle; includes the abdominal cavity for the digestive organs and the pelvic cavity that houses the reproductive organs, bladder, and rectum

abduction   an action that moves a limb laterally away from the side of the body

absolute risk   ratio of the number of people who have a medical event to those who could have the event because of a medical condition

absorption   the act of taking up a substance into a tissue, such as the movement of nutrients from the small intestines into the bloodstream

abuse   an act that inflicts physical or emotional harm

accessory organs   organs attached to the alimentary canal, including the salivary glands, pancreas, and liver

accreditation   official recognition from a professional association that an educational program meets minimum educational standards for an occupation

acculturation   the process by which immigrants learn the beliefs and customs of the dominant culture and adopt some of them, while maintaining beliefs and customs of their own culture

acronyms   an abbreviation in which each letter stands for a word

addendum   a note that is added to correct an error, explains the new or corrected information, and gives a reason for the change

adduction   an action that returns a limb to the side of the body

adenoids   lymphatic tissues located behind the nose, which help protect against infection

adrenal glands   glands that are located just above the kidneys and contain two parts, the adrenal cortex and the adrenal medulla

advance directive   a legal document prepared by a patient before a health crisis occurs to guide healthcare decisions in situations when the patient is unable to speak for himself or herself

advocate   to promote or support

afferent   term that describes sensory transmitters that send impulses from receptors in the skin, muscles, and joints to the central nervous system

Affordable Care Act (ACA)   healthcare reform legislation that encourages the use of electronic health records and the electronic exchange of information and aims to extend coverage to uninsured Americans

Age Discrimination in Employment Act (ADEA)   a federal law that extends civil rights protection to workers 40 years of age and older

airborne precautions   practices used when an infection can be spread over a long distance and through air

algorithms   sets of rules that computers follow to process and analyze information

alimentary canal   a long, hollow tube that is made up of digestive organs and runs from the mouth to the anus

alternative, complementary, integrative therapies   healthcare practices and treatments that minimize or avoid the use of surgery and drugs

alveoli   tiny, hollow air sacs clustered like bunches of grapes at the ends of the bronchioles, which exchange gas with the surrounding capillaries

ambulatory care   nonemergency or outpatient services provided at walk-in clinics

Americans with Disabilities Act (ADA)   a federal law that extends civil rights protection to workers with physical or mental disabilities

amino acids   substances in proteins that provide the building blocks for the body to repair and make new cells

amputate   to cut off a limb or extremity, usually by surgical operation

anatomy   the physical structures or parts of the body

aneurysms   conditions characterized by weakened blood vessels, which can then burst

anterior   a directional term that refers to the front side of the body

antibiotics   medications used to control bacterial infections

antibodies   proteins produced by leukocytes that bind with and disable antigens

antigen   a foreign substance that causes the body to make antibodies

antioxidant   a substance that promotes good health by reducing cell deterioration and may contribute to disease prevention

apical pulse   a pulse measurement taken by listening over the apex (lower tip) of the heart using a stethoscope

apothecary system a system of measurement used by early pharmacists, or *apothecaries*, that is sometimes still used for herbal medicines

appendicular skeleton term that describes the bones of the arms and legs, including the shoulder and hip bones where they are attached

apps applications; software that is accessed through the Internet and runs on a computer, smartphone, tablet, or other mobile device

aptitude natural inclination

aqueous humor a clear fluid in the front of the eye that maintains pressure and nourishes the cornea and lens

artery a major blood vessel that moves blood from the heart out to the body tissues

aseptic techniques practices used by healthcare professionals to maintain a pathogen-free environment and prevent the transmission of disease

aspiration the inhalation of a liquid into the lungs

assault any words or actions that lead an individual to fear that another person intends to harm him or her

assay analysis done to determine the presence and amount of a substance or to determine the potency of a drug

assertive communication a communication style characterized by confidence and consideration for others

assess to evaluate

assessment evaluation

assignment of benefits the process in which adult patients sign a claim form, granting permission to release their medical information to the insurance company; the person carrying the insurance also signs the form, allowing payments to be made directly to the medical office

assimilation the process by which members of a new cultural group adopt all the beliefs and customs of the majority group

atrium a chamber at the top of the heart that receives blood from the veins

audiologist a professional who diagnoses hearing and balance problems and plans treatment

audiometer a machine that makes sounds at different frequencies to test hearing

auditory learner a person who uses sounds, rhythm, and music to store and recall information

auscultation the use of a stethoscope to listen to sounds made by a patient's internal organs to make a diagnosis

authenticate to give legal authority to

autoclaves chambers for sterilizing items with steam under pressure

automated analyzer a piece of equipment that can automatically sort and prepare samples for analysis

automated external defibrillator (AED) a device that delivers an electric shock to the heart to restore its normal rhythm

axial skeleton term that applies to the skull, spine, and rib cage, which rotate around an imaginary center line of the body

axon a long, tail-like projection on a neuron, which takes information from the cell body out to the muscles

B

Background Information Disclosure (BID) form an application that collects a prospective employee's past history

bacteria one-celled microorganisms that are so small they can only be seen under a microscope

ball-and-socket joint a joint that consists of the rounded head of a bone that fits into the cup-shaped cavity of another bone

bar code scanner a device that captures a printed series of numbered black bars and spaces, translates them into numbers and letters, and sends the data to a computer to access information about a patient or product

bar graph a chart that shows comparisons between categories of data

barred prevented

base rates measures that help researchers see the significance of a change that is given in percentages

battery the act of touching a person without his or her consent

benchmark a performance standard

benefits advantages or profits

bias a systematic error that produces a research finding that deviates from a valid finding

bile substance that helps mix fat with digestive enzymes so that it breaks down in the intestines

bioassay analysis done to determine the potency of a substance by measuring its effect on living tissues

bioethics the study of ethical practices in medical research and the use of advanced technology to treat patients

biohazard term that describes a biological agent, infectious organism, or insecure laboratory procedure that constitutes a danger to humans or the environment

bioinformatics a scientific discipline that combines the tools and techniques of mathematics, computer science, and biology to understand the biological significance of data

bioinformatics scientists researchers who use their computer skills to organize the expanding overload of data created by improved DNA sequencing technologies

biological safety cabinet (BSC) an enclosed laboratory workspace that filters and controls airflow to prevent chemical and biological material from being released into the air

biomedical engineer a person who applies his or her combined knowledge of biology and engineering to the design and development of products such as artificial organs, prostheses, and machines for diagnosing medical problems

bioreactor an apparatus in which a biological process is carried out

biorepositories libraries of biological information that may be accessed for medical research

biotechnology the manipulation of living organisms to produce useful products

biotechnology research laboratories research facilities that develop new products or treatments and are located on college campuses, in hospitals, and in private biotechnology companies

bladder a hollow, muscular organ that stores urine

blastocyst a fluid-filled cavity that develops in a morula

Bloodborne Pathogens Standard an OSHA regulation that protects employees from exposure to blood and other potentially infectious materials

blood pressure the force of blood pushing against the inside of the blood vessel (artery) walls

body alignment term used to describe a position of the body in which the spine is not crooked or twisted

body cavity a hollow space within the body that is lined by a membrane and contains bodily organs

body language nonverbal communication that occurs through conscious or unconscious gestures and movements

body mass index (BMI) a method of relating weight to height used to define normal weight, overweight, and obesity

body mechanics specific positions for muscles and joints that help a person avoid injury during a physical task

body plane a flat or level surface seen by cutting away part of the body through surgery or medical imaging to serve as a point of reference when discussing anatomy

body region an area of the body with a specific name, which is used as a reference point when discussing anatomy

body system a group of organs working together to perform a vital function in the body

brainstem area of the brain that controls the smooth muscles of the heart and lungs; also known as the *vital functions center*

breach access, use, or disclosure of protected health information that compromises the security or privacy of that information

bronchi tubes that branch out from the trachea into the right and left lungs

bronchioles tubes that branch out from the bronchi and travel down to the air sacs in the lungs

business letters formal letters written to people outside one's healthcare facility for a variety of purposes

business-to-business selling exchanging goods between businesses rather than between businesses and individuals

C

calibration the adjustment of a piece of equipment so that it operates within its intended standards of performance

calories the units used to measure energy gained from digestion

cancer uncontrolled cell growth

capillary bed a network of very small, thin-walled blood vessels (capillaries) located in body tissues

carcinogenic cancer-causing

cardiac arrest a condition in which a person's heart stops beating or does not beat well enough to circulate blood to the brain and other vital organs

cardiac muscle an involuntary, striated muscle tissue located in the walls of the heart

cardiopulmonary resuscitation (CPR) a procedure that keeps the brain and other vital organs supplied with oxygen until advanced medical care arrives

cardiovascular related to the heart and blood vessels

cardiovascular technologists healthcare workers who assist physicians in diagnosing heart and blood vessel disorders

career assessments tools such as questionnaires and surveys that you can use to find careers that will match your individual needs

career clusters groups of similar occupations and industries that share a core set of basic knowledge and skills for all workers

career ladder a sequence of job positions progressing from entry-level to higher levels of responsibility and authority based on education, experience, and performance

career pathways smaller groups of specialized occupations within a career cluster that require more specific sets of knowledge, skills, and training

career portfolio a written record of career planning and preparation

caregiver background form an application that collects information about a prospective healthcare employee's past

cartilage firm, whitish, flexible connective tissue found in various body parts, including where two bones meet to form a joint

case manager an RN who develops a care plan along with the client and his or her family and supervises the care being provided

catheters tube-shaped medical devices that can be inserted into blood vessels or body cavities for diagnostic and therapeutic purposes

caudal a directional term used to reference a point closer to the tailbone

cell a small group of organelles that fulfill a specific purpose and are held together by a membrane

cell body part of a neuron that contains the nucleus

cell membrane a semipermeable outer covering of a cell with holes that act as its doors and windows

Celsius scale a method of measuring temperature that is used in most healthcare facilities around the world (including many US facilities); also called the *Centigrade scale*

Centers for Disease Control and Prevention (CDC) a division of the HHS that focuses on disease outbreaks and prevention in the United States

Centers for Medicare and Medicaid Services (CMS) a division of the HHS provides health insurance for 100 million Americans under the Medicare program for the elderly and the Medicaid program for the poor

central nervous system (CNS) the brain and spinal cord

central services term for the hospital department responsible for receiving, storing, cleaning, disinfecting, sterilizing, and distributing medical and surgical supplies and equipment

centrifuge a machine with a rapidly rotating container, which is used to separate fluids

cerebellum the second-largest area of the brain, which coordinates incoming and outgoing messages to produce smooth skeletal movements

cerebral cortex the outer surface of the cerebrum, which has many bumps and grooves

cerebrum the largest part of the brain, which is formed by the four lobes of the cerebral cortex

certification a credential that is typically voluntary and is created by a professional association

certified nursing assistant (CNA) a healthcare worker who completes a nursing assisting class and passes a certification test; works under the supervision of a nurse

cervix the narrow neck at the bottom of the uterus that connects to the vagina

chain of command term for the hierarchy of authority that establishes the flow of decision making and directives

chain of infection the elements required for an infection to spread from one source to another

charting the process of recording observations and information about patients

choroid a membrane that supplies blood to the eye and controls the light reflected to the retina

chronic refers to a disease or condition that is long-lasting and potentially lifelong

chyme a mixture of food and acid

cilia tiny hairs in the mucous membranes that filter out dirt and foreign material, sweeping it toward the throat

circle graph a chart that shows the relationship of parts of a data set to the whole; also known as *pie chart*

circumduction a motion that makes circles rather than twisting

civil law the branch of law that establishes rules for business relationships between people or between individuals and businesses

Civil Rights Act a federal law that bans employment discrimination based on a person's race, color, religion, gender, or national origin

claims process the procedure for submitting costs for medical services so that payment can be collected or denial can be determined

clean technique the practice of disinfecting any object or surface that has come into contact with pathogens

clear writing written work that avoids wordiness and uses simple language to explain ideas that may be complex

clients people who receive treatment in privately owned offices and treatment facilities, as well as in their own homes

clinical data the clinical information found in various forms in a patient chart

clinical engineer a worker who uses medical technology to improve healthcare delivery

clinical information section of a patient's chart that begins with the patient's medical history and includes all of the information about his or her health, medical conditions, and treatment

clinical laboratories facilities that examine materials taken from the human body to discover information related to diagnosis, prognosis, prevention, or treatment of disease

Clinical Laboratory Improvement Act (CLIA) a government act that regulates how a laboratory test should be performed and how the test results should be interpreted and reported

clinical training term that describes hands-on work with patients that students do under the supervision of a licensed healthcare provider

clinical trial an experiment performed on human beings to evaluate the comparative effectiveness of two or more treatments

cochlea a fluid-filled chamber of the inner ear that is used for hearing

code of ethics formal statement of expected ethical behaviors; describes the standards of conduct expected of members of the profession

cognitive impairments conditions that occur when a patient's ability to think is affected by pain or medication, when the patient is confused or disoriented, and when the patient suffers from dementia

coinsurance an individual's share of healthcare costs compared to the insurance company's share

collaborate to work together; to consult with each other

collagen a protein fiber that connects, supports, and gives strength to body tissues such as the skin, muscle tendons, and bone ligaments

colonoscopy a screening test that examines the inner surface of the colon

combining vowel a letter used to connect root words together when the next root or suffix does not begin with a vowel

commode hat   a measuring device for urine that is placed under the toilet seat before the patient urinates

Common Rule   a set of regulations adopted in common by a number of federal agencies to ensure the safety of testing on human subjects

communication   the act of sharing a message, thought, or idea so that it is accurately received and understood

communication barrier   anything that blocks or interferes with the exchange of information

communication style   a person's preferred method for exchanging information, which includes words, tone of voice, and nonverbal signals

compact bone   dense structure made of bone cells lined up close together to withstand stress

compassion   sympathy for the distress of others accompanied by a desire to help

compensation time   time off given to an employee in place of overtime pay

competent   capable

complementary and alternative medicine (CAM)   a term that describes healthcare practices, products, and supplements that are not a part of Western medicine

compliance   adherence and observation of guidelines

computerized patient record   an early version of the EHR that contains patient information for a single organization

concentration   a term that describes how much of a drug is in a specific volume of liquid

condylar   term that describes joints that can bend, straighten, and move side to side

confidentiality   the legally protected right of patients to have their personal and medical information kept private

congenital   a term that describes a disorder present from birth

conscious   being aware of surroundings or of different attitudes

consistency   degree of firmness, density, viscosity, or resistance to movement or separation of parts

consultant   a person who provides professional advice

contact precautions   practices used when an infection can be spread by direct or indirect contact with a patient or his or her environment

contagious   able to spread easily from one person to another

contamination   the unwanted presence of harmful substances or microorganisms

continuing education units (CEUs)   measures used to quantify the time spent on additional coursework that an individual must complete to renew his or her license

continuity of care record (CCR)   record that contains a standardized summary of the most relevant and timely health information about a patient

continuous compression resuscitation (CCR)   a type of CPR that involves using only chest compressions

contract   a legally binding agreement between two or more people or agencies

contraindicated   a term that means that a patient has a particular condition that makes normal care tasks uncomfortable or dangerous for him or her

controlled substance   a powerful medication that must be dispensed according to strict rules from the government

conversion factor   a numerical value that represents how much ingredients must be adjusted for a revised recipe; new yield ÷ old yield = conversion factor

copay   an out-of-pocket fee paid by a person with health insurance at the time a covered service, such as an office visit or a prescription, is received

cornea   a transparent tissue through which light enters the eye

coronary   relating to the arteries that supply blood to the heart

cover letter   a message sent with a résumé to introduce the job applicant and give the reasons he or she is applying for a particular job; also called *a letter of application*

cranial   a directional term used to talk about a point closer to the head

cranial cavity   the part of the dorsal cavity that contains the brain

cranial nerves   12 pairs of nerves that provide connections from the brain to the head and neck

credentials   documents proving a person's qualifications for a particular occupation

criminal law   the branch of law that aims to protect individuals and society by defining certain actions as crimes, or offenses against society

cross-contamination   the transfer of harmful substances from one object or surface to another

cultural competence   the ability to interact effectively with people of different cultures

cultural differences   variations among people that arise from nationality, ethnicity, race, and family backgrounds and which affect beliefs, practices, behavior, and expectations

cultural diversity   term that describes differences in age, gender, physical and intellectual abilities, sexual orientation, race, or ethnicity that influence what we believe, the way we think, and what we do

customer objections   concerns, doubts, or other reasons a customer gives for not making a purchase

cytoplasm   a semifluid structure contained within the walls of a cell in which chemical reactions take place

D

danger zone   the range of temperature from 40°F to 140°F at which bacteria grow most rapidly to the levels that cause food poisoning

data   facts about a specific topic, which are used for reference or analysis

de-identified information   health documents from which specified personal data has been removed

deductible   the minimum amount a patient must pay out-of-pocket before the insurance company will pay for healthcare

deep   a directional term that refers to body structures farther below the surface of the body

defamation   a term that means damaging someone's good name or reputation

dehydration   a condition caused by too little fluid in the body tissues

delegate   to direct another healthcare worker to perform a care task that is within that worker's training and experience and within the scope of practice of the licensed provider giving the direction

delegation   the act of assigning tasks to each member of a team

dementia   a condition characterized by memory loss and the decline of other thinking skills

dendrites   branches of a neuron that collect stimuli and transport them to the cell body

deoxyribonucleic acid (DNA)   material present in a cell that contains complete plans for items the cell builds; carries cell's genetic information

Department of Health and Human Services (HHS)   a government agency with 11 divisions that oversee many programs focused on improving the health of Americans

deposit slip   a form used to record the total amount of cash and checks in a bank deposit

dermis   the middle layer of the skin, which contains most of the skin's structures

diagnostic   pertaining to the identification of a disease or syndrome

diaphysis   the long shaft of bone between the two epiphyses

dictation   a verbal recording describing a patient's symptoms and the treatment given

dietetic technician   a worker who plans and produces meals based on established guidelines, teaches principles of food and nutrition, and helps clients make healthy food choices

dietitians   food and nutrition experts who advise patients on what foods to eat to improve their particular health condition

differential diagnosis   a determination made by a doctor that distinguishes a disease or condition from others that have similar symptoms

digestion   term for the mechanical and chemical breakdown of food into nutrients that can be absorbed and used by the body

Digital Imaging Communications in Medicine (DICOM)   a standard for handling, storing, printing, and transmitting information that enhances the distribution and viewing of medical images

dilemma   a problem that requires a person to choose between two conflicting obligations

dilution ratio   the amount of solvent as compared to the amount of solute in a solution

direct contact   physical interaction with an infected patient, surface, fluid, or object that can cause infection transmission

discretion   the ability to know when to keep sensitive information private

discrimination   unfair treatment of individuals on the basis of their membership in a specific group, such as age, ethnicity, gender, nationality, or religion

disinfection   the use of chemicals to kill pathogens that are present on nonliving objects

distal   a directional term that refers to a part that is farther away from the attachment site on the body; can also be used to describe internal organs

dorsal   a directional term used to describe surfaces are located on the back of the body

dorsal cavity   the cavity in the back of the body that is protected by the bones of the skull and vertebrae

dosage   the total quantity of medicine that is to be administered

dose   the portion of medicine to be administered at one time

droplet precautions   practices used when a pathogen can be transmitted through close contact with the respiratory system or mucous membranes of a patient

drug-resistant bacteria   strains of a bacterium that have adapted and are no longer controlled or killed by normal antibiotic treatment

E

edema   a condition caused by too much fluid in the body tissues

efferent   term that describes motor transmitters that carry impulses from the central nervous system out to the muscles and glands

electronic balances   measuring instruments that display the weight of a substance digitally and are used to weigh chemicals in labs

electronic health record (EHR)   a medical document that contains information from all of the clinicians involved in a patient's care and which can be created and managed by authorized clinicians and staff across more than one healthcare organization

electronic medical record (EMR)   an earlier version of the EHR that allowed physician's offices and outpatient clinics to convert their paper records to electronic formats

embryo   the developing human from the time of implantation to the end of the eighth week after conception

emergency medical services (EMS)   a system that provides rapid response care for those experiencing sudden illness and injury

empathy   the ability to identify with another person's feelings and thoughts

employability skills   skills related to choosing a career, acquiring and keeping a job, changing jobs, and advancing in a career

Employee Assistant Program (EAP)　an employer-sponsored service designed to help employees with personal or family problems, including mental health, substance abuse, addiction, marital problems, parenting problems, emotional problems, or financial or legal concerns

employment at will　a principle that describes employment as a mutual agreement between employer and employee that either party can end whenever they wish

endoplasmic reticulum (ER)　the organelle that moves ribosomes in and out of the nucleus as they are assembled; can be rough (covered with ribosomes from the nucleus for building proteins) or smooth (builds and stores fats and carbohydrates and detoxifies harmful substances)

environment　the factor of a system that involves the setting in which the system operates; can be internal or external

environmental barriers　distractions in the surrounding area that cause a person's attention to wander

environmental engineer　a worker who ensures the health of the public, such as by monitoring safe drinking water and air quality

Environmental Protection Agency (EPA)　a government agency that recommends practices for maintaining the environment and determines appropriate chemicals for reducing the spread of infection in healthcare facilities while minimizing environmental risks

environmental services　the hospital department responsible for housekeeping, laundry, and facility maintenance

e-prescribing　electronic generation, transmission, and filling of a medical prescription

epidemiologists　scientists who study the spread of diseases

epidermis　the thin, outer layer of the skin

epididymis　the structure where sperm mature

epiglottis　a flap of cartilage that helps direct food and air down the correct tubes

epiphysis　the knob at the end of a long bone, which is made up of mostly spongy bone

Equal Employment Opportunity Commission (EEOC)　a federal agency that enforces various employee protection acts and has the power to bring lawsuits on behalf of workers who believe they have been discriminated against

Equal Pay Act　a federal law that requires employers to pay men and women equally for performing the same job under the same conditions

erythrocyte　a red blood cell that transports oxygen and carbon dioxide to and from body tissues

esophagus　the digestive tube that runs from the throat to the stomach

estrogen　a hormone that is responsible for the development of female characteristics during puberty

ethical　a term used to describe an action that fits with someone's personal morals or professional rules of conduct

ethics board　a committee that meets to discuss unusual or controversial cases and advises professionals on ethical dilemmas

etiquette　term for a code of polite behavior among members of a profession or group

eugenics　a movement that attempts to promote desirable genetic characteristics

evidence-based practices　methods of diagnosis and treatment based on the best available current research, clinical expertise, and a patient's needs and preferences

exclusive provider organization (EPO)　insurance plan that charges an access fee for a network of healthcare providers at reduced rates; premiums are usually lower than those of an HMO, but the choice of covered providers is more limited

excretion　the removal of waste products from the body

executive summary　an overview of a technical document

explanation of benefits (EOB)　a detailed account of each claim processed by an insurance plan, which is sent to the patient as notification of claim payment or denial

exposure control plan　a detailed set of standards that explains how specimens, contaminated equipment, contaminated work surfaces, and contaminated waste materials can be handled safely

expressed　a term that means the terms are spelled out in detail

extension　an action that moves a dorsal surface toward a dorsal surface and increases the angle of the ventral surfaces of a joint

F

face page　part of a patient's electronic health record that shows contact information, insurance information, and medical history; also called the *summary screen*

facsimile machine　a machine used to transmit pictures or written documents using the public telephone network

Fahrenheit scale　a method of measuring temperature that is sometimes used in US healthcare facilities

Fair Labor Standards Act (FLSA)　a federal law that restricts work settings and hours for workers younger than 18 years of age

fallopian tubes　tubes that carry the ovum to the uterus

false imprisonment　that act of holding people against their will or limiting their movement without the right to do so

Family and Medical Leave Act (FMLA)　a federal law that grants workers the right to up to 12 weeks off work in a 12-month period to give birth to a child, care for a newborn or newly adopted child, care for a seriously ill family member, or recover from a personal illness or injury

family medical history a record that includes major illnesses and surgeries of a patient's close relatives, including parents, grandparents, aunts and uncles, and siblings

fascicle a bundle of structures, such as nerve or muscle fibers

FAST (Face, Arm, Speech, Time) a mnemonic that can be used to identify a stroke

Federal Insurance Contributions Act (FICA) a government act that established a tax to fund Social Security

Federal Needlestick Safety and Prevention Act a government act that requires healthcare facilities to use needles specially engineered for safer injections and blood draws

federal withholding tax a tax on personal income

feedback the response of an audience to a message

feedback loop the factor of a system that involves responses to the functions that are used to keep the system going

fellowship highly specialized program or subspecialty, such as endocrinology or pediatric cardiology, that requires even more training than other fields

fermentor a machine that maintains optimal conditions for the growth of microorganisms and is used to produce drugs or enzymes for use in the biotechnology industry

fertilization a process that occurs when the chromosomes of the ovum and sperm unite to produce a zygote

fetus a developing human from eight weeks after conception to birth

filtration the process of separating substances, such as solid from liquid, large from small, or impure from pure

fire triangle term that describes the three elements of a fire, which include oxygen, fuel, and a heat source

first aid emergency treatment given before regular medical services can be obtained

flat bone a thin bone that is effective as a protective shell

flexion an action that moves a ventral surface toward a ventral surface, decreasing the angle of the joint

fluid balance term for a state in which the amount of fluid taken into the body equals the amount of fluid that leaves the body

fomites contaminated objects

fontanel the soft spot on an infant's head where the bones have not grown together yet

Food and Drug Administration (FDA) a government agency that regulates products in the food and drug industries and develops nutrition facts labels to help consumers make informed food choices

foramen an opening or hole, especially in a bone

forebrain the largest part of the brain, which includes the cerebrum, basal ganglia, and limbic system

forensic DNA analyst a person who works in a crime lab to extract and match DNA from samples that are used as evidence to solve crimes

Fowler's an inclined position in which the patient's body is elevated at 45 degrees

fracture a break

frontal lobes lobes of the brain that are located at the forehead and are responsible for voluntary muscle control, thinking, memory, language, judgment, creativity, and personality

frontal plane the body plane that divides the body (or organ) into its front and back sections; also called the *coronal plane*

functional nursing a care model in which each nurse is responsible for completing a set of assigned tasks for every patient or resident

fungi parasitic microbes that live in soil and on plants

G

gallbladder the organ that stores bile and delivers it to the duodenum when needed

gametes reproductive cells that have half the normal number of chromosomes and unite during fertilization; sperm in males and ova in females

ganglion a swelling located between two neurons

gene term for a combination of DNA found on the 46 chromosomes inside each human cell that determine the unique genetic makeup of an individual and carry the code for building human cells, tissues, and organs

gene therapy insertion of a new gene to replace an abnormal or defective gene

generic drug a medication that is chemically identical to a brand-name product and meets the same standards for quality and performance, but is usually less expensive

genetic counselors people who meet with clients to gather medical information and help them understand genetic disorders

genetic discrimination the use of genetic information by employers and insurance companies to deny employment or insurance coverage or to treat individuals differently because of a genetic condition

genetic disorder a disease or condition that results from damaged, incorrectly located, or abnormal genes

genetic engineering the deliberate manipulation of genetic materials to eliminate harmful traits or to ensure the presence of desirable traits

Genetic Information Nondiscrimination Act (GINA) a federal law that protects employees from discrimination based on genetic information

geneticists medical scientists who study genes, heredity, and the variation of organisms

genetic test the examination of a person's cells to analyze his or her genes and identify possible genetic disorders

genomic medicine   personalized medical care that uses a patient's unique combination of genes and chromosomes to prevent illness and maintain health

Golgi apparatus   an organelle made up of layers of membrane in the cytoplasm; inspects, sorts, and packages proteins for use within or removal from the cell.

gonads   the primary reproductive organs; testes in males and ovaries in females

goniometer   an instrument for measuring angles

good laboratory practices (GLPs)   regulations that describe how laboratories must operate

good manufacturing practices (GMPs)   regulations that describe how manufacturers must operate

graduated cylinder   a tall container used for measuring the volume of liquids

gross pay   the total amount of money earned in a pay period

grounding   the act of carrying current safely away from an electrical circuit to prevent shocks from occurring in the event of a problem with the circuit

gurney   a wheeled stretcher

H

hair follicle   a tube within the skin's surface that surrounds the root of a hair

hand hygiene   procedure that includes regular hand washing using plain or antibacterial soap and the use of alcohol-based gels

handoff care report   report used during a shift change or change in the level of patient care to explain a patient's current situation

harassment   unwelcome, offensive, and repeated language or actions based on race, color, religion, sex, national origin, age, disability, or genetic information that affect an employee's job performance or advancement opportunities or create an uncomfortable working environment

harms   damages or injuries

Hazard Communication Standard (HCS)   an OSHA regulation aimed at promoting awareness of hazardous substances and understanding of safe handling practices

hazardous   dangerous; risky

healthcare-associated infection (HAI)   an infection that is not present when a patient is admitted to a hospital or healthcare facility but develops 48 hours or more after admission

health informatics (HI)   a group of careers that combines health information management and health information technology; workers design and develop information systems that improve the quality, effectiveness, and efficiency of patient care

health informatics services   career pathway that involves methods, devices, and resources used to acquire, store, retrieve, and work with healthcare and biomedical information

health information management (HIM)   a field of health informatics services that is responsible for assembling and organizing a patient's health information to create a medical record

health information technology (HIT)   a field of health informatics services that focuses on the systems that are used to manage health information and the secure exchange of health information in a digital format

Health Information Technology for Economic and Clinical Health (HITECH) Act   a law that made significant changes to the HIPAA privacy and security regulations and seeks to increase the nationwide use of electronic health records

Health Insurance Portability and Accountability Act (HIPAA)   a federal law that makes it easier to obtain healthcare coverage and protects personal health information

health literacy   a person's ability to obtain and understand health-related information and make informed decisions using that information

health maintenance organization (HMO)   insurance organization that employs doctors, pharmacists, dentists, laboratories, and hospitals in an integrated and patient-focused network to cover all aspects of medical care for insured individuals

hemoglobin   a protein that helps red blood cells carry oxygen and gives them their red color

heredity   the passing of traits (such as eye color, height, and some diseases) from parent or ancestor to offspring through chromosomes

hierarchy   a term that describes the levels of authority within an organization

high Fowler's   an inclined position in which the patient's body is elevated at 90 degrees

hindbrain   the part of the brain that includes the cerebellum and brainstem

hinge joint   a joint that only bends and straightens or opens and closes with no side-to-side movement

holistic care   therapies that treat the patient as a whole person after assessing the individual's physical, social, mental, and spiritual well being

home health care   healthcare provided for frail, elderly, or disabled people who live at home; care is provided by nurses, home health aides, clergy, and professionals who provide rehabilitation services

homeostasis   a state of balance between interdependent elements

hormone   a chemical used to send messages from an endocrine gland to a target organ

HOSA–Future Health Professionals   a career and technical student organization for future healthcare workers

hospice care   healthcare available for clients who have been diagnosed with a terminal disease and generally have less than six months to live

hospital   typically a large facility that offers a wide range of services from inpatient care, surgery, and critical care to physical therapy, radiology, and laboratory services

Human Genome Project an international scientific research project with the goal of determining the sequence of chemical base pairs which make up human DNA

human resources term that describes workers who specialize in maximizing workers' effectiveness and productivity

hypertension a condition in which blood pressure is too high

hypodermis the innermost layer of the skin, which stores fat

hypotension a condition in which blood pressure is too low

hypothalamus the brain's center for emotions and instincts, which controls pleasure, pain, sleep, hunger, and thirst

hypothesis a theory or proposed explanation that serves as the starting point for further investigation

I

Illness and Injury Prevention Program (I2P2) a proactive, systemic approach to finding and fixing hazards before people are injured

immunization the injection of a harmless form of a pathogen into the body, which trains the body to protect itself against a disease

implied a term that means an agreement is assumed based on the actions of both parties

incident report a form used to record the details of an unusual event, such as an accident or injury

incompetence a lack of qualifications or ability to perform job tasks

indirect contact interaction with fomites, droplets, and other objects that can cause infection transmission

indispensable absolutely necessary

industrial engineer a worker who identifies the most efficient ways to use space, time, workers, and other resources

infectious able to live in a host and cause disease

infectious agent a pathogen that can cause infection

inferior a directional term that means lower down on the body

informed consent a patient's choice to accept or reject a procedure after receiving information on available options and possible consequences

infrastructure term that describes the internal systems that a facility needs to operate, such as power supplies; electrical, plumbing, and heating and cooling systems; water; waste management; and phones and computer systems

infusion injection of drugs or another solution directly into a vein

ingestion the stage of digestion in which food is taken into the body through the mouth

ingredient cost a numerical value representing the total cost of one ingredient in a recipe

initiative the ability to decide independently what to do and when to do it

innervate to provide an area with a nerve connection to the brain

input the factor of a system that includes the population being served and why they need or want service through this system; also includes the resources the system needs to function, such as workers, equipment, and financial resources

inspection visual examination used to assess parts of the body by looking for abnormal color, shape, size, or texture

intake and output (I&O) term for measurements of all the fluids that enter and leave the body

integrity adherence to ethical principles and professional standards

integumentary related to the skin

interdisciplinary healthcare team a group of professionals from different health science training backgrounds working in coordination toward a common goal for the patient

intern a term that describes a student doctor when he or she is completing rotations through various specialties in the first year of residency

International Classification of Diseases Clinical Modifications (ICD-CM) a system published by the Department of Health and Human Services that contains the coding system for diagnoses based on information from the World Health Organization

International Units (IU) a system of measurement that describes the effect or potency of manufactured drugs and vitamins

internship practical work or training experience that allows students to apply what they have learned in class

interoperability the ability to exchange and use computer information within and across networks

interview etiquette accepted appearance and behavior for the interview process

invasion of privacy intrusion on a person's privacy; applies to personal information as well as a person's body

invasive procedure a test or treatment that requires incisions to the skin or the insertion of instruments or other materials into the body

inventory a count of disposable and durable medical equipment

in vitro a fertilization process that takes place in a test tube, or otherwise outside the body

involuntary seclusion the practice of isolating a person and preventing him or her from interacting with others

irregular bone a bone that is a complex shape and contains mostly spongy bone with a covering of compact bone

islets of Langerhans clusters of cells located on the pancreas that make the hormones insulin and glucagon

isolation confinement to a private room to prevent the spread of infection

K

ketoacidosis a serious condition that can lead to diabetic coma and needs further medical care

kidneys organs that filter, concentrate, and remove waste from the blood to form urine

kinesthetic learner a person who uses his or her body, hands, and sense of touch to learn

L

lab information system (LIS) a computer system that manages data about patients, lab test requests, and lab test results

laboratory documentation written records of observable, measurable, and reproducible findings obtained through examination, testing, research studies, and experiments

lacteal a specialized lymphatic vessel that picks up digested fats and fat-soluble vitamins in the villi of the small intestine

laparoscopic pertaining to operations that use tubes with cameras and tools attached to them and require very small incisions

larynx a space near the pharynx that aids in voice production; also known as the *voice box*

lateral a directional term that refers to a point toward the side of the body

learning style an individual's preferred way of gaining or processing new information

legal a term used to describe issues that are defined by laws that are enforced by the government

legal disability a condition that results in a person being unable to enter a contract, such as being under the age of consent, being ruled mentally incompetent, or having an altered mental state due to drugs or semi-consciousness

lens a transparent, flexible structure that focuses light at the back of the eye

letter of resignation a written document that formally states an employee's decision to leave a job

leukocyte a white blood cell that is involved in fighting infection

liable legally responsible

libel written defamation

licensed practical nurse (LPN) a healthcare worker who completes a one-year technical training program and can perform basic nursing tasks such as giving injections, monitoring catheters, and dressing wounds

licensed vocational nurse (LVN) a healthcare worker who completes a one-year technical training program and can perform basic nursing tasks such as giving injections, monitoring catheters, and dressing wounds

licensure a credential that is required by law for some professions to protect public health, safety, and welfare

ligament a tough, fibrous tissue that connects bones to other bones and holds organs in place

line graph a chart that shows the changes in data over time

lines of authority term that describes the hierarchy of command from the top down through all the different ranks of employees

liver the organ that breaks down and removes toxic substances, drugs, bacteria, and dead red blood cells from the body

living will a patient's written document giving instructions about which procedures may or may not be used to sustain or prolong his or her life, such as feeding tubes or ventilation

long bone a bone that is longer than it is wide and has a hollow diaphysis

long-term care facility healthcare facility that provides skilled nursing care and rehabilitation services for residents who will live in the facility for many months or years

lymph blood plasma that remains between cells after delivering its oxygen, nutrients, and hormones

lymphatic related to or containing the watery fluid (lymph) collected from body tissues

lymph node a small capsule where lymphocytes collect to remove dead cells, destroy pathogens, and create antibodies against infection

lymphocyte a cell that makes antibodies to mark and destroy invading pathogens

lysosomes organelles that use digestive enzymes to destroy used, dead, and foreign materials that are left behind after energy is used up

M

malpractice term for actions that violate a professional's scope of practice or standard of care and result in injury to a patient that could reasonably have been expected

mammogram X-rays that test for breast cancer

managed care a system that limits access to and use of healthcare to control costs

mandatory overtime required hours of work outside an employee's typical schedule

mandatory reporting the legal requirement for certain health issues to be reported to authorities

marketing term that describes a field specializing in making others aware of a company's or individual's products and services

mean the mathematical average of a set of data

meaningful use the use of electronic health records that follows a series of stages with sets of objectives for healthcare providers to meet in each stage

medial a directional term that refers to a point closer to the center of the body

median term that describes the number found exactly in the middle when a data is listed in numerical order

Medicaid a government-provided health insurance program that provides hospital and medical insurance for people with low incomes, children in low-income families, and those who are disabled and cannot work

medical coding the act of assigning numbers to descriptions of a patient's diseases, injuries, and treatments according to established codes

medical diagnosis a determination made by a doctor that identifies the cause of a patient's illness

medical documentation written reports of observable, measurable, and reproducible findings from examinations, supporting laboratory or diagnostic tests, and assessments of a patient

medical errors preventable mistakes that can occur at any point in the healthcare process and may potentially cause harm to the patient

medical history a list all of the diseases and surgeries a patient has had, his or her current symptoms, results of examinations and diagnostic tests, treatments, and other health services

medical interpreter an individual who translates for a patient with limited English proficiency to ensure that the patient's needs are being met

medical record a file that contains documents that describe a specific patient's medical history and medical care within one healthcare organization; also known as a *chart* or *file*

medical terminology special vocabulary that is used in healthcare and is often formed from Latin and Greek word parts

Medical Waste Tracking Act a government act that empowers OSHA to investigate workplaces' storage and disposal methods for medical waste

Medicare a government-provided health insurance program that provides coverage for people 65 years of age and older; helps with the cost of healthcare, but doesn't pay for all medical expenses or long-term care

medication a substance or mixture of substances that have been proven through research to have a clear value in the prevention, diagnosis, or treatment of diseases

Medigap private health insurance policies that individuals must purchase to cover costs not paid by Medicare

meiosis the sexual process of cell division that produces four new haploid cells, each with a unique combination of 23 chromosomes

melanin the brownish-black pigment produced by melanocytes

memorandum short, informal messages that are sent between people within an organization

meninges three tough layers of tissue covering the brain and spinal cord, including the dura mater, arachnoid mater, and pia mater

meniscus curve at the surface of a liquid caused when it sticks to the walls of a graduated cylinder

menopause term for the end of fertility and monthly menstruation, which usually begins around 50 years of age

mental health a component of wellness that combines emotional, psychological, and social well-being

metabolize to process a substance through metabolism

methicillin-resistant *Staphylococcus aureus* **(MRSA)** a type of staph, or *bacterial*, infection caused by the bacterium *S. aureus*, which is most common in healthcare settings but is increasingly found in the community at large

metric system the decimal measurement system based on the meter, liter, and gram as its primary units of length, volume, and weight or mass respectively

mHealth a term that refers to mobile health apps

micropipette an instrument designed for the measurement of very small volumes

midbrain the section of the brain that includes the thalamus, hypothalamus, pituitary gland, and pineal gland

midsagittal plane the body plane that divides the body exactly down the midline

minimum data set (MDS) a comprehensive evaluation of the functional capabilities of each resident in a long-term care facility

minimum wage the lowest hourly earnings that an employer can legally pay a worker

misappropriation the unauthorized use of something that belongs to someone else

misidentification the failure to match the correct patient to the correct treatment before beginning a procedure, which is a significant cause of medical errors

mitered corner a neat corner fold used for making beds in hospitals

mitochondria organelles that function as power stations for cells

mitosis the asexual process of cellular reproduction that creates two identical copies of a cell, each with a full set of 46 chromosomes

mnemonic device a learning tool that helps students memorize information

mode the number that occurs most frequently in a data set

mode of transmission the way in which a pathogen moves from its reservoir to a new host

molecular imaging a technique that provides detailed pictures of what is happening inside the body at the molecular and cellular level

morticians workers who manage funeral homes and arrange the details of a funeral

morula a solid ball of 16 cells that results when a zygote divides

mucous membranes thin layers of tissue that line body cavities to provide a natural barrier against pathogens

multidisciplinary healthcare team a group of healthcare workers from different healthcare specialties, each providing specific services to the patient

multi-drug resistant organisms microorganisms that are relatively unaffected by infection-battling drugs

muscle tone the normal, partly contracted state of skeletal muscles in the trunk and limbs, which helps maintain the body's balance

myelin a fatty layer that protects the axons of some nerves

N

nail bed term for the sensitive layer of cells beneath the nail plate at the tips of a person's fingers and toes

nanotechnology a field of science that manipulates individual atoms and molecules to create devices that are thousands of times smaller than current technologies allow

National Healthcare Skill Standards standards determined by the National Consortium for Health Science Education, which describe the skills that workers need to succeed in healthcare careers

National Institutes of Health (NIH) a division of the HHS that conducts research and provides information toward improving public health through 27 different agencies

National Labor Relations Act (NLRA) a federal law that gives workers the right to join together, with or without a union, to discuss ways of improving working conditions

negative feedback system mechanism that reduces a body function in response to a stimulus, such as a hormone

negligence the failure to do something a person with training should have known enough to do

nephron the fundamental excretory unit of each kidney

net pay the amount of money received in a pay period after all deductions have been taken out; also known as *take-home pay*

network the group of people who work in healthcare that someone might know

neuron a nerve cell

neurotransmitter a chemical used to carry a signal from an axon to a receptor cell to pass along a message

non-intact skin broken skin, including rashes

noninvasive procedure a test or treatment that does not require incisions to the skin or the insertion of instruments or other materials into the body

nonprofit organization business entity that uses any profits to achieve its charitable goals, such as research, education, and low-cost care

nosocomial infections infections acquired in hospitals or other healthcare facilities

nourishments healthy snacks for residents in a healthcare facility

nuclear medicine technologists healthcare workers who administer radioactive substances as part of the imaging process

nucleolus the organelle located at the center of the nucleus, which uses ribosomes to build proteins

nucleus the organelle that contains genetic material controls the cell's activity

number needed to harm (NNH) the number of patients who must be treated over a specific period to cause harm in an average of one patient who would not otherwise have been harmed

number needed to treat (NNT) the number of patients who must be treated to prevent the occurrence of the condition under examination

nursing diagnosis the description of a client's health problem that a nurse is licensed and competent to treat

nutrients molecules such as carbohydrates, proteins, fats, vitamins, and minerals used by the body to grow and maintain body processes

O

objective observation an indication of a health condition that can be clearly observed; also called a *sign*

objective writing written work that draws a conclusion from the facts and makes no assumptions

occipital lobes the smallest of the brain's lobes, which are located in the back of the skull and control sight, visual-spatial processes, memory, and storage

occupational exposure term for the reasonable expectation for contact with blood or other potentially infectious materials during the performance of job duties

Occupational Safety and Health Administration (OSHA) a government agency that creates regulations to prevent work-related injuries, illnesses, and deaths

Office of the National Coordinator as Authorized Testing and Certification Body (ONC-ATCB) an agency that certifies bodies for evaluating electronic health record systems and verifying their compliance with the US Department of Health and Human Services' standards

off-label term that describes a type of prescribing in which a doctor uses a medication in a way that is not specified in the product information

olfactory bulb the thickened end of the olfactory nerve that sends sensory impulses to the olfactory region of the brain

ombudsman a person who addresses complaints and advocates for improvements in the long-term healthcare system

Omnibus Budget Reconciliation Act (OBRA) a law that requires certified nursing assistants (CNAs) to have at least 75 hours of training and to pass written and skill tests

open-ended question a question that requires more than a one- or two-word response

ophthalmologist an eye specialist

opportunistic infections diseases that take advantage of an already weakened immune system

optometrist   a professional who performs vision testing and prescribes routine vision corrections

organ   a distinct body structure made of different tissues working together for the same purpose

organelle   a part of a cell that has a specific task

organizational chart   a diagram that shows how departments in an organization are related to one another

orthopedic surgeon   a medical doctor who focuses on the surgical treatment of musculoskeletal conditions

ossicles   bones that transfer vibrations from the middle ear to the inner ear, including the malleus, incus, and stapes

ossification   the process of taking calcium from any ingested food and drink and depositing it into cartilage to form bone

osteoblast   a specialized bone-forming cell that begins the mineralization process

osteoclast   a cell that breaks down bone during exercise so it can be remodeled into new bone cells

osteoporosis   a condition characterized by loss of bone mass, which weakens the bones so they break easily

other potentially infectious material (OPIM)   term that describes body tissues and bodily fluids other than blood

otolaryngologist   an ear specialist

outpatient procedures   surgeries that allow patients to leave the hospital shortly after a procedure has been completed

output   the factor of a system that refers to the results produced by the system's functioning

outsource   to contract out jobs to workers in a foreign country

ova   the female gametes, also known as *eggs*

ovaries   the female gonads

overtime pay   payment at one and a half times the regular wage for each hour an employee works beyond 40 hours in a week

P

pacemakers   devices used to regulate heartbeats

pain scale   a tool used to help patients describe and identify their pain

palpation   a medical examination that uses touch to detect growths, changes in the size of organs, or tissue reactions to pressure

pancreas   the organ that produces enzymes to digest carbohydrates, fats, and proteins

papillae   tiny bumps on the tongue that house taste buds

paralysis   a condition that limits the ability to move certain parts of the body

paraphrase   to summarize important information in your own words

parathyroid glands   four tiny glands that are located on the back of the thyroid and which secrete a hormone that triggers the release of calcium from bones

parietal lobes   lobes of the brain that are located behind the frontal lobes and integrate sensory information from the skin, internal organs, muscles, and joints

pasteurization   a process that uses heat to kill pathogens that can cause foodborne illnesses

patents   licenses that give researchers or inventors the sole right to produce and sell a product for a set time

pathogen   a disease-causing microorganism

patient interview   a structured communication between a patient and a healthcare worker for the purpose of collecting subjective data such as a medical history

penis   the male reproductive organ, which delivers sperm to the female reproductive tract

percentiles   measures used to indicate how close to the average a person's height and weight fall

percussion   a medical examination that includes tapping various body parts and using resulting sounds to assess the condition of internal organs

peripheral devices   pieces of equipment that are used to gather information and upload it to computer systems

peripheral nervous system (PNS)   term for the sensory and motor nerves that go out to the body's extremities

peristalsis   muscle contractions

personal and professional development   term that describes steps taken to improve personal, educational, and career-related performance

personal bias   an unfair preference for, or dislike of, something or someone

personal data page   a document that contains personal data and can be used to complete job applications; contains contact information, education, work experience, skills, and references

personal health record (PHR)   a file that contains information about your own health that you store electronically for easy reference

personal identifying information   information that is used to connect a patient to the correct record

personalized medicine   term for medical treatments that are tailored to a person's genetic makeup and individual needs

personal leadership style   an individual approach to giving directions, implementing plans, and motivating people

personal protective equipment (PPE)   equipment such as gloves, masks, gowns, respirators, and eyewear worn to protect skin, clothing, and the respiratory tract from infectious agents

personal traits   an individual's unique combination of qualities and characteristics

pharynx   the passageway between the nasal cavity and mouth and the esophagus; also known as the *throat*

phlebotomist   a medical assistant who helps draw blood and receives specimens for testing

physician assistant (PA) healthcare workers who practice medicine under the supervision of a physician; can diagnose, treat, and prescribe medication for patients

Physician's Current Procedural Terminology (CPT) a system created by the American Medical Association that contains the codes used to report procedures and services to public and private insurance companies

physiology the functions or inner workings of the body

pictograph a chart that presents data using images

pigment color

pituitary gland gland that releases hormones that affect the operation of many other glands in the body; also called the *master gland*

placebo a harmless substance that contains no medication

placenta an organ that grows in the uterus to meet the nutritional needs of the embryo and fetus

plasma a yellowish liquid containing mostly water, which carries nutrients, hormones, and waste for other body systems

pleura membranes that line the surfaces of the lungs

plexus an interwoven combination of spinal nerve roots through which messages pass

plural a term that means more than one in number

pluripotent capable of becoming many different cell types

point-of-care testing medical diagnostic testing that is performed outside of a laboratory, closer to where a patient is receiving care

point of service (POS) insurance plans that have smaller deductibles and copays than a PPO, but require a referral from a patient's primary care provider before seeing a specialist, like an HMO does

portal of entry a natural body opening or break in the skin that provides a way for pathogens to enter the body

portal of exit a natural body opening or break in the skin that provides a way for pathogens to leave the body

portion the amount of food in one serving

posterior a directional term that refers to the back side of the body

postgraduate term that describes education and training completed after receiving a bachelor's degree

postsecondary education education past high school that can be obtained at community colleges, vocational or technical colleges, public and private colleges and universities, institutes of technology, and career colleges

posture an important part of body mechanics that describes the position of a person's body while performing a task

power of attorney (POA) the appointment of a person to make healthcare decisions for someone in the event that he or she is unable to make his or her own choices

precise writing written work that uses concrete rather than figurative language and is as specific as possible to avoid confusion

preferred provider organization (PPO) insurance organization in which insurers contract with private physicians and hospitals to provide treatment and care at a reduced cost in return for an increased number of patients

prefix a word part that appears at the beginning of a word

prejudice a strong feeling or belief about a person or subject that is not based on reason or actual experience

premium the monthly fees individuals pay into a shared money pool to receive insurance coverage

primary care teams groups of healthcare providers that include the primary care physician along with physician assistants and nurse practitioners who see the patient in the clinic setting; may also include nutritionists, pharmacists, social workers, or others

primary motor cortex an area of the frontal lobe that directs muscle movement through efferent neurons to muscles in the body

primary nursing a care model in which one RN, LPN, or LVN is assigned several patients or residents and is responsible for planning and carrying out all aspects of care for as long as the patients are in the care unit

primary research articles scientific papers that provide the original data and conclusions of researchers who conducted experiments

primary sensory cortex an area of the parietal lobe dedicated to gathering and interpreting information regarding the five senses of the body from afferent neurons

primary source a document that describes research in which the authors directly participated

privileged communication any private conversations between a healthcare professional and a patient, which cannot be disclosed in court

probability the likelihood of something happening

problem-oriented medical record (POMR) a record organized under a system in which information in a medical record appears according to the patient's problem

professional distance term used to describe the act of showing a caring attitude toward patients without trying to become friends

professional look the standards of appearance normally expected of a qualified person in a work environment

professional organization an association formed to unite and inform people who work in the same occupation

progesterone a hormone that prepares the uterine lining for an egg to implant

proposals documents that propose or suggest something

proprietary privately owned and managed

prostatectomy   surgical removal of the prostate gland

prostheses   custom-built artificial limbs

protected health information (PHI)   all individually identifiable personal information obtained through healthcare

protocol   the appropriate conduct, etiquette, or procedures for communication

proximal   a directional term that indicates that the part being discussed is closer to the point of attachment to the body; can also be used to describe internal organs

public health laboratory professionals   highly educated specialists who have knowledge of one or more scientific disciplines

public relations   term that describes a field specializing in communication between an organization and the public

Pull, Aim, Squeeze, Sweep (PASS)   acronym that describes how to correctly operate a fire extinguisher

pulmonary loop   the flow of blood from the heart to the lungs and back to pick up oxygen and drop off carbon dioxide

pupil   the opening through which light rays enter the eye

Q

qualitative   term that describes data that cannot be measured

quality improvement (QI)   a formal approach to the analysis of a healthcare team's performance and systematic efforts to improve it

quantitative   term for a type of information or data that is based on quantities; also called *statistics*

quantitative data   information that can be measured

quick response(QR) code   a two-dimensional bar code that is used to provide easy access to information through a smartphone; also known as *quick read code*

R

radial pulse   a pulse measurement taken by placing two or three fingers over the radial artery on the inside of the wrist

radiation therapist   a healthcare worker who uses CT or other imaging techniques to pinpoint a tumor's location and consults a treatment plan to position the patient for radiation treatment

radio frequency identification (RFID)   a data collection technology that uses electronic tags for storing data

radiographers   healthcare professionals who create medical images or treat diseases by passing radiation, such as X-rays or gamma rays, through an object

range of motion (ROM)   the full extent of movement for a joint

rapport   an understanding between people

reabsorption   the act of returning a substance to the part of the body from which it was previously filtered out

reagents   chemicals often used in diagnostic tests to trigger desired chemical reactions

receptor   a nerve cell that receives stimuli

recipe cost   a numerical value representing the total cost of all ingredients in a recipe

recombinant DNA   genetically engineered DNA that usually includes segments from two or more different genetic sources

recommendation reports   documents that provide a way to meet a need in the workplace

rectal temperature   a body temperature taken by placing the thermometer in the rectum

rectum   a short segment whose lower end comprises the anal canal

recurrence   the return of something after a period of time, such as the return of cancer

references   people who are willing to discuss someone's skills and job qualifications with potential employers

reflex   an involuntary response of the nervous system

regenerative medicine   a form of medical care that creates living tissue to replace tissue or organ functions lost due to age, disease, injury, or birth disorder

regenerative therapy   treatment that uses stem cells to combat a variety of diseases and conditions at a cellular level

regimens   plans for medical treatment

registered nurse (RN)   a healthcare worker with either an associate's degree in nursing (ADN) or a bachelor's of science in nursing (BSN)

registration   placement on an official list, or registry, of qualified workers

registry   an archive in which data, records, and other information are kept

regulate   to control

Rehabilitation Act   a federal law that prohibits discrimination on the basis of disability in programs conducted by federal agencies, in programs receiving federal financial assistance, in federal employment, and in the employment practices of federal contractors

relative risk   ratio of the chance of a disease developing among people who are exposed to a specific factor compared with those who are not exposed

reproductive cloning   the creation of exact genetic duplicates

Rescue, Alarm, Contain, Extinguish/Evacuate (RACE)   acronym that describes the steps to take when there is a fire

reservoir   a place where the pathogen can live, such as the human body, animals, food, or fomites

residents   (1) individuals living in long-term care facilities; (2) medical school graduates who are completing the last portion of their medical training before becoming licensed physicians

resistant   not susceptible; able to survive in negative conditions

respiration   one breath in (inhalation) and one breath out (exhalation)

respiratory   related to the act of or organs involved in breathing

respiratory hygiene   practices that seek to protect people from airborne infectious particles; also called *cough etiquette*

résumé   a short, one-page document that contains your accomplishments and experiences and explains how these relate to a job in which you are interested

review articles   scientific papers that give an overview of a specific topic by summarizing the data and conclusions from several different studies

ribosomes   organelles that build proteins for the cell; may be free in the cytoplasm or attached to rough endoplasmic reticulum

risk assessments   methods used to calculate and describe a person's chance of becoming ill or dying of a specified condition

root   the part of a hair where growth begins, which is embedded at the bottom of a hair follicle

root word   the foundation of a medical term; carries the term's meaning

rotation   the action of turning on an axis

S

safety check   the process of looking for and removing potential hazards that could cause injury or harm

Safety Data Sheet (SDS)   an OSHA-required document that explains the hazards of a chemical product

safety precautions   information about the safe operation of a piece of equipment, which is usually found in the instruction manual or on equipment labels

sagittal plane   the body plane that divides the body, organ, or appendage into right and left sections

sales presentation   a prearranged meeting in which a salesperson presents detailed information and often a demonstration of a product

salivary glands   glands in the mouth that secrete saliva

sanitation   term that describes procedures and practices that maintain cleanliness and preserve public health

SBAR system   a method that helps healthcare workers communicate with each other more clearly by using a standardized communication format for reporting changes in a patient's status; stands for *Situation, Background, Assessment,* and *Recommendation*

scientific communication   a type of technical communication used by scientists and nonscientists to provide information and promote understanding

sclera   the tough, fibrous outer layer of the eye; also known as the *white of the eye*

scope of practice   tasks that an employee is legally allowed to perform based on his or her training and certification

scrotum   a sac that holds the testes on the outside of the body

sebaceous gland   a small gland in the skin that provides an oily secretion that coats the hair and skin with a softening, waterproof film

secondary care teams   groups of healthcare providers that deliver specialized services to hospital patients

secondary source   a document that summarizes the results of several studies

secretion   the release of a liquid substance from blood, cells, or tissues

select agent   a highly dangerous and strictly controlled substance that can potentially be used to develop biological or chemical weapons

semen   a thick, milky white fluid that supports sperm on their way to the uterus

semi-Fowler's   an inclined position in which the patient's body is elevated at 30 degrees

sensory impairments   conditions such as hearing loss, vision loss, or speech difficulties that may create communication barriers

service learning   an educational experience that integrates academic achievement with community service

sharps   needles, scalpels, or other sharp-edged objects found in healthcare settings that can puncture the skin

shift report   a statement that tells oncoming staff the information necessary for a smooth continuation of patient care

short bone   a bone that is as long as it is wide and which is made of spongy bone covered by a layer of compact bone

sign   evidence of a health condition that can be seen or measured

simulate   to imitate an action

sinus cavities   air-filled spaces around the nose that contain mucous membranes that help defend against infection

skeletal muscle   a voluntary, striated muscle that connects to bones and is responsible for movement

slander   verbal defamation

sleep deficit   a lack of sufficient sleep

smooth muscle   an involuntary muscle located in the body's visceral organs and blood vessels; also known as *visceral muscle*

social media   a group of online communication tools that allow people to share information and resources via the Internet

Social Security   a government program that provides retirement income, disability, and survivors' benefits

soft skills   employability skills related to communication, attitude, teamwork, and problem solving that are difficult to teach but critical to workplace success

solute   a chemical in a solution

solutions   uniform mixtures of two or more substances, which may be solids, liquids, gases, or a combination of these

solvent   a liquid that is used to dissolve a chemical in a solution

sonographers   healthcare professionals who create medical images or treat diseases through the use of high-frequency sound waves

source-oriented medical record (SOMR)   a record organized under a system in which information in a medical record is categorized behind tabs such as *imaging*, *laboratory*, and *pharmacy*

sperm   male gametes

sphygmomanometer   a medical instrument that measures blood pressure and which may be mercury, aneroid, or digital

spinal cavity   the part of the dorsal cavity that contains the spinal cord

spinal nerves   31 pairs of nerves that connect the spinal cord to the rest of the body

spleen   a lymphatic organ located just below the diaphragm that makes lymphocytes, filters the blood, and removes old red blood cells

spongy bone   a lighter and less dense structure than compact bone

stamina   endurance

standard anatomical position (SAP)   the agreed-upon reference for body position when studying anatomy; standing erect on two legs, facing frontward, with the arms at the sides and palms facing forward

standard of care   the level of service that a healthcare professional is expected to provide to a patient based on that professional's position and the patient's condition

standard operating procedures (SOPs)   established methods that describe the exact steps to be followed when completing a laboratory task

standard precautions   steps that a healthcare worker takes with all patients to prevent the spread of infection

standards of care   best practice guidelines for diagnostic and treatment processes a clinician should follow for a certain type of patient, illness, or clinical circumstance

statistical data   numerical information gathered through research that is used to draw conclusions about research findings

statistics   term for the science that includes the collection, organization, and interpretation of numerical data

stem cell   a cell that can duplicate itself many times and has the ability to develop into many different types of cells

stent   a tubular support that is used to keep arteries, blood vessels, canals, or ducts open to aid healing or prevent an obstruction

stereotype   the assumption that everyone in a particular group is the same

sterile technique   the practice of using sterilization to prevent the introduction of pathogens during invasive procedures

sterilize   to make something free from bacteria or other microorganisms

stethoscope   a medical instrument that amplifies sounds within the body

stomach   a reservoir in which food is broken down before it enters the small intestine

stool   waste material released during a bowel movement

stress   the body's attempt to adjust to a change

striated   arranged in a striped pattern

stroke   a medical emergency in which blood flow to a part of the brain is cut off

study limitations   restrictions or circumstances involved in a study that might mean its results cannot be generalized to a larger population

subcutaneous fat   fat below the skin that provides padding to absorb shock, holds in body heat, and stores energy

subjective observation   an indication of a health condition that is experienced by the patient; also called a *symptom*

sudoriferous glands   glands in the dermis that secrete sweat

suffix   a word part that appears at the end of a word

superficial   a directional term that refers to the outside surface of the body

superior   a directional term that means above or higher up on the body

support services   the career pathway that focuses on creating a therapeutic environment for providing patient care

susceptible host   anyone who can contract a disease

sutured   term that describes the way cranial bones grow together to form a strong and immovable joint

symptom   an indication of a disease or disorder experienced by the patient, such as pain

synapse   a tiny gap between an axon and a receptor cell

synergist   functional group of muscles that work together to provide body movement

system   an organized structure composed of many parts that work together and depend on each other to carry out a set of functions

systemic loop   the flow of blood from the heart to the body systems and back to drop off nutrients and pick up waste

T

table   a chart that arranges data in rows or columns

tact   the ability to communicate difficult or embarrassing information without giving offense

tare weight   the weight of an empty container

target audience   a specific group of people for whom a technical document is written

taste bud   a sensory cell that converts flavors into electrical signals

team nursing   a care model in which an RN functions as a team leader and has a group of nursing staff members who report to him or her; together the group divides the nursing care tasks

technical reading   a skill used to comprehend science, business, or technology publications

technical skills   the ability to perform tasks in a specific healthcare discipline or department

technical training   education lasting two years or less and leading to an industry certificate, a technical diploma, or an associate's degree

technical writing   a type of writing used in the workplace to inform or persuade a specific audience

teleconferencing   the use of telephones to hold meetings that allows healthcare professionals to interact and collaborate over long distances

telehealth   the use of electronic information and telecommunications technologies to support long-distance clinical healthcare, health-related education, public health, and health administration

telemedicine   a field of medicine in which communication and information technologies are used to provide medical services to patients in remote locations

telesurgery   a surgical technique that combines a reliable telephone line and multimedia image communication with robotic equipment and a skilled surgeon who is a considerable distance from the patient

temporal lobes   lobes of the brain that lie near the ears and control hearing, balance, emotions, speech planning, and memory associations

tendon   a tough, fibrous tissue that connects muscles to bones

terminal branches   branches located at the end of an axon, which connect to other cells

terminal cleaning   procedure for cleaning and disinfecting a patient hospital room in preparation for a newly admitted patient

tertiary source   a document compiled from primary and secondary sources that gives an overview of a specific topic

testes   the male sex organs

testosterone   a hormone that is responsible for development of male characteristics during puberty

thalamus   area of the brain that acts as a relay station for sorting, interpreting, and directing sensory signals to the appropriate area of the cerebral cortex

therapeutic   term that describes treatment given to maintain or restore health

therapeutic diet   a special food plan ordered by a physician to help treat a disease

third-party payer   an insurance company that pays the healthcare service provider for services rendered to a patient

thoracic cavity   the part of the ventral cavity that lies above the diaphragm muscle; includes the pericardial cavity and two pleural cavities

thrombocyte   a cell fragment that helps form blood clots to repair injured blood vessels

throughput   the factor of a system that refers to how the system processes or uses the inputs

thymus   a butterfly-shaped organ in the chest that helps program lymphocytes to respond to infection

thyroid gland   the largest endocrine gland in the body, which controls energy, metabolism, and calcium levels in the blood

tier   one of two or more rows, levels, or ranks arranged one above another

tissue   a group of cells of the same type working together for the same purpose

tonsils   lymphatic tissues located near the back of the throat that help protect against infection

tort   an action that harms another person's body or property or takes away his or her freedom of action in some way

total lung capacity   the amount of air the lungs can hold during the deepest possible breath

toxic   poisonous or harmful

trachea   the tube that leads from the larynx to the lungs; also known as the *windpipe*

transcriptionist   a health information technician who types medical record information from a physician's recorded dictation

transmission-based precautions   heightened care techniques that are performed in addition to standard precautions based on how a patient's infection is spread

transport technicians   healthcare workers who take patients to and from diagnostic imaging appointments and maintain transportation devices

transverse plane   the body plane that divides the body into top and bottom sections

triage   an evaluation process in which a group of patients is sorted according to the urgency of their need for care

tuberculosis (TB)   a very serious bacterial infection that most commonly affects the lungs and, before the development of antibiotics, was generally fatal

tympanic membrane   thin membrane that divides the outer and middle ear and changes sound waves into vibrations; also known as the *eardrum*

U

ultrasonic cleaners   devices that use sound waves to create millions of water jets that gently remove debris from lab equipment

unconscious   being unaware of surroundings or of different attitudes

unions   organizations that bring together workers from the same company or region to bargain collectively

unit cost   the price of one measurable unit of a food item, such as 1 pound, 1 ounce, or 1 piece

United States Department of Agriculture (USDA) a government agency that regulates the agriculture industry and researches and recommends diets for maintaining and improving general health

ureter a tube that leads from the kidney to the bladder

urethra a thin tube that leads from the bladder to outside of the body

urinals measuring devices for urine that are used by males confined to a bed

urinalysis the examination of urine's physical, chemical, and microscopic properties

US customary units the main system of weights and measures used in the United States based on the yard, pound, and gallon as units of length, weight, and liquid volume respectively; also known as *household measurements*

uterus a hollow, muscular organ whose purpose is to receive and nourish a fertilized egg

V

vacuole an organelle that allows larger enzymes and waste molecule packages to pass through the cell membrane

validity the quality of being legitimate, accurate, and factually sound

valve a part of a vein that prevents backflow as blood moves against gravity toward the heart

vancomycin-resistant *Enterococcus* **(VRE)** a bacterial infection caused by the bacterium *Enterococcus*, which is most often contracted in healthcare settings

vas deferens a duct through which sperm leave a testicle; also called the *ductus deferens*

vein a main blood vessel that moves blood from body tissues toward the heart

ventral a directional term used to describe surfaces move closer together when you bend a joint

ventral cavity the cavity in the front of the body that is surrounded by the ribs and pelvic bones

ventricle a chamber at the bottom of the heart that pumps blood out to the rest of the body

vestibular canals chamber in the ear that senses movement of fluid

villi finger-like projections in the intestines that increase their surface area

virus a very small pathogen that invades and reproduces inside other cells

visual learner a person who prefers to learn through pictures and has a good understanding of direction, spacing, and location

vital signs the key measurements that provide information about a person's health, including temperature, pulse, respiration, and blood pressure

vitreous humor a clear fluid that maintains the eye's shape

W

waived tests simple tests with little risk of error

Western medicine the most common form of medical care in the United States, which uses medication and surgery to treat the signs and symptoms of illness

worker's compensation government healthcare program in which plans cover injuries that happen to people while they are working on a job

work ethic a belief in the benefits of working hard, demonstrating initiative, and being personally accountable for the work you do

workplace violence acts of verbal abuse, threats, physical assault, or homicide that occur at work

work styles different methods that individuals might prefer to complete a job task

World Health Organization (WHO) an agency of the United Nations that is concerned with international public health

wrongful discharge dismissal from a job without cause

Y

yield the number of portions a recipe will produce

Z

zero-tolerance policy a policy in which threats and harassment are never acceptable behavior

zygote the genetically unique cell that results from fertilization and contains 46 chromosomes

Index